THE CALORIEKING®
Calorie, Fat & Carbohydrate Counter

Alcoholic Drinks (w. Alcohol Counts)
Baking Ingredients
Bars (Breakfast, Granola, Nutrition) — 136
Beverages: Cocoa, Hot Chocolate
   ..., Turkey, Duck, Goose) — 138
Coffee & Coffee Drinks — **Rice & Rice Dishes** — 140
Energy, Protein, Diet Shakes — 38 — Salads — 141
Fruit & Vegetable Juices — 41 — Salad Dressings — 142
Milk (Plain, Flavored, Mixes) — 47 — Sauces & Gravy — 144
Non-Dairy (Soy, Rice/Cereal/Nut) — 49 — Seasonings, Flavorings, Spices — 147
Soda/Soft Drinks — 51 — Snacks (Popcorn, Chips, Pretzels) — 148
Tea & Iced Tea Drinks — 53 — Soups — 152
Bread & Bread Products, Bagels — 54 — Soy, Tofu, Supplements/Cough Syrup — 156
Breakfast Cereals (Hot & Cold) — 57 — Sugar, Sweeteners, Honey, Jam — 157
Cakes, Donuts, Muffins, Pastries — 62 — Syrups, Dessert Toppings — 157
Candy, Chocolate, Gum — 68 — Vegetables (Fresh, Frozen, Canned) — 158
Cheese & Cheese Products/Dips — 76 — Yogurt, Yogurt Drinks & Probiotics — 162
Chicken ~ See Poultry

Eating Out:

Condiments, Salsa, Pickles — 80 — Cafeteria, Sandwiches — 165
Cookies, Crackers — 81 — Fair/Carnival/Stadium Foods — 166
Crispbreads, Matzo — 88 — Restaurant & International Foods — 168
Cream & Creamers — 89
Desserts (Puddings, Gelatin Desserts) — 90
Eggs, Egg Substitutes, Egg Dishes — 91 — *Fast-Food Chains & Restaurants* — 175-258
Fats, Butter, Spreads, Oils, Mayonnaise — 93
Fish, Shellfish — 95
Flour, Grains — 98 — **A-Z Food Index** — 282-287
Fruit (Fresh/Packaged/Dried/Snacks) — 99
Ice Cream & Frozen Yogurt/Novelties — 103

Meals, Entrees, Sides:

Cans/Packaged/Frozen — 111
Meats: Beef, Lamb, Pork, Game — 123
Sausages/Franks/Hot Dogs — 127
Lunch/Deli Meats & Sausages — 128
Milk ~ See Beverages
Nuts, Seeds, Peanut Butter — 130
Pancakes & Waffles — 132
Pasta & Noodles, Macaroni — 133

EXTRA DIET GUIDES & COUNTERS

Diabetes Guide 16-21
Alcohol Guide & Counter 23-29
Caffeine Guide & Counter 37
Fats & Cholesterol Guide 259-263
Fiber Guide & Counter 264-269
Protein Guide & Counter 270-274
Salt/Sodium Counter with
  High Blood Pressure Guide 275-281
Weight Control Guide 2-15

Weight Control Tips

✔ Eat & Drink Sensibly

- Avoid fad diets. Eat 3 sensible portion-controlled meals daily.
- Limit fats, high-fat foods/snacks and sugar. Eat adequate fresh fruit & vegetables.
- Limit soft drinks, energy drinks, fruit juice and alcohol. Quench your thirst on water.
(See Sample Meal Plan ~ Page 11)

✔ Exercise Daily

- Aim for at least 30 minutes daily – even in 5-10 minute lots. For motivation, find an exercise buddy, personal trainer or join a gym. *(Extra Notes ~ Page 12)*

✔ Reshape Eating Behaviors

- Be aware of eating and shopping behaviors that lead to overeating.
- Also focus on social and emotional situations that may trigger compulsive eating. *(Extra Notes ~ Page 14)*

✔ Keep a Food & Exercise Journal

- A journal helps you see exactly what you eat and drink, and how much you exercise.
(Extra Notes ~ Page 15)
- An excellent motivator and proven weight loss aid. Keeps you honest!

✔ Arrange Moral Support

- Gain the support of family and friends.
- Get extra professional help if required, from your doctor, dietitian, psychologist, exercise trainer, or slimming group.
- Beware of family saboteurs who discourage you from adopting a healthier lifestyle!

DOCTOR CHECK-UP

Ask your doctor to check your blood pressure, blood sugar and blood cholesterol levels.

HEALTHY WEIGHTS
~ MEN & WOMEN ~
(Over 18 Years)

Based on weights with least risk of disease or death from heart disease, diabetes, stroke and cancer.

Based on Body Mass Index of 20-25

BMI calculated as: $\dfrac{\text{Weight (kg)}}{\text{Height (m)}^2}$

Height (No Shoes) Ft Ins		Healthy Weight Range (Pounds)
4'7"	~	86-108
4'8"	~	88-110
4'9"	~	92-114
4'10"	~	97-121
4'11"	~	99-123
5'0"	~	101-127
5'1"	~	105-132
5'2"	~	110-136
5'3"	~	112-140
5'4"	~	114-145
5'5"	~	119-149
5'6"	~	123-156
5'7"	~	127-158
5'8"	~	129-162
5'9"	~	134-167
5'10"	~	138-173
5'11"	~	143-178
6'0"	~	145-182
6'1"	~	149-187
6'2"	~	156-193
6'3"	~	158-198
6'4"	~	162-202
6'5"	~	170-211
6'6"	~	172-215
6'7"	~	175-220

Body Fat Distribution & Health

Moderate amounts of body fat do not compromise health. However, excess fat above the hips carries a far greater health risk than fat on or below the hips - better to be a 'pear-shape' than an 'apple-shape'.

Abdominal obesity greatly increases the risk of developing diabetes, heart disease, high blood fats, hypertension, stroke, sleep apnea, arthritis and some cancers. So-called 'cellulite' carries no extra health risk.

Waist Circumference directly reflects the increased health risk of abdominal obesity. Waist size associated with a high health risk:

Men ~ Over 40 inches   **Women** ~ Over 35 inches

Body Mass Index (BMI)

BMI is a general (but not specific) indicator of body fatness. Although BMI alone is not diagnostic, the higher the BMI, the greater the health risk of developing diabetes, high blood pressure and heart disease. BMI does not apply to heavily muscled persons. BMI is used in a different way for children.

Abdominal obesity greatly increases the risk of ill-health and earlier death.

Check Your BMI: Find your height (no shoes) - look across the row to the weight nearest your own. Then track down to BMI.

Ht	☺		WEIGHT (LBS) ~ ADULTS											☺	
5'1"	100	106	111	116	122	127	132	137	143	148	153	158	185	211
5'2"	104	109	115	120	126	131	136	142	147	153	158	164	191	218
5'3"	107	113	118	124	130	135	141	146	152	158	163	169	197	225
5'4"	110	116	122	128	134	140	145	151	157	163	169	174	204	232
5'5"	114	120	126	132	138	144	150	156	162	168	174	180	210	240
5'6"	118	124	130	136	142	148	155	161	167	173	179	186	216	247
5'7"	121	127	134	140	146	153	159	166	172	178	185	191	223	255
5'8"	125	131	138	144	151	158	164	171	177	184	190	197	230	262
5'9"	128	135	142	149	155	162	169	176	182	189	196	206	236	270
5'10"	132	139	146	153	160	167	174	181	188	195	202	207	243	278
5'11"	136	143	150	157	165	172	179	186	193	200	208	215	250	286
6'0"	140	147	154	162	169	177	184	191	199	206	213	221	258	294
6'1"	144	151	159	166	174	182	189	197	204	212	219	227	265	302
6'2"	148	155	163	171	179	186	194	202	210	218	225	233	272	311
6'3"	152	160	168	176	184	192	200	208	216	224	232	240	279	319
6'4"	156	164	172	180	189	197	205	213	221	230	238	246	287	328

| BMI | 19 | 20 | 21 | 22 | 23 | 24 | 25 | 26 | 27 | 28 | 29 | 30 | 35 | 40 |

BMI Classification:

BMI Below 19
Underweight

BMI 19-24.9
Healthy Weight
(Low Health Risk)

BMI 25-29.9
Overweight
(Moderate Health Risk)

BMI 30-40
Obese (High Health Risk)

BMI Over 40
Morbid Obesity
(Very High Risk)

Interactive BMI Calculator
www.calorieking.com

Recommended Fat Intake

▶ Fat in the Diet

Fats in the diet are essential for good health. However, too much fat can contribute to obesity and a higher risk of heart disease, high blood pressure, diabetes, gallstone and certain cancers.

Dietary fat and oils have over double the calories of carbohydrates and protein. (Example: Changing from whole-milk to non-fat milk halves the calories.)

MAXIMUM DESIRABLE FAT INTAKE (DAILY)	
Calories	**Fat**
1200 cals	30g fat
1500 cals	40g fat
1800 cals	50g fat
2000 cals	60g fat
2200 cals	70g fat
2500 cals	80g fat
3000 cals	110g fat

ZERO GRAMS TRANS FAT

*Don't be fooled by **Zero Grams Trans Fat** boldly displayed on some high-fat snacks. They are still high in fat and calories.*

Examples: Cheetos 99c pkg ~ 24g fat, 380 cals
Lay's Chips (2¾ oz pkg) ~ 27g fat, 430 calories

0 grams
Trans Fat

▶ Beware low-fat foods

It is a mistake to think that eating low-fat or fat-free foods allows you to eat double the quantity. You can end up with even more calories than eating smaller amounts of regular-fat products.

Food products which are fat-free but high in calories include soda drinks, fruit juices, beer, alcoholic spirits, sugar and candy. Bread, rice and pasta also have negligible fat but need to be eaten in controlled amounts.

Ultimately, **it is food portion size as well as total calories that count** whether from fat, carbohydrate or protein. Remember, cows get fat on grass!

Reduced fat and fat-free foods are not necessarily low calorie. Portion size is still important.

3 Cookies
140 Calories

6 oz Fat-Free Muffin:
450 calories

FOOD LABEL MEANINGS

FDA Nutrition Claim Definitions
(All are on a Per Serving Basis)

Low Calorie: 40 Calories or less
Light or Lite: One third fewer calories or, 50% or less fat than regular product
Fat-Free: Less than half a gram of fat
Low-Fat: 3 grams or less of fat
Reduced Fat: 25% less fat than regular product
Fewer or Less Calories: At least 25% fewer calories than regular product

▶ **Meats, Poultry, Fish**

- **Choose lean cuts** of meat with little marbling. **Trim all visible fat** from meat and remove the skin from poultry. Removal of fat after cooking, is okay (to prevent dryness). Choose 'extra lean' ground beef.
- **Avoid high-fat meat products** such as salami, bacon, sausage and franks.
- **Broil or bake. Avoid frying in oil.** Allow casseroles to cool and skim off surface fat.
- **Avoid fried fish,** frozen fish in batter and canned fish in oil.

▶ **Fats & Oils**

- **Use minimal amounts** of all types of fat and oil. All are high in calories.
- **Choose** 'light' and 'reduced fat' spreads but still use sparingly.
- Use minimal amounts of oil when stir-frying. Use no-stick sprays like Pam.

▶ **Salad Dressings & Sauces**

- **Avoid regular mayonnaise and oil dressings.** Choose 'light', 'reduced fat' or 'fat-free' brands.
- **Choose low-fat or fat-free sauces** (mainly tomato-based). Avoid 'pesto', 'alfredo', 'cheese' and 'creamy' sauces.

▶ **Milk, Cheese**

- **Choose low-fat or nonfat milks and yogurts.** Avoid full-cream milk, cream, Half & Half.
- **Cheese:** Choose fat-free, and low-fat cheese. Part-skim ricotta is still high in fat. Low-fat cottage cheese is a good choice. Cheese substitutes can still be high in fat.

▶ **Snacks, Cookies, Candy**

- **Avoid** high-fat snacks such as potato chips, corn/tortilla chips, cheese puffs, buttered popcorn, chocolate and carob bars.

▶ **Desserts/Sweets**

- **Avoid high-fat desserts,** such as cake, pie, pastries, cheesecake, full-fat puddings.
- **Choose** fresh fruits, fresh fruit salad, canned fruit in water pack, low-fat ice cream. Use low-fat yogurt in place of cream.

▶ **Fast-Foods & Take-Out**

Check the Fast-Foods Section of this book for actual fat and calorie counts.

- **Avoid deep-fried foods such as** chicken, french fries and onion rings.
- **Pizzas:** Avoid sausage/pepperoni. Choose vegetarian topping and modest quantity of cheese. Eat a moderate serving. Eat extra salad and fresh fruit.
- **Hamburgers:** Choose medium size, lower fat burgers. Avoid bacon. Have a side salad (with fat-free dressing).
- **Delis:** Choose sandwiches/bread rolls, pitas with low-fat fillings and plain salad. Limit meat/cheese to small portions.
- **Coffees:** Avoid large sizes of latte and frappuccino. Request nonfat milk and no whipped cream. Avoid cookies and pastries.

Extra Information: www.CalorieKing.com

FRYING ADDS FAT!

The greater the surface area of potato exposed to fat or oil, the higher the fat content and calories.

 Whole Potato (3 oz)
`0g Fat` 65 Cals

 Roasted Potato (3 oz)
`5g Fat` 155 Cals

 Fries (Large cut, 3 oz)
`12g Fat` 220 Cals

 Fries (Small, 3 oz)
`15g Fat` 265 Cals

 Potato Chips (3 oz)
`30g Fat` 450 Cals

Naturally-Friendly Carbs

- **Carbohydrate foods in their more natural forms** (not overly processed) are essential to good health. They are the main source of fuel for the body, and also provide important vitamins, minerals, antioxidants and fiber – all of which help protect against heart disease, diabetes, hypertension, constipation-related ailments and many other diseases.

- Carbohydrates even help the body produce serotonin, the 'feel good' brain chemical that helps control appetite and overeating. Too little serotonin can lead to mood swings and depression.

Carbohydrates are found in different forms in food as:

- Sugars in fruit, sugar cane, milk
- Starches in whole grains, legumes, nuts, seeds and vegetables
- Dietary fiber (See Fiber Guide ~ Page 264)

Glycemic Index & Diabetes ~ Page 21

Carbohydrate foods (minimally processed) are essential to good health.

Be sure to eat adequate fruit and vegetables (5 - 7 servings) every day.

RECOMMENDED CARBOHYDRATE INTAKE

Calories (Daily)	Carbohydrate (Grams)	Percent Carbohydrate Calories
1200 cals	100-120g	35-40%
1500 cals	140-170g	40-45%
1800 cals	180-200g	40-45%
2000 cals	200-250g	40-50%
2500 cals	310-350g	50-55%
3000 cals	410-450g	55-65%

How Much Do We Need?

- As shown in the chart, well-balanced diets above 2000 calories contain 50-60% of total calories from carbohydrates.
- At lower calorie levels used for weight control (1200-1500 calories), carbohydrates account for as little as 40% of total calories. This is because protein calories have nutritional priority.
- Carbohydrates & Diabetes ~ See Page 21

Low-Carbohydrate Diets

- Popular low-carbohydrate diets are extreme in their recommendations to initially cut carb intake to as little as 20 grams per day – the amount in 1 thick slice of bread, or 1 medium apple, or 1 small potato.

  This greatly increases the risk of nutritional deficiencies and compromises health, particularly if fat intake is excessive through fatty meats, high-fat dairy products, and fried foods.

- While overweight Americans do need to reduce carbohydrate intake, it should be done **sensibly as part of reducing portion size and total calories.**

- Simply eating 'low-carb' food products without regard to portion size, calories or fats, will do little to promote weight loss or good health.

- **Low-carb diets (and indeed any diet) only work if total calories are reduced.**

- Refined sugars should be one of the first targets in reducing carb intake.

Extra Info ~ www.CalorieKing.com

FAT MATTERS
CARBS COUNT
BUT CALORIES ARE KING!

Sugar-free & lower carb products may still be high in calories and fat.

- Many overweight, inactive people consume over 500 calories of refined sugars per day, either self-added or as part of food products. This is equivalent to over 30 level teaspoons – a significant amount in weight control terms. Halving this amount would be reasonable and worthwhile.

Note: Naturally occurring sugars in fruits, vegetables and milk are fine when consumed in normal recommended amounts. These foods are also rich in other nutrients.

Refined sugar is referred to as having 'empty calories' because it supplies calories but negligible nutrients and no fiber.

- Most sugar in our diet is 'hidden' in processed foods such as soft drinks, fruit drinks, candy, cookies, cake, jam, sauces, ice cream, desserts, canned foods, and breakfast cereals.

Certainly enjoy moderate quantities of these foods, but for serious weight control, look for 'low calorie', 'diet' or 'sugar-free'.

However, be careful not to substitute sugar-rich foods with high-fat foods which might boost calories even more!

- Be aware that sugar comes in different forms such as sucrose, glucose, fructose, malt, high-fructose corn syrup, molasses, honey and maple syrup. Check the label.

- **Sugar alcohols such as sorbitol,** mannitol and maltitol are carb-based and have ½ - ¾ the calories of regular sugar. While not counted as sugar on food labels, they do add to the carb count. Excess amounts can cause bloating, gas and diarrhea.

- **Sugar-free sweeteners** such as *Equal, DiabetiSweet, NutraSweet, Splenda, Sweet'n Low* and *Stevia* make it easy to reduce sugar in drinks and recipes. Use only in moderation. Note: Most recipes can be adapted to contain less sugar with little effect on taste or quality.

Extra Info ~ www.CalorieKing.com

Sugar-free snacks and foods may be higher in fat and calories than the regular product.

Example	~ Creme Wafers (3):
Regular	~ 115 cals, 6g fat
Sugar-Free	~ 160 cals, 10g fat

SUGAR CONTENT OF SOME COMMON FOODS

Teaspoons of Sugar	
Coca Cola or *Pepsi,* 12 fl.oz	10
20 fl.oz size	17
Iced Tea, sweetened, 12 fl.oz	8
Chocolate Milk, 12 fl.oz	6
Honey Smacks Cereal, ¾ cup, 1 oz	4
Popcorn, caramel, 1 cup	3.5
Chocolate Bar, 1.5 oz	6
M&M's 1.7 oz pkg	7
Muffin, large, 4 oz	6
Choc Chip Cookie, 1 oz	2
Donut, iced	6
Apple Pie, 1 piece	7
Jell-O, ½ cup	4.5
Jam, 1 Tbsp, ¾ oz	2.5
Syrup, maple, 1 Tbsp	3

Reach for fresh fruit when you want to snack instead of candy or snack products rich in sugar and fat.

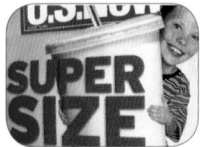

The XL Generation

Some 15% of American kids and adolescents are overweight; and childhood obesity has doubled over the last 20 years. Diabetes, high blood pressure and high cholesterol are major problem areas for overweight children and adolescents, as are depression, low self-esteem, sleep apnea and bone joint problems.

To address this problem, cooperation is required between kids, parents, schools and government. Weight control is a family and community affair.

Five Simple Tips To Get Started:

❶ Watch Soda Intake

Limit soda and sugary drinks to one serving on the weekends. Soda should not be an everyday beverage – water should be. When at restaurants or using a soda fountain, choose small servings with ice or choose diet soda instead. Schools should provide water and restrict access to soda as should parents when eating out or in the home!

❷ Cut back on Fast-Foods and Eating Out

Many more calories are consumed when you eat out. Healthy meals prepared at home are best for the whole family.

❸ Say "No" to Super-Sizing

When meals are upsized, loads more calories are consumed. Choose sensible portion sizes when eating out and at home. Use smaller plates and choose smaller packages.

❹ Limit Between-Meal Snacking

Watch out for high-fat and high-calorie snacks – they can have more calories than a meal! Keep your eye on portion sizes and limit salty snack foods and candy to parties and special occasions. Choose fresh fruit, vegetables, nuts and low-fat milk instead.

❺ Get Moving ~ Watch Less TV

Kids need at least 60 minutes of physical activity every day. It's critical for their fitness, and greatly lessens the risk of obesity.

Encourage kids to be active out of school hours. Wearing a pedometer can be highly motivational for kids to move more – as can playing dance video games such as *Dance Dance Revolution. Dance Central* (XBox360) and *Wii Fit* (Nintendo) are also excellent fitness motivators.

Limit TV and non-active computer games to just one hour per day. Also limit the accompanying snacks! Include exercise in family activities.

Extra information and tips ~ www.CalorieKing.com

**For Healthy, Overweight Persons ~ Not for Persons With Any Medical Condition
~ Please Check With Your Doctor & Dietitian ~**

 Breakfast (approx. 300 cal)

	1 Small Fruit or ½ oz Dried Fruit
Plus	Cereal: 1½ oz Dry (high fiber)
	or 1 cup cooked Oatmeal
Plus	½ oz Almonds/Seeds
Plus	Milk (from daily allowance) or Yogurt (low-fat)

Daily Milk Allowance (approx.160 calories)
2 cups Non-Fat Milk or 1½ cups Low-fat (1%) Milk
or equivalent Soy Drink, Yogurt, Cheese, Tofu

Fat Allowance (140 calories; 15g Fat)
4 tsp Fat or 6-8 tsp Diet Margarine or 3 tsp Oil
or 1½ Tbsp Mayonnaise or ½ medium Avocado
or 1½ Tbsp Peanut Butter or 30g Nuts/Seeds

 Lunch (approx. 440 calories)

	2 slices Wholegrain Bread (2 oz)
	or 4 Crispbreads/Crackers or 6" Pita
Plus	2 oz lean Meat, Chicken or Turkey
	or 3½oz Tuna (in water) or 2½ oz Salmon
	or 1 oz Cheese or ½ cup (4 oz) Cottage Cheese
	or ½ cup (4 oz) Ricotta Cheese (low-fat)
	or ½ cup (4 oz) Fruit Yogurt (low-fat)
	or ½ cup (4 oz) Bean Salad
Plus	Large Salad (Oil-free dressing)
Plus	1 small Fruit or ½ oz Dried Fruit

 Dinner (approx. 360 calories)

	Soup (fat-free)
Plus	3 oz lean Meat (cooked weight)
	or 4 oz Chicken Breast (no skin)
	or 3 oz Chicken Thigh/Leg (no skin)
	or 5 oz Fish (grilled, no fat)
	or ¾ cup (6 oz) Beans (Soy, Kidney, Pinto etc)/Lentils
	or Low-fat Entree (e.g. Lean Cuisine)
Plus	1 small Potato
	or ½ cup Rice/Pasta/Sweet Corn
	or 1 slice Wholegrain Bread
Plus	2-3 servings Vegetables/Salad
Plus	1 small Fruit + Diet Gelatin Dessert

 Breakfast ~ Choice 2

	1 Small Fruit
Plus	2 Eggs (no added fat)
	or 2 oz Cheese (low-fat)
	or 4 oz Cottage Cheese (low-fat)
	or 2 oz Lean/Canadian Bacon
Plus	1 Tomato
Plus	1 Slice Wholegrain Toast

 Between Meals

Water, Coffee, Tea, Diet drinks,
Fruit from main meals; Raw vegetable
pieces, Milk from Daily Allowance

Exercise & Weight Control

- **Persons who exercise regularly lose more weight** and keep it off longer than non-exercisers.
- **Exercise also improves general health and well-being.** Mood, confidence and self-esteem are enhanced by a sense of control and accomplishment.
- **Exercise is a good way to 'wake up' a sluggish metabolism** and burn extra fat tissue.
- **Aerobic (huff and puff) exercise most days** is great for burning calories and for cardiovascular fitness. But, it is strength training that mainly builds the muscles that burn calories even while we sleep.
- **Strength training is the key to retaining or rebuilding muscles.** As we age, we lose some 6 pounds of muscle per decade. This results in a lower metabolism and fewer calories being burnt.

  Muscles are the furnaces that burn calories. The more muscle you have, the more calories you will burn.

- **Regular strength training (2-3 times weekly)** can increase our metabolic rate for several days following exercise – and an extra 100 calories per day being burnt. While 2-3 pounds of muscle may be gained in the first 8-10 weeks, weight from exercised muscles is okay. It is excess fat (particularly abdominal fat) that is a potential health hazard. Gaining muscle and losing fat also helps body reshaping – even if the scales don't show it.
- **Avoid injury** by beginning with walking, low impact aerobics, or weight-supported exercise (e.g. swimming, cycling). Avoid competitive sports. Allow 2-3 days of recovery between strength training sessions. Get professional advice ~ particularly if you have a medical condition.
- **How Much?** Start with 10-20 minutes per day and progress to 30-60 minutes per day.

  Also walk up stairs instead of using elevators. Take a brisk walk at lunch. Use an exercise bike, treadmill or stair machine while watching TV. Walk the dog.

- **How Often?** While aerobic fitness requires only 3-4 sessions weekly, **weight control is a daily event which requires daily exercise to burn calories.** Add in strength training 2-3 times weekly.
- **For motivation,** find an exercise buddy, personal trainer or join a gym.

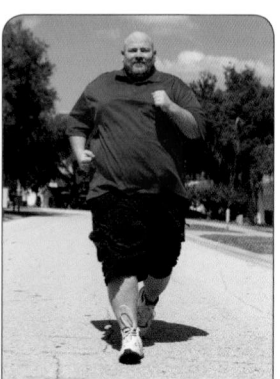

Brisk walking each day is a safe and effective way to burn calories and keep fit.
Try it – you'll like it!

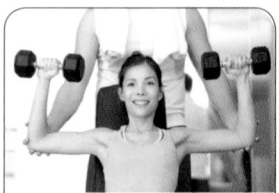

Strength training is the key to retain or rebuild muscles.
Muscles burn extra calories even while you sleep.
For extra guidance, seek a qualified trainer or join a gym.

Calories Used in Exercise

LIGHT	MODERATE	HEAVY
130 lbs ~ 3 Cals/Min	130 lbs ~ 5 Cals/Min	130 lbs ~ 8 Cals/Min
170 lbs ~ 4 Cals/Min	170 lbs ~ 6 Cals/Min	220 lbs ~ 12 Cals/Min
220 lbs ~ 5 Cals/Min	220 lbs ~ 7 Cals/Min	170 lbs ~ 10 Cals/Min
▼	▼	▼
Walking, slow	Walking, brisk	Walking (power), Jogging
Cycling, light	Cycling, moderate	Cycling (vigorous), Spinning
Frisbee playing	Swimming, crawl	Swimming, strenuous
Gardening, light	Weight-training, light	Weight-training, heavy
Golf, social	Tennis, moderate	Wrestling/Judo, advanced
Tennis, doubles	Racquetball, beginners	Racquetball, advanced
Housework, cleaning	Aerobics, light	Tae Bo, Kick Boxing
Calisthenics, light	Football, touch	Football, training
Bowling	Basketball, Baseball	Basketball (Pro)
Ping-pong, social	Walking Downstairs	Climbing Stairs
Ice Skating, light	Snow Skiing (downhill)	Skipping Rope
Aquarobics, light	Shovelling snow	Skiing (cross country)
Skate Boarding	Dancing (ballroom)	Aquarobics, advanced
Line/Square Dancing	Rowing, moderate	Dancing (strenuous), Zumba
Tai Chi, Yoga	Volleyball, competitive	Rowing, vigorous
Volleyball		Martial Arts

Note: Only those sports or activities that are sustained over a period of time (e.g running) qualify for heavy exercise. Stop-start sports such as tennis are considered 'moderate'.

Interactive Calculations ~ www.CalorieKing.com/tools

WALKING PROGRAM

USE DISTANCE, STEPS OR TIME

Weeks	Distance	Steps Pedometer	Time
▼	▼	▼	▼
1-2	1 mile	2000	20 mins
3-5	1.5 miles	3000	28 mins
6-8	2 miles	3500	35 mins
9-10	2.5 miles	4500	45 mins
11+	3.5 miles	6000	60 mins

10,000 STEPS PER DAY

A pedometer can motivate you to be more active. It clips to your belt or waist band and registers each step.

Aim for 8,000 - 10,000 steps per day, instead of an average of only 3,000 - 4,000 steps.

For Extra Information:
www.CalorieKing.com

Reshaping Eating Behaviors

- Eating is a behavior that is largely controlled by people with whom we live or socialize, places in which we carry out our lives, and our emotions. Become aware of those situations that commonly lead to extra food being eaten.

- We may also be unaware of 'bad' eating habits that can lead to excess calorie intake; e.g. eating quickly, large mouthfuls, eating when tense or bored, finishing a large serving of food when not hungry.

Tips to help uncover and correct those 'bad' or problem eating habits:

- **Don't eat while engaged in other activities;** for example, watching TV, reading. Eat only at the table, not at the fridge or while standing.

- **Don't eat quickly.** Chewing slowly allows time to register a feeling of fullness. Don't use fingers, only utensils. Cut food into smaller pieces. Don't load your fork until the previous mouthful is finished.

Practice saying 'NO' politely but assertively.

- **Don't purchase problem high calorie foods.** Shop from a set list to prevent impulse buying. Avoid shopping with children.

- **Buy snack foods** in the smallest package. The larger the serving size or package, the more you are likely to eat or drink.

- **Plan meals in advance. Stick to a set menu.**

- **Plan a strategy to avoid uncontrolled eating** and drinking at social events, or when your emotions urge you to binge.

  Rehearse repeatedly in your mind exactly what you will do in such situations. Remind yourself several times each day that you are in charge of your actions and that you can be strong-willed. Seek counseling or coaching on various strategies.

- **Distract yourself** when you feel the urge to snack impulsively. Engage in some activity that will distract you from thinking about food. Examples: go for a walk, brush your teeth, phone a friend.

  If you eat out of boredom, find some new hobby or interest that gets you out of the house. Even enrol in an adult education class.

Do you use food as an emotional crutch? If so, professional counseling may be helpful.

The food journal is the most powerful proven aid for dieters. Persons who keep a food and exercise journal not only lose more weight, they also keep it off. Here are some of the reasons:

- **Recording your eating and exercise habits** jolts you into realizing just what you do eat and drink each day; and also whether you exercise sufficiently.

- **Helps you identify problem foods** and drinks with excessive calories and fat.

- **Helps identify moods,** situations and events that lead to excessive eating of unwanted calories. You can then plan to overcome or avoid them.

- **Prevents 'calorie amnesia',** the forgetfulness that leads to rebound weight gain after successful weight loss. Recording puts you back on the right track.

- **Helps you develop greater self-discipline.** You will think twice about overindulging if you have to record it - especially if someone checks your journal regularly. It certainly keeps you honest!

- **Motivates you** to carefully plan your meals and to exercise each day.

- **Serves as a check system** for your doctor, dietitian or counselor to assess your progress and make recommendations.

Write It Down!

"Keeping a journal gives me feedback on exactly what I eat and drink each day.

It helps prevent 'calorie amnesia' and reminds me to exercise each day.

It's a 'must' for successful weight control!"

3 Easy Ways to Track Your Food & Exercise Calories!

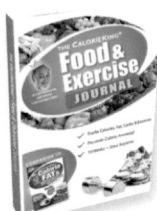

CalorieKing Online
Part of a comprehensive personalized program that includes tools, reports and a supportive community.

iPhone
Make smart food choices wherever you are! ControlMyWeight is easy to use & always with you.

Book
A 10-week journal that fits in your pocket. Includes Weekly Summary page and Progress Checklist

Extra Information ~ CalorieKing.com

Diabetes Guide
(In Association with Joslin Diabetes Center)

What is Diabetes?
Diabetes occurs when the body has difficulty processing glucose sugar in the blood.

- **After digestion,** sugar and starches are changed into **glucose** – the simplest form of sugar vital for body energy and growth.
- Insulin is the hormone which acts like a key that opens the door to body cells and allows glucose to enter.
- **Without enough insulin,** glucose builds up in the blood and passes into the urine. High blood glucose levels lead to frequent urination, extreme thirst, and tiredness.
- **Untreated diabetes increases the risk of damage to nerves and blood vessels.** This, in turn, increases the risk of heart disease, stroke, blindness, kidney damage, foot ulcers and gangrene (with amputation), impotence and other complications.

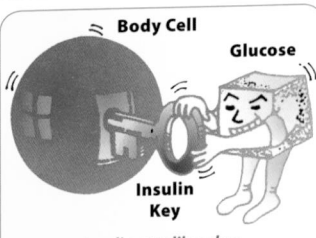

Insulin acts like a key. It opens the door to body cells and allows glucose to enter.

People with type 1 diabetes and some with type 2 have too few or no keys and require insulin injections.

Others (primarily type 2) make enough insulin but the body doesn't use it as well as it should – particularly if obese and inactive.

SYMPTOMS OF DIABETES

- Frequent urination
- Extreme thirst
- Unusual hunger
- Rapid weight loss
- Extreme fatigue
- Blurred vision
- Skin infections that are slow to heal
- Tingling/numbness in feet

Note: Diabetes can be present even with no symptoms.

DON'T IGNORE DIABETES
IT'S A SERIOUS DISEASE!

TYPE 2 DIABETES

- Occurs in 90% of diabetes cases
- Occurs mainly in adults - particularly in overweight and inactive persons
- Insulin is produced but body cells resist its action and glucose cannot enter cells
- Usually treated with meal planning and physical activity. Sometimes requires medication (pills or insulin)

TYPE 1 DIABETES

- Occurs in 10% of diabetes cases
- Usually in children and young adults
- Pancreas produces little or no insulin. Daily insulin injections (or use of an insulin pump) are necessary, as well as:
  - matching pre-meal insulin to the amount of carbohydrate eaten
  - weight control and regular physical activity

GESTATIONAL DIABETES

- Occurs in some women during pregnancy. It usually disappears after the baby's birth.
- Women who have had gestational diabetes still have a high risk of developing type 2 diabetes within 5 to 10 years.
- Requires weight control, a healthy lifestyle and regular medical checks

Are You At Risk for Diabetes?

Pre-Diabetes ~ An Early Warning!

Pre-diabetes means that your blood glucose levels are higher than normal, but not high enough to be called diabetes.

If you have pre-diabetes, you have a higher risk for getting diabetes later on.

The good news is that you can start taking steps to prevent diabetes by making healthy lifestyle changes – such as losing weight if overweight, and being more physically active.

WHAT'S YOUR RISK?

Find out if you're at risk for diabetes by answering the following questions:

- ☐ I have been told I have pre-diabetes
- ☐ I have a family history of diabetes
- ☐ I am African American, Latino American, Asian American, Native American or a Pacific Islander
- ☐ I have had gestational diabetes (diabetes during pregnancy)
- ☐ I am over age 45
- ☐ I am overweight
- ☐ My waist is larger than: 35 inches (for a woman) or 40 inches (for a man)
- ☐ I get little or no physical activity
- ☐ My blood pressure is higher than 130 over 85
- ☐ My HDL (good cholesterol) is too low
- ☐ My triglycerides (blood fats) are too high

✔ CHECK YOUR RESULT

- If you've put a check mark in two or more of the boxes, you may be more likely to develop type 2 diabetes.
- Talk with your healthcare provider to see if you should have a blood test for diabetes.

BLOOD GLUCOSE CLASSIFICATION OF DIABETES

Normal:	Below 100 mg/dl*
Pre-Diabetes:	100-125 mg/dl*
Diabetes:	Over 125 mg/dl*

(*Fasting Blood Glucose)

KNOW YOUR BGL
(Blood Glucose Level)
Everyone over the age of 45 should have a blood glucose test every three years

Importance of Weight Control

- **Type 2 diabetes** is more common in people who are overweight.
- **Being overweight** means that your insulin doesn't work as well to control blood glucose levels.
- **Losing just 10 to 20 pounds** can help you better manage your diabetes and lower your risk for heart disease.
- **Keys to weight control include:**
- Following a healthy eating plan
- Controlling food portions
- Being physically active most days of the week
- Keeping food records
- Setting realistic goals
- **Work with a registered dietitian** who can help you reach a weight that's ideal for you.

KEEP MOVING!
Every day, do at least 30 minutes of moderate intensity exercise.
(even in 5-minute sets)

It's the key to improving insulin action. Add muscle strength training 3-4 times a week to double the benefits.

Managing Diabetes

Don't battle diabetes alone. Establish a partnership with your doctor, dietitian, certified diabetes educator, and pharmacist.

Extra Support: • *Joslin Diabetes Center*
- *American Diabetes Association*
- *American Association of Diabetes Educators*
- *Juvenile Diabetes Research Foundation*
- *National Diabetes Education Program*

Hints to keep blood glucose within safe limits:

- **Control your food intake.** Know what and when you will eat. Seek referral to a dietitian for expert advice.
- **Exercise regularly.** It assists weight control and can improve sensitivity of body cells to insulin. Plan physical activity into your daily routine.
- **Monitor your blood glucose** at home and work with a blood glucose meter. It will help you become familiar with your blood glucose patterns, and the effects of food, activity and medication.
- **Take insulin or oral medication as prescribed.** If on insulin, know what action to take if hypoglycemia (low blood glucose) occurs. Also educate your family and friends. More Info: www.joslin.org

Be Heart Smart ~ Know Your ABC's

If you have diabetes, you are at a higher risk for heart attack and stroke than someone without diabetes. But you can fight back!

Be smart about your heart!

Take control of the ABC's of diabetes and live a long and healthy life. Talk to your healthcare provider about your ABC targets.

 is for A1C
The A1C (A-one-C) test – short for hemoglobin A1C. It reflects your average blood glucose (sugar) over the last 3 months.
Suggested Target: Below 7%

is for Blood Pressure
High blood pressure makes your heart work too hard.
Suggested Target: Below 130/80

is for Cholesterol
Bad cholesterol, or LDL, can build up and clog your arteries. **Suggested Target: Below 100**

Be Smart About Your **Heart**
Control the **Diabetes**
ABCs of

➤ A1C
➤ Blood Pressure
➤ Cholesterol

National Diabetes Education Program

Be smart about your heart!

Take control of the ABC's of diabetes and live a long and healthy life.

Talk to your healthcare provider about your ABC targets.

Take action now to lower your risk for heart attack, stroke and other diabetes problems.

* * *

◄ *Note: These targets are suggested by the National Institutes for Health and the American Diabetes Association*

Guidelines for choosing a healthy diet apply equally to people with or without diabetes. Eating a wide variety of foods that are mainly low in fat, low in refined sugars, and high in fiber, is recommended.

However, actual food quantities, as well as when you eat, will also influence control of blood glucose. Your dietitian will individualize a meal plan to suit your food preferences, lifestyle and medical status.

Here are a few tips:

- **Maintain a healthy weight.** If overweight, even a modest weight loss plus daily physical activity can help manage blood glucose in type 2 diabetes.

- **Don't skip meals.** If you take insulin or an oral hypoglycemic agent, regular meals are important.

  If on insulin, eat meals at the same time each day. Eat a similar amount of food at each meal. Eating about the same amount of carbohydrate over the day will make best use of insulin and prevent wide variations in blood glucose levels.

- **Know which foods contain carbohydrate;** and learn how to check the *Nutrition Facts Label* on foods. Check the serving size, total fat and total carbohydrate – not just the sugar content. All carbohydrate breaks down to sugars after digestion.

- **Choose wholegrain breads, cereals and pasta.** Eat fresh fruits, vegetables and legumes. These foods contain more fiber and slow the release of glucose into your blood after a meal.

- **Limit foods high in saturated fat, trans fat and cholesterol.** Enjoy fish, soy foods, and other foods rich in omega-3 fats. *(Extra Notes: Page 259)*

- **Limit sugars and foods high in added sugar** particularly if overweight. Small amounts of sugar as part of a meal may occasionally be okay. Check with your dietitian. *(Extra Notes: Page 9)*

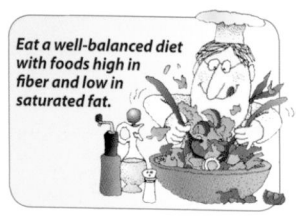

Eat a well-balanced diet with foods high in fiber and low in saturated fat.

The Plate Method is an easy way to eat healthfully. (See next page)

MAIN MEAL

Vegetables & Salad Greens

Bread · Starch · Grain | Meat · Protein

ALCOHOL TIPS

- **If you drink alcohol, have only moderate amounts:**
  Men ~ 1-2 drinks/day
  Women ~ 1 drink/day
  For some people, safe drinking will mean no alcoholic drinks at all.

  (Also see Alcohol Guide ~ Page 23)

- **Drink along with your food** – especially if you use insulin or diabetes pills.

- **Do not omit any carb food** in exchange for an alcoholic drink. However, non-alcoholic beers (12 fl oz) count as one carb exchange.

- **Alcohol increases the risk of hypoglycemia** (low blood sugar) and drug interactions if you take insulin and certain types of diabetes pills.

- **Check with your doctor and dietitian.**
  Extra Info: www.joslin.org

Diabetes Guide ~ The Plate Method

The Plate Method – An Easy Way to Eat Healthfully

The plate method is a helpful tool to guide your food choices until you see a dietitian for your own meal plan.

For a healthy meal:

- Fill half of your plate with non-starchy vegetables (broccoli, green beans, carrots).
- Fill a quarter of your plate with carbohydrate (wholegrain bread, pasta, potato, brown rice).
- Fill the other quarter of your plate with 3-4 ounces of lean meat, poultry, or fish.
- Use 1-2 teaspoons of tub margarine or a heart-healthy vegetable oil.
- Add a small piece of fruit or 8 ounces of skim/low-fat milk or yogurt.

MAIN MEAL

Vegetables & Salad Greens

Bread · Starch · Grain   Meat · Protein

PLUS ONE CHOICE

Milk, Fruit, Dessert or other Carb Food

How Much Carbohydrate Should You Eat?

A dietitian can best determine how much carbohydrate you need at each of your meals, based on your lifestyle, food preferences, and overall diabetes control.

Until you see a dietitian, aim to keep the amount of carbohydrate you eat the same at each of your meals.

CARB CHOICES MEAL PLAN
One Carb Choice = 15 Grams of Carb

The amount in: 1 slice Bread
or ¾ cup Cereal (unsweetened)
or 1 small Potato **or** 1 small Fruit

Breakfast
- Eat 2-3 carb choices (30-45 grams)
- Include a low-fat protein source such as egg whites or skim milk.

Lunch and Dinner
- Eat 3-4 carb choices (45-60 grams carb)
- Include fruit and non-starchy vegetables. Choose small portions of low-fat protein foods.

Snacks: If needed, eat 1-2 carb choices (15-30 grams carb).

Note: Above plan is for adults. Carbohydrate amounts will vary with physical activity level.

Carb Type Affects Blood Glucose

The various forms of carbohydrate affect blood glucose levels in different ways. It is difficult to predict the effect of particular foods, sugars, or meals, simply by their carbohydrate content.

Thus the same amount of carbohydrate from different foods may affect blood sugar levels very differently. Many factors affect the rate of digestion and absorption such as:

- the type of sugar, starch, and fiber
- the degree of processing and cooking (which increases digestion rate)
- the amount of protein and fat (which slow stomach emptying and digestion).

Glycemic Index (GI)

The GI is a method of ranking carbohydrate foods on a scale (0-100) according to how they affect blood glucose levels. (See next column.)

The higher the GI value, the greater the food's ability to rapidly raise blood glucose levels, and the more insulin needed by the body (not desirable).

Eating low-GI foods may lead to better control of blood glucose and insulin levels (which in turn lowers the risk of damage to blood vessels and nerves). The slower digestion of low-GI foods may also help to delay hunger pangs and benefit weight control.

Cautionary Notes on GI

Choosing low-GI foods is not a license to eat unlimited amounts. Calorie restriction and portion control for weight control is of prime importance.

Also remember, Low-GI foods are carbohydrate foods and must still be counted as part of any dietetic carbohydrate plan.

GI is not meant to be used by itself without regard to portion size, and other dietary recommendations for healthy eating. Foods are not good or bad on the basis of their GI.

While GI may be a helpful tool for some people with diabetes, what is most important is to control the total amount of carbohydrate that you eat.

LOWER-GLYCEMIC FOODS

Slower-Acting Carbohydrates

These foods are more slowly digested and absorbed. They help maintain more even blood glucose levels, as long as excessive amounts are not eaten. Use these foods regularly but still limit portion size for weight control.

Examples:

- Dried beans, peas, lentils
- Nuts and seeds
- Wholegrain breads
- Bran cereals, oats
- Sweet corn, barley, buckwheat
- Wholegrain pasta, basmati rice
- Fresh fruit: apples, avocados, bananas (firm), cherries, grapefruit, grapes, olives, oranges, peaches, pears, plums. Fresh juices.
- Vegetables: broccoli, yam, sweet potatoes, salad greens
- Milk, yogurt, soy drinks
- Dark chocolate
- Sugar alcohols (sorbitol, maltitol)

HIGHER-GLYCEMIC FOODS

Quicker-Acting Carbohydrates

These foods are more rapidly raise blood glucose levels. Eat only in moderation.

- White bread, rice cakes, bagels, croissants, doughnuts
- Low-fiber cereals: Cornflakes, *Rice Krispies, Froot Loops*
- White potatoes, white rice
- Watermelon, ripe bananas, cantaloupe, pineapple
- Soda, sugar-sweetened sports and energy drinks
- Sugar, candy, popcorn (plain)
- Ice cream (low-fat), frozen yogurt

High-GI fruits and potatoes are still healthy choices when eaten in moderate amounts.

Notes ◆ Abbreviations ◆ Disclaimer

⟫ Calorie and fat values have been rounded off. **Calories** ~ to the nearest 5 or 10 calories. **Fat** ~ to nearest half gram. **Note:** Trace amounts of fat (less than 0.3 grams) have been treated as zero.

⟫ **Carbohydrate figures** in this book are for total carbohydrate, and **not Net Carbs** (which deducts fiber, polydextrose and sugar alcohols from total carbs).

⟫ Because manufacturers' figures on labels are rounded off, figures in this book may differ slightly from the label. Serving sizes may also vary.

C ~ Calories
F ~ Fat (grams)
Cb ~ Carbohydrate (grams)

Abbreviations

tsp = teaspoon
Tbsp or T = Tablespoon
oz = ounce(s)
c = cup
fl.oz = fluid ounce(s)
g = gram(s)
avg = average
pkg = package

Volume Measures

(All measures are level)
3 tsp = 1 Tbsp
2 Tbsp = 1 fl.oz
½ cup = 4 fl.oz
1 cup = 8 fl.oz
2 cups = 1 Pint
2 Pints = 1 Quart

Note: 8 oz weight is not the same as 8 fl oz volume (space occupied). Dense foods weigh more per set volume. Examples:
1 cup popcorn weighs ½ oz
1 cup milk weighs 8½ oz
1 cup pudding weighs 10 oz

Metric Conversion

½ oz = 14 grams
1 oz = 28.4 grams
2 oz = 57 grams
3½ oz = 100 grams
1 fl.oz = 30 mls
1 cup (8 fl.oz) = 240 mls
33 fl.oz = 1 liter (volume)

IMPORTANT DISCLAIMER

* The authors and publishers of this book are not physicians and are not licensed to give medical advice. This book is not a substitute for professional advice. Users should consult their medical professional before making any health, medical or other decisions based on the material contained herein.

* This book is a compilation of original material from other sources intended for educational purposes only. Because food manufacturers constantly change their products, only they are the authoritative source for food's most current nutritional information.

* Persons using the information herein for any medical purposes, such as matching insulin dosage to carbohydrate intake, should not rely solely on the accuracy of figures herein and should independently check food labels or contact the food manufacturer for the latest data.

Canadian Readers:

Please note that figures in this book are based on U.S. food products and restaurants. Equivalent Canadian foods may vary and should be checked independently.

* WARRANTY DISCLAIMER:

THE AUTHOR AND PUBLISHER DISCLAIM ANY LIABILITY ARISING DIRECTLY OR INDIRECTLY FROM THE USE OF THIS BOOK. THE INFORMATION HEREIN IS PROVIDED "AS IS" AND WITHOUT ANY WARRANTY EXPRESSED OR IMPLIED. ALL DIRECT, INDIRECT, SPECIAL, INCIDENTAL, CONSEQUENTIAL OR PUNITIVE DAMAGES ARISING FROM ANY USE OF THIS INFORMATION IS DISCLAIMED AND EXCLUDED.

This information is also provided subject to Family Health Publications' Terms and Conditions found at the website, www.calorieking.com/terms and incorporated herein.

INFORMATION SOURCES

• U.S. Dept. of Agriculture
• U.S. Food Manufacturers
• Food Industry Boards & Councils
• Author extrapolations

FEEDBACK WELCOME!

Please contact the author with your queries and suggestions.
feedback@calorieking.com

- **Health Hazards: Excessive alcohol intake** contributes to obesity, high blood pressure, stroke, heart and liver disease, some cancers, and even impotence. **Concentration and short-term memory** are reduced as well as athletic performance.

  Other alcohol hazards include: Fetal Alcohol Syndrome, stomach upsets, menstrual problems, depression, snoring, sleep problems, work absenteeism, impaired judgement, risky behaviors and social/family problems.

- **Alcohol contributes to obesity** through its high calories and by lessening the body's ability to burn fat. Fat storage is promoted, particularly in the belly – a health danger zone. Alcohol can also stimulate the appetite; and weaken the dieter's resolve!

- **Alcohol is potentially more harmful while dieting:** Blood sugar levels may drop with resultant fatigue and further impairment of concentration, reflexes and driving skills.

Excess alcohol contributes to obesity, high blood pressure and many other health problems

---

LOWER RISK ALCOHOL LIMITS

 WOMEN:
No more than
1 drink per day

 MEN:
No more than
2 drinks per day
(Over 65 y.o. ~ 1 drink)

(At least 2 days a week should be alcohol-free)

1 DRINK CONTAINS 14 GRAMS ALCOHOL
→ 12 fl.oz Regular Beer (5% Alc.)
OR 14 fl.oz Light Beer (4.2% Alc.)
OR 5 fl.oz Wine (12% Alc.)
OR 1½ fl.oz Spirits (80 Proof)

Note: You cannot save daily drinks for one occasion.
Binge drinking is particularly harmful:
4 drinks for males or 3 drinks for females (within 2 hours).

For some people, safe drinking means no alcohol at all. Even one drink may impair driving skills, particularly if tired. For women who drink frequently, breast cancer risk is increased by 9% for each drink after the first drink. In men, just 2 drinks a day doubles the risk of cancers of the mouth and throat.

It is advisable not to drink at all if you are:

- pregnant, trying to conceive or breastfeeding
- taking medication or have liver or heart disease (unless approved by your doctor or pharmacist)
- planning to drive, use machinery or play sports
- studying or needing to concentrate
- a child or adolescent

 Women and adolescents are more prone to alcohol's ill-effects due to their lower body weight, smaller livers and lesser capacity to metabolize alcohol. As we age, our ability to handle alcohol decreases.

HOW TO CALCULATE ALCOHOL CONTENT

Percent alcohol on label refers to alcohol volume (ml alcohol/100ml).
Note: 100ml = 3½ fl.oz

To convert to grams (weight) of alcohol, multiply the alcohol volume by 0.8 – since 1 ml of alcohol weighs only 0.8 grams.

EXAMPLE:
12 fl.oz Can Beer
(5% alcohol)

5% alc. volume
= 5% of 12 fl.oz = 0.6 fl.oz
= 18ml alcohol (Note: 1 fl.oz = 30ml)
Weight (18ml x 0.8) = 14.4g alcohol

GOVERNMENT WARNINGS!

(1) According to the Surgeon General, women should not drink alcoholic beverages during pregnancy because of the risk of birth defects.

(2) Consumption of alcoholic beverages impairs your ability to drive a car or operate machinery, and may cause health problems.

EXTRA INFORMATION

Alcohol & Diabetes ~ See Page 19
Alcohol & The Heart ~ See Page 18
Tips to Avoid Harmful Drinking ~ Page 19

Quick Guide   **Alc** ~ Alcohol (Grams)

Beer: **Cb** ~ Carbohydrate

Beer Contains Zero Fat:

	C	Alc	Cb
Regular Beer (5% Alc. Vol.):			
7 fl.oz Glass	80	8.5	4
12 fl.oz Bottle/Can/Glass	140	14	10
16 fl.oz Bottle/Can	185	19	13
22 fl.oz Bottle	260	26	18
24 fl.oz Can	280	28	20
32 fl.oz Bottle	370	38	28
40 fl.oz Bottle	470	47	35
50 fl.oz Football	590	59	50
Light Beer (4.2% Alc. Vol.):			
7 fl.oz Glass	65	7	4
12 fl.oz Bottle/Can/Glass	110	12	7
16 fl.oz Bottle/Can	145	16	9
22 fl.oz Bottle	200	22	13
24 fl.oz Can	220	24	14
Non-Alcoholic Brews:			
(Less than 0.5% alcohol by volume)			
Average all Brands, 12 fl.oz	70	1	14

Beer ~ Brands

Note: Figures shown are for the United States except for the states of Utah, Colorado, Kansas and Oklahoma who have certain restrictions limiting the alcohol content to not more than 4% by volume (3.2% by weight).

Percentage alcohol listed is by volume - not by weight.

Per 12 fl.oz Serving

	C	Alc	Cb
Amstel, Light (3.5%)	95	10	6
Anchor: Porter (5.6%)	210	15	23
Steam (4.9%)	165	14	14
Asahi: Kuronama (5.3%)	165	14	14
Select (4.7%)	140	13	11
Super Dry (4.9%)	150	14	14
Bass, Pale Ale (5.1%)	155	14	12
Beck's: Original (5%)	145	14	10
Premier Light (2.3%)	65	7	4
Big Sky: Original IPA (6.2%)	195	18	17
Moose Drool (5.3%)	175	15	16
Scape Goat (4.7%)	155	14	14
Trout Slayer Ale (4.7%)	145	14	12
Blatz: Original (4.6%)	145	13	13
Light (3.9%)	110	11	8
Blue Moon: Belgian (5.4%)	165	15	13
Grand Cru Ale (8.2%)	230	21	19
Harvest Pumpkin Ale (5.8%)	180	17	14
Spring Ale (5.7%)	180	16	15
Summer Ale (5.2%)	150	15	13
Winter Abbey Ale (5.7%)	180	14	14
Bohemia (4.73%)	140	14	12

Brands (Cont)   **Alc** ~ Alcohol (Grams)

Per 12 fl.oz Serving

	C	Alc	Cb
Bud Ice, (5.5%)	120	16	4
Bud Light: Regular (4.2%)	110	12	7
& Clamato Chelada (4.2%)	150	12	16
Platinum (6%)	140	17	5
Lime (4.2%)	115	12	8
Lime-A-Rita (8%), 8 oz	220	15	29
Straw-Ber-Rita (8%), 8 oz	200	15	24
Budweiser: Lager (5%)	145	14	11
Black Crown (6%)	165	17	11
Clamato Chelada (5%)	185	14	20
Picante (5%)	200	14	23
Select (4.3%)	100	12	3
Select 55 (2.4%)	55	7	2
Busch: Original (4.3%)	115	12	7
Ice (5.9%)	135	17	4
Light (4.1%)	95	12	3
Carlsberg, Pilsner (5%)	135	14	10
Carta Blanca (4.6%)	145	13	11
Castlemaine XXXX,			
Bitter (4.6%)	140	14	10
Cerveza, Aquila (4%)	125	11	11
Colt 45, Malt Liquor (5.6%)	155	16	11
Coors: Banquet (5%)	150	14	12
Extra Gold (5%)	150	14	13
Light (4.2%)	100	12	5
Corona: Extra (4.6%)	150	13	14
Light (4.1%)	100	12	5
Dos Equis XX: Amber (4.6%)	145	13	12
Lager (4.6%)	140	13	11
Fosters: Lager (5%)	145	14	11
Premium Ale (5.5%)	145	16	12
Genesee: Lager (4.5%)	150	13	14
Genny Light Lager (3.6%)	95	10	6
George Killian's, Irish Red (5%)	160	14	15
Grolsch: Blonde (2.8%)	120	8	16
Light (3.6%)	95	11	6
Premium (5%)	145	14	10
Guinness: Draught (4%)	125	10	10
Extra Stout (6%)	175	17	14
Hamm's: Original (4.7%)	145	13	12
Special Light (3.9%)	110	12	8
Heineken: Lager (5%)	150	14	12
Special Dark (5%)	165	14	15
Premium Light (3.5%)	100	10	7
Hurricane: Malt Liquor (5.9%)	135	17	4
High Gravity (8.1%)	185	23	6
Icehouse: Original (5.5%)	150	16	10
Light (5%)	125	14	7
Keystone: Ice (5.9%)	140	17	6
Light (4.2%)	105	12	5
Killian's, Irish Red (5%)	165	14	14
King Cobra (6%)	135	17	4

Brands (Cont) — Alc ~ Alcohol (Grams) / Cb ~ Carbohydrate

Per 12 fl.oz Serving Unless Indicated

	C	Alc	Cb
Beer Contains Zero Fat:			
Per 12 fl.oz Serving			
Kirin: Ichiban (5%)	145	14	10
Light (3.2%)	95	9	4
Kokanee Glacier, (5%)	145	14	11
Labatt: Blue (4.7%)	135	14	10
Blue Light (4%)	110	11	8
Landshark, Lager (4.6%)	150	13	13
Leinenkugel's: Original (4.6%)	150	13	14
Summer Shandy (4.2%)	130	12	12
Lone Star: Pale Lager (4.7%)	135	13	12
Light (3.9%)	110	11	9
Lowenbrau, Original (5%)	140	14	12
Magic Hat, #9 (5.1% alc)	155	15	14
Magnum, Malt Liquor (5.6%)	160	16	11
Michelob: Lager (4.8%)	160	14	14
Light (4.1%)	120	12	9
Amber Bock (5.1%)	150	14	12
Golden Draft (4.6%)	120	13	7
Golden Draft Light (4.1%)	110	12	7
Ultra (4.2%)	95	12	2.5
Ultra Amber (3.9%)	90	11	3
Ultra Fruit Flavors (4%)	95	11	5
Mickey's, Malt Liquor (5.6%)	160	16	11
Miller: Chill, 100 Calorie (4.2%)	100	12	4
Genuine Draft /High Life (4.7%)	145	13	13
High Life Light (4.2%)	110	12	7
Lite (4.2%)	95	12	3
MGD 64 (2.8%)	65	8	2.5
Milwaukee's Best:			
Premium (4.3%)	130	12	11
Ice (5.9%)	145	17	7
Light (4.2%)	100	12	4
Minnesota's Best, Original (4.9%)	140	14	10
Modelo, Especial (4.4%)	145	13	13
Molson Canadian: Lager (5%)	135	14	11
'67' Light (3%)	70	9	2
Light (4%)	115	11	10
Moosehead, Lager (5%)	140	14	14
Natural: Ice (5.9%)	130	17	4
Light (4.2%)	95	12	3
Negra Modelo (5.4%)	170	15	15
Newcastle, Brown Ale (4.7%)	140	13	10
Old English "800",			
Malt (5.9%)	160	17	11
Old Milwaukee:			
Lager (4.5%)	150	13	15
Light (4.3%)	125	12	10
Ice (5.5%)	150	16	10
Old Style: Lager (4.7%)	145	13	12
Light (4.2%)	115	12	7
Pabst: Blue Ribbon (4.7%)	145	13	12
Light (3.9%)	110	11	8

	C	Alc	Cb
Pacifico, Clara (4.4%)	145	13	13
Piels, Lager (4.3%)	125	12	9
Pilsner Urquell, Lager (4.4%)	155	13	16
Point: Amber Classic (4.7%)	160	14	11
Special Lager (4.6%)	150	13	9
Redbridge, Lager (4%)	135	12	12
Red Dog, Lager (5%)	150	14	14
Red Hook: ESB (5.8%)	185	16	16
India Pale Ale (4.7%)	190	13	19
Red Stripe, Jamaican Ale (5%)	155	14	14
Redd's, Apple Ale (5%)	165	14	17
Samuel Adams:			
Boston Lager (4.9%)	175	14	19
Sam Adams, Light Lager (4%)	125	13	10
Sapporo, Prem. Lager (4.9%)	140	14	10
Schaefer: Lager (4.6%)	145	13	12
Light (3.9%)	110	11	8
Schell's: Deer (4.8%)	135	14	8
Light (4%)	100	11	7
Schlitz: Pale Lager (4.6%)	145	13	12
Light (3.8%)	110	11	8
Schmidt's: Pale Lager (4.6%)	145	13	12
Light (3.8%)	110	11	8
Sheaf, Stout (5.8%)	190	16	19
Shock Top: Belgian White (5.2%)	165	15	15
Lemon Shandy (4.2%)	130	12	10
Sierra Nevada: Bigfoot (9.6%)	330	28	32
Pale Ale (5.6%)	175	16	14
Glissade Golden Bock (6.4%)	205	18	16
Porter (5.6%)	195	16	18
Sol (4.2%)	130	12	11
Southpaw, Light (5%)	125	14	7
Sparks, Lager (6%)	255	17	35
Steel Reserve:			
High Gravity Malt Liquor (8.1%)	220	23	16
Steel 6 (6%)	160	17	11
Stella Artois: Pale Lager (5.2%)	155	15	12
Cidre (4.5%)	170	13	21
Stroh's: Pale Lager (4.6%)	145	13	12
Light (3.9%)	115	11	7
Tecate: Pale Lager (4.6%)	140	13	11
Light (4%)	110	10	8
Third Shift, Amber Lager (5.3%)	185	15	18
Trader Jose:			
Premium Lager (5%), 11.2 fl.oz	145	14	14
Light (3.8%), 11.2 fl.oz	105	14	8
Weinhard's:			
Private Reserve (4.8%)	150	14	13
Widmer, Hefewéizen (4.9%)	165	14	13
ZeigenBock, Amber (4.9%)	145	14	11

Alc ~ Alcohol (Grams)   **Cb** ~ Carbohydrate

Cider ~ Alcoholic/Hard

Per 12 fl.oz Unless Indicated

	C	Alc	Cb
Ace: Cider (5%), average all flavors	155	14	12
Joker (6.9%)	135	20	12
Angry Orchard: Apple Ginger (5%)	200	14	26
Crisp Apple (5%)	220	14	31
Traditional Dry (5.5%)	180	16	20
Crispin: Original (5%)	150	14	15
Blackberry (5%)	160	14	16
Brut (5.5%)	130	16	14
Pacific Pear (4.5%)	160	13	17
Hornsby's:			
Amber (5.5%), 11.2 oz	165	15	16
Crisp (5.5%), 11.2 fl.oz	200	15	24
Johnny Appleseed, (5.5%)	210	16	26
Magners, (4.5%)	125	13	9
Michelob, Ultra Light Cider (4%)	120	10	10
Smith & Forge, (6%)	220	17	26
Stella Artois Cidre, (4.5%)	160	13	17
Strongbow:			
Gold Apple (5%), 11.2 oz	170	13	20
Honey & Apple (5%), 11.2 fl.oz	195	13	26
Woodchuck: Amber (5%)	200	14	21
802 (5%)	180	14	16
Granny Smith (5%)	160	14	11
Pear (4%)	150	12	18
Raspberry (4%)	170	12	22
Wyder's: Pear (4%)	140	12	22
Raspberry (4%)	120	12	17

Quick Guide

Table Wines:
Average all Varieties (11.5% Alc.)
(Wine Contains Zero Fat)

	C	Alc	Cb
4 fl.oz, 1 small wine glass OR ½ large wine glass	100	12	3
6 fl.oz, (¾ large wine glass)	145	18	5
8 fl.oz, (1 large wine glass)	195	25	7
½ Carafe/Bottle, 12 fl.oz	295	37	10
1 Bottle, 750ml, 25.4 fl.oz	620	78	21

Table Wines

Red: *Per 4 fl.oz*

	C	Alc	Cb
Burgundy/Cabernet/Merlot, av.	100	11	4
White: *Per 4 fl.oz*			
Dry (Chenin; Fume Blanc; Chardonnay)	95	11	4
Sparkling, (4%)	95	11	4
Zinfandel Sweet, (Moselle/Sauterne), 4 fl.oz	85	11	2

Table Wines (Cont)

Champagne: *Per 4 fl.oz*

	C	Alc	Cb
Average all types, 1 glass	85	11	2
with Orange Jce (3:1 orange)	75	8	4
with Orange Jce (1:1 orange)	65	5	7
Mulled Wine (Gluhwein), 4 fl.oz	180	14	20
Non-Alcoholic Wine: *Less than 0.5% Alcohol*			
Ariel: White varieties, average, 4 fl.oz	35	0.5	8
Red varieties, average, 4 fl.oz	25	0.5	5
Reduced Alcohol Wine:			
Average all types, (6%), 4 fl.oz	80	6	10
Skinnygirl, Red/White, (8.5%), 5 fl.oz	100	10	5
Sake (Gekkeikan), (16%), 4 fl.oz	120	15	5
Sangria (Skinnygirl), (4%), 5 fl.oz	130	12	23

Flavored Wines

Average All Brands (6% alcohol)
(Arbor Mist, Wild Vines, Boone's Farm):

	C	Alc	Cb
1 small wine glass, 4 fl.oz	80	6	10
1 large wine glass, 8 fl.oz	160	11	20
1 bottle, 750 ml (25.4 fl.oz)	510	35	64

Dessert Wines

	C	Alc	Cb
Madeira (18%), 2 oz	85	9	5
Marsala (18%), 2 oz	110	9	11
Port, Muscatel (18%), 2 oz	85	9	5
Sherry (15%), 2 oz:			
Dry, 1 Sherry glass	90	7	7
Sweet/Cream, average	90	7	8
Vermouth (Martini & Rossi):			
Extra Dry (18%), 2 oz	65	9	2
Martini Rosso (16%), 2 oz	90	8	8

Cooking Wines

Holland House:

	C	Alc	Cb
Marsala, (14%), 2 T., 1 fl.oz	45	4	4
Red/White, (10%): 2 T., 1 fl.oz	20	2	1
1 cup, 8 fl.oz	160	24	8
Sherry, (17%), 2 Tbsp, 1 fl.oz	45	5	2

Cooking with Wine:
For alcohol to evaporate, sufficient heat and cooking time (at least 30 minutes) is required.
Red and white table wines would then contain negligible residual calories.
Sweetened wines (marsala/sherry) would contain 10 calories per 1 fl.oz.
Flambé Desserts: Only surface alcohol is burned off, so negligible reduction in alcohol or calories.

Quick Guide — Alc ~ Alcohol (Grams)

Spirits/Liquors:
Includes Bourbon, Brandy, Gin, Rum, Scotch, Tequila, Vodka, Whiskey.

Note: All spirits with same alcohol proof have similar calories and zero fat.

Average All Brands	C	Alc	Cb
80 Proof (40% Alcohol by Volume):			
1 fl.oz	65	9.5	0
1.5 fl.oz (1 shot)	100	14	0
3 fl.oz (Double shot)	195	28	0
½ Bottle, 350 ml (12 fl.oz)	770	113	0
1 Bottle, 700 ml (24 fl.oz)	1540	227	0
86 Proof (43% Alc):			
1 fl.oz	70	10	0
1.5 fl.oz (1 shot)	105	15	0
1 Bottle (24 fl.oz)	1670	247	0
100 Proof (50% Alc),			
1.5 fl.oz	125	18	0
Shochu (Soju),			
average all types (25% alc), 2 fl.oz	65	12	0

Flavored Spirits

Captain Morgan: Per 1.5 fl.oz			
Original (35%)	85	12	0.5
Black Spiced (47.3%)	115	14	1
Parrot Bay (21%), average	90	7.5	10
Silver Spiced (35%)	95	12	2
Malibu Rum,			
Original/Fruit Flavors (21%), 1.5 fl.oz	80	8	8
Southern Comfort (35%), 1.5 fl.oz	100	13	3

Hard Lemonade, Sodas & Tea

Margaritaville: Per 12 fl.oz			
Lime Margarita (8%)	310	23	30
Paradise Punch (8%)	340	23	46
Mike's:			
Lemonade: Hard (5%), 11.2 fl.oz	220	13	33
Harder (8%) average, 16 fl.oz	395	31	44
Margarita (5%), 11.2 fl.oz	220	14	34
Punch:			
Hard Mango (5.5%), 11.2 fl.oz	230	15	33
Harder (8%), 12 fl.oz	300	23	36
Sparks: Per 16 fl.oz Can			
Blackberry (8%)	385	31	44
Iced Tea (8%)	375	31	41
Lemonade (8%)	345	31	36
Original (6%)	335	23	45
Twisted Tea: Original (5%)	220	14	31
Half & Half (5%)	260	14	34

Coolers & Premix Cocktails

Ready-To-Drink:
Zero Fat Unless Indicated

	C	Alc	Cb
Bacardi: Per 4 fl.oz			
Party Drinks (Ready To Pour):			
Bahama Mama; Mai Tai (10%)	130	9	16
Mojito (15%)	160	14	16
Rum Island Ice Tea (12.5%)	150	12	16
Bacardi Silver: Per 12 fl.oz			
Lemonade/Sangria (6%), av.	270	17	41
Raz/Strawberry (5%)	240	14	36
Mojito (5%)	240	14	36
Bartles & Jaymes: Per 11.2 fl.oz			
Malt Based Coolers (3.2%):			
Exotic Berry	195	9	31
Margarita	245	9	43
Pina Colada	250	9	45
Sangria	240	9	40
Strawberry Daiquiri	205	9	34
Captain Morgan's,			
Parrot Bay (4.1%), all var. av., 11.2 fl.oz	210	10	35
Chi Chi's: Long Is. Iced Tea, 4 fl.oz	145	12	17
Mexican Mudslide, 4 fl.oz (8g fat)	240	1.5	42
Mojito, 4 fl.oz	160	11	21
Pina Colada, 4 fl.oz (6g fat)	240	4	42
White Russian, 4 fl.oz (7g fat)	245	1.5	43
Daily's, Frozen Pouches (6.9%),			
average all flavors, 10 fl.oz	280	0	46
Jack Daniels, Country Cocktails (4.8%),			
average all varieties, 10 fl.oz	200	9	30
Jose Cuervo:			
Margaritas:			
Classic Lime (10%), 6 fl.oz	210	14	29
Golden (12.7%), 4.7 fl.oz	170	14	19
Seagram's:			
Escapes Coolers (3.2%):			
Bahama Mama, 11.2 fl.oz	200	9	36
Strawb. Daiquiri, 11.2 fl.oz	225	9	41
Skinnygirl:			
Vodka with flavors (30%), 1.5 fl.oz	75	11	0
Cocktails (10%), av., 3 fl.oz	70	8	4
Smirnoff,			
Frozen Lemonades (5%), av,, 10 oz	285	12	53
Ice, 4.5%:			
Cherry Lime, 12 oz	250	13	30
Mango/Pineapple, 12 oz	220	13	35
Raspberry/Tropical Fruit, 12 oz	230	13	38
TGI Friday's:			
On The Rocks: Per 6 fl.oz			
Long Island Ice Tea (15%)	250	21	28
Margarita (7.5%)	185	11	29
Mudslide (10%)	365	14	31
Blenders (12.5%),			
Mudslide, 6 fl.oz	365	18	31

Coolers & Premix Cocktails (Cont)

Ready-To-Drink:
The Club Premix Cocktails: Per 3.4 oz Serving (½ can)

	C	Alc	Cb
Censored on Beach; Margarita (7.5%)	105	6	17
Gin/Vodka Martini (21%), average	155	17	0.2
Long Island Ice Tea (15%)	145	12	17
Manhattan (17%)	115	13	5
Mudslide/Pina Colada (10%), average	200	8	16
Screwdriver (7.5%)	95	6	14
Whiskey Sour (10%)	95	8	11

Shooters

Alc ~ Alcohol (Grams)

Alabama Slammer	110	14	2
Amaretto Sour	120	6	19
B52	145	14	11
Beam Me Up Scotty	145	13	13
Blue Tequila	160	18	6
Jager Bomb	205	8	30
Jager Bomb, w/ Sugar-Free Red Bull	155	8	18
Jell-O Shot: 3 oz, With 1.5 oz Vodka	180	14	19
With Diet Jell-O	110	14	0
Kamikaze	75	8	3
Kool-Aid	160	15	14
Orgasm	100	12	6
Peppermint Patty	195	8	11
Stinger	170	18	12
Surfer on Acid	90	7	11

Cocktail Mixers ~ Non-Alcoholic

Bacardi: Per 8 fl.oz, Prepared from 2 fl.oz Concentrate

Daiquiris; Rum Runner	120	0	32
Margarita	90	0	25
Mojito	110	0	30
Pina Colada	170	0	36

Baja Bob's: Per 4 fl.oz

Cranberry Cosmo Martini	10	0	2
Pina Colada	30	0	4

Jose Cuervo:

Margaritas: Av. all flav., 4 oz	85	0	21
Light (Sugar Free), Lime, 4 oz	5	0	1

Mr & Mrs T:

Bloody Mary: Original, 5 oz	30	0	7
Bold & Spicy, 4 oz	35	0	7
Mai Tai	130	0	32
Margarita	100	0	26
Pina Colada	200	0	44
Strawberry Daiquiri	180	0	46

TGI Friday's:

Mudslide, 2.3 fl.oz	110	0	23
Cosmo; Berrytini, 2 fl.oz	80	0	20
Strawb. Daiquiri; Marg., 4 fl.oz	190	0	46

Cocktails

Alc ~ Alcohol (Grams)

Made to Standard Recipes (Standard Size):
(Main Reference: The New American Bartender's Guide)
Zero Fat Unless Indicated

	C	Alc	Cb
Adios Mother F.	260	23	23
Bacardi & Coke (with 1.5 oz Bacardi)	160	14	17
Bellini, 4.5 fl.oz	95	11	7
Bloody Mary (with 1.5 oz Vodka)	125	10	7
Blushin' Russian (20g fat)	405	14	23
Bourbon & Soda (with 2 oz Bourbon)	130	19	0
Brandy Alexander (10g fat)	300	20	15
Chupa Naranjas (with 1.5 oz Tequila)	150	16	8
Cosmopolitan	215	24	12
Daiquiri (w/ 2 oz Rum), av. all types	140	19	4
Frozen Daiquiri (with 2 oz Rum):			
Without fruit	155	19	6
With fruit (with 1.5 oz Rum)	145	14	11
Grasshopper	260	17	28
Greyhound (with 1.5 oz Vodka)	170	14	17
Harvey Wallbanger (2 oz)	200	19	17
Highball (1.5 oz Whiskey)	100	14	0
Irish Coffee (10g fat)	205	14	2
Kahlua Mudslide: with milk (3g fat)	145	11	12
With cream (12g fat)	230	11	10
Lemon Drop, 4 fl.oz	130	14	10
Long Island Iced Tea (with 3 oz Cola)	270	19	32
With 3 oz Diet Cola	235	19	22
Mai Tai (with 2 oz Rum)	290	24	33
Manhattan	130	17	5
Margarita	160	18	7
Martini: Dry, with 1.5 oz gin	100	14	0
Sour Apple, w/ 2 oz Vodka/1 oz Schnapps	250	31	10
Mint Julep (with 2½ oz Bourbon)	180	24	4
Mojito (with 2 oz rum)	170	19	9
Moscow Mule	185	14	24
Pina Colada (10g fat), 6 oz	250	15	28
Red Bull & Vodka (with 1.5 oz vodka)	210	14	28
With Sugar Free Red Bull	105	14	3
Rum & Coke (with 1.5 oz Rum)	160	14	17
Sangria: With 1 oz Fruit Juice, 5 oz	120	12	9
With 0.5 oz Brandy, 5.5 oz	150	17	9
Screwdriver	160	14	15
Sex On The Beach	235	19	25
Spritzer (with 3 oz Wine)	65	8	2
Tequila Sunrise	200	14	25
Tom Collins (with 2 oz Gin)	210	19	18
Vodka Soda (with 1.5 oz Vodka)	100	14	0
Vodka Tonic (with 1.5 oz Vodka)	165	14	18
Whiskey Sour (w/ 2 oz Whiskey)	155	19	7
White Russian (10g fat)	240	19	7
Non-Alcoholic:			
Cinderella	45	0	11
Shirley Temple (with 6 oz Ginger Ale)	140	0	34

Liqueurs/Cordials

Per 1 fl.oz

	C	Alc	Cb
Advocaat (36 Proof; 2g fat)	85	4	9
Alizé: Cognac (80 Proof)	70	9	2
Gold/Red Passion (32 Proof)	105	4	11
Amaretto (56 Proof)	110	7	17
Baileys Irish Cream (34 Proof; 4g fat)	100	4	8
Benedictine (80 Proof)	90	9	5
Chambord (33 Proof)	105	4	11
Chartreuse (80 Proof)	100	9	9
Cherry Brandy (48 Proof)	80	6	9
Coffee Liqueur (53 Proof)	115	7	16
Cointreau (80 Proof)	95	9	7
Creme de Cacao (54 Proof)	100	6	15
Creme de Menthe (72 Proof)	125	9	14
Curacao (70 Proof)	95	8	6
Drambuie (80 Proof)	105	9	9
Frangelico (40 Proof)	65	5	12
Galliano (86 Proof)	100	10	8
Grand Marnier (80 Proof)	100	9	7
Kahlua (40 Proof)	85	5	14
Kirsch (68 Proof)	80	8	6
Midori (42 Proof)	80	5	11
Ouzo (80 Proof)	105	9	11
Pernod (80 Proof)	75	9	11
Sambuca (84 Proof)	100	10	11
Schnapps (100 Proof)	115	12	9
Southern Comfort (70 Proof)	65	8	3

Liqueur Coffee & Hot Drinks

Per Standard Drink

Liqueur Coffee: Av. all types	200	10	10
Irish, 1.5 oz Whiskey & 1 oz whip	205	9	4
Hot Toddy, with 1½ oz liquor, av. all	170	9	19
Mulled Wine (Glühwein), 4 fl.oz, av	195	14	25

"The doctor told him to cut down to just one glass a day."

TEN TIPS TO AVOID HARMFUL DRINKING

1. **Add up the alcohol** you typically drink each day and on social occasions. How does this compare with 'low risk' amounts? *(See page 23)*

2. **Compare the alcohol content of** different drinks and select the lowest. Request half shots of alcohol in cocktails and mixed drinks. Dilute them and keep topping off with non-alcoholic drinks.

3. **Go easy on 'Light' beers.** At 4% alcohol, on average, they are still high in alcohol compared to regular beer (5% alcohol).

4. **Try low alcohol or non-alcohol** alternatives such as fruit juices and mineral water. Take your own to parties.

5. **Before drinking alcohol,** quench your thirst with water and non-alcoholic drinks – particularly after vigorous exercise or sports.

6. **Slow the rate of drinking.** Chugging or drinking fast is the major cause of illness and death from alcohol poisoning.

7. **Avoid drinking in 'rounds'.**

8. **Have a non-alcohol 'spacer'** between drinks (e.g. mineral water, orange juice).

9. **Don't drink on an empty stomach.** Food slows the rate of alcohol absorption.

10. **Keep track of the number of drinks** and know when to stop. Stick to a set limit.

Note: Alcohol can be very dangerous when taken with prescription or street drugs, or when you are very tired.

Extra Info: www.CalorieKing.com

Cocktail Mixers & Extracts

	C	Alc	Cb
Angostura Bitters, ¼ tsp	2	0	0.5
Grenadine, ½ tsp	6	0	2
Lime/Lemon Juice, 2 Tbsp, 1 oz	10	0	2
Maraschino Cherry, 1 small	8	0	2
Simple Syrup, 1 Tbsp, av.	50	0	14
Sweet & Sour Mix, 2 Tbsp, 1 oz	30	0	7
Tonic Water, 8 fl.oz	80	0	22
Flavor Extracts *(McCormick):*			
Pure Lemon (83%), 1 tsp	0	3.5	0
Pure Vanilla (35%), 1tsp	0	1.5	0

Baking Ingredients	C	F	Cb
Almond Paste,			
(Marzipan), 2 Tbsp	170	7	24
Apple Pie Filling,			
Sweetened, 9.4 oz	290	0	69
Baking Powder: Regular, 1 tsp	5	0	1
Cream of Tartar, 1 tsp	10	0	2
Baking Mix (Bisquick):			
Original, ⅓ cup, 1.5 oz	160	5	26
Heart Smart, 1.5 oz	140	2.5	27
Batter Mix (Golden Dipt),			
All Purpose, ¼ cup	100	0	20
Blueberries, 1 cup, 5 oz	90	0.5	21
Butter/Margarine, ½ cup, 4 oz	800	88	1
Stick (Land O' Lakes), 0.5 oz	100	11	0
Carob Flour, ½ cup	115	0.5	46
Chocolate Baking Bars: Average all Brands			
Sweet (Baker's):			
1 oz portion	120	7	16
4 oz bar	470	28	64
Semi-sweet, 1 oz	140	9	16
Bittersweet, 1 oz	140	12	14
White Baking, 1 oz	160	9	16
Unsweetened: 1 oz	140	14	8
Grated, 1 cup, 4.5 oz	660	69	39
Chocolate Baking Chips: Average all Brands			
Milk Choc./Semi Sweet, 1 oz	140	8	18
½ cup, 3 oz	420	24	54
1 cup, 6 oz	840	48	108
Dark, 1 Tbsp, 0.5 oz	70	5	3
Mini Kisses (Hershey), 1 piece	5	0.5	1
Cocoa Powder:			
Hershey's: 1 Tbsp	20	0.5	3
⅓ cup, 1 oz	115	3	17
Nestle: 1 Tbsp	15	1	3
⅓ cup, 1 oz	85	5	17
Coconut, dried:			
Sweetened/Flaked:			
1 oz	130	8	15
½ cup, 1.3 oz	195	12	22
Toasted (Baker's), 1 oz	170	13	13
Unsweetened, 1 oz	190	18	7
Coconut Cream/Milk ~ See Page 89			
Coconut Manna (Nutiva), 1 Tbsp	100	9	3
Cornstarch, 1 Tbsp	30	0	7
Eggs: Large (1)	75	5	0
Jumbo (1)	90	6	0.5
Egg White: 1 Egg White	15	0	0
½ cup (4 egg whites), 4 oz	60	0	1
Flour:			
White: 1 Tbsp, 0.3 oz	25	0	5.5
1 cup, 4.2 oz	400	1	88
Whole Wheat, 1 cup, 4.2 oz	400	2	84

	C	F	Cb
Flavor Extracts: Av. all Brands			
Imitation, 1 tsp	10	0	2
Pure Extract, 1 tsp	10	0	0.5
Almond; Vanilla, 1 tsp	10	0	0.5
Fruit Pectin: Swtnd, ¼ tsp	5	0	1
Unsweetened, ¼ tsp	0	0	0
Gelatin, dry, unsweetened, 0.3 oz	20	0	0
Glaze (Duncan Hines): Choc., 2 T.	150	7	21
Vanilla, 2 Tbsp	140	6	22
Golden Dipt, Batter Mix			
¼ cup, 1 oz	100	0	23
Honey, ½ cup, 6 oz	515	0	140
Lemon/Orange Peel, ¼ cup	25	0	6
Lighter Bake (Sunsweet):			
(Butter & Oil replacement)			
1 Tbsp, ½ oz	35	0	9
¼ Cup, 2.7 oz	140	0	36
Milk: Whole, 1 cup, 8 fl.oz	150	8	12
2%, 1 cup, 8 fl.oz	120	5	12
1%, 1 cup, 8 fl.oz	100	2.5	12
Fat-Free, 1 cup, 8 fl.oz	90	0.5	13
Pastry ~ See Page 134			
Pie Crusts ~ See Page 134			
Pie Fillings, Fruits ~ See Page 134			
Lemon Creme, ⅓ cup	130	1.5	28
Mincemeat, 3.5 oz	190	5	45
Pumpkin, 1 cup, 9.3 oz	270	1.5	60
Prune Puree, ¼ cup, 3 oz	220	0	55
Raisins, ½ cup, 2.8 oz	240	0.5	63
Rennin, 0.4 oz pkt	10	0	2
Soy Milk ~ See Pages 49-50			
Sprinkles, all types, 1 tsp	20	1	3
Sugar: 1 Tbsp, 0.5 oz	55	0	14
1 oz	110	0	28
1 cup, 7 oz	775	0	195
1 lb, 16 oz	1760	0.5	454
Sweeteners & Sugar Substitutes ~ See Page 156			
Vinegar, average all types, 1 oz	5	0	1
Whey, sweet, dry, 1 oz	100	0.5	21
Yeast: Active, dry, 0.3 oz pkg	25	0.5	3
Bakers, compressed, 1 oz	30	0.5	5
Fleischmann's, 0.6 oz pkg	0	0	0

ℱor **Full Nutritional Data**
& Product Updates
~ See Author's Website
www.CalorieKing.com

Note: Actual weight of bars is usually 5-10% more than label Net Weight. Weigh bar and allow extra calories.

Bars ~ Brands	C	F	Cb

Per Bar

ABB,

    Steel Bar, av. all varieties, 2.5 oz | 255 | 5 | 35

AdvantEdge ~ *See EAS*

Annie's Homegrown:

Organic Granola Bars: *Per 1 oz Bar*

Berry Berry	120	3.5	20
Chocolate Chip	120	4	19
PB & J; Peanut Butter	120	4.5	18

Atkins:

Advantage Meal:

Chocolate Chip Cookie Dough, 2 oz	240	11	29
Chocolate Chip Granola, 1.7 oz	200	9	19
Choc. Peanut Butter, 2 oz	250	14	23
Cookies 'n Crème, 1.7 oz	180	9	20
Strawberry Alm., 1.7 oz	200	9	20

Note: Carb figures include 7-15g sugar alcohol

Advantage: *Per 1.6 oz Bar*

Caramel varieties, average	175	10	20
Coconut Almond Delight	200	15	18
Dark Choc. Decadence	150	6	23

Note: Carb figures include 9g sugar alcohol

Day Break: *Per 1.3 oz Bar*

Apple Crisp	150	7	16
Choc. Chip Crisp; Cranb. Alm., av.	145	6	16
Peanut Butter Fudge Crisp	150	7	14

Note: Carbs figures include 5-9g sugar alcohol

Endulge:

Caramel Nut Chew, 1.2 oz	130	8	17
Chocolate Caramel Mousse, 1.2 oz	120	4.5	23
Nutty Fudge Brownie, 1.4 oz	170	12	18
Peanut Caramel Cluster, 1.2 oz	140	9	12

Note Carb figures include 4-12g sugar alcohol

Attune Bars:

Probiotic Bars: *Per 0.7 oz Bar*

Dark Chocolate	80	6	11
Milk Chocolate Crisp	90	6	12
Mint Chocolate	90	6	12

Balance: *Per 1.8 oz Bars*

Original/Bare varieties, average	200	7	21
Dark varieties	180	6	20
Gold varieties, average	200	7	23

Cascadian Farms *(General Mills):*

| Chewy Granola, av. all var., 1.2 oz bar | 135 | 3 | 26 |
| Crunchy Granola, all var., 2 bars, 1.4 oz | 185 | 8 | 27 |

Per Bar | C | F | Cb

Clif:

Original,

    average all varieties., 2.4 oz | 240 | 5 | 45

Builder's: Av. all varieties, 2.4 oz | 270 | 8 | 30

Max, average all varieties, 3.4 oz | 385 | 13 | 40

Kid, ZBar, av. all varieties, 1.3 oz | 125 | 3.5 | 23

Mojo, average, 1.6 oz | 190 | 11 | 21

Corazonas:

Oatmeal Squares: *Per 1.8 oz Bar*

| White Chocolate Macadamia | 200 | 8 | 29 |
| Av. other varieties | 185 | 7 | 28 |

Detour:

Original, Caramel Peanut, 3 oz | 350 | 11 | 32

Lean Muscle: Av. all var., 1.6 oz | 190 | 7 | 17

    Average all varieties, 3.2 oz | 395 | 15 | 33

Lower Sugar, average all varieties:

| 1.4 oz Bar | 170 | 5.5 | 16 |
| 2.8 oz Bar | 340 | 11 | 33 |

Note: Carb figures include 12-28g sugar alcohol

Oatmeal, av. all varieties, 4.3 oz | 455 | 11 | 61

dotFIT:

dotBAR:

Chocolate Mint, 2 oz	160	5	15
Choc. Peanut Butter Crunch, 2 oz	190	5	23
Iced Mochaccino, 2 oz	200	5	24

Note: Carb figures include 5.5g sugar alcohol

dotSTICK, Iced, av. all var., 2 oz | 190 | 6 | 26

Note: Carb figure includes 7g sugar alcohol

EAS:

AdvantEDGE:

Carb Control: Crisp Bars, 2 oz | 240 | 8 | 27

    Other varieties, 2 oz | 230 | 8 | 27

Note: Carb figures include 17-19g sugar alcohol

Myoplex 30, average all varieties | 350 | 10 | 36

Extend Bar: Crunch, av., 1.4 oz | 150 | 2.5 | 30

    Delight, av. all varieties, 1.4 oz | 150 | 3 | 21

Noe: Carb figures include 4-6g sugar alcohol

Fiber One: Chewy, av. all, 1 oz | 105 | 3.5 | 21

    90-Calorie Bar, average all, 0.8 oz | 90 | 3 | 18

FiberPlus *(Kellogg's):*

Antioxidants: Choc. Chip, 1.3 oz | 120 | 4 | 26

    Nutty Delights, av. all var., 1.3 oz | 150 | 8 | 22

    Other varieties, 1.3 oz | 130 | 5 | 25

Bars ~ Brands (Cont)	C	F	Cb

Per Bar

	C	F	Cb
Full Bar, Regular, av. all, 1.6 oz	170	4	28
GeniSoy: *Per 2 oz Bar*			
Protein: Chunky PB Fudge	220	6	30
Crispy Choc. Mint	210	4.5	33
Other varieties	220	6	32
General Mills: *Per 1.6 oz Bar*			
Milk 'n Cereal Bar,			
Honey Nut Cheerios	160	4	28
Glenny's: *Per 1 oz Bar*			
Cashew/Cranberry & Almond, av.	145	7	17
Cherry & Almond	130	6	18
Classic Fruit & Nut	140	6	18
Peanuts & Peanut Butter	170	13	10
Glucerna:			
Crispy Delights Nutrition Bars,			
Peanut/Choc. Chip, av., 1.4 oz	145	5	20
Note: Carb figure includes 7-8g sugar alcohol			
Mini Snack Bar, average, 0.7 oz	80	3	11
Note: Carb figures include 5 g sugar alcohol			
Gnu Foods: *Per 1.6 oz Bar*			
Banana Walnut; Cinnamon Brownie	140	4	30
Cinnamon Raisin; Orange Cranberry	130	3	32
Great Value *(Walmart):*			
90 Calories, average all, 0.8 oz	90	1.5	19
Fiber, Oats & Peanut Butter, 1.4 oz	150	4.5	29
Fruit & Grain, low fat,			
average all varieties, 1.3 oz	135	2.5	26
Fruit & Nut, Trail Mix Bar, 1.3 oz	140	4	24
Granola: Choc Chunk, 0.9 oz	90	2	18
Crunchy Oats & Honey, 1.5 oz	200	7	29
Sweet & Salty, Almond, 1.3 oz	160	8	20
Health Valley,			
Cobbler Cereal Bars, av. 1.3 oz	130	2.5	27
Herbalife,			
Protein Deluxe!, average, 1.3 oz	160	6	17
HMR, Benefit Bars, av. all, 1.4 oz	155	4	24
Jenny Craig: S'mores, 1.3 oz	140	4	22
Chocolate Caramel P'nut, 1.3 oz	140	5	19
Choc. Chip Snack Bar, 1.2 oz	140	3	23
Yogurt Dream Bar, 1.2 oz	130	4.5	20
Kashi:			
Cereal Bars, av. all var., 1.3 oz	125	3	24
Granola & Seed Bars (2), av., 1.4 oz	180	7	27
Granola Bars:			
Chewy, av. all var., 1.3 oz	135	4	21
Layered,			
average all varieties, 1 oz	125	4	21

Per Bar

	C	F	Cb
Kashi *(Cont):*			
Go Lean:			
Crisp!:			
Chocolate Caramel, 1.6 oz	150	3	28
Chocolate Peanut, 1.8 oz	180	5	30
Average other varieties, 1.6 oz	165	4	27
Dipped, average all, 1.9 oz	195	5	32
Soft & Chewy, average all, 1.4 oz	130	3	24
Kellogg's,			
Cinnabon Bar, Original, 1.3 oz	150	4.5	26
Fiber Plus ~ *See page 31*			
Nutrigrain ~ *See page 33*			
Special K ~ *See page 34*			
Kind: *Per 1.4 oz Bar*			
Fruit & Nut:			
Almond & Apricot	180	10	23
Apple Cinnamon & Pecan	190	12	20
Nut Delight	210	16	14
Peanut Butter & Strawberry	190	11	19
Nuts & Spices:			
Cashew & Ginger Spices	200	14	16
Dark Chocolate, all varieties	200	13	16
Madagascar Vanilla Almond	210	16	14
Plus, average all varieties	185	12	18
Kudos, av. all varieties, 0.9 oz	100	3	17
Labrada:			
Protein Bars:			
Lean Body, S'mores Delight,	360	14	33
Cookie Roll, Choc. Chip, 2.8 oz	330	11	34
Larabar:			
Apple Pie, 1.6 oz	190	10	24
Cherry Pie, 1.7 oz	200	8	30
Chocolate Chip Brownie, 1.6 oz	200	9	31
Peanut Butter & Jelly, 1.7 oz	210	10	27
Lindora, av. all varieties, 1.6 oz	155	5	17
Luna:			
Bars For Women,			
average all varieties, 1.7 oz	180	4.5	27
Protein, av. all varieties, 1.6 oz	180	7	21
Marathon *(Snickers):*			
Energy: Chewy, av. all var., 2 oz	210	8	26
Crunchy, Dark Chocolate, 1.6 oz	150	4.5	22
Protein, average all, 2.8 oz	285	9	40

Bars ~ Brands (Cont)	C	F	Cb

Per Bar

Market Pantry (Target):

Crunchy Gran., Oat & Honey, 1.5 oz	180	6	28
Cereal Bars: PB Choc Chip, 0.8 oz	100	3	17
Average other varieties	150	5	23
Chewy Bars: Choc Chip, 0.8 oz	100	2.5	18
Choc. Chunk; S'Mores, 0.8 oz	90	1.5	18
Fiber Dark Choc. & Alm., 1.3 oz	140	5	25

Mariani: *Per 1.4 oz Bar*

Honey Bars: Cranb.; Granola, av.	170	8	23
Sesame	200	14	16
Medifast: Crunch, av., 1.2 oz	110	3	13

Note: Carb figures include 2-3g sugar alcohol

Maintenance, C'rmel Nut, 1.5 oz	170	5	22

Met-Rx: *Per 3.5 oz Bar Unless Indicated*

Big 100, average all varieties	375	6	49

Big 100 Colossal:

Brownie, Super Choc Fudge	390	12	40
Chocolate Toasted Almond	410	13	46
Crispy Apple Pie	400	10	47
Protein Plus, Mud Pie Fusion, 3 oz	300	9	32

Mojo Bars ~ *See Clif*

Muscle Milk (Cytosport):

High Protein:

Choc. P'nut Caramel, 2.6 oz	320	11	30
Vanilla Toffee Crunch, 2.6 oz	310	11	29
Protein Crunch, Choc. PB, 2.9 oz	360	13	30

MuscleTech:

Nitro-Tech Hardcore, 2.8 oz	310	8	29

Smart Protein:

Peanut Caramel Crunch, 2.2 oz	290	12	26
Triple Choc., 2.2 oz	270	9	26

Nature's Path:

Granola Bars:

5 Bar Box, 1 bar, av., 1.3 oz	145	4	23
10 Bar Box, 2 bars, av, 1.4 oz	195	7	28

Nature Valley:

Crunchy Granola Bars:

Apple Crisp (2), 1.5 oz	160	6	26
Average other var. (2), 1.5 oz	185	7	28
Chewy, Yogurt coating, av., 1.2 oz	140	3.5	26
Granola Thins, av. all var., 0.6 oz	85	4.5	11
Protein, all varieties, 1.4 oz	190	12	14
Trail Mix, Chewy, av. all, 1.3 oz	135	4	25

Nutri-Grain (Kellogg's):

Cereal Bars: Fruit Flav., av. all, 1.3 oz	120	3	24
Yogurt Bar, Strawberry, 1.3 oz	130	3.5	25
Crunch, (2), all varieties, 1.5 oz	190	7	29

Per Bar

Nutrilite (Amway Global):

Meal Bars, all varieties, 1.8 oz	200	7	26

Snack Bar:

Chocolate Caramel, 0.9 oz	100	3	16
Fudgy Brownie w/ Almds., 0.9 oz	100	3	9

NutriSystem:

Granola Breakfast Bars:

Chewy Chocolate Chip	150	2	27
Peanut Butter	160	5	25

Snack Bar: Chewy Peanut | 180 | 9 | 19 |

Chocolate Caramel	150	3.5	23

Odwalla:

Chewy:

Choc. Alm. Coconut, 1.6 oz	200	8	29

Nourishing: *Per 2 oz Bar*

Choco-walla	210	5	39
Dark Chocolate Chip Walnut	220	7	36
White Chocolate Macadamia	210	10	27
Protein, Choc. Chip Peanut, 2 oz	230	8	33

Superfood: *Per 2 oz Bar*

Original	200	3.5	39
Berries GoMega	210	6	36
Blueberry Swirl	200	3	41
Strawberry Pomegranate	200	2	42

Oh Yeah! (ISS),

Orig., Almond Fudge Brownie, 3 oz	350	13	27
Optifast, 800 Bars, av., 1.6 oz	165	4	20

PowerBar:

Harvest Energy: Fruit & Nut/Nut	210	10	21
Average other varieties	245	5	42
Performance Energy, av. all var.	240	4	45

Protein & Recovery:

10G Protein, Triple Threat, av. all	230	9	30
20g Protein Plus, av. all flavors	210	5	27
30g Protein Plus, av. all flavors	360	11	34

Power Crunch (BNRG),

Protein Bar, av. all var., 1.4 oz	205	12	10
PR Bar: Double Chocolate, 1.8 oz	200	6	22
Yogurt Berry, 1.8 oz	210	7	22
Granola, Oatmeal Raisin, 1.8 oz	210	7	22

Premier Nutrition:

Premier Protein:

Crisp Bars, average all var.,1.8 oz	190	6	26
Protein Bars, average all var., 2.5 oz	280	7	24

Promax:

Gluten-Free:

Chocolate Peanut Crunch, 2.6 oz	300	8	37
Double Fudge Brownie, 2.6 oz	280	7	37
Lower Sugar, av. all var., 2.4 oz	230	7	33

Proti Bars (Bariatrix),

average all varieties, 1.5 oz	160	5.5	16

Note: Actual weight of bars is usually 5-10% more than label Net Weight. Weigh bar and allow extra calories.

Bars ~ Brands (Cont)

Per Bar

	C	F	Cb
PureFit, av. all varieties, 2 oz	220	7	25
Pure Protein:			
Baked, all varieties, 1.6 oz	190	8	14
Hi Protein, average all varietie:			
1.8 oz bar	190	5	18
2.8 oz bar	305	10	30
Quaker:			
Chewy Granola Bars:			
25% Less Sugar,			
Choc. Chip, 08 oz	100	3.5	17
90 Calories, av. all varieties, 1 oz	90	2	19
Big, average all varieties, 1.5 oz	170	6	29
Dipps, Caramel Nut	140	6	21
School Days,			
Amazing Apple; Best Berry, 1 oz	100	2	20
Yogurt, all varieties, 1.2 oz	150	4.5	25
Oatmeal To Go:			
Regular, average all varieties, 2 oz	220	4	43
High Fiber, Maple Brown Sugar, 2 oz	210	4	43
Soft Baked, av. all varieties, 1.5 oz	140	3.5	26
Quest Bar:			
Protein Bar:			
No Sugar Added, av. all var., 2.2 oz	180	5	23
Note: Carb figures include 17-20g fiber/xylitol			
Revival Soy *(Direct):*			
Apple Cinnamon	230	3	30
Chocolate Temptation	270	7	32
Peanut Pal	240	6	28
Low Carb, all varieties, average	235	8	31
Slim-Fast:			
Meal Bars:			
Chewy Chocolate Crisp, 1.7 oz	200	6	25
Chocolate P'nut Caramel, 1.6 oz	200	7	21
Sweet & Salty Choc. Almond, 1.6 oz	200	8	21
Snack Bars, average all flavors	100	3	16
SoyJoy Bars, av. all var., 1 oz	135	6	16
Solo, GI, av. all, 1.8 oz	200	7	26
Special K:			
Cereal Bars, av. all varieties, 0.8 oz	90	1.5	18
Protein Meal, all varieties, 1.6 oz	175	5	25
Protein Snack Bars,			
average all varieties, 0.9 oz	110	3	16
Steel Bar *(ABB),* average all var., 2.5 oz	250	4	36

Per Bar

	C	F	Cb
Supreme Protein:			
High Protein:			
Caramel Nut Chocolate, 3.4 oz	390	15	36
Peanut Butter & Jelly, 3.4 oz	390	15	35
Peanut Butter Crunch, 3 oz	390	18	26
Note: Carb figures include 14-20g sugar alcohol			
thinkThin:			
High Protein:			
Choc. Covered Strawberries, 1.8 oz	200	7	23
2 oz Bars, average	235	8	24
Note: Carb figures include 18-22g sugar alcohol			
Bites, averge all varieties, 0.9 oz	100	4	12
Note: Carb figure includes 10g sugar alcohol			
Tiger's Milk:			
Protein Rich, 1.2 oz	140	5	18
Peanut Butter Crunch, 1.2 oz	150	6	18
King Size, average all varieties, 2 oz	225	9	28
Toaster Strudel ~ *see page 64*			
Trader Joe's:			
Chewy Coated Granola Bars, 6-Packs:			
Chocolate Chip, 1.3 oz	150	4	26
Peanut Butter, 1.3 oz	170	8	19
Vanilla Almond, 1.3 oz	150	6	22
Fruit Bars: Fig 1.5 oz	120	2	24
Average other varieties, 1.5 oz	140	2.5	27
Granola Bars, 6-packs:			
Fiberful, 1.3 oz	120	3.5	22
Trail Mix, 1.3 oz	150	5	23
Tri-O-Plex *(Chef Jay's):*			
High Protein, Ban. Walnut, 4.2 oz	405	14	40
Duo: Caramel Peanut Butter	340	8	45
Bursting Peanut Butter	395	17	35
Usana:			
Choco Chip, 1.4 oz	160	5	17
Go Nuts 'n' Berries, 1.2 oz	150	7	18
Peanutt Bliss, 1.2 oz	160	5	17
Zoe's, Omega-3's, Choc. Delight	190	7	27
Zone Perfect:			
Blueberry Pomegranate, 1.8 oz	210	6	24
Choc, Chip Cookie Dough, 1.5 oz	180	5	24
Dark Chocolate, av. all varieties, 1.5 oz	185	6	22
Fudge Graham, 1.8 oz	210	7	23
Strawberry Yogurt, 1.8 oz	200	6	25
Sweet & Salty, Cashew Pretzel, 1.6 oz	200	7	23

Cocoa & Hot Chocolate C F Cb

	C	F	Cb
Cocoa:			
Small (8 fl.oz):			
With Whole Milk	205	8.5	22
With Nonfat Milk	145	1	23
Tall (12 fl.oz): With Whole Milk	280	12	26
With Nonfat Milk	185	1	28
Hot Chocolate:			
Small (8 fl.oz): With Whole Milk	180	7	26
With Nonfat Milk	140	2	27
Tall (12 fl.oz): With Whole Milk	260	10	36
With Nonfat Milk	190	2	37
Cinnabon, Mochalatta Chill, 16 oz	420	17	63
Swiss Miss, Mixes, av., 1 packet	120	2.5	22

Cocoa - Chocolate Mixes

Add extra cals/fat/carbohydrate for milk
Carnation Breakfast Drinks ~ *See Page 38*

	C	F	Cb
Carnation: *Per 3 Tbsp*			
Malted Milk: Original	90	2	15
Chocolate	90	1	18
Ghirardelli:			
Chocolate Mocha, 3 Tbsp, 1.2 oz	120	1.5	29
Double Chocolate, 3 Tbsp, 1.3 oz	120	1.5	30
Hershey's, Cocoa,			
Natural, unsweetened,			
1 Tbsp, 0.2 oz	10	0.5	3
Land O Lakes:			
Arctic White Cocoa, 1.3 oz	160	6	26
Other varieties, 1.3 oz	140	3.5	26
Nestle: *Per Per Single Serve Envelope*			
Chocolate Caramel	100	3	19
Dark Chocolate	100	3	19
Rich Milk Chocolate:			
Regular	80	3	14
Fat Free	25	0	5
No Sugar Added	50	0	9
Nesquik Powder: *Per 2 Tbsp*			
Chocolate; Strawberry	60	0.5	15
Chocolate; Strawb., No Added Sugar	35	1	7
Ovaltine, All Natural Cocoa Mixes,			
average all varieties, 2 Tbsp	40	0	10
Swiss Miss: *Per Single Serve Envelope*			
Breakfast Blends: Great Start	60	1	11
Pick Me Up	110	2	23
Classics:			
Average all flavors	120	2	23
Fat-Free: Original	50	0	10
Marshmallow Lovers	70	0	13

Instant Coffee C F Cb

	C	F	Cb
Powder/Granules: *Regular or Decaffeinated,*			
1 level tsp	2	0	0.5
1 rounded tsp	4	0	1
Ground, 3 tsp	7	0	2
Brewed/Percolated, 1 cup, 8 fl.oz	4	0	1
Coffee With Milk/Cream/Creamers: *Per 8 oz Cup*			
Black:	4	0	1
With Whole Milk: Dash, 1 Tbsp	15	0.5	1
2 Tbsp, 1 fl.oz	25	1	2.5
With 2% Milk, 2 Tbsp	20	0.5	2.5
With 1% Milk, 2 Tbsp	20	0.5	2.5
With Fat Free Milk, 2 Tbsp	15	0	2.5
With Soy Milk: 1 Tbsp	10	0	1.5
2 Tbsp, 1 oz	15	0.5	2
With Half & Half: 2 Tbsp	50	3	3
¼ cup, 2 fl.oz	90	6	4
With Cream (light coffee), 2 Tbsp	65	6	2
With Coffee Mate: Liquid, reg., 1 T.	20	1	3
Liquid Fat Free, 1 Tbsp	25	0	2
Powder, 1 heaping tsp	15	1	2
Sugar ~ Add Extra: 1 heaping tsp	25	0	6
Single portion, 1 package	25	0	6
Sweeteners, *(Equal/Splenda/Sweet N Low),*			
Powder, 1 package	0	0	0

Flavored Coffee Mixes

	C	F	Cb
Chicory:			
Instant Coffee, 1 tsp	5	0	1
Coffee Essence, 1 tsp	15	0	4
Caffé D'Vita:			
Mixes, average all varieties, 3 tsp,	60	1.5	11
Sugar Free Mixes, 2 tsp	35	2	3
General Foods International:			
Average all varieties, 0.5 oz	60	3	10
Sugar-free, av. all varieties, 1 tsp	30	2.5	2
Cappuccino Coolers, all varieties, 0.5 oz	60	0	15
Hills Bros: *Per 3 Tbsp, 1 oz*			
Cappuccino: French Vanilla	120	4.5	19
Chocolate Hazelnut	110	3.5	19
Classic Cappuccino	120	5	17
Dark Chocolate	110	4	19
Mocha Mint	120	4	20
Nescafe, Memento, 1 stick,			
average all varieties	100	2.5	19
Starbucks, VIA, Iced Coffee,			
all varieties, 1 stick/packet	100	0	24

Coffee Shops/Restaurants

Per 8 fl.oz Cup (Unless Indicated)

	C	F	Cb
Coffee, Regular/Percolated/Filtered	5	0	0
Americano Drip Coffee, 1 cup	7.5	0	1
Cafe Au Lait: 1 cup, 8 fl.oz	60	3.5	5
Nonfat Milk, 1 cup, 8 fl.oz	35	0	5
Caffe Latté:			
8 fl.oz cup: With Whole Milk	110	6	9
With 2% Milk	100	3.5	9
With Nonfat Milk	70	0	10
12 fl.oz: With Whole Milk	180	9	14
With Nonfat Milk	100	0	15
16 fl.oz: With Whole Milk	220	11	18
With Nonfat Milk	130	0	19
Cafe Mocha (Mochaccino): 8 fl.oz	150	6	20
12 fl.oz	230	9	31
16 fl.oz	290	12	41
Cappuccino:			
8 fl.oz cup: With Whole Milk	90	3.5	7
With 2% Milk	80	3	8
With Nonfat Milk	50	0	8
12 fl.oz: With Whole Milk	110	6	9
With 2% Milk	90	3.5	9
With Nonfat Milk	60	0	9
16 fl.oz: With Whole Milk	140	7	11
With 2% Milk	120	3.5	11
With Nonfat Milk	80	0	12
Mocha: *With Cream*			
8 fl.oz: With Whole Milk	200	11	22
With Nonfat Milk	160	6	22
12 fl.oz: Whole Milk	290	15	33
With Nonfat Milk	230	8	34
Iced Mocha: *Without Cream*			
12 fl.oz: With Whole Milk	170	6	26
With Nonfat Milk	130	2	27
Espresso: Single (Solo), 1 fl.oz	5	0	1
Double (Doppio), 2 fl.oz	10	0	2
Espresso con Panna,			
(w/ dollop wh. cream), solo, 1 fl.oz	30	2.5	1
Espresso Macchiato, solo, 1 fl.oz	5	0	1
Frappuccino: Tall, 12 fl.oz	180	2.5	37
Grande, 16 fl.oz	240	3	48
Frappuccino Mocha:			
(With Cream): Tall, 12 fl.oz	280	11	43
Grande, 16 fl.oz	380	15	57
Iced Latte, Similar to Caffe Latte			

McCafe (McDonald's) ~ *See Fast Food, Page 216*
Starbucks ~ *See Fast-Foods Section , Page 243*

Coffee Substitute Mixes C F Cb

Roasted Cereal Beverages ~ *(No Caffeine)*

	C	F	Cb
Cafix, Instant Beverage, 1 tsp	5	0	1
Kaffree Roma, Instant Beverage, 1 tsp	10	0	2
Teeccino, Herbal Coffees, 1 tsp	10	0	2

Irish & Liqueur Coffees

	C	F	Cb
Irish Coffee, without sugar	175	10	0
Liqueur Coffee, with cream, all varieties, av., 1 fl.oz	100	5	7

Coffee Extras

	C	F	Cb
Chocolate (Cocoa) Topping, ½ tsp	5	0	1
Flavored Syrups: Regular, 2 Tbsp	80	0	20
Sugar-free, 2 Tbsp	0	0	0
Half & Half Cream: 2 Tbsp	40	3.5	1
Single serve pkg, ⅜ fl.oz	15	1.5	0.5
Light whipped cream, 2 Tbsp	15	1.5	1
Marshmallows, miniature (2)	5	0	1
Sugar:			
1 single portion package	20	0	5
1 level tsp	15	0	4
1 heaping tsp	25	0	6
Equal/Splenda/Sweet 'N Low	0	0	0

Coffee Shop ~ Cakes, Cookies

	C	F	Cb
Cookies:			
Biscotti, 1 oz	140	6.5	18
Chocolate Chip, 3 oz	350	15	54
Oatmeal Raisin, 3 oz	350	12	56
Peanut Butter, 3 oz	410	25	39
White Chocolate Macadamia, 3.33 oz	420	20	55
Cakes/Pastries:			
Almond Croissant, 5 oz	620	35	67
Apple Danish, 5 oz	450	18	67
Banana Walnut, 4.5 oz	410	17	60
Brownie, 3 oz	390	24	42
Bundt, Chocolate, 4 oz	440	21	61
Carrot Cake, 4 oz	400	22	45
Chocolate Cake, 5 oz	530	28	65
Crumble Coffee Cake, 4.5 oz	500	25	65
Cupcake, 3 oz	330	16	43
Pound Cake, av., 3 oz	330	17	40
Cinnamon Roll, 6 oz	500	15	83
Donuts:			
Sugared, 1.8 oz	220	11	27
Glazed, 2 oz	250	12	34
Pretzel, large, 4 oz	290	5	52

Starbucks Bakery Items ~ *See Page 244*

Ready To Drink Coffee C F Cb

Chilled:

Adina: *Per 8 fl.oz Can*

Double XXpresso	100	2	18
Mayan Mocha	130	2.5	24
Mocha Madness	110	2.5	20

Full Throttle Coffee & Energy ~ *See Page 38*

International Delight,
Iced, all varieties, 8 fl.oz	150	2.5	29

Java Monster Energy ~ *See Page 39*

Kahlua, Cappuccino Shake, 10.5 fl.oz	130	2	24

RealBeanz: *Per 9.5 fl.oz*

Iced Coffee:
All varieties	140	2	27
Diet, Trim & Fit, Cappuccino	60	2	16

Shock Coffee:
Triple Latte, 8 fl.oz can	150	3.5	27
Triple Mocha, 8 fl.oz can	150	3.5	28

Starbucks:

Discoveries,
all flavors	120	2	20

DoubleShots: *Per 6.f fl.oz*

Espresso & Cream:
Regular	140	6	18
Light	70	4	6

Frappuccino: *Per 9.5 fl.oz Bottle Unless Indicated*

Caramel/Coffee/ Vanilla	200	3	37
Dark Chocolate Mocha, 13.7 fl.oz			
Mocha	180	3	33
Light, Mocha/Vanilla	100	3	12
Iced Coffee, Caramel, 11 fl.oz	110	0.5	21

Starbucks Energy Drink ~ *See Page 40*

Caffeine Counter

Moderate caffeine intake is not harmful to healthy adults. However, frequent large amounts (over 350mg/day) may cause dependency ('caffeinism') and adversely affect health. To be safe, limit caffeine to 200mg/day. Avoid if pregnant, breast feeding, a child under 8, have sleep problems, an overactive bladder or heart arrhythmia.

Caffeine (mg)

Coffee: Instant, weak, 1 level teaspoon	30
Medium, 1 rounded teaspoon	60
Strong, 1 heaping teaspoon	100
Decaffeinated, 1 round teaspoon	2
Bags (Folgers), 1 bag (6-8 cups)	115
Ground, 1 Tbsp, 0.2 oz	60
Bottled (Ready-To-Drink), 9.5 fl.oz	70
Coffee Shop: Brewed, 8 fl.oz	110 -150
Cappuccino: 1 cup, 8 fl.oz	75
Tall, 12 fl.oz	110
Large, 16 fl.oz	150
Decappuccino, decaffeinated	5
Espresso: Regular/Solo	75
Double, (Doppio)	150
Iced Coffee, 12 fl.oz	140
Latte, 1 cup, 8 fl.oz	75
Mocha, 1 cup, 8 fl.oz	90
Hot Chocolate, 8 fl.oz	15
Tea (Black/Green): Weak, 1 cup	20
Medium Strength, 1 cup	40
Strong, 1 cup	70
Decaffeinated Tea, 1 cup	0-5
Herbal Tea, 1 cup	0
Iced Tea, tall glass/can, 12 fl.oz	25-30
Soft Drinks: *Per 12 fl.oz Can*	
Coca-Cola; Pepsi (Regular/Diet)	35
Diet Coke; TAB; RC Cola (Regular)	45
Dr. Pepper; Sunkist Orange	40
Pepsi One; Mountain Dew; Mellow Yellow; Surge	55
Pepsi Max (Regular/Diet) Sun Drop (Reg/Diet)	70
7-Up, Fanta, Sprite, Fresca, Diet Rite Cola	0
Energy Drinks (with added caffeine):	
(AMP, Adrenaline Rush, Full Throttle	
Monster, No Fear, Red Bull, Rockstar)	
Average all brands: 8 fl.oz	80
16 fl.oz	160
NOS Energy, 16 fl.oz	260
Chocolate Bars: Milk Chocolate, 2 oz	20
Dark Chocolate, 2 oz	30
Choc Chip Cookies, 2 medium, 2 oz	6
Chocolate Syrup, 2 Tbsp, 1.4 oz	5
Medicinals: Excedrin, Extra Strength (2)	130
NoDoz Maximum, 1 tablet	200

Energy/Protein Drinks

	C	F	Cb
5-hour Energy, 2 fl.oz	4	0	1
ABB:			
Energy: Speed Shot, 8.5 fl.oz	0	0	0
Ripped Force, 18 fl.oz	90	0	23
Hi-Pro:			
Pure Pro 35 Shake, all flav., 12 fl.oz	160	0.5	5
Pure Pro 50, all flavors, 14.5 fl.oz	240	1.5	7
Recovery,			
Maxx Recovery, all flavors, 18 fl.oz	400	0.5	60
AdvantEDGE (EAS),			
Carb Control, av. all flavors, 11 fl.oz	100	2.5	3
AllSport,			
Body Quencher, all flavors, 20 fl.oz	150	0	40
AMP: Per 16 fl.oz Can			
Active: Lemonade	130	0	31
Lemonade, Sugar Free	15	0	0.5
Boost: Original	220	0	58
Original, Sugar Free	10	0	0.5
Cherry; Grape	130	0	31
Focus: Mixed Berry	130	0	31
Arizona,			
Caution Extreme Performance, 11 fl.oz	160	0	40
Atkins, Advantage Shakes, av., 11 oz	155	9	4
Bariatrix, Proti-Max,			
Anytime Shakes, av., 8 oz	100	4	4
Bawls:			
Guarana: Original, 10 fl.oz	120	0	32
Cherry, 10 fl.oz	90	0	32
Blue Sky, Blue Energy, 8.3 fl.oz	120	0	29
Bolthouse: Per 8 fl.oz			
Protein Plus:			
Blended Coffee	190	2.5	26
Choc.; Mango; Vanilla, av.	200	2	30
Boost: Per 8 fl.oz			
Original, all flavors	240	4	41
Glucose Control, all flavors	190	7	16
High Protein, all flavors	240	6	33
Plus, all flavors	360	14	45
Carnation:			
Breakfast, Essentials Powder:			
All flavors, 1 envelope, 1.3 oz	130	1	27
No Sugar Added, all flav., av., 0.7 oz	60	1	12
Ready To Drink,			
Rich Milk Chocolate, 8 fl.oz	240	4	41
Celestial Seasoning, Shots,			
Kombucha, 2 fl.oz	30	0	8
CeraSport, EX1 powder, 1 pkt, 8.4 oz	40	0	10
Champion Lyte, Sports Drink	0	0	0

Champion Nutrition:	C	F	Cb
Heavywt Gainer 900, av., 4 scps, 5.4 oz	600	7	102
Ultramet, Original, 1 packet, 2.7 oz	280	2	24
Clif Shot,			
Energy Gel, all flavors, 1.2 oz pkt	110	1.5	21
Cocaine, Energy, 8.4 fl.oz can	70	0	18
Curves, Protein Drink,			
Choc.; Vanilla, 2 scps, 1 oz	120	1	12
CytoSport:			
Muscle Milk:			
Powder, all flavors, av., 2 scoops	310	12	18
Ready To Drink: Chocolate, 11 fl.oz	240	11	12
17 fl.oz	320	16	12
Drank, Anti Energy, 16 fl.oz bottle	220	0	54
EAS ~ See AdvantEDGE/Myoplex			
Ensure: Per Bottle			
Clear, 10 fl.oz	180	0	35
High Protein Shake, 14 fl.oz	210	2.5	23
Nutrition Shake,			
all flavors, 8 fl.oz	250	6	40
Plus, 8 fl.oz bottle	350	11	50
Enterex, Diabetic, all flavors, 8 fl.oz	240	9	27
FRS, Energy, Wild Berry; Cherry Limeade			
average, 12 fl.oz	90	0	22
Fruit:O (Veryfine), 20 fl.oz bottle	0	0	0
Full Throttle: Per 16 fl.oz			
Energy: Citrus	220	0	58
Blue Agave; Red Berry	230	0	58
Fuze:			
Blends average, 16.9 fl.oz	185	0.5	43
Juice: Berry Punch, 8 fl.oz	80	0	20
Strawb. Lemonade, 8 fl.oz	100	0	25
Gatorade:			
G Series: Ready To Drink			
Endurance, Thirst Quencher: 12 fl oz	80	0	21
32 fl oz bottle	215	0	56
G2 Low Calorie Thirst Quencher:			
12 fl oz	30	0	7
32 fl oz	80	0	19
Prime, Sports Fuel,			
4 fl oz pouch	100	0	25
Recover:			
Post-Game Prot. Drink, 16.9 fl oz	230	0	41
Protein Shake, 330 ml carton	270	1.5	45
Genisoy,			
Protein Powder, Chocolate; Vanilla,			
average, 1.3 oz scoop	125	0	18
Glaceau:			
Smartwater, 8 fl.oz	0	0	0
Vitaminwater, all flav., 20 fl.oz	125	0	33
Glucerna,			
Shakes, all flavors, 8 fl.oz	200	7	27

GNC:	C	F	Cb
Lean Shake: Powder, all flav., 2 scoops	200	3	17
Drinks, av. all flavors, 14 fl.oz bottle	170	6	6
Pro Performance:			
100% Whey Protin Powder, Natural Vanilla, 1 scoop, 1 oz	150	2.5	8
Amplified: Mass XXX, Strawberry, 4 level scoops	750	6	124
Wheybolic Extreme 60, all flavors, 3 scoops	280	1	7
Golazo:			
Sports Energy: Av. all flavors, 12 fl.oz	95	0	22
Sugar Free, Mango Lime, 12 fl.oz	10	0	5
Sports Hydration, 20 fl.oz bottle:			
Mandarin; Mango Limon, average	95	0	33
Other flavors	130	0	33
GU, Energy Gel, av. all flavors, 1 packet	100	1	25
Guru, Energy: Regular, 8.3 oz can	100	0	25
Lite,12 oz can	10	0	2
Hammer, Gel, av. all, 1.7 Tbsp, 1.2 oz	90	0	22
Hansen's: Energy Pro, 8 fl.oz	130	0	34
Energy Diet Red, 8 fl.oz	20	0	6
Vidration, all flavors, 8 fl.oz	0	0	0
Herbalife: Nutr. Shake, 1 pkt	90	1	13
With 8 fl.oz non-fat milk	170	1	26
Hollywood Miracle Diet, 4 fl.oz	100	0	15
Hype:			
Energy: Regular/ Organic/MFP, all flavors, 8.4 fl.oz	120	0	28
Enlite, 8.4 fl.oz	25	0	4
Shot, 3.5 fl.oz	45	0	10
Jarrow:			
Whey Protein: Unflavored, 0.8 oz	95	2	2
Chocolate; Vanilla, average, 1 oz	105	1	6
Muscle Optimeal, 2 scoops, 1.5 oz	160	1	15
Java Monster: Per 15 fl.oz Can			
Regular, average all flavors	190	3	33
Light, Vanilla	95	3	13
Kellogg's:			
To Go, Breakfast Shakes:			
RTD, all flavors, av., 10 fl.oz bottle	185	5	29
Shake Mix, all flavors, av., 1 pkt	130	0.5	27
Knudsen: Recharge, average, 8 fl.oz	70	0	23
Simply Nutritious, av. all, 8 fl.oz	120	0	30
Kombucha, Wonder Drink, 8.5 fl.oz	60	0	16
La Brada:			
Powders: Lean Body, 2.8 oz	330	8	24
Lean Body, Mass 60, 6 oz	615	7	76
Carb Watchers, 2.3 oz	250	4.5	12
RTD, Lean Body, 17 fl.oz	260	9	9
Lipovitan, B3, 8.6 fl.oz	130	0	30
Liquid Ice: Regular, 8.3 fl.oz	130	0	32
Sugar Free, 8.3 fl oz	15	0	0

	C	F	Cb
Liquid Lightning, Regular, 8.5 fl.oz	90	0	22
Max Velocity:			
Regular: 8.5 fl.oz can	130	0	33
16 fl.oz can	240	0	62
Sugar Free, 16 fl.oz can	15	0	1
Met-Rx:			
Protein Plus:			
Powder, Choc., 2 scoops	220	1.5	7
Ready To Drink 51, av. all flav.,15 fl.oz	235	2	6
Metabol: Endurance, 2 scoop,1.8 oz	200	5	24
GlyProXTS, 1 scoop, 0.2 oz	20	0	5
Met, 2 scoops, 2.3 oz	260	3	40
Met Max, mix, 2 scoops, 2.2 oz	230	2.5	11
MiO Energy, 1 serving	0	0	0
MLO, Mus-L Blast, Chocolate, 4 scoops	570	3.5	112
Monster, Energy: 16 fl.oz can	200	0	54
Lo-Carb, 16 fl.oz	20	0	6
M-80, 16 fl.oz	180	0	46
Mixxd (with Juice), 16 fl.oz	220	0	54
MRM: All Natural Whey, 1 scoop, 0.9 oz	85	1	1.5
Low Carb Protein, average, 1 scoop	115	2.5	2
Muscle Milk ~ See Cytosport			
Muscle Tech: Dry Powder Only			
100% Ultra Premium, Mass Gainer, 2 scoops, 11.6 oz	1290	4	261
Mass-Tech Advantage, Milk Chocolate, 5 scoops, 9 oz	1000	9	168
Nitro Tech Lean Muscle, Van., 1.3 oz	140	1.5	1
Myoplex (EAS):			
Original Shakes, av. all flavors, 17 fl.oz	300	7	19
Lite, all flavors, 11 fl.oz	170	2	20
Powder: Original Choc. 1 pkt	290	4.5	22
Lite, 1 packet, 1.9 oz	180	2	24
Nature's Best:			
Carbo Power, all flavors, 16 fl.oz	400	0	100
Isopure: Alpine Punch, 20 fl.oz	260	0	25
Mass, all flavors, 20 fl.oz	350	0	53
Zero Carb, all flavors, 20 fl.oz	160	0	0
JavaPro Powders, average all flavors, 1.5 scoops, 1 oz	110	1.5	2
No-Fear: Regular, 16 fl.oz	260	0	72
Sugar Free, 16 fl.oz	20	0	2
Noni, Tahitian, 2 Tbsp	15	0	3
NOS:			
Energy: All flavors, 16 fl.oz can	210	0	54
Sugar Free, all flav., 22 fl.oz bottle	20	0	2
Natural Caffeine & Electrolytes, all flavors, 12 fl.oz	10	0	1
Nutrament (Nestle), 12 fl.oz	360	10	52
Nutrilite (Amway):			
Meal Replacement Shakes, all, 11 fl.oz	140	3	15
Whey Protein Powder, av., all, 1.3 oz	150	1	9

Energy/Protein Drinks (Cont)

	C	F	Cb
Optifast 800 (Nestle):			
High Protein Powder, 1 pkg	200	6	10
Powder 800 Formula, 1 pkg	160	3	20
Ready To Drink Shakes, 8 fl.oz	160	3	20
Optimum Nutrition:			
100%: Whey, 1 oz scoop	120	1	3
Oats & Whey, 1.9 oz scoop	200	1.5	22
Soy Protein, 1 oz scoop	120	1.5	1
Optisource (Nestle),			
Very High Protein Drink, 8 fl.oz	200	6	12
Powerade:			
Sports Drink:			
Regular, av. all flav.,12 fl.oz	80	0	22
Zero, 12 fl.oz	0	0	0
PowerBar:			
Performance Energy, 1 pouch	80	0	21
Power Gel, av. all flavors, 1.5 oz pkg	110	0	27
Propel, Workout Water,			
all flavors, 12 fl.oz	0	0	0
Radioactive:			
Regular: 10.5 oz	150	0	37
16 oz	220	0	56
Sugar Free, all sizes	0	0	0
Red Bull:			
Energy Drink, all flavors:			
8.4 fl.oz	110	0	28
12 fl.oz can	160	0	40
Simply Cola, 12 fl.oz	130	0	31
Sugar-Free, 8.4 fl.oz	10	0	3
Zero Calories, 8.4 fl.oz	0	0	0
Resource (Nestle):			
Breeze, 8 fl.oz	250	0	54
Diabetishield, 8 fl.oz	150	0	30
Health Shake: 4 fl.oz	200	4	35
No Added Sugar, 4 fl.oz	200	9	22
Shake Plus, 8 fl.oz	480	16	69
Revenge (Champion Nutrition):			
Sport, Choc., Vanilla, av., 0.9 oz scoop	125	1.5	6
Strength, Choc.; Vanilla, av., 1.3 oz scp	145	2	8
Revival, Soy Mix, unsweetened:			
Plain, 2 scoops, 0.95 oz	105	1	4
Chocolate Day Dream, 1 package	120	2.5	7
Rhino's, Energy Drink, 100ml	50	0	11
Rip It, Energy Fuel, Citrus X, 16 fl.oz	260	0	66
Rockstar: Per 16 fl.oz Can			
Energy Drink: Punched, av.	270	0	62
Sugar Free	20	0	0
Rush: Per 8 fl.oz			
Energy Drink: Regular	140	0	31
Lite	0	0	0
SK Energy, Energy Shot, all flavors, 2 oz	0	0	0

	C	F	Cb
Slim-Fast:			
Protein Meal Shakes: 10 fl.oz			
Ready to Drink,			
average all flavors	190	6	25
Protein Shake Mixes,			
French Vanilla, 0.9 oz scoop	200	4	30
SoBe: Per 20 fl.oz Can/Bottle			
Energize, Citrus Energy	270	0	67
Lifewater: Average all flavors	100	0	25
O-Cal, average all flavors	0	0	9
Note: Carb figures inlude 7-10g sugar alcohol			
Vita Boom: Cranberry Grapefruit	250	0	64
Orange-Carrot	220	0	57
Solixir, Energy Drink, av. all, 12 fl.oz	55	0	13
Spiru-Tein: Per 1.2 oz			
Energy Meal:			
Banana; Cappuccino	100	0	10
Black Cherry Chocolate	110	1	13
Starbucks,			
Refreshers, av. all flav.,12 fl.oz	60	0	19
Steaz: Energy, 12 fl.oz	135	0	35
Zero Calorie, Berry, 12 fl.oz	0	0	0
The Sports Club/LA:			
Beachbody Whey Protein Powder,			
Chocolate; Vanilla, 2 scoops, 1.4 oz	130	4	7
Twin Lab:			
Endurance Fuel, 1.1 oz scoop	110	0	20
Energy Fuel, 250ml can	0	0	0
Venom: Mojave Rattler, 16 fl.oz	50	0	8
Average other varieties, 16 fl.oz	235	0	57
Verve: Energy, 8.3 fl.oz can	70	0	18
Sugar Free	5	0	1
Weider:			
Creatine ATP, powder, ½ cup, 1.7 oz	210	0	37
Dynamic Weight Gainer, pdr, 4.5 oz	450	2.5	94
Mega Mass 2000, powder, av., 3.5 oz	400	7	62
Training Whey, 1.2 oz scoop	140	1.5	2
Worldwide:			
Carbo Rush, average, 20 fl.oz	270	0	68
Pure Protein Shakes,			
35g Protein, 11 fl.oz	160	1	2
Worx, Energy,			
Original; Extra Strength, 2 fl.oz	0	0	0
XS (Quixtar), Energy Drink, 8.4 oz	10	0	0
Zola, Acai, Original Juice, 12 fl.oz	185	3	39

Quick Guide	C	F	Cb

Orange Juice
Average ~ Fresh

	C	F	Cb
½ Cup, 4 fl.oz	55	0	13
Small Glass, 6 fl.oz	85	0	19
Regular Cup 8 fl.oz	110	0.5	26
Regular Glass, 12 fl.oz	160	0.5	39
10 fl.oz Bottle	140	0.5	32
11.5 fl.oz Can	160	0.5	37
16 fl.oz Bottle	225	1	52
20 fl.oz Bottle	280	1	64

Juices ~ Generic

Average All Brands:

	C	F	Cb
Aloe Vera Juice, unsweetened, 2 oz	10	0	0
Apple Juice: 8 fl.oz	120	0	29
10 fl.oz Bottle	145	0.5	36
16 fl.oz	235	0.5	58
Carrot Juice: Fresh, 6 fl.oz	35	0	8
Sweetened, 6 fl.oz	75	0	17
Coconut Water, 8 fl.oz	50	0.5	9
Cranberry Juice, Cocktail/Blend	140	0	34
Fruit Blends, average all, 8 fl.oz	110	0	27
Fruit Nectars, average all, 8 fl.oz	140	0	36
Grape Juice, 8 fl.oz	155	0	38
Grapefruit Juice, 8 fl.oz	95	0	22
Lemon/Lime Juice: 1 Tbsp	5	0	1
1 cup, 8 fl.oz	50	0.5	16
Concentrate, 1 tsp	0	0	0
Noni Juice:			
Tahitian, 2 Tbsp, 1 fl.oz	15	0	3
Tahiti Traders, 1 fl.oz	20	0	5
Passion Fruit Juice, Fresh:			
Purple, 1 cup, 8 fl.oz	125	0	34
Yellow, 1 cup, 8 fl.oz	80	1.5	14
Papaya/Peach Nectar, av., 8 fl.oz	140	0	36
Pear Nectar, 8 fl.oz	150	0	40
Pineapple Juice, 8 fl.oz	130	0	32
Pomegranate Juice, 8 fl.oz	160	0	40
Prune Juice, 8 fl.oz	180	0	45
Strawb./Raspberry Juice, 8 fl.oz	100	0	23
Tangerine Juice, 8 fl.oz	105	0.5	25
Tomato Juice, 8 fl.oz	40	0	10
Vegetable Juice, 8 fl.oz	45	0	11
Wheat Grass Juice:			
1 fl.oz 'Shot'	10	0	1.5
2 fl.oz 'Shot'	20	0	3

Quick Guide	C	F	Cb

Fruit Smoothies (Jamba Juice; Smoothie King)
Average All Brands

	C	F	Cb
Fruit Only: 8 fl.oz	115	0.5	29
12 fl.oz	175	1	43
16 fl.oz	230	1	58
24 fl.oz	350	1	78
Fruit + Non-Fat Milk/Soy:			
12 fl.oz	135	0	29
16 fl.oz	155	0	37
24 fl.oz	265	1	59
Fruit + Non-Fat Frozen Yogurt/Sherbet:			
12 fl.oz	200	0.5	47
16 fl.oz	265	1	63
24 fl.oz	395	1.5	95

Juice ~ Brands

Per 8 fl.oz Unless Indicated

	C	F	Cb
Apple & Eve:			
Cranberry Grape/Pommeg.	140	0	34
Naturally Cranberry	130	0	32
Fruitables, av. all flavors, 6.75 fl.oz	60	0	14
Bolthouse Farms: *Per 8 fl.oz*			
Juice: 100% Carrot	70	0	14
Orange & Carrot	120	0	27
Fruit Smoothies:			
Berry Boost	130	0	30
Blue Goodness	160	0	34
C-Boost	120	0	29
Green Goodness	140	0	33
Strawberry Banana	130	0	32
Bom Dia: *Per 8 fl.oz*			
Acai: Original	110	0	27
+ 10 Superblend	120	0	31
Mango Coconut Splash	60	0	15
Pomegranate	170	0	42
Bright & Early *(Minute Maid)*,			
Orange Juice (Chilled/Frozen)	110	0	30
Campbell's:			
Tomato Juice: 5.5 fl.oz can	30	0	7
8 fl.oz	50	0	10
Cactus Cooler, Orange Pineapple Blast,			
12 fl oz can	150	0	40

Juice Brands (Cont)

	C	F	Cb

Per 8 fl.oz Unless Indicated

Capri Sun: *Per 6 fl.oz*

	C	F	Cb
100% Juice: Citrus	100	0	23
Average other flavors	85	0	21
Juice Drinks, (25% Less Sugar), average all flavors	60	0	17
Roarin' Waters, all flavors, 6 fl.oz	30	0	8

Clamato:

Original Tomato Cocktail	60	0	12
Picante	60	0	13

Crystal Geyser:
Juice Squeeze: *Per 12 fl.oz Bottle*

Blackberry Pomegranate	170	0	43
Ruby Grapefruit	150	0	36
Average other flavors	135	0	32

Dole: *Per 8 fl.oz*

Aguas Frescas, average all flavors	110	0	26
Blended Juices:			
Orange Peach Mango	120	0	29
Pina Colada	120	0	29
Pineapple-Orange Banana	120	0	30
Strawberry Kiwi	120	0	31
Fruit Squish'ems, all flavors, 3.2 oz	60	0	14

Florida's Natural: *Per 8 fl.oz*

Apple Juice	120	0	29
Cranberry Ruby Red	130	0	32
Lemonade, Home Squeezed	110	0	28
Orange: Premium	110	0	26
Mango	110	0	27
Pineapple	130	0	31
Strawberry	110	0	26
Ruby Red Grapefruit, Original	90	0	22

Fuze: *Per 16.9 fl.oz Bottle*

Banana Colada	180	0.5	43
Other Fruit Flavors	180	0	45
Slenderize, average all flavors	15	0	3

Goya: *Per 12 fl.oz Can*

Nectar: Guava; Tamarind	240	0	59
Mango	230	0	56
Papaya	220	0	56
Peach	220	0	54
Pear & Passion Fruit	230	0	57
Pineapple & Passion Fruit	220	0	55

Per 8 fl.oz Unless Indicated

Hansen's:
Juice Box: *Per 6.75 fl.oz Box*

	C	F	Cb
Awesome Apple; Loud Lemonade, av.	90	0	23
Burstin Berry; Totally Tropical	100	0	24
Strawberry Banana	110	0	27
Other flavors	100	0	24

Junior Juice,

100% Juice, all flavors, 4.23 oz box	60	0	15

Natural, (64 fl.oz Bottles): *Per 8 fl.oz*

Apple	120	0	28
Apple Strawberry	110	0	27
Grape	120	0	33
Ruby Red Grapefruit	100	0	25
White Grape	140	0	36
Smoothie Nectar, average, 12 fl.oz	180	0	46

Hawaii's Own, Frozen Concentrate,

100% Juice, all varieties, av., 8 fl.oz	110	0	28

Hi-C Juice Drinks: *Per 6.75 fl.oz Box*

Flashin' Fruit Punch	90	0	26
Orange Lavaburst	90	0	26
Poppin' Lemonade	100	0	27

Hood: *Per 8 fl.oz*

Apple	120	0	31
Fruit Punch; Orange	120	0	30
Lemonade	110	0	28

Jamba Juice ~ *See Fast-Foods Section*

Juicy Juice *(Nestle):*
Average all flavors:

4.23 fl.oz box	60	0	15
6.75 fl.oz box	100	0	24

Kerns:
Nectars: *Per 11.5 fl.oz Can*

Guava	210	0	53
Pear; Strawb. Banana, av.	220	0	53
Pineapple Coconut	280	8	53
Strawberry	210	0	52

Kool Aid: *Per 6 fl.oz Containers*
Jammers: Grape; Cherry

Grape; Cherry	80	0	20
Average other flavors	70	0	19

L & A: *Per 8 fl.oz*

All Cherry	180	0	45
All Cranberry	60	0	14
Papaya Delight	130	0	32
Pineapple Coconut	140	3	28

Juice Brands (Cont)	C	F	Cb

Per 8 fl.oz Unless Indicated

Lakewood Organic: *Per 8 fl.oz*

	C	F	Cb
Blends: Acai Amazon Berry	125	3.5	27
Banana Strawberry	110	0	27
Blueberry Blend	110	0	27
Cranberry Lemonade	80	0	20
Lemonade	80	0	20
Pomegranate Blend	125	0	31
Super Veggie	60	0	13
Pure: Apple	110	0	28
Blueberry	100	0	22
Carrot	80	0	19
Pink Grapefruit	90	0	22
Prune	170	0	42
Light: Lemonade	40	0	10
Average other flavors	55	0	13

Langers: *Per 8 fl.oz*

100% Juice (No Sugar Added):

	C	F	Cb
All Pomegranate	140	0	35
Apple Cider	120	0	28
Apple Juice	120	0	28
Mixed Berry	120	0	30
Pineapple Coconut	140	3	28
Red/White Grape Juice	160	0	40

Juice Cocktails (27% Juice):

	C	F	Cb
Blueberry Cranberry	135	0	34
Cranberry	140	0	35
Cranberry Grape	165	0	41
Cranberry Raspberry	150	0	36
Pomegranate	140	0	34
Pomeg. Blueb./Cranberry	140	0	34
White Cranberry	120	0	28
White Cran-Raspberry	120	0	28
20% Juice, Strawberry Peach	120	0	30

Martinelli's: *Per 8 fl.oz*

	C	F	Cb
Sparkling: Apple-Cranberry	110	0	27
Apple-Grape/Raspberry, av.	120	0	31
Apple-Mango/Pomegranate	150	0	38
Apple-Pear/Marionberry, av.	130	0	32
Apple-Wild Berry	150	0	36

Per 8 fl.oz Unless Indicated

Minute Maid:

15.2 fl.oz Bottles:

	C	F	Cb
Apple Juice	210	0	52
Cranb. Apple Raspberry	230	0	61
Fruit Punch	220	0	58
Orange Juice, 100% Squeezed, Orig.	220	0	51
Pineapple Orange	220	0	55
Coolers, Clear Cherry; Orange Strawb., average, 6.75 fl.oz Pouch	100	0	27
Juice Boxes, all flavors, 6 fl.oz	90	0	22
Soft Frozen, Limeade, 1.5 fl.oz	90	0	26
MonaVie, Acai Blends, Active; Pulse, 2 fl.oz	45	0.5	10

Mott's:

100% Juice:

	C	F	Cb
Original: Apple, 8 fl.oz	120	0	29
Apple White Grape, 6.75 fl.oz	110	0	26
Fruit Punch, 4.23 fl.oz	60	0	15
Light, Apple, 8 fl.oz	50	0	12

Juice Drink:

	C	F	Cb
Fruit Punch Rush, 8 fl.oz	140	0	32
Strawberry Boom, 8 fl.oz	60	0	15
Wild Grape Surge, 8 fl.oz	60	0	16

Medleys:

	C	F	Cb
Apple & Carrot, 8 fl.oz	110	0	25
Grape, Apple & Carrot, 8 fl.oz	140	0	33
Tropical, 8 fl.oz	140	0	32

Mott's For Tots (47-54% Juice):

	C	F	Cb
40% Less Sugar: Average all flavors, 6.75 fl.oz	55	0	13
Grape, 8 fl.oz	70	0	17
Average other flavors, 8 fl.oz	60	0	16

Naked Juice: *Per 8 fl.oz*

100% Juice, No Sugar Added:

	C	F	Cb
O-J	110	0	27
Orange Mango	130	0	31
Pomegranate Acai	160	1	31
Pomegranate Blueberry	150	0	36

100% Juice Smoothie, No Sugar Added:

	C	F	Cb
Berry Blast; Strawb. Banana	130	0	30
Mighty Mango	150	0	36
Orange Carrot	120	0	29
Boosted: Acai Machine	160	3	31
Blue Machine	170	0	40
Green Machine	140	0	33
Power-C Machine	120	0	29
Red Machine	170	4.5	31
Coconut Water, Pure, 11.2 fl.oz	60	0	14

Juice Brands (Cont)

	C	F	Cb

Per 8 fl.oz Unless Indicated

Nantucket Nectars:

100% Juice: *Per 8 fl.oz*

	C	F	Cb
Peach Orange	130	0	32
Pineapple Orange Banana	140	0	34
Pomegranate Cherry	120	0	29
Premium Orange Juice	110	0	26
Pressed Apple	120	0	30
Juice Cocktail, Cranberry	130	0	33

Juice Drinks: *Per 8 fl.oz*

	C	F	Cb
Orange Mango	120	0	31
Pineapple Orange Guava	120	0	29
Pomegranate Pear	110	0	28
Red Plum Juice	130	0	31
Watermelon Strawberry	110	0	28
Lemonade, Squeezed	110	0	28

Newman's Own: *Per 8 fl.oz*

	C	F	Cb
Lemonade, Regular; Pink	110	0	27
Limeade	140	0	34

Fruit Juice Cocktail:

	C	F	Cb
Gorilla Grape	140	0	34
Orange Mango Tango	130	0	33

Northland,

100% Juice,

	C	F	Cb
Cranb. Blackberry/Raspberry/Grape, average	140	0	36

Ocean Spray: *Per 8 fl.oz*

Juice Cocktails:

	C	F	Cb
Blueberry	110	0	28
Cranberry	120	0	30
With Calcium	130	0	31
Ruby Red Grapefruit	110	0	28
White Cranberry	110	0	27

100% Juice Blends:

	C	F	Cb
Citrus Tangerine Orange	110	0	28
Cranberry Concord Grape	150	0	37
Cranberry Raspberry	140	0	34
White Grapefruit	90	0	21

Juice Drinks:

	C	F	Cb
Cran-Apple	130	0	32
Cran-Grape	120	0	31
CranRaspberry/Strawberry, av.	110	0	28
Diet Juice Drinks, all flavors	5	0	2
Light Juice Drinks, av. all flavors	50	0	13

Per 8 fl.oz Unless Indicated

	C	F	Cb

Odwalla: *Per 12 fl.oz Bottle*

	C	F	Cb
Blueberry B	210	0	50
Carrot Juice	100	0	22
Chocolate Protein Monster	320	6	40
Mango Tango	220	1	50
Mo'Beta	170	0	40
Orange Honey Passion Wellness	220	0	53
Original Super Food	190	0.5	44
Original Super Protein	290	1	52
Pomegranate Limeade	180	0	44
Strawberry C Monster	240	0	56

Orange Julius:

Originals, Orange:

	C	F	Cb
Small, 16 fl.oz	210	0	52
Medium, 17.5 fl.oz	270	0	68
Large, 26 fl.oz	420	0	103

Smoothies ~ *See Fast-Foods Section*

	C	F	Cb
Orangina, 10 fl.oz bottle	130	0	32

Pom Wonderful: *Per 8 fl.oz*

100% Juice,

	C	F	Cb
Blueberry; Cherry; Pomegranate	150	0	36

Juice Blends: Coconut

	C	F	Cb
Coconut	140	0	33
Hula	140	0	35
Mango	140	0	34

R.W. Knudsen: *Per 8 fl.oz*

Organic, 100% Juice: Apple

	C	F	Cb
Apple	120	0	30
Concord Grape	150	0	39
Cranberry Blueberry	120	0	30

Natural, 100% Juice:

	C	F	Cb
Mango Peach	120	0	30
Cranberry Raspberry	130	0	32
Kiwi Strawberry	120	0	30
Razzleberry	120	0	30
Rio Red Grapefruit	140	0	34
85% Juice, Hibiscus Cooler	100	0	25

Just Juice:

	C	F	Cb
Just Black Currant	100	0	15
Just Black Cherry	160	0	37
Just Blueberry	100	0	24
Simply Nutritious: Mega C	140	0	34
Average other flavors	125	0	30

Sparkling Essence,

	C	F	Cb
average all flavors, 10.5 fl.oz	0	0	0

Juice Brands (Cont)

C F Cb

Per 8 fl.oz Unless Indicated

R.W. Knudsen (Cont):

Spritzers: *Per 10.5 fl.oz Cans*

	C	F	Cb
Black Cherry	120	0	29
Mango Fandango	110	0	28
Red Raspberry	110	0	27
Very Veggie, Original, 8 fl.oz	60	0	12

ReaLemon – ReaLime:

Lemon/Lime Juice (from concentrate):

	C	F	Cb
1 teaspoon	0	0	0
2Tbsp, 1 fl.oz	10	0	2.5

Santa Cruz: *Per 8 fl.oz*

Organic, 100% Juice:

	C	F	Cb
Apple Juice	120	0	30
Concord Grape; White Grape	160	0	39
Orange Mango	130	0	32
Strawberry Kiwi	120	0	30

25% Juice Drink Boxes:

	C	F	Cb
Lemon	120	0	29
Grape	100	0	23

Carbonated Beverages: *Per 10.5 fl.oz Can*

	C	F	Cb
Lemon Lime	130	0	32
Root Beer	130	0	32

Celebratory Style:

	C	F	Cb
Sparkling Lemonade	110	0	27
Sparkling Limeade	100	0	26

Nectars: Berry

	C	F	Cb
Berry	120	0	29
Cranberry	120	0	30
Passionfruit	160	0	38

Seismic *(Amway):*

Super Juices: *Per 10 fl.oz Bottle*

	C	F	Cb
Citrus; Berry	180	0	44
Low Sugar Cherry	100	0	26

Simply Orange Juice Company:

	C	F	Cb
Lemonade; Limeade	120	0	30

Orange Juice,

	C	F	Cb
with or without pulp	110	0	26

Snap•E•Tom,

Tomato & Chili Cocktail,

	C	F	Cb
11.5 fl.oz can	70	0	15

Snapple: *Per 16 fl.oz Bottle*

Juice Drink Blends:

	C	F	Cb
Go Bananas; Raspb Peach, average	220	0	55
Grapeade; Lemonade; Orangeade	190	0	46
Fruit Punch	200	0	48
Diet, Cranberry Raspberry	20	0	4

Per 8 fl.oz Unless Indicated

Ssips, Juice Boxes,

	C	F	Cb
average all flavors, 6 fl.oz box	80	0	21

Stonyfield Farm: *Per 10 fl.oz Bottle*

Smoothies: Strawberry; Wild Berry

	C	F	Cb
Strawberry; Wild Berry	230	3	39
Peach; Strawb. Banana, av.	230	3	41

SunnyD:

Original: *Per 64 fl.oz Ctn*

	C	F	Cb
Smooth/Tangy Orange, 8 fl.oz	50	0	14

Blends, 64 fl.oz Containers,

	C	F	Cb
average all flavors, 8 fl.oz	60	0	15

Baja Juice: *Per 12 fl.oz Bottles*

	C	F	Cb
Red Punch	170	0	43
Other flavors	190	0	46

Sunsweet: *Per 8 fl.oz*

Plum Smart: Original

	C	F	Cb
Original	160	0	36
Light	60	0	15

Prune Juice: Original

	C	F	Cb
Original	180	0	42
With Pulp	150	0	44
Light	100	0	26

Trader Joe's:

All Natural Pasteurized, 32/64 fl.oz Bottle: *Per 8 fl.oz*

	C	F	Cb
100% Cranberry	70	0	16
Blueberry Pomegranate	140	0	34
Just Blueberry	100	0	24
Just Pomegranate	150	0	37
Mango PassionFruit	130	0	32
Omega Orange Carrot	110	0	26

Organic, 32/64 fl.oz Bottle: *Per 8 fl.oz*

	C	F	Cb
100% Pomegranate	140	0	35
Apple Juice	120	0	30
Concord Grape Juice	160	0	39
Cranberry	70	0	18
Grapefruit Sunset; Lemonade	120	0	30
Mango Nectar	130	0	32
Pink Lemonade	130	0	32
Strawberry Lemonade	120	0	29
White Grape Juice	160	0	40

Joe's Kids: *Per 6.75 fl.oz Box*

From Concentrate: Apple

	C	F	Cb
From Concentrate: Apple	90	0	23
Apple Grape	100	0	24
White Grape	120	0	30
10% Juice, Lemonade	90	0	22

Sparkling Juices: 25.4 fl.oz Botle:

	C	F	Cb
Blueberry, 8 fl.oz	120	0	30
Cranberry, 8 fl.oz	140	0	35
Pomegranate, 8 fl.oz	130	0	31

Updated Nutrition Data ~ www.CalorieKing.com
Persons with Diabetes ~ See Disclaimer (Page 22)

Juice Brands (Cont) | C | F | Cb |

Per 8 fl.oz Unless Indicated

	C	F	Cb
Tree Top:			
100% Juice Concentrates:			
64 fl.oz Bottle: *Per 8 fl.oz*			
Apple Berry/Grape, average	125	0	32
Apple Cranb.; Blueberry Pomegr.	120	0	30
11.5 fl.oz Can: *Per Can*			
Apple Berry/Grape, av.	180	0	46
Fruit Punch	170	0	42
6.75 fl.oz Box: *Per Box*			
Apple Pear	100	0	25
Fruit Punch	110	0	26
Grape Juice	110	0	27
Tropicana: *Per 8 fl.oz*			
Chilled:			
Orangeade	130	0	33
Punch, average all flavors	125	0	31
Non-Refrigerated:			
100% juice, 10 fl.oz bottles: Apple	170	0	40
Fruit Medley	170	0	42
20% Juice, 15.2 fl.oz Bottle,			
Cranberry	270	0	67
Farmstand, 46 fl.oz bottle,			
average all flavors, 8 fl.oz	120	0	30
Trop50, 50% less sugar, 59 fl.oz bottle,			
average all flavors, 8 fl.oz	50	0	13
Tropics, 59 fl.oz container,			
average all flavors, 8 fl.oz	120	0	30
Twisters, 20 fl.oz bottle,			
average all flavors	300	0	74
V8 Juices & Drinks:			
Original/Spicy 100% Vegetable Juice:			
5.5 fl.oz can	35	0	7
8 fl.oz cup	50	0	10
11.5 fl.oz can	70	0	14
12 fl.oz bottle	75	0	15
Splash: Average all flavors	70	0	19
Diet Splash, all flavors	10	0	3
Smoothies: Strawberry Banana	90	0	20
Tropical Colada	100	0	21
V-Fusion: Grape Raspberry	140	0	33
Av. other flavors	110	0	27
Light Varieties, av. all flav.	50	0	13
Refreshers, average all flavors	100	0	25
Smoothies, average all flavors	125	0	31
Sparkling, av. all flavors, 8.4 fl.oz	55	0	13

Per 8 fl.oz Unless Indicated

	C	F	Cb
Veryfine:			
100%: Apple Juice	120	0	29
Orange Juice	120	0	30
Walnut Acres: *Per 8 fl.oz*			
Organic: Apple	110	0	29
Apricot; Raspberry	130	0	32
Cherry	140	0	34
Cranberry	110	0	26
Incredible Vegetable	50	0	12
Mango Nectar	120	0	29
Welch's: *Per 8 fl.oz*			
100% Juice: Grape Juice	140	0	36
Red Grape juice	160	0	41
White Grape	140	0	38
White Grape Cherry/Peach	140	0	34
Cocktails, 100% Juice,			
Grape; White Grape, 2 fl.oz	140	0	38
Cocktails, Refrigerated, 64 fl.oz Ctn:			
Dragon Fruit Mango	140	0	35
Mango Twist	150	0	38
Strawberry Breeze	130	0	33
Concentrates, 100% Juice,			
Grape; White Grape, 2 fl.oz	140	0	38
Light Juice, 52 fl.oz Bottle			
Concord/WhiteGrape	45	0	12
Sparkling Juice Cocktail,			
all varieties, average	140	0	34
Zola: *Per 12 fl.oz Bottle*			
Acai: Original	185	3	39
With Blueberry Juice	180	3	38

CALORIEKING PORTION WATCH

ORANGE JUICE	C	Cb
8 fl.oz	110	26
16 fl.oz	220	52
24 fl.oz	330	78
32 fl.oz	440	104

Quick Guide   **C** **F** **Cb**

Cow's Milk ~ Average All Brands

Whole (3.25% fat):

	C	F	Cb
2 Tbsp, 1 fl.oz	20	1	1.5
1 Cup, 8 fl.oz	150	8	12
1 Large Glass, 12 fl.oz	220	12	17
1 Pint, 16 fl.oz	295	16	22
1 Quart, 946 ml	590	32	44

Reduced-Fat (2% fat):

	C	F	Cb
2 Tbsp, 1 fl.oz	15	0.5	1.5
1 Cup, 8 fl.oz	120	5	12
1 Large Glass, 12 fl.oz	180	7.5	18
1 Pint, 16 fl.oz	245	10	23
1 Quart, 946 ml	490	20	46

Light/Low-Fat (1% fat):

	C	F	Cb
2 Tbsp, 1 fl.oz	15	0.3	1.5
1 Cup, 8 fl.oz	100	2.5	12
1 Large Glass, 12 fl.oz	150	4	18
1 Pint, 16 fl.oz	205	5	25
1 Quart, 946 ml	410	10	49

Fat Free/Skim:

	C	F	Cb
2 Tbsp, 1 fl.oz	10	0	1.5
1 Cup, 8 fl.oz	90	0.5	13
1 Pint, 16 fl.oz	180	1	26

Protein Fortified,

	C	F	Cb
1 cup	100	0.5	14

Buttermilk: *Average All Brands*

	C	F	Cb
Reduced-Fat (2%), 1 cup, 8 fl.oz	120	5	10
Low-Fat (1%), 1 cup, 8 fl.oz	100	2.5	12

Lactose-Free: *Per 8 fl.oz*

	C	F	Cb
Dairy Ease: Whole	160	9	11
2% Reduced-Fat	130	5	12
Fat-Free	90	0	12
Lactaid 100: Whole	150	8	12
2% Reduced-Fat	130	5	12
1% Low-Fat	110	2.5	13
Fat-Free; Calcium Fort.	80	0	13
Real Goodness, 2% Fat	120	5	7
Smart Balance,			
FF + Omega-3s & Vit. E	110	1	14

Lower Calorie Dairy Drinks: *Per 8 fl.oz Cup*

Calorie Countdown (*Hood*):

	C	F	Cb
2% Reduced-Fat	90	5	3
2% Reduced-Fat, Chocolate	90	5	5
Fat-Free	45	0	3

Goat/Sheep Milk, Kefir   **C** **F** **Cb**

Goat's Milk *(Meyenberg):*

	C	F	Cb
Whole, 1 cup, 8 fl.oz	140	7	11
Light/Low-Fat (1%), 8 fl.oz	100	2.5	11
Evaporated, reconst., 8 fl.oz	150	8	11

Kefir: *Per 8 fl.oz*

Lifeway: Original

	C	F	Cb
Original	150	8	12
Greek Style	210	14	12
Green	170	2	25
Lowfat, average all flavors	140	1.5	20
Nancy's: Plain	110	3	14
Fruit flavors, average	180	2.5	34
Trader Joe's: Plain, 1%	110	2.5	8
Strawberry	160	2	21
Sheep's Milk, Whole, 1 cup	265	17	13

Canned & Dried Milk

Condensed: Sweetened, 2 T., 1 fl.oz

	C	F	Cb
Sweetened, 2 T., 1 fl.oz	130	3	23
Low Fat, 2 Tbsp	120	1.5	23
Fat-Free, 2 Tbsp	110	0	24

Evaporated: Whole, 2 Tbsp

	C	F	Cb
Whole, 2 Tbsp	40	3	3
Whole, ½ cup, 4 fl.oz	170	10	13
Carnation: Low Fat, 2 Tbsp, 1 oz	25	0.5	3
½ cup, 4 fl.oz	115	2.5	14
Fat-Free, 2 Tbsp, 1 oz	25	0	4

Dried: Whole, ¼ cup, 1 oz

	C	F	Cb
Whole, ¼ cup, 1 oz	160	9	12
Skim/Non-Fat, ⅓ cup	80	0	12
Made-up, 1 cup, 8 fl.oz	80	0	12
Buttermilk (sweet cream): 1 oz	110	2	14
Non-Fat, 1 Tbsp	25	0	3
Carnation, Malted, dry, 1 Tbsp	30	0.5	6
Horlick's, Malt Powder, dry, 1 oz	180	4	27

Soy/Non-Dairy Drinks ~ See Page 49

'Whatever happened to sensible portion size?!'

Quick Guide   **C** **F** **Cb**

Chocolate Milk:
Average All Brands:

	C	F	Cb
Whole Milk, (3.3%):			
8 fl.oz cup	250	9	35
1 Pint, 16 fl.oz	415	17	52
Reduced-Fat, (2%):			
8 fl.oz cup	190	5	30
1 Pint, 16 fl.oz	380	10	60
Low-Fat, (1%):			
8 fl.oz cup	160	3	26
1 Pint, 16 fl.oz	315	5	52

Flavored Milk ~ Brands

Ready-To-Drink: *Per 8 fl.oz Cup Unless Indicated*

	C	F	Cb
Albertson's, Choc Milk	180	2.5	29
Hood: Chocolate	230	9	31
Low-Fat (1%), Chocolate	170	3	28
Horizon Organic:			
Low-Fat: Chocolate with Omega 3	160	2.5	26
Vanilla with Omega 3	150	2.5	23
Kellogg's:			
To Go, Breakfast Shakes: *Per 10 fl.oz*			
Milk Chocolate	190	5	29
Strawberry; Vanilla	180	5	29
Mixes, average all flavors,			
1 packet	130	0	26
Kroger, Simple Truth,			
Choc Milk, Low-Fat, 1%	150	2.5	22
Grip 'n Go:			
Swiss Chocolate (2% red-fat)	190	5	26
Strawberry (whole milk)	190	8	22
Muscle Milk ~ *See Energy Protein Drinks*			
Nesquik: *Per 8 fl.oz*			
Chocolate: Low Fat	150	2.5	25
No Sugar Added	100	2	13
Strawberry, Low Fat	180	2.5	31
Prairie Farms: *Per 8 fl.oz*			
Chocolate, 2% Reduced Fat	180	5	26
Strawberry, 1% Low Fat	160	2.5	28

Flavored Milk ~ Brands (Cont)

C **F** **Cb**

Ready-To-Drink: *Per 8 fl.oz Cup Unless Indicated*

	C	F	Cb
Ralphs, Chocolate, Low-Fat, 8 fl.oz	210	2.5	36
Skinny Cow, Chocolate, Fat-Free	150	0	26
TruMoo, Choc.; Strawb. av., 8 fl.oz	145	2.5	22
Yoo-Hoo, Chocolate,15.5 fl.oz bottle	230	2	51

Bottled Coffee Drinks ~ *See Page 37*

Shakes

	C	F	Cb
Arby's:			
Chocolate; Jamocha, 16 oz	440	12	76
Vanilla, 16 oz	380	12	60
Burger King:			
Chocolate:			
Small, 12 fl.oz	580	17	97
Medium, 16 fl.oz	760	21	131
Large, 20 fl.oz	980	24	174
Other flavors ~ *See Fast Food Section*			
Denny's: *Per 14 oz*			
Chocolate	680	31	90
Strawberry	580	25	78
Vanilla	640	31	80
Hardees, all varieties, av., 16 oz	710	33	86
McDonalds, McCafe Shakes:			
Chocolate & Strawberry:			
12 fl.oz cup	555	16	91
16 fl.oz cup	695	20	114
22 fl.oz cup	850	24	141
Other Restaurants ~ *See Fast-Foods Section*			

Smoothies

Made Up Ready-To-Drink:
8 fl. oz Milk/Soy + Fruit: *Per 12 fl.oz*
Average all flavors:

	C	F	Cb
With Whole Milk	300	8	50
+ Ice Cream, 1 scoop	400	13	62
With Non-Fat Milk	240	0	50
Kroger/Ralph's Smoothies: *Per 8 fl.oz*			
Mixed Berry	210	2.5	40
Strawberry Banana	200	2.5	37
LALA: *Per 7 fl.oz Bottle*			
Frusion C-Charged Smoothie,			
average all flavors	180	2.5	35
Freshens; Jamba Juice; TCBY ~ *See Fast-Foods*			

Nut, Rice & Cereal Drinks

Per 8 fl.oz Cup Unless Indicated

	C	F	Cb
Almond Breeze *(Blue Diamond)*:			
Refrigerated/Shelf Stable, average:			
Original	60	2.5	8
Chocolate	120	3	22
Vanilla	80	2.5	14
Unsweetened, Orig; Van.	30	2.5	1
Almond Dream:			
Shelf Stable, Enriched:			
Original	70	3	12
Unsweetened	50	3.5	3
Alpina:			
Oat Based Smoothies: *Per 8.4 oz*			
Original; Cinnamon	180	4	29
Light, Original	110	1.5	19
Amazake, Oh So Original,			
Rice Shake	150	0	34
Better Than Milk:			
Rice Vegan Powder Mix,			
Original; Vanilla, 2 Tbsp, 0.7 oz	70	0	17
Cacique,			
Horchata Rice Drink	160	3.5	31
Don Jose:			
Cereal Match	100	3	17
Horchata Rice Drink	140	4	25
Pacific:			
Rice Drinks, Plain; Vanilla	130	2	27
Organic Oat, Original/Vanilla, av.	130	2.5	25
Nut Drinks:			
Hazelnut, Original	110	3.5	19
Chocolate	120	5	19
Organic Almond:			
Original; Vanilla, av.	65	2.5	10
Chocolate, single serve container	100	3	19
Rice Dream:			
Refrigerated, Enriched, Original	120	2.5	23
Shelf Stable:			
Classic Carob	150	2.5	30
Classic/Enriched Van., av.	130	2.5	27
Horchata	160	2.5	32
Silk:			
True Almond: Original	60	2.5	8
Dark Chocolate	120	3	23
Unswt'nd, Orig.; Vanilla	30	2.5	1
Trader Joe's:			
Rice Drinks:			
Unsweetened: Original, Organic	120	2.5	23
Vanilla	130	2.5	26
WestSoy, Rice, Plain; Vanilla	110	2.5	20

Note: Rice/Oat/Nut drinks are very low in protein.
Unless enriched with protein (and calcium), they
are not suitable for infants as a substitute for milk
or calcium-enriched soy drinks.

Soy Milk ~ Ready-To-Drink

Per 8 fl.oz Cup Unless Indicated

	C	F	Cb
365 Organic *(Whole Foods)*:			
Original, unsweetened	70	4	4
Chocolate	140	3.5	22
Vanilla	90	3.5	10
Light: Original	70	1.5	9
Vanilla	70	1.5	10
8th Continent:			
Original	80	2.5	7
Complete Vanilla	80	2.5	8
Vanilla	100	2.5	11
Fat-Free: Original	60	0	8
Vanilla	70	0	11
Light: Original	50	2	2
Chocolate	90	1.5	12
Vanilla	60	2	5
Better Than Milk, Original	90	1.5	17
Bolthouse Farms:			
Perfectly Protein Cafe Drinks:			
Green Tea Soy Latte	150	3	25
Vanilla Chai Tea	180	4	27
Edensoy: *Per 32 fl.oz Container*			
Organic: Original	140	5	14
Unswseetened	120	6	5
Carob; Chocolate, av.	175	4	28
Vanilla	160	3	25
Extra: Original	130	4	13
Vanilla	150	3	24
Kidz Dream:			
Smoothies: Berry Blast	100	2	17
Orange Cream	120	2	21
O Organics *(Safeway)*:			
Plain	90	3.5	8
Chocolate	150	4	23
Vanilla	90	3	9
Odwalla: *Per 12 fl.oz Bottle*			
Protein Monster:			
Strawberry	240	5	28
Vanilla	290	5	36
Pacific:			
Super Protein:			
Original	290	1	52
Mango	260	1	42
Pumpkin	240	5	33
Vanilla Al'Mondo	290	8	37
Organic, Original, Unsweetened	90	4.5	4
Select Soy: Original	70	2.5	9
Vanilla	80	2.5	11
Ultra: Original	140	5	12
Vanilla	140	5	14

Soy Milk ~ Ready-To-Drink (Cont)

Per 8 fl.oz Unless Indicated

	C	F	Cb
Silk:			
Original	110	4.5	9
Chocolate	120	3	19
Vanilla	100	3.5	10
Very Vanilla	130	3.5	18
Light: Original	60	1.5	5
Chocolate	90	1.5	16
Vanilla	70	1.5	7
Organic: Original	100	4	8
Unsweetened	80	4	4
Slim-Fast ~ See Page 40			
Soy Dream:			
Enriched: Original	100	3.5	9
Vanilla	120	3.5	14
Shelf Stable:			
Classic Vanilla	140	4	18
Enriched: Original	100	4	8
Chocolate	150	4	21
Vanilla	120	4	14
Soy Slender,			
average all varieties	70	3	4
Trader Joe's:			
Soy Milk: Original	110	2	13
Chocolate	130	2.5	23
Vanilla	100	2	16
Organic: Original	130	3	17
Chocolate	120	3	17
Vanilla	130	3	19
WestSoy:			
Organic Plus, (25% Less Sugar):			
Plain	110	4.5	11
Vanilla	110	4.5	11
Low-Fat: Plain	90	2	15
Vanilla	120	2	23
Non-Fat: Plain	70	0	10
Vanilla	80	0	12
Unsweetened: Plain	90	4.5	5
Chocolate; Vanilla, average	100	4.5	6

Soy Powder Mix

	C	F	Cb

1 oz (¼ cup) mix makes 8 fl.oz Cup

	C	F	Cb
Soy Protein Isolate, dry, 1 oz	95	1	2
Better Than Milk:			
Original, 2 Tbsp	90	1.5	18
Vanilla, 2 Tbsp	90	1.5	18
Genisoy: *Per Scoop*			
Protein Shake Powder:			
Natural, 1 oz	100	0	0
Chocolate, 1.2 oz	120	0	17
Vanilla, 1.2 oz	130	0	18
Now:			
Soy Protein Isolate:			
Plain, ⅓ cup, 0.8 oz	90	0.5	0.5
Natural:			
Chocolate, 1 level scoop, 1.6 oz	160	1.5	9
Vanilla, 1 level scoop, 1.6 oz	180	2.5	13
Revival: *Per Packet*			
Unsweetened Shakes: Plain	105	1	4
Cappuccino; Strawberry Smile	115	2	4
Chocolate	120	2.5	7
Vanilla Pleasure	120	2	6
Average other flavors	115	2	4
Whole Foods:			
Chocolate, with Spirulina, 1 oz	100	1	10
Vanilla, with Spirulina, 1 oz	100	0	11

Coconut Milk Drink

	C	F	Cb
So Delicious: *Per 8 fl.oz cup*			
Original	70	4.5	8
Vanilla	80	4.5	10
Unsweetened,Orig., Vanilla	45	4.5	2
Trader Joes: *Per 8 fl.oz cup*			
Unsweetened	60	5	1
Vanilla	90	5	9
(Enriched with calcium + vitamins D & B12)			

Confucious say:

"*Man who eat with one chopstick never have problem with obesity*"

Quick Guide

C **F** **Cb**

Cola:

Drinks: *Average all Brands*

		C	F	Cb
8 fl.oz Cup/Can		100	0	26
12 fl.oz Can		150	0	39
16 fl.oz Bottle		200	0	52
20 fl.oz Bottle		250	0	65
24 fl.oz (Pepsi)		300	0	84
1-Liter Bottle (34 fl.oz)		400	0	100
2-Liter Bottle (68 fl.oz)		800	0	200

Other Soda Drinks: *Per 12 fl.oz, average all brands*

	C	F	Cb
Club Soda	0	0	0
Cream Soda	190	0	48
Ginger Ale	125	0	31
Lemonade, Regular/Pink	180	0	45
Orange	180	0	45
Root Beer	150	0	39
Tonic Water	125	0	32
Mineral Water: Plain	0	0	0
Sweetened/flavored	150	0	37
With Fruit Juice	120	0	30
Soda Water/Seltzer: Plain/Diet	0	0	0
Sweetened/flavored	155	0	39
With Fruit Juice	160	0	40

Fountain, Movie Theater & Take-Out

Average All Flavors

	C	F	Cb
Small Cup, 12 fl.oz: No Ice	160	0	40
With ⅓ Ice	120	0	30
Regular, 16 fl.oz: No Ice	215	0	53
With ⅓ Ice	160	0	40
Medium, 22 fl.oz: No Ice	295	0	73
With ⅓ Ice	220	0	55
Large, 32 fl.oz: No Ice	430	0	105
With ⅓ Ice	320	0	80

Note: ⅓ Cup of Ice = ¼ Cup Liquid

Soft Drink ~ Brands

Per 12 fl.oz Unless Indicated

	C	F	Cb
365 Organic *(Whole Foods),*			
Spritzers, all flavors	110	0	28
A&W: Root Beer	175	0	47
Ten	10	0	3
Albertson's:			
Super Chill: Cola	160	0	43
Root Beer	180	0	48
Barq's, Root Beer	160	0	42
Big Red, Soda, 20 fl.oz	250	0	63
Blue Sky, Natural Soda, Cola	160	0	42

Soft Drink Brands (Cont)

Per 12 fl.oz Unless Indicated

	C	F	Cb
Bubble Up, Lemon-Lime Soda,			
8 fl.oz	110	0	28
Cactus Cooler	150	0	40
Canada Dry: *Per 8 fl.oz*			
Club Soda; Diet Ginger Ale	0	0	0
Ginger Ale; Tonic Water, average	90	0	25
Cheerwine	150	0	42
Coca-Cola:			
Classic; Caffeine Free	140	0	39
Diet Coke, all varieties	0	0	0
Cherry Coke; Vanilla Coke	150	0	42
Country Time *(Dr Pepper/Snapple),*			
Lemonade, all varieties, 20 fl.oz	230	0	58
Crush: *Per 20 fl.oz Bottle*			
Grape; Orange	270	0	72
Peach; Pineapple, average	315	0	85
Strawberry	290	0	77
Dad's: Orange Cream Soda	180	0	46
Root Beer	165	0	41
Diet Rite, Pure Zero	0	0	0
Dr Pepper: *Per 12 fl.oz Can*			
Regular	150	0	40
Cherry	160	0	43
Ten	10	0	3
Fanta: Orange	160	0	44
Other flavors	180	0	48
Fresca, all flavors	0	0	0
GuS, average all flavors	95	0	23
Hansen's:			
Natural Cane Sugar:			
Creamy Root Beer	160	0	43
Original Cola	160	0	41
Pomegranate	130	0	35
Hawaiian Punch: *Per 12 fl.oz Can*			
Aloha Morning, 40% less sugar,			
all flavors	90	0	20
Maizin Melon Mix; Wild Purple Splash	165	0	44
Average other flavors	100	0	27
Henry Weinhard's: Root Beer	170	0	43
Orange/Vanilla Cream, average	180	0	44
Hires, Root Beer	170	0	44
IBC: Root Beer	160	0	43
Cream Soda; Black Cherry	180	0	48
Icee: Coca-Cola; Orange Fanta	100	0	27
Lemon Lime Fanta	90	0	24
Minute Maid, Raspberry Lemonade	100	0	27
Jarritos, all flavors, 8 fl.oz	110	0	28
Jelly Belly, all flavors	180	0	42
Jolt, Cola	150	0	41

Soft Drink Brands (Cont)

Per 12 fl.oz Unless Indicated

	C	F	Cb
Jones Soda: Cola	170	0	43
Whoopass, 16 fl.oz	200	0	52
Average other flavors	185	0	46
Kool Aid, Bursts, av., 6.75 fl.oz	35	0	9
Mello Yello, Regular	170	0	46
Mountain Dew:			
All flavors	170	0	46
Diet varieties	0	0	0
Mug, Root Beer	160	0	43
Natural Brew:			
Draft Root Beer	170	0	43
Outrageous Ginger Ale	180	0	44
Vanilla Cream Soda	160	0	39
Nehi, Royal Crown Peach	190	0	51
Pepsi:			
Regular; Caffeine Free	150	0	41
Diet Pepsi; Jazz; Pepsi One	0	0	0
Pepsi Next	60	0	16
Perrier, Carbonated Water	0	0	0
Pibb, Xtra	140	0	39
RC Cola: Regular	160	0	43
Ten	10	0	3
Reed's, Ginger Brew, all varieties	145	0	38
7•UP: Lemon Lime; Cherry	140	0	39
Diet flavors	0	0	0
Ten, Lemon Lime	10	0	3
Safeway: *Per 8 fl.oz*			
Refreshe: Cola	110	0	29
Grape	140	0	36
Lemon Lime	110	0	27
Mtn Breeze; Strawberry	120	0	30
Santa Cruz: Or. Mango, 10.5 fl.oz	120	0	29
Raspberry Lemonade, 10.5 fl.oz	100	0	26
Average other varieties, 10.5 fl.oz	135	0	33
Schweppes: Ginger Ale	120	0	33
Tonic Water	130	0	33
Shasta: Cream Soda	190	0	47
Cherry Cola	180	0	45
Club Soda; Diet, all flavors	0	0	0
Dr. Shasta	150	0	38
Ginger Ale	130	0	33
Tiki Punch; Pineapple; Orange	200	0	50
Average other flavors	170	0	41
Sierra Mist, Lemon Lime	140	0	37
Slurpee ~ *See Page 236*			
Sprite: Regular, 8 fl.oz	100	0	26
Zero	0	0	0

Per 12 fl.oz Unless Indicated

	C	F	Cb
Squirt, Ruby Red	170	0	45
Stewarts: Root Beer	160	0	41
Grape; Orange 'n Cream	190	0	48
Sun Drop: Citrus Soda, 20 fl.oz	290	0	76
Diet Citrus Soda	10	0	1
Sunkist: Orange	170	0	44
Ten, Orange	10	0	2
TAB	0	0	0
Tampico:			
64 fl.oz Container:			
Blue Raspberry Punch	45	0	21
Pineapple Coconut	105	0	25
Average other flavors	90	0	21
Thomas Kemper:			
Black Cherry	170	0	44
Ginger Ale; Vanilla Cream	150	0	36
Root Beer	160	0	41
Trader Joe's:			
Sparkling:			
French Berry Lemonade:			
1 cup, 8 fl.oz	130	0	31
1 bottle, 33.8 fl.oz	520	0	124
Lime Ade: 1 cup, 8 fl.oz	110	0	28
1 bottle, 33.8 fl.oz	440	0	108
Pink Lemonade: 1 cup, 8 fl.oz	130	0	31
1 Bottle, 33.8 fl.oz	520	0	124
Vernors, Ginger Soda	140	0	39
Virgil's, Root Beer	160	0	42
Walgreens: *Per 20 fl.oz*			
Orchard Grape Soda	300	0	84
Cola; Zesty Lemon Lime, av.	225	0	65
Root Beer	225	0	75
Zevia, average all flavors	0	0	6
(Contains between 4-7g Erythritol)			

Powdered Soft Drink Mixes

Per 8 fl.oz Prepared, Unless Indicated

	C	F	Cb
Country Time:			
Lemonade; Pink Lemonade	60	0	16
Strawberry Lemonade	80	0	19
Crystal Light *(Kraft):*			
Fruit Drinks, all flavors, ½ tsp	5	0	0
Pure Fitness, average all flavors, 1 pkt	15	0	4
Flavor Aid, ⅛ package	0	0	0
Kool-Aid, sweetened, 0.6 oz	60	0	16
Tang, Regular, 2 Tbsp, 1 oz	90	0	24

Quick Guide

C F Cb

Teas

Regular: Bag, Loose or Instant

	C	F	Cb
Brewed, 1 cup, 8 fl.oz	2	0	0.5
(Add extra for sugar/milk)			
Herbal: All flavors, average, 1 cup	2	0	0.5
Bigelow, all flavors	0	0	0
Celestial Seasonings, all flavors	0	0	0
Bubble Milk Tea, w/ Pearls, 8 fl.oz	175	0	41
Chai Tea, 2 Tbsp	120	3.5	21
Starbucks ~ See Fast-Foods Section			

Iced Tea

Average All Brands

	C	F	Cb
Sweetened: 8 fl.oz cup	90	0	22
12 fl.oz glass/can	140	0	35
16 fl.oz bottle	180	0	45
20 fl.oz bottle	225	0	55
Unsweetened, 8 fl.oz	0	0	0

Iced Tea Mixes

Per 8 fl.oz Made-Up

4C Iced Tea:

	C	F	Cb
Average all flavors, 0.67 oz	70	0	18
Totally Light, all flavors	0	0	0
Crystal Light, sugar free	5	0	0
Lipton:			
Sweetened: Lemon	70	0	18
Mango; Peach	80	0	19
Unsweetened	0	0	0
Diet, all varieties	5	0	1

Bottled & Canned Teas

Arizona: *Per 8 fl.oz*

	C	F	Cb
Black: Cranberry	80	0	22
Sweet	90	0	23
With Ginseng	60	0	15
Green Tea, average all flavors	70	0	18
Fuze, Iced Lemon	70	0	19
Gold Peak, Lemon, 12 fl.oz	120	0	30
Honest Tea: *Per 16 fl.oz Bottle*			
Just Black/Green	0	0	0
Assam Black	35	0	9
Community/Jasmin			

Bottled & Canned Teas (Cont)

Lipton:
Iced Tea: *Per 8 fl.oz*

	C	F	Cb
Natural: With Lemon	50	0	13
With Pomegr. Blueberry	50	0	13
Natural Green Tea: With Citrus	70	0	19
With Passionfruit Mango	50	0	13
White Tea, with Raspberry	50	0	14
Diet, all flavors	0	0	0
Sparkling,			
Strawberry Kiwi, Diet	0	0	0
Sweet Iced Tea	80	0	23
Minute Maid, Pomeg. Tea, 8 fl.oz	40	0	9
Nestea:			
Iced Tea, with Lemon:			
8 fl.oz	50	0	12
20 fl.oz bottle	125	0	30
Diet, Green/Lemon	0	0	0
POM:			
Antioxidant Super Tea: *Per 16 fl.oz*			
Pomegranate:			
Lychee Green Tea	140	0	36
Peach Passion White Tea	160	0	38
Snapple: *Per 16 fl.oz*			
Green Tea	120	0	31
Diet Green Tea	0	0	0
Lemon/ Raspberry Tea	150	0	37
Diet Lemon/Raspberry Tea	10	0	0
SnapTea: Lemon	120	0	31
Peach Green Tea	160	0	42
Sweet Tea	170	0	46
SoBe, Energize, Green Tea, 20 fl.oz	200	0	52
Ssips, Lemon Iced, 6 fl.oz	70	0	18
Steaz, Green Tea,			
average all flavors, 16 fl.oz	80	0	20
Tazo, Org. Iced Black Tea, 13.8 fl oz	60	0	15
TeaZazz: Original; Peach, 20 fl.oz	50	0	12
Green Tea Lemon, 20 fl.oz	60	0	17
Trader Joe's: *Per 8 fl.oz*			
Organic Tea & Lemonade	100	0	25
Pomegranate Green Tea	60	0	15
Unsweetened *(Kettle/Green)*	0	0	0
Turkey Hill: Iced Tea, 16 fl.oz	180	0	42
Fruit flavors, av., 16 fl.oz	205	0	50
Green Tea, Mango	180	0	42
365 Organic *(Whole Foods):*			
Unsweetened: Black Tea	0	0	0
Green Tea	0	0	0

Note: Most breads have similar calories on a weight basis. However, volume may vary.

For example, 1 oz of bread may equal 1 slice regular bread or 2 slices of a lighter bread. It is best to weigh bread used and calculate using: 1 oz bread = 70 calories, 14g carb.

Quick Guide   C F Cb

Bread

White or Wheat: *Average Per Slice*

	C	F	Cb
Thin or Light, 0.75 oz	50	0.5	9
Sandwich slice, 1 oz	70	1	12
Thick or Large, 1.5 oz	105	1.5	18
Thick, 2 oz	140	2	28
Extra Thick, 3 oz	210	3	35
Whole Loaf: 16 oz	1120	15	185
24 oz Loaf	1680	24	280

Multi Grain/Whole Grain: *Per Slice*

	C	F	Cb
Sandwich Slice, 1 oz	75	1.5	12
Thick Slice, 2 oz	150	2.5	25

Toast: *Based on same counts as White/Wheat as above*

1 Slice (1 oz fresh):

	C	F	Cb
With 1 tsp butter/margarine	105	5	12
With 1 tsp "light" butter/marg.	90	3.5	12
With 2 tsp butter/margarine	140	9	12
With 2 tsp "light" butter/marg.	110	6	12

Breads

Per Slice Unless Indicated

	C	F	Cb
12-Grain, 1.5 oz	110	1.5	22
Bran style/Dark, 1 oz	70	1	14
Buttermilk, average, 1.5 oz	110	1	22
Challah, 0.75 oz	85	1.5	17
Chapati, 1 oz	110	3	18
Ciabatta, 2 oz	130	1	26
Cornbread, average, 3 oz	220	6	37
Cracked Wheat Sourdough, 1.5 oz	130	0.5	27
Croissants ~ *See Page 134*			
Crustless Bread, regular, slice, 0.75 oz	40	0.5	8.5
Crusts Only, regular slice, 0.25 oz	30	0	7
English Toasting, 2 oz	140	1.5	27
Flax & Grain, 1.5 oz	120	3	19
Foccacia: Plain, 2 oz serve	150	2.5	28
Cheese & Garlic; Pesto, 2 oz serve	160	6	21
Tomato & Olive, 2 oz serve	150	5	21

Per Slice Unless Indicated

	C	F	Cb
French Stick/Baguette, 1 oz	70	1	15
French Toast: Slices, 1.5 oz	140	2	26
Aunt Jemima, Sticks, av., 2 oz	110	2	18
Garlic Bread/Toast:			
Small slice + 1 tsp spread, 0.75 oz	80	5	7
Medium slice + 2 tsp spread, 1.5 oz	160	10	14
Thick slice + 3 tsp spread, 1.8 oz	220	14	20
Pepperidge Farm, 1 slice, 1.4 oz	160	10	15
Hawaiian Sweet Bread, 1.5 oz	110	2	19
Hemp Bread, 1.2 oz	95	2	12
Italian Bread, 2 oz	140	1	28
Lower Carb, (higher protein/fiber), average all brands, 1 oz	60	1.5	9
MultiGrain, 1.5 oz	100	2	21
Naan Flatbread, 2 oz	160	3.5	29
Nut/Health Nut, 1.35 oz	90	1.5	18
Oatmeal/Oatbran Bread, 1.5 oz	90	0.5	19
Pita, average all types:			
Small (4" diam), 1 oz	90	0	18
Large (6½" diam), 2 oz	140	1.5	27
Extra Large (9" diam), 4 oz	300	1.5	60
Popovers, (1), without butter	130	2	18
Pumpernickel:			
Cocktail/Party size	30	0.5	6
Large slice, 1.35 oz	80	0	15
Raisin Bread, 1 oz	80	1	15
Rye: 1 thin slice, av., 1 oz	80	1	14
1 thick slice, 2 oz	150	2	25
Cocktail size, 0.4 oz	25	0.5	4
Sandwich Pockets, 2 oz	140	1.5	27
Sourdough: Regular, 1.5 oz	120	1	25
French Style, 1 oz	75	0	14
Spelt, 1.6 oz	130	1	26
Sprouted 7-Grain, 1.5 oz	110	0.5	18
Squaw, 1.1 oz	85	0.5	13
Tacos/Tortillas ~ *See Page 172*			
Turkish/Middle Eastern, 1 oz	80	1.5	16
Wheat-Free Breads: Spelt, 1.6 oz	130	1	26
Rice, with Fruit Juice, 1.5 oz	110	2	21
Healthseed Rye, 1.6 oz	90	1	20
Millet, 1.5 oz	100	1	20

Bread ~ Brands

C F Cb

Per Slice Unless Indicated

Ener-G, Gluten-Free Breads:

	C	F	Cb
Brown Rice Loaf, Regular, 1.3 oz	100	3	16
High Fiber Loaf, 1.4oz	90	4.5	16
Tapioca, regular, sliced,1 oz	80	3	11

Ezekiel:

7 Sprouted Grains, 1.2 oz	80	0.5	15
Sesame, 1.2 oz	80	0.5	14
Whole Grain, 1.3 oz	80	0.5	15

French Meadow: *Per Slice*

Flax & Sunflower, 1.2 oz	90	1.5	15
Hemp, 1.2 oz	100	2.5	12
Spelt, 1.2 oz	85	0.5	15

Francisco International:

Extra Sourdough Loaf, 1 slice, 1.7 oz	130	1	24
French, 2 slices, 1.6 oz	120	1	22

Oroweat:

3 Seed Oatnut, 1.35 oz	110	2.5	18
100% Whole Wheat, 1.3 oz	90	1	18
Country Buttermilk, 1.3 oz	100	1	19
Honey Wheat Berry, 1.2 oz	80	1	17

Pepperidge Farm: *Per Slice Unless Indicated*

100% Whole Wheat, Very Thin, 3 slices	110	2	20
15 Grain	100	2	20
Farmhouse, Hearty White	110	1.5	22
Goldfish: White/100% Whole Wheat, average, 2 slices	100	1.5	23
Italian, with Sesame Seeds	90	1	15
Light Style, average all varieties	130	1	26

Frozen Breads:

Garlic Bread:

Five Cheese, 2.2 oz	200	10	20
Parmesan, 2.5"	180	8	21
Premium: Roasted Garlic Bread	150	7	18
Tuscan Inspired Sourdough	170	7	22
Roman Meal: Orig. Multigr., 2 slices	110	1.5	20
Honey Oat Bran, 1.5 oz	110	1.5	20
Sara Lee: Honey Wheat, 1 oz	75	1	15
100% Whole Wheat, 1 oz	70	1	14
45 Cals & Delightful Wheat	45	0.5	9

Schwan's, Frozen:

Cheese Stuffed Breadsticks, 1.7 oz	130	5	15
French Baguette, half, 1.7 oz	130	0.5	26
Trader Joe's: Gourmet White, 1.5 oz	120	3.5	15
Soft 10 Grain, 1.5 oz	90	1.5	16
Sprouted Rye, 1.2 oz	90	1	15

Biscuits, Bread Rolls & Buns

Biscuits: *Average, 2½ diameter*   **C F Cb**

Plain/Butter Milk:

	C	F	Cb
Prepared from Recipe	210	10	27
Refrig. Dough, Baked	95	4	13
Brown 'n Serve, av., 1 oz	70	1	13

Refrigerated Dough:

Pillsbury, Buttermilk Biscuit, (3), 2.25 oz	150	2	30

Buns:

Frankfurter/Hot Dog: 1.25 oz	110	1.5	21
1.5 oz	130	2	25
Hamburger: Regular, 1.5 oz	110	1.5	22
Large, 3 oz	210	3	40
Hoagie/Submarine, Plain, 2.3 oz	200	1	38

Rolls:

Ciabatta Roll, 3.5 oz	230	4	41
Crescent Roll, Original, 1 oz	100	6	11
Dinner: 1 small, 1 oz	90	1.5	17
1 medium (3" diam),1.5 oz	110	1	23
French: 1 med, 1.3 oz	110	1.5	22
1 large, 3 oz	230	2.5	42
Kaiser: Small, 2 oz	200	2.5	35
Large, 3.5 oz	350	4	61
Plain, 6", average all, 2.5 oz	200	1	38
Sourdough, 1.3 oz	110	1	21
Wheat Rolls: Small, 1.2 oz	100	1	17
Medium, 1.8 oz	130	1.5	23
Large, 3.5 oz	260	3	46

Breadsticks, Croutons

Breadsticks:

	C	F	Cb
Salt Sticks, plain, 1 oz	110	1	20
Fresh baked (1), 2 oz	180	2.5	34
Stella D'oro: Original (1)	45	1	7
Sesame (1)	50	2	7
Croutons: Seasoned, 2 Tbsp, 0.3 oz	35	1.5	4
Pepp. Farm, Zesty Italian, 6 croutons	30	1	5

Bread Products

Bread Crumbs, dry:

	C	F	Cb
Plain or seasoned: 1 oz	110	1	20
1 cup, 3.5 oz	385	5	70
Corn Flake Crumbs, 1 oz	120	0	29
Graham Cracker Crumbs (Keebler),1 oz	110	2.5	20

Bread Dough, average:

Frozen, 1 slice, 2 oz	140	2	26
Refrigerated: French, 1" sl.	60	1	13
Wheat; White, 1" slice	80	2	14
Coating Mixes, av., 1 oz	100	0.5	20
Stuffing: Dry mix, average all,1 oz	110	1	20
Prepared, ½ cup, 4 oz	180	9	11

Quick Guide | C | F | Cb

Bagels
Average All Brands

Plain/Onion:

	C	F	Cb
1 mini/bagelette, 1 oz	65	0.5	13
1 small bagel, 2 oz	145	1	29
1 medium bagel, 3 oz	220	1.5	43
1 large bagel, 4 oz	290	2	57
Bagel Chips, 1 oz	130	4.5	19
Pizza Bagel Bites (Bagel Bites), average all varieties.. 4 pieces, 3 oz	190	5.5	27
Bagel Crisps (New York Style), average all varieties, 6 crisps, 1 oz	130	5	17
Bagel Thins (Thomas'), 1, 1.5 oz	110	1	25

Bagel ~ Brands

Per Bagel

	C	F	Cb
Bubba's: Plain; Onion, average	240	2	48
Blueberry	150	0.5	32
Cinnamon Raisin	250	1.5	51
Costco Bakery: Plain	330	1.5	70
Cinnamon Raisin	340	1.5	73
Whole Grain	300	5	56
Lender's, Fresh, NY Style:			
Plain, 3.3 oz	240	2	46
Blueberry, 2 oz	150	0.5	32
Whole Grain, 3.3 oz	250	1.5	49
Whole Wheat, 3.3 oz	210	1.5	41
Panera Bread: Plain	290	1.5	59
Cinnamon & Raisin Swirl, 3.8 oz	320	2	65
Everything, 4 oz	300	2.5	59
Whole Grain, 4.3 oz	340	2.5	67
Sara Lee: Mini, average, 1.3 oz	100	0.5	20
Plain, 3.4 oz	260	1	50
Blueberry, 3.7 oz	280	1	54
Cinnamon Raisin, 3.7 oz	270	1	54
Everything, 3.7 oz	280	3.5	50
Onion, 3 oz	270	1	52
Western, The Alternatives, av., 2 oz	120	0.5	29

Bagel Spreads

Cream Cheese:

	C	F	Cb
Plain: 2 Tbsp, 1 oz	100	9	1
2 oz mini-tub	200	18	2
Reduced Fat: 2 Tbsp, 1 oz	60	5	2
2 oz mini-tub	120	10	4
Flavors: Lox, 1 oz	90	8	2
Honey Nut, 1 oz	80	7	4
Strawberry, 1 oz	90	7	5
Sundried Tomato, 1 oz	80	7	2
Vegetable, 1 oz	90	8	2

English Muffins | C | F | Cb

Average All Brands

Plain/Whole Wheat:

	C	F	Cb
Regular, 2 oz	135	1.5	26
Heavier, 2.5 oz	155	2	31
Super, 3.2 oz	190	2	38
Raisin-Cinnamon, 2.2 oz	150	1	30

Note: Actual weight of packaged muffins can be 10-15% heavier than stated weight.

Rice Cakes

	C	F	Cb
Regular size (1), average, 0.3 oz	35	0.5	7.5
Hain, Mini, Mild Cheddar (10)	70	2.5	11
Lundberg, all varieties, 0.4 oz	70	0.5	14
Quaker, Apple Cinn., 0.5 oz	50	0	11

Tortillas & Shells

Tortillas: *Per Tortilla*

	C	F	Cb
Corn Flour:			
White/Yellow: 6", 1 oz	55	1	11
7", 1.2 oz	75	1	14
Wheat Flour:			
6", 1.2 oz	100	3	16
8", 1.4 oz	130	4	20
10", 2.3 oz	200	6	31

Shells: *Per Shell, Without Fillings*

	C	F	Cb
Corn Taco Shells:			
Mini, 3", 0.2 oz	25	1	3
Medium, 5", 0.5 oz	60	2.5	8
Large, 6½", 0.7 oz	100	4.5	13
Salad Shell, 10"	310	17	34
Tostada Shells, fried:			
White Corn, 5½" diam., 0.4 oz	55	2.5	8
Yellow Corn, 5½" diam., 0.5 oz	80	3.5	11
Sopes, 1 shell, 4" 2 oz	110	1.5	23
La Tortilla Factory: *Per Tortilla*			
Corn: *Hand Made Style*			
Regular, 1.4 oz	90	1	14
Grande, 2.5 oz	150	2	25
Wheat/Flour:			
Low Carb:			
Original size, 1.3 oz	50	2	10
Large size, 2.2 oz	80	3	18
100 Calorie, 2 oz	100	1.5	24
Burrito size, 2 oz	170	4.5	24
Mission Foods:			
Corn: *Yellow/White*			
Regular size, 0.8 oz	40	0.5	8
Super size, 1 Tortilla, 1.2 oz	70	1	14
Flour: Estilo Casero, 1 Tortilla, 1.8 oz	170	6	24
Homestyle, 1 Tortilla, 2.2 oz	190	4.5	32

Quick Guide

	C	**F**	**Cb**
Cooked Cereals			
Barley, pearled, cooked, 1 cup	195	0.5	44
Buckwheat Groats, roasted:			
Dry, ½ cup, 3 oz	285	2	61
Cooked, 1 cup, 6 oz	155	1	34
Bulgur: Dry, ½ cup, 2.5 oz	240	1	53
Cooked, 1 cup, 6.5 oz	150	0.5	34
Corn/Hominy Grits:			
Dry: Regular, ¼ cup, 1.4 oz	140	0.5	32
Instant: 0.8 oz packet	75	0	18
W/ Imitation Bacon Bits, 1 oz	100	0.5	22
Cooked, ¾ cup, 6.5 oz	110	0.5	24
Cream of Rice, cooked, ¾ cup, 6.5 oz	95	0	21
Cream of Wheat:			
Cooked: Regular, ¾ cup, 6.5 oz	95	0.5	20
Instant, ¾ cup, 6.5 oz	105	0.5	21
Quick, ¾ cup, 6.5 oz	100	0.5	22
Farina, cooked, ¾ cup, 6 oz	95	0.5	19
Millet, dry, ¼ cup, 1.8 oz	190	2	36
Oat Bran: Raw, ⅓ cup, 1 oz	70	2	19
Cooked, ½ cup, 3.8 oz	45	1	13
Oatmeal:			
Dry: Regular, ⅓ cup, 1 oz	100	1.5	18
Instant: Regular, average, 1 oz	105	1.5	18
Flavored, average, 1.5 oz	165	2	34
Cooked: Regular, ¾ cup, 6 oz	125	2.5	21
1 cup, 8 oz	165	3.5	28
Whole Wheat, cooked, ¾ cup, 6.5 oz	115	1	25

Brans, Wheat Germ, Add-Ons

	C	**F**	**Cb**
Bee Pollen Granules, 1 Tbsp, 0.3 oz	25	1	2
Bran:			
Oat Bran: Raw, 1 Tbsp, 0.2 oz	20	0.5	3
⅓ cup, 1 oz	100	2	17
Rice Bran: Raw, 1 tbsp, 0.2 oz	15	1	2.5
¼ cup, 1 oz	95	6	15
Fruit: Dried, average, 1 oz	70	0	18
Banana, ½ medium	55	0	14
Prunes in Syrup (5), 3 oz	90	0	23
Honey, 1 Tbsp, 0.75 oz	65	0	17
Lecithin Granules, 1 Tbsp, 0.4 oz	55	4	0.5
Nuts, Almonds (6), 0.3 oz	40	4	1.5
Psyllium Husks, 1 Tbsp, 0.2 oz	10	0	4
Wheat, unprocessed, 1 Tbsp	5	0	2
Wheat Germ: Raw, 1 Tbsp, 0.3 oz	25	0.5	4
¼ cup, 1 oz	105	3	15

Hot/Cooked Cereals ~ Brands

Per Serving, Dry Mix only

	C	**F**	**Cb**
Albers,			
Quick Grits, ¼ cup, 1.4 oz	140	0.5	31
B&G:			
Cream of Wheat Instant:			
Orig., 1 oz	100	0	20
Maple Brown Sugar, 1.3 oz	130	0	28
Bobs Red Mill,			
10 Grain, ¼ cup, 1.6 oz	140	1	28
Country Choice,			
Quick Oats, ½ cup, 1.5 oz	150	3	27
Dr. McDougall's:			
Big Cup Oatmeal, Organic:			
Apple Flax, 2.3 oz	250	3.5	48
Cranberry Almond & Grains, 3 oz	330	4	64
Hemp Peach, 3 oz	330	5	63
Maple, 2.5 oz	270	3.5	55
Great Value *(Walmart):*			
Instant Oatmeal:			
Maple & Brown Sugar, 1.5 oz	160	2	32
Peaches & Cream, 1.3 oz pkg	130	2.5	27
McCann's:			
Instant Irish Oatmeal:			
Regular, 1 oz package	100	2	19
Apple & Cinn., 1.3 oz	130	1.5	27
Maple & Brown Sugar, 1.5 oz	160	2	32
Malt-O-Meal: Orig., 3Tbsp, 1.2 oz	130	0.5	27
Maple Brown Sugar, ¼ cup	170	0	37
Natures Path:			
Oatmeal:			
Apple Cinnamon, 1.7 oz	210	2.5	40
Hemp Plus, 1 pkt, 1.4 oz	160	2.5	30
Maple Nut, 1.7 oz	210	4	38
NutriSystem,			
Oatmeal, Apple Cinnamon, 1 pkt	130	1.5	26
Quaker:			
Grits:			
Instant, average all flavors, 1 oz	100	0	22
Quick, Original, ¼ cup, 1.3 oz	130	0.5	29
Instant Oatmeal:			
Original, Organic 1 oz	100	2	19
Cinnamon & Spice, 1.5 oz	160	2	32
Maple Brown Sugar, 1.5 oz	160	2	32
Peaches & Cream, 1.3 oz	130	2	27
Old Fash'nd/Quick Oats, ½ c., 1.4 oz	150	3	27
Real Medleys: Blueb. Hazelnut, 2.5 oz	270	7	49
Summer Berry, 2.5. oz	250	3	51
Average other flavors, 2.6 oz	290	8	49
Wegmans:			
Food You Feel Good About:			
Instant Oatmeal: Original, 1oz pkg	100	2	19
Maple & Brown Sugar, 1.5 oz pkt	160	2	32

Quick Guide | C | F | Cb

Cold Cereals
Average All Brands

	C	F	Cb
Bran Flakes, ¾ cup, 1 oz	95	0.5	24
Corn Flakes, 1 cup, 1 oz	100	0	22
Frosted Flakes, ¾ cup, 1 oz	110	0	27
Granola, 100% Nat., ½ cup, 1.7 oz	205	6	35
Oat Bran Cereal, ½ cup, 1.5 oz	145	3	25
Puffed Rice, 1 cup, 0.5 oz	55	0	13
Puffed Wheat, 1 cup, 0.5 oz	45	1	10
Raisin Bran, ½ cup, 1 oz	90	0.5	22
Rice Crisps, 1 cup, 1 oz	105	0.5	24
Shredded Wheat, 1 biscuit, 1 oz	85	0.5	20
Wheat Flakes, ¾ cup, 1 oz	105	1	24

Breakfast/Cereal Bars ~ *See Page 31*

Ready-To-Eat Cereal ~ Brands

Arrowhead Mills:

	C	F	Cb
Flakes: Amaranth, 1.2 oz	140	2	26
Kamut, 1 oz	120	1	25
Oat Bran, 1.2 oz	140	2.5	24
Spelt, 1 oz	120	1	24
Sprouted Multigrain, 1.3 oz	120	1	26
Breadshop Granola:			
Crunchy Oat Bran,			
with Almonds & Raisins., 1.8 oz	210	8	33
Raspberry 'n Cream, ½ cup, 1.8 oz	220	8	34
Puffed: Corn, 0.5 oz	60	1	12
Kamut, 0.5 oz	50	0	11
Millet, 0.5 oz	60	0.5	11
Rice, 0.5 oz	60	0	14
Wheat, 0.5 oz	60	0	12
Shredded Wheat:			
Bite Size:			
Regular, 1.7 oz	190	1	38
Sweetened, 1.8 oz	200	1	42

Back to Nature: *Per ½ Cup, Unless Indicated*

	C	F	Cb
Granola: Apple Blueberry, 1.8 oz	200	2.5	39
Blueberry Walnut, 1.5 oz	190	6	30
Chocolate Delight, 1.8 oz	220	6	37
Classic, 1.8 oz	200	3	39
Cranb. Pecan, 1.6 oz	180	4.5	34
Honey Almond, 1.5 oz	190	7	29
Organic Cherry Vanilla, 1.8 oz	200	4	38
Sunflower & Pumpkin Seed, 1.8 oz	210	7	30

Barbara's Bakery:

	C	F	Cb
Classics, Organic & Sweetened:			
Brown Rice Crisps, 1 oz	120	1	25
Corn Flakes, 1 cup, 1 oz	110	1	25
Honest O's, Original, 1 oz	120	2	22
High Fiber:			
Original, 12 oz	180	1.5	42
Cranberry, 2 oz	190	1.5	42
Flax & Granola, 1 c., 2 oz	200	3	42
Puffins:			
Original, ¾ cup, 1 oz	90	1	23
Cinnamon, ⅔ cup, 1 oz	90	1	26
Multigrain, ¾ cup, 1 oz	110	0	25
PB/PB & Choc., av., ¾ cup, 1 oz	110	2	24
Puffs: Crunchy Cocoa, ¾ cup, 1 oz	120	1	24
Fruit Medley, ¾ cup , 1.1 oz	120	1	26
Morning Oat Crunch:			
Original, 1 cup, 2 oz	210	2	44
Cinn. Crunch, 1 cup, 2 oz	230	3	43
Vanilla Almond, 1 cup, 2 oz	220	3	42
Shredded Wheat, 2 biscuits, 1.4 oz	140	1	31
Spoonfuls, Multigrain, ¾ cup, 1 oz	120	1.5	24

Cascadian Farm:

	C	F	Cb
Cinnamon Crunch, 1 cup, 1 oz	110	2.5	22
Graham Crunch, ¾ cup, 1 oz	110	2	23
Granola: Ancient Grains, 1cup, 2 oz	210	5	38
French Vanilla Almond, ¾ c.,1.8 oz	210	5	38
Oats & Honey, ⅔ cup, 2 oz	230	6	42
Av. other varieties, ¾ cup, 1.8 oz	210	5	39
Honey Nut O's, 1 cup, 1 oz	110	1	25
Multi Grain Squares,			
1 cup, 1.9 oz	210	1	44
Raisin Bran, 1 cup, 1.8 oz	180	1	41

EnviroKidz: *Per 1 oz*

	C	F	Cb
Amazon Frosted Flakes, ⅔ cup	120	0	26
Gorilla Munch, ¾ cup	120	1	26
Koala Crisp, ¾ cup	110	1	25
Leapin' Lemurs, ¾ cup	120	1.5	25
Panda Puffs, ¾ cup	130	3.5	23

Erewhon:

	C	F	Cb
Corn Flakes, 1 cup, 1.2 oz	130	0	30
Crispy Brown Rice: Original, 1 oz	110	0.5	25
W/ Mixed Berries, 1 cup, 1 oz	120	0.5	27
Raisin Bran, 1 cup, 1.8 oz	180	1	40
Rice Twice, ¾ cup, 1 oz	120	0	26
Strawb. Crisps, ¾ cup, 1 oz	120	0.5	28

Ready-To-Eat Cereal (Cont)

	C	F	Cb
Ezekiel 4.9:			
Sprouted Whole Grain Cereals:			
Original, ½ cup, 2 oz	190	1	40
Almond, ½ cup, 2 oz	200	3	38
Cinnamon Raisin, 2 oz	190	1	41
Golden Flax, ½ cup, 2 oz	180	2.5	37
F-Factor, Skinnys'n Fruit, ½ c., 1.2 oz	70	1	27
General Mills:			
Cheerios: *Per ¾ Cup Unless Indicated*			
Original, 1 cup, 1 oz	100	2	20
Apple Cinn., ¾ cup, 1 oz	120	1.5	24
Banana Nut, ¾ cup, 1 oz	100	1	24
Cinnamon Burst, 1 c., 1.2 oz	120	2	27
Chocolate; Fruity, ¾ cup, 1 oz	100	1.5	22
Dulce de Leche; Frosted, ¾ cup, 1 oz	110	1.5	24
Honey Nut, ¾ cup, 1 oz	110	1.5	22
Yogurt Burst, Strawberry, ¾ c., 1 oz	120	1.5	24
Multigrain:			
Regular, 1 oz	110	1	24
Dark Choc. Crunch, ¾ cup, 1 oz	110	2	23
Peanut Butter, ¾ cup, 1 oz	110	1.5	23
Protein: Honey & Cinn. Alm.,1¼ c.	210	3	42
Oats & Honey, 1¼ cups, 2 oz	220	4.5	40
Chex: Corn, 1 cup, 1 oz	120	0.5	26
Apple Cinn; Choc., average, 1 oz	130	2.5	26
Honey Nut, ¾ cup, 1 oz	120	0.5	28
Rice, 1 cup, 1 oz	100	0	24
Vanilla, ¾ cup, 1 oz	120	2	25
Wheat, ¾ cup, 1.7 oz	160	1	39
Cinnamon Toast Crunch, ¾ cup, 1.1 oz	130	3	25
Count Chocula, ¾ cup, 1 oz	100	1.5	23
Fiber One: Original, ½ cup, 1 oz	60	1	25
80 Calorie Honey Squares, ¾ cup, 1 oz	80	1	25
Honey Clusters, 1 cup, 1.8 oz	170	1.5	44
Protein, av. all flavors, 1 cup, 2 oz	220	5	41
Kix: Original, 1¼ cups, 1 oz	110	1	25
Berry Berry; Honey, 1¼ cups, 1.2 oz	120	1.5	28
Lucky Charms, all varieties, average, ¾ cup, 1 oz	110	1.5	23
Total: Original, ¾ cup, 1 oz	100	0.5	22
Raisin Bran, 1 cup, 2 oz	160	1	40
Trix, 1 cup, 1 oz	120	1.5	27
Wheaties: Original, ¾ cup, 1 oz	100	1.5	22
Fuel, ¾ cup, 2 oz	190	3	46

	C	F	Cb
Great Value *(Walmart):*			
Apple Blasts, 1 cup, 1.2 oz	120	0	29
Crunch Honey Oats, with Almonds, ¾ cup, 1 oz	130	2	26
Frosted Shredded Wheat, 1.9 oz	180	1	42
Fruit Spins, 1 cup, 1 oz	110	1	25
Honey Crunch, ¾ cup, 1 oz	100	0	24
Raisin Bran, 1 cup, 2 oz	210	1	45
Health Valley:			
Crunch-Ems!: Corn, 1 cup, 1 oz	110	0	27
Rice, 1¼ cups, 1 oz	110	0	26
Organic Flakes:			
Amaranth, 1¼ cups, 2 oz	210	2	43
Fiber 7, Multigrain , 1 cup, 1.8 oz	160	1	37
Oat Bran, 1 cup, 1.8 oz	190	1.5	39
With Raisins, 1 cup, 1.9 oz	200	1.5	43
Heartland:			
Granola:			
Original, ½ cup, 2.3 oz	240	6	40
Harvest Spice, ½ cup, 1.8 oz	210	5	37
Low-Fat Raisin, ½ cup, 2 oz	200	3	40
Hershey's, Cookies'n'Creme, 1 oz	110	3	21
Kashi:			
7 Whole Grain: Flakes, 1 c., 1.8 oz	170	0.5	41
Honey Puffs, 1 cup, 1 oz	120	1	25
Nuggets, ½ cup, 2 oz	210	1.5	47
Puffs, 1 cup, 0.7 oz	70	0.5	15
GoLEAN: Original, 1 cup, 1.8 oz	160	1	35
Crunch!: Original, 1 cup, 1.9 oz	200	3	38
Honey Almond Flax, ⅔ cup, 2 oz	200	5	35
Good Friends, Orig., 1 cup, 2 oz	160	1.5	42
Heart to Heart:			
Honey Toasted Oat, ¾ cup, 1.2 oz	120	1.5	26
Oat Flakes & Blueb. Clusters, 1 c., 2 oz	200	2	44
Organic Promise:			
Berry Fruitful, 29 bisc., 1.8 oz	170	0.5	42
Indigo Morning, ¾ cup	100	1	22
Raisin Vineyard, ¾ c., 1.8 oz	170	0	40
Simply Maize, ¾ cup, 1 oz	100	1	23
Whole Wheat Biscuit:			
Av. all varieties, 30 biscuits, 2 oz	180	1	43
Kellogg's:			
All-Bran:			
Original, ½ cup, 1 oz	80	1	23
Bran Buds, ⅓ cup, 1 oz	80	1	24
Compl. Wheat Flakes, 1 oz	90	0.5	24
Apple Jacks, 1 cup, 1 oz	110	1	25
Cinnabon, 1 cup, 1 oz	120	2	25

continued next page...

Ready-To-Eat Cereal (Cont)

	C	F	Cb
Kellogg's (Cont):			
Cinnabon, 1 cup, 1 oz	120	2	25
Cocoa Crispies, ¾ cup, 1 oz	120	1	27
Corn Flakes, Original, 1 cup, 1 oz	100	0	24
Corn Pops, 1 cup, 1 oz	120	0	27
Cracklin' Oat Bran, ¾ cup, 1.8 oz	200	7	34
Crispix, Original, 1 cup, 1 oz	110	0	25
Crunchy Nut:			
Golden Honey Nut Flakes, ¾ cup, 1 oz	120	1	26
Roasted Nut & Honey, ¾ cup, 1 oz	100	1	23
Fiber Plus,			
Cinnamon Oat Crunch, ¾ cup, 1 oz	170	1.5	43
Froot Loops: Original, 1 cup, 1 oz	110	1	26
Marshmallow, 1 cup, 1 oz	110	1	26
Frosted Flakes:			
Original, ¾ cup, 1 oz	110	0	27
Reduced Sugar with Fiber, 1 cup, 1 oz	110	0	26
Honey Smacks, ¾ cup, 1 oz	100	0.5	24
Krave:			
Chocolate, ¾ cup, 1.1 oz	120	3.5	24
Double Choc., ¾ c., 1.1 oz	120	3.5	23
Mini-Wheats, Frosted:			
Big Bites (7), 2 oz	200	1	49
Bite Size, Orig. (21), 2 oz	190	1	46
Little Bites:			
Original, 1 cup, 2 oz	200	1	47
Chocolate, 1 cup, 2 oz	200	2	46
Touch of Fruit In Middle, Raspberry (24), 2 oz	190	1	45
Mini Wheats, Unfrosted,			
Bite Size (30), 2 oz	190	1	45
Mueslix, ⅔ cup, 2 oz	200	3	41
Nutri-Grain Bars ~ See Page 31			
Product 19, 1 cup, 1 oz	110	0	25
Raisin Bran:			
Regular, 1 cup, 2 oz	190	1	46
Crunch, 1 cup, 2 oz	190	1	45
Rice Krispies:			
Original, 1¼ cups, 1.2 oz	130	0	29
Frosted, ¾ cup, 1 oz	120	0	27
Treats, ¾ cup, 1 oz	120	1	26

	C	F	Cb
Kellogg's (Cont):			
Scooby-Doo, 1 cup, 1.1 oz	120	1.5	27
Smart Start,			
Antioxidants, 1 cup, 1.8 oz	190	1	44
Special K: Original, 1 cup, 1 oz	120	0.5	23
Fruit & Yogurt, ¾ cup, 1 oz	120	1	27
Low Fat Granola, Touch of Honey, ½ cup, 1.8 oz	190	3	39
Red Berries, 1 cup, 1 oz	110	0	27
Vanilla Almond, ¾ cup	110	1.5	25
Malt-O-Meal:			
Apple Zings, 1 cup, 1.2 oz	130	1	30
Cocoa Dyno-Bites, ¾ cup	120	1	26
Coco Roos, ¾ cup, 1 oz	120	1.5	26
Colossal/Berry Crunch, ¾ cup, 1 oz	120	1.5	26
Frosted Flakes, ¾ cup, 1 oz	120	0	28
Frosted Mini Spooners, 1 cup	190	1	45
Golden Puffs, ¾ cup, 1 oz	100	0	24
Honey Nut Scooters, 1 cup, 1 oz	110	1	24
Raisin Bran, 1 cup, 2 oz	220	1.5	45
Nature's Path:			
Flax Plus:			
Maple Pecan Crunch, ¾ cup	220	7	38
Pumpkin Raisin Crunch, ¾ c.	210	4.5	40
Raisin Bran Flakes, ¾ c., 2 oz	190	2.5	41
Heritage Flakes, ¾ cup, 1 oz	120	1	23
Honey'd Cornflakes, ¾ cup, 1 oz	120	0	27
Kamut Puffs, 1 cup, 0.5 oz	50	0	11
Multigrain Oatbran Flakes, ¾ cup, 1 oz	110	1	24
Qi'a, all varieties, av., 2Tbsp, 1 oz	135	6.5	14
Optimum Power, Blueb. Cinn. Flax, 2 oz	200	3	38
New England Natural Bakers:			
Granola Pouches:			
All Natural:			
Banana Walnut, ½ cup, 2 oz	260	12	34
Honey Nut Cinn., ½ cup, 2 oz	270	12	35
Probiotic Raspb., ½ cup, 1.7 oz	200	3	37
Organic:,			
Crispy Fruity Cereal, Gluen Free, ⅔ cup, 2 oz	250	9	39
Muesli, ½ cup, 2 oz	220	5	40
New Morning:			
Fruit-e-O's, Organic, 1 cup, 1 oz	120	1.5	25
Oatios, Original, 1 cup, 1 oz	110	2	22

Ready-To-Eat Cereal ~ Brands (Cont)

	C	F	Cb
NutriSystem: Per Packet			
Granola, Low-Fat	160	2.5	31
NutriFlakes	110	1	23
Sweetened O's	110	1.5	21
Peace:			
Clusters & Flakes:			
Honey Almond, 2 oz	210	4	40
Average other varieties, 2 oz	235	5	43
Low Fat, Hearty Raisin Bran, 2 oz	190	2	44
Crispy Rice & Flakes,			
Blueberry Pomegranate, 2 oz	240	6	41
Granola, average all varieties, ⅔ cup	240	6	41
Post:			
Alpha Bits, 1 cup, 1 oz	120	1.5	24
Bran Flakes, ¾ cup, 1 oz	100	0.5	24
Good Mornings, average, 1 oz	120	1.5	25
Grape-Nuts: Original, 2 oz	210	1	45
Fit, ⅔ cup, 2 oz	220	3	44
Flakes, 1 cup, 1 oz	110	1	24
Great Grains:			
Banana Nut Crunch, 1 cup, 2 oz	230	5	42
Cranb. Alm. Crunch, ¾ cup, 1.7 oz	180	3	37
Honey, Oats & Seeds, 1 cup, 2 oz	220	5	37
Protein Blend, av. all varieties, 2oz	230	5	38
Honey Bunches of Oats:			
With Almonds, ¾ cup, 1 oz	130	2.5	26
With Van. Bunches, 2 oz	220	3	46
Honeycomb, 1½ cups, 1 oz	130	1	28
Mini Cinnamon Churros, 1 cup, 1.2 oz	130	3	26
Morning Energy,			
Chocolate Almond Crunch, 2 oz	220	4.5	43
Pebbles, average all varieties, ¾ cup, 1 oz	120	1	24
Raisin Bran, 1 cup, 2 oz	190	1	46
Selects, Blueberry Morning, 1¼ cups, 2 oz	220	3	45
Shredded Wheat, Spoon Size:			
Original, 1 cup, 1 oz	170	1	40
Honey Wheat, 2.1 oz	220	2	49
Waffle Crisp, 1 cup, 1 oz	120	2.5	25
Quaker:			
Honey Graham Oh's, 1 oz	110	2	23
King Vitaman, 1½ cups, 1 oz	120	1	26
Life, all types, ¾ cup, 1 oz	120	1.5	25
Natural Granola:			
Apple Cranberry Almond, 1.7 oz	200	6	35
Oats, Honey, & Alm., ½ cup, 1.7 oz	210	5	38
Oatmeal Squares, Honey Nut, 1 cup, 2 oz	210	2.5	44
Whole Hearts, ¾ cup, 1 oz	110	1.5	23

	C	F	Cb
Sweet Home Farm:			
Honey Nut Granola, 1.9 oz	250	10	37
Other varieties, 2 oz	250	8	40
Low-Fat Granola,			
½ cup, 1.9 oz	210	3	44
Stop & Shop:			
Oats & O's, ½ cup, 1.8 oz	110	1.5	22
Raisin Bran, 1 cup, 2 oz	190	1	46
Trader Joe's:			
Clusters: Raisin Bran, 1 cup, 2 oz	190	3	41
Super Nutty Toffee, ¾ cup, 2 oz	250	9	38
Average other varieties,			
⅔ cup, 1.3 oz	145	3.5	26
Corn Flakes, 1 cup, 1 oz	110	0	26
Golden Flax Cereal, 1.7 oz	200	3.5	37
Granola: Mango Passion, 2 oz	240	7	38
Pecan Praline, ½ cup, 1.6 oz	210	7	31
Trek Mix, ⅔ cup, 2 oz	240	8	37
High Fiber, ⅔ cup, 2 oz	80	0.5	23
Honey Nut O's, ¾ cup, 1 oz	120	1.5	24
Joe's O's, 1 cup, 1 oz	110	1.5	22
Shredded Wheats, Bite Size, 1 cup, 1.7 oz	180	1	38
Triple Berry O's, ¾ cup, 1 oz	110	1	25
Toasted Oatmeal Flakes, ¾ cup, 1 oz	110	1	23
Wheats, average all var., 1 cup, 2 oz	200	1	42
Uncle Sam:			
Original, ¾ cup, 2 oz	190	5	38
Raisin Bran, 1 cup, 2 oz	190	1	42
Weetabix,			
2 biscuits, 1.3 oz	130	1	29
Wegmans:			
Blueberry Muffin Squares, ¾ cup, 1 oz	130	3.5	24
Cinnamon Oat Crisps, ¾ cup, 1 oz	120	1	26
Chocolaty Rice Crisps, 1 oz	120	1	26
Corn Flakes, 1 cup, 1 oz	100	0	24
Frosted Flakes, 1 oz	120	0	28
Granola, Vanilla, ⅔ cup	240	6	41
Raisin Bran, 1 cup, 2 oz	190	1	46
Whole Foods (365):			
Corn Flakes, 1 cup, 1 oz	110	0	26
Frosted Flakes, ¾ cup, 1 oz	110	0	27
Hon. Flakes & Oat Clusters,			
¾ cup, 1 oz	120	1	25
Protein & Fiber Crunch, 1 cup, 1.8 oz	190	1	33
Raisin Bran, 1 cup, 2 oz	180	1	44
Wheat Squares:			
Bite Sized, 1.7 oz	180	1	38
Frosted, 1 cup, 1.9 oz	210	1	45

Ready-to-Eat

C **F** **Cb**

Per Piece/Slice

	C	F	Cb
Angel Food, Plain: Without oil, 2 oz	145	0	33
With oil, 2 oz	145	1	27
With Cream Frosting	255	7	45
Almond Croissant, 5 oz	620	35	67
Apple Danish, 5 oz	450	18	67
Apple Pie ~ See Pies/Tarts Page 134			
Baklava, 1½" square, 1.75 oz	200	10	27
Banana Cake, with Butter Cream, 2 oz	230	9	37
Banana Walnut Cake, 3 oz	270	11	40
Bear Claw, 4.5 oz	540	24	71
Black Forest, 3 oz	345	11	59
Brownie: Small, 2" Square, 1 oz	130	8	14
Large, 3 oz	390	24	42
Bundt Cakes, average all types:			
3 oz slice	300	13	42
Mini-Bundt, 5 oz	500	22	70
Cannoli's: Mini, 1 oz	85	3	11
Regular, 2.5 oz	215	8	28
Carrot Cake: Plain, 3 oz	300	16	37
With Cream Cheese Frosting	400	22	48
Cheesecake:			
Small serving, 3 oz	240	13	26
Large serving, 5 oz	400	21	44
With Low-Fat Cheese/Fruit, 3 oz	170	4	28
Denny's, NY Style, 5oz	510	34	43
Chocolate Cake:			
With Chocolate Frosting, 4 oz	415	18	62
Without Frosting, ½₂ of 9", 3.5 oz	340	14	51
Chocolate Croissant, 4.25 oz	470	26	54
Chocolate Eclair, w/ custard, 3.5 oz	260	16	24
Chocolate Fudge Cake, 3 oz	270	12	40
Chocolate Meringue, 2.5 oz	320	13	48
Churros, 1 stick, 1.5 oz	165	8	21
Cinnamon Crumb Cake, 2.5 oz	260	9	40
Cinnamon Rolls: Small, 2 oz	220	8	34
Regular, 4 oz	440	16	68
Large, 6 oz	660	24	102
Brands ~ See Page 67			
Coffee Cake, 2 oz	180	6	30
Concha: Small, 2 oz	240	9	33
Large (5" diameter), 5.5 oz	615	23	85
Cream Puff, custard filled, 4.6 oz	335	20	30
Cream Horn, 3 oz	210	5	36
Crumble Coffee Cake, 4.5 oz	500	25	65
Danish Pastries:			
Small, 2.5 oz	250	14	25
Large, 5 oz	500	28	50
Donuts ~ See Page 66			
Eclair, Chocolate, custard filled, 3.5 oz	260	16	24
Fig Bars, average	160	3	31

Ready-to-Eat (Cont)

C **F** **Cb**

Per Piece/Slice

	C	F	Cb
Fruit Cake, Dark/Light, 2 oz	185	5	34
Fudge Nut Brownie, 3.5 oz	380	18	54
Gingerbread, from mix, 3" square	210	4	41
Honey Bun, 2.7 oz	310	15	39
Jelly Roll, ½ roll, 1.8 oz	150	2	31
Key Lime Pie, 4.3 oz	400	25	41
Lady Finger, 1 oz	310	4.5	57
Lemon Cake, 4 oz	440	24	49
Lemon Poppy Seed Creme, 1.6 oz	180	9	23
Marble Cake, 4 oz	430	23	50
Mississippi Mud Pie, 4 oz	480	22	67
Mud Cake, 4.5 oz	380	20	44
Muffins ~ See Page 67			
Palmier Cookie, large, 4.5 oz	490	25	62
Pineapple Upside Down Cake,			
2.5 oz	230	9	36
Peach Melba, 3.5 oz	300	8	52
Pecan Sticky Roll, 6.5 oz	690	22	91
Pecan Twirls, 1.3 oz	170	7	26
Pies & Tarts ~ See Page 134			
Pound Cakes: Iced Lemon, 3.5 oz	360	17	50
Marble, 3.75 oz	350	13	53
Raspberry Rugulah,			
1.2 oz	110	9	7
Scone, fruit, 2 oz	200	9	30
Sponge Cake: Plain, 2.5 oz	220	10	33
With Chocolate Frosting	290	12	45
With Cream & Strawberry Jam	390	12	69
Starbucks Cakes ~ Page 244			
Strawberry Creme Cake, 4.7 oz	400	27	33
Strudel Bites, 0.75 oz	60	2.5	9
Strudel, fruit, av., 4.5 oz	300	17	32
Swiss Rolls, 1 oz	135	6	19
Tiramisu, 4.5 oz	440	22	34
Turnovers, fruit, average, 3 oz	290	15	35

Cupcakes

Average all Varieties

	C	F	Cb
Regular:			
Cake only, 1.5 oz	140	5.5	20
Cake + Icing, 2.5 oz	260	13	34
Large, (Muffin Size):			
Cake only, 3 oz	235	9	34
Cake + Icing, 5 oz	520	27	67
Mini, (2-Bite):			
Cake only, 0.4 oz	40	1.5	5.5
Cake + Icing, 1 oz	110	5.5	13
Icing Only: Per 1 oz	115	7	13
Thick/Tall amount, 2.5 oz	290	17	32

Cakes ~ Brands | C | F | Cb
	C	F	Cb

Albertson's Bakery:

Ring Cakes: *Per ⅛ Cake*

Angel Food, 2 oz	160	0	36
Butter; Chocolate, av., 3 oz	305	15	39

Cake Slices: *Per Slice Unless Indicated*

Banana Nut Loaf	330	17	39
Butter Creme	110	6	20
Creme Cake (2), 3.2 oz	300	12	43
Cinnamon Streusel (2), 3.2 oz	350	18	43

Bimbo Bakery:

Concha, Vanilla, 2 oz	260	11	35

Pound Cakes: *Per Slice*

Panquecitos, 1.8 oz	170	4.5	29
Pecan, 2.3 oz	260	11	36
Raisin, 2.3 oz	240	7	38

Bon Appetit Bakery:

Banana Bread, 4 oz	440	25	49
Cream Cheese Cake, 4 oz slice	430	24	49

Danish:

Apple (1), 5 oz	210	11	25
Bear Claw (1), 5 oz	240	13	27
Cheese & Berries (1), 5 oz	250	14	26
Vienna Cream (1), 5 oz	240	14	27

Slices:

Cheesecake, 4 oz	430	24	49
Lemon Cake, 4 oz	430	24	49
Marble Cake, 4 oz	430	24	50

Walnut Brownie, 3.5 oz	380	18	54

Cheesecake Factory ~ *See Fast-Foods Section*

Entenmann's: *Per Slice*

Crumb Cakes:

All Butter French, 1.8 oz	210	10	29
Chocolate, ⅛ cake	270	12	39

Danish:

Pecan Danish Twist, ⅙ cake	260	16	27
Cheese-Filled Crumb Coffee, 2 oz	200	10	25
Raspberry Danish Twist, 2 oz	220	11	29

Dessert Cakes:

Banana, 2.3 oz	270	14	36
Carrot, Iced, 2.4 oz	260	12	37
Chocolate Fudge, 2.3 oz	240	10	37
Red Velvet, Iced, ⅛ cake	270	14	36

Loaf Cakes:

Chocolate, ⅙ loaf	190	8	29
Cinnamon Crunch, ⅙ loaf	270	14	33

Glenny's:

100 Calorie:

Blondie, Choc. Chip, 1.5 oz	100	4	15
Brownies: Chocolate Chip, 1.5 oz	100	4	12
Peanut Butter, 1.5 oz	100	4	15

Muffins/Sweet Rolls ~ *See Page 67*

Great American Cookies:

Cookie Cakes: *Per Slice*

By the Slice, 4.5 oz	580	27	83
Heart Shaped, 3.5 oz	440	21	64
M&M, 4 oz	500	24	73

Great Value (Walmart):

Devil's Food Cake (1), 1.4 oz	160	7	23
Swiss Rolls (2), 2.2 oz	250	10	38

Hostess:

Twinkies, (1)	135	4.5	23

Cup Cakes:

100 Calorie, Lemon Golden (1)	100	2.5	21
Chocolate, 8-pack, 1 cupcake, 1.5 oz	160	6	26

Ding Dongs, (1), 2.8 oz	350	18	46

Donettes ~ *See Page 66*

Little Debbie:

100 Calories:

Choc. Cake (1), 1 oz	100	3	17
Yellow Cake with Icing (1), 1 oz	100	3	18

Brownie:

Choc Chip (1), 2.2 oz	270	11	41
Fudge (1), 2.2 oz	280	12	40

Chocolate Cup Cake (1)	210	8	33
Cocoa Creme (1), 1.5 oz	170	8	24
Coffee Cake (1)	190	5	35
Devil Creme (1), 1.7 oz	200	9	29
Devil Squares (2), 2.2 oz	260	11	38
Fancy Cake (2)	300	13	44
Frosted Fudge Cake, 1.5 oz	190	9	27
Star Crunch (1)	150	6	22
S'mores (1)	190	7	30
Strawberry Shortcake Roll, 2 oz	240	9	40
Swiss Cake Roll (2), 2.2 oz	270	12	38
Zebra Cake (2), 2.5 oz	320	14	48

Nemo's:

Brookie (1), 1.5 oz	160	7	26

Cake Squares:

Banana, 3 oz	300	12	45
Carrot, 3.6 oz	390	21	47
Chocolate, 3 oz	300	12	44

Crumble Cake:

Blueberry (1), 4 oz	390	17	54
Cinnamon Streusel (1), 4 oz	420	18	59
Lemon Rasp. (1), 4 oz	400	19	55

Oreo:

Brownie,

Creme Filled, 1.5 oz	190	9	25

Soft Cakesters:

Chocolate (2), 2 oz	250	12	36
Double Stuf (2), 2.6 oz package	350	18	48
Golden (2), 1.8 oz	220	10	32

Cakes ~ Brands (Cont)

	C	F	Cb
Pepperidge Farm:			
3-Layer Cakes: *Per ⅛ Cake*			
Devil's Food	220	9	34
Key Lime	230	11	31
Orange Cream	210	9	32
Average other varieties	240	11	33
Cookie Cakes: Choc. Chunk, ⅛ cake	250	12	33
Milano, ⅛ cake	250	15	28
Turnovers (Frozen):			
Apple; Cherry (1)	260	13	31
Peach; Raspberry (1)	270	13	34
Pop Tarts (Kellogg's):			
Fruit/Frosted/Unfrosted, av.	200	5	36
Gone Nutty; Oatmeal Delights,			
average all varieties, 1.8 oz	200	5	35
Mini Crisps, all flavors, 1 pouch, 0.5 oz	60	1.5	11
Safeway Select,			
Molten Chocolate Lava Cake, 4.5 oz	440	26	50
Sara Lee:			
Carrot Cake, ⅙ cake	340	18	41
Cheesecakes:			
Classic: French, 4.7 oz slice	410	26	38
Strawberry, 4.3 oz slice	320	18	37
New York Style, 5 oz slice	480	29	48
Limited Edition,			
NY Style, Chocolate, 5 oz slice	500	29	55
Original Cream:			
Cherry, 4.8 oz slice	320	11	50
Classic, 4.3 oz slice	340	18	38
Strawberry, 4.7 oz slice	330	12	51
Coffee Cake, Butter Streusel, ⅙ cake	190	9	24
Pound Cakes:			
All Butter,1.9 oz slice	260	9	42
Lemon, 2.7 oz slice	270	9	42
Individual Slices:			
All Butter, 1 oz	100	3	15
Double Choc, 1.8 oz	180	7	28
Lemon, 1 oz	100	3.5	15
Original, 1.6 oz	160	5	25
Smart Ones (Weight Watchers):			
Smart Delights: *4 Pack*			
Brownie à la Mode, 2.2 oz	120	2	36
Chocolate Fudge Brownie, 2 oz	140	3.5	24
Double Fudge Cake, 2 oz	140	3	26
Key Lime Pie, 3 oz	150	3	28
Raspberry Cheesecake	130	3.5	22
Strawberry Shortcake, 2.4 oz	120	4	19
Sundaes, average all varieties	140	3	24
Special K, Pastry Crisps (2),			
all varieties, 1 oz	100	2	20

Tastykake: *Per 3 Cakes*

	C	F	Cb
Chocolate Creme Cups (2), 1.9 oz	210	8	32
Kandy Kake, Peanut Butter, 1.7 oz	230	12	26
Krimpets, Butterscotch,			
Iced Vanilla, 2 oz	220	6	39
Toaster Strudel (Pillsbury): *Per 2 oz*			
Boston Cream Pie	180	7	25
Cream Cheese,			
average all varieties	185	9	24
Fruit flavors, all varieties	170	7	25
Trader Joe's:			
Bakery Fresh:			
Apricot Almond Tart,			
4 oz slice	450	24	56
Cheesecake Brownie Bites (1)	110	7	9
Chocolate Ganache Cake, 3 oz slice	390	22	44
Flourless Chocolate Cake,			
1 slice, 2 oz	260	17	23
Lemon Cake, 3.3oz slice	350	19	43
Mini Bundt, Triple Choc., ½ cake	340	21	41
Mini Carrot Cake, 5 oz	450	19	68
Whoopie Pie (1), 2.5 oz	350	14	54
Bread Cake:			
Banana Bonanza, 2.6 oz slice	250	9	39
Pumpkin Nut, 2.6 oz slice	270	10	43
Walnut Streusel Coffee, 2 oz slice	180	8	25
Zucchini Carrot, 2 oz slice	200	7	32
Loaf Cake:			
Cranberry Pumpkin, 2 oz slice	140	2	30
Pumpkin Nut, 2.6 oz slice	270	10	43
Frozen:			
Apple Raspberry Turnover, 3.2 oz	280	14	34
Chocolate Dilemma Cheesecake:			
Plain, 3.5 oz	320	19	30
Choc. Chip; Triple Choc, av., 3.5 oz	345	20	35
Tuxedo, 3.5 oz	320	17	34
Choc Lava Cake (1), 4 oz	360	23	40
Karat Cake, 3 oz slice	320	19	37
N.Y. Style Cheesecake, 4.5 oz slicce	400	28	32
Tiramisu Torte, 3.2 oz slice	230	12	24
Tarts:			
Pear, 3.5 oz slice	250	9	39
Raspberry, 5 oz slice	290	10	51
Wild Blueberry, 3.5 oz slice	260	6	52

Cakes ~ Mixes

C F Cb

Prepared as Directed

Arrowhead Mills:

Brownie Mix:

	C	F	Cb
Regular, 1/20 package, 1 oz	150	7	21
Gluten Free, 1/20 package, 1 oz	160	8	21

Cake Mix:

	C	F	Cb
Chocolate, organic, 1/12 pkg., 1.5 oz	260	11	39
Vanilla, 1/12 package, 1.8 oz	260	10	41

Betty Crocker:

Bars:

	C	F	Cb
Caramelita, 1/16 pkg	190	8	28
Reese's, 1/15 package	180	13	20
Sunkist Lemon, 1/16 pkg	140	4	24

Brownie Mix:

	C	F	Cb
Dark Chocolate Fudge, 1/20 package	160	7	24
Fudge, 1/20 package	170	8	23
Low-Fat Fudge, 1/18 package	140	3	28
Premium:			
Choc. Chunk, 1/16 package	170	7	26
Original Supreme, 1/16 package	190	8	27
P'nut Butter/Walnut, av., 1/16 pkg	170	7	24
Triple Chunk, 1/16 package	180	7	28
Ultimate Fudge, 1/16 package	170	6.5	26

Cake Mixes: *Per 1/10 Package*

SuperMoist:

	C	F	Cb
Butter Recipe Yellow	240	9	36
Carrot	310	18	35
Cherry Chip	280	14	36
Devil's Food	280	14	35
French Vanilla	280	14	35
Milk Chocolate	250	10	35
Average other Chocolate varieties	280	14	35

If using No-Cholesterol Recipe, deduct 40 cals and 4g fat.

Cupcakes: *Per 0.8 oz Mix & 0.4 oz Filling*

FUN da-middles:

	C	F	Cb
Chocolate Cake, Vanilla Filling	200	9	27
Yellow Cake, Chocolate Filling	190	9	25

Duncan Hines:

Brownie Mix: *Per 1/20 Pkg Unless Indicated*

	C	F	Cb
Decadent, Caramel Turtle, 1/16 pkg	150	7	23
Premium: Chewy Fudge	180	8	24
Snack Size, 1/12 pkg	140	7	20
Milk Chocolate	160	8	21

Cake Mix,

	C	F	Cb
Classic, Dark Choc. Fudge, 1/20 pkg	220	11	28

Prepared as Directed

Duncan Hines (Cont):

C F Cb

Decadent: *Per 1/12 Package*

	C	F	Cb
Apple Caramel	280	12	39
Classic Carrot	265	11	39

Signature:

	C	F	Cb
Banana Supreme	270	12	36
Coconut Supreme	250	11	34
French Vanilla	270	12	34

Jell-O:

No Bake Cheesecake:

	C	F	Cb
Cherry, 1/9 pkg, 2.4 oz	290	11	48
Real Cheesecake, 1/8 pkg, 2.1 oz	360	21	42

Krusteaz: Cinnamon Crumb Cake, 2"

	C	F	Cb
Cinnamon Crumb Cake, 2"	210	5	39
Lemon; Key Lime Bar, 2½x2" bar	160	4.5	29

Pillsbury:

Brownies, Premium Mix: *Dry Mix Only*

	C	F	Cb
Caramel Swirl, 1/12 packet, 1.2 oz	130	3	26
Cheesecake Swirl, 1/18 pkt, 0.9 oz	100	2.5	19
Chocolate Extreme, 1/12 pkg, 1.2 oz	110	3	22
Double Chocolate, 1/16 pkg, 1 oz	110	2	23

Cakes, Moist Supreme: *Per 1/10 Pkg, Dry Mix Only*

	C	F	Cb
Classic White/Yellow, 1.5 oz	160	4	33
Devils Food, Regular, 1.5 oz	160	3	34

Supreme Collection: *Per 1/12 Pkg, Dry Mix Only*

	C	F	Cb
Apple Spice, 1.8 oz	160	3.5	33
Fudge Truffle, 1.8 oz	200	4.5	40
Red Velvet, 1.8 oz	200	5	41

Cake Frostings

Betty Crocker:

	C	F	Cb
Rich & Creamy, av., 2 T., 1.2 oz	140	6	23
Whipped, av. all var.,2 T., 0.9 oz	100	4.5	15
Cool Whip, all varieties, 0.5 oz	60	3.5	8

Duncan Hines:

	C	F	Cb
Creamy Homestyle, av. all var., 2T.	140	6	23
Whipped, av. all varieties, 3 Tbsp	155	8	23

Pillsbury: *Per 2 Tbsp*

Creamy Supreme:

	C	F	Cb
Choc Fudge; Milk Choc., 1.2 oz	130	6	20
Classic White, 1.2 oz	140	5	22
Vanilla; Vanilla Funfetti, 1.2 oz	140	5	22
Sugar Free, Chocolate Fudge	100	6	16
Whipped Supreme, av. all varieties	100	5	14

Quick Guide

C **F** **Cb**

Donuts
Average All Brands

	C	F	Cb
Cake: Plain, 1.8 oz	205	12	23
Chocolate Iced, 2 oz	255	14	29
Sugared, 0.8 oz	205	10	29
Non-Cake, Glazed, 2 oz	225	11	29

Croissant-Donuts
(Includes Cronuts/Frissants)
Average all Brands

	C	F	Cb
Cream-filled, 3.5 oz	430	26	45
Custard-filled, 3.5 oz	360	19	45

Extra Listings ~ See CalorieKing.com
(Cronut is a trademark of Dominique Ansel Bakery, New York)

Donuts ~ Brands

	C	F	Cb
Albertson's:			
Donut Holes:			
Glazed Old Fashioned (4)	240	12	31
Powdered Sugar (4)	210	12	24
Gem Donuts: Plain Cake (3)	190	12	20
Cinnamon Sugar (3)	240	15	23
Glazed (1)	140	6	21
Bon Appetit:			
Mini Donuts:			
Chocolate (4)	270	16	29
Crumb (4)	240	12	32
Powdered (4)	250	12	34
Dunkin' Donuts:			
Apple Crumb	490	18	80
Apple N' Spice	270	14	32
Barvarian Kreme	270	15	31
Blueberry Cake	340	17	44
Blueberry Crumb	500	18	84
Boston Kreme	310	16	39
Chocolate Frosted Cake	370	23	45
Chocolate Glazed Cake	370	24	35
Cocoa Boston Kreme	300	16	37
Glazed Cake	360	22	44
Jelly Filled	270	14	32
Powdered Cake	340	22	38
Vanilla Kreme Filled	380	23	42

Extra Listings ~ See Fast Food Section

Donuts ~ Brands (Cont)

C **F** **Cb**

	C	F	Cb
Entenmann's:			
8 Pack: *Per Donut*			
Chocolate Lovers, 2 oz	300	20	31
Crumb, 2 oz	250	12	36
Frosted Devil's, 2.4 oz	310	18	36
Glazed, 2.3 oz	210	10	32
Rich Frosted, 2 oz	300	20	30
Pop'ems:			
Frosted (4), 2 oz	320	23	28
Powdered (4), 2 oz	250	12	32
Great Value (Walmart):			
Minis: Chocolate Frosted (4)	280	16	32
Powdered (4)	210	10	30
Hostess:			
Mini Donettes: Crumb, 6-pack, 4 oz	430	18	63
Frosted, 6-pack, 3 oz	360	22	38
Powdered, 6-pack, 3 oz	340	17	43
Krispy Kreme:			
Apple Fritter, 3 oz	210	14	18
Baseball Donut, 2.4 oz	290	17	33
Chocolate: Iced Cake, 2.5 oz	280	15	34
Iced Custard Filled, 3.2 oz	310	17	36
Iced Glazed Cruller, 2.5 oz	260	12	38
Iced Glazed, 2.3	240	11	33
Iced Kreme Filled, 3.2 oz	360	21	40
Iced Glazed w/ Sprinkles, 2.3 oz	250	12	35
Cinnamon Twist, 2 oz	240	15	23
Glazed Cruller, 2 oz	220	12	27
Glazed Doughnut Holes:			
Original (4)	200	11	26
Blueberry (4)	190	8	26
Chocolate Cake (4)	190	9	25
Glazed Kreme Filled, 3 oz	340	20	38
Maple Iced Glazed, 2.3 oz	230	11	32
New York Cheesecake, 3.4 oz	350	21	36
Original Glazed, 1.7 oz	190	11	21
Powdered Cake, 1.9 oz	220	11	27
Traditional Cake, 2 oz	190	12	19
Little Debbie,			
Donut Sticks (1), 1.7 oz	230	14	25
Tastykake:			
Cinnamon, 1.8 oz	210	11	26
Mini: Coated, 3 oz	380	22	42
Powdered Sugar (6), 2.5 oz	280	13	37

Quick Guide   **C** **F** **Cb**

Muffins: Ready-To-Eat
Average All Brands

		C	F	Cb
Small, 1 oz		90	3.5	14
Medium, 2 oz		185	6.5	28
Large, 3 oz		275	10	42
Extra Large, 4 oz		365	13	57
Giant, 6 oz		550	20	84
Super Size, 8 oz		730	27	112

Muffins Ready-To-Eat ~ Brands

	C	F	Cb
Albertsons:			
Minis: Banana Nut (2)	200	12	20
Blueberry (2)	180	10	21
Honey Raisin Bran (2)	170	7	24
Entenmann's: *Per Muffin*			
Single Serve: Powdered Pop'ems (4)	250	12	33
Softee, Frosted Donuts (1)	250	17	24
Great Value *(Walmart),*			
Double Blueberry (1), 4 oz	430	16	65
Little Debbie: Banana Nut (1), 1.9 oz	210	9	30
Blueberry (1), 1.9 oz	190	8	27
Chocolate Chip (1), 1.9 oz	210	9	28
My Favorite Muffin: *Per 6 oz Muffin*			
Banana Nut	585	33	63
Blueberry	505	24	66
Boston Cream Pie	530	21	78
Chocolate Chip	635	33	81
Lemon Poppyseed	605	30	75
Otis Spunkmeyer:			
Banana Nut, 3.3 oz	360	18	48
Chocolate Chip, 2 oz	230	12	29
Wild Blueberry, 2 oz	200	8	28
Starbucks ~ *See Fast-Foods Section*			
Trader Joe's: *Per Muffin*			
Apple Cranberry, 4.8 oz	220	5	38
Banana Chocolate Chip, 4 oz	400	18	57
Carrot, 4 oz	320	11	52
Triple Berry, 4 oz	310	11	49
Vitalicious:			
VitaMuffins: Average all., 2 oz	100	1	24
Large, average all varieties., 4 oz	200	2	50
Sugar-Free, Banana Nut, 2 oz	90	2.5	21
VitaTops: Average all varieties, 2 oz	100	1.5	25
Sugar free, av. all varieties, 2 oz	90	1	22
Weight Watchers,			
Blueb.; Double Choc, av., 2.5 oz	185	2.5	42

Muffin Mixes   **C** **F** **Cb**

Per Muffin, Prepared

	C	F	Cb
Betty Crocker: Banana Nut	170	8	22
Cinnamon Streusel	180	8	26
Wild Blueberry	160	6.5	24
Pouch Mix:			
Banana Nut	120	3	22
Blueberry; Triple Berry	120	2.5	23
Chocolate Chip	130	3.5	22
Fiber One:			
Apple Cinnamon; Blueberry, average	160	6	29
Banana Nut	160	6.5	27
Krusteaz: Banana Nut	250	13	29
Choc Chunk	260	13	29
Lemon Poppyseed	170	4	31
Oat Bran	180	4.5	32
Trader Joe's, Triple Berry	150	2	28

Sweet Rolls & Buns   **C** **F** **Cb**

Note: It is best to weigh for accuracy as actual weight can be 10-50% higher than label weight·
Per Sweet Roll or Bun Unless Indicated

	C	F	Cb
Bimbo, Bimbolete, 2.2 oz	250	10	36
Bon Appetit,			
Cinnamon Roll, 2.5 oz	230	8	34
Cinnabon: Classic	880	36	127
Caramel Pecanbon	1080	50	147
Cloverhill Bakery,			
Jumbo Honey Bun, 4.8 oz	600	35	64
Entenmann's,			
Cinnamon Swirl Bun, 3 oz	320	14	44
Little Debbie: Honey Buns, 1.8 oz	230	13	26
Pecan Spinwheels, 1 oz	100	3.5	17
McDonald's,			
Cinnamon Melts, 4 oz	460	19	66
Pillsbury			
Sweet Rolls, Refrigerated: *Per Roll Unless Indicated*			
Cinnamon, w/ Icing	140	5	23
Reduced Fat	130	3.5	24
Mini-Bites, with Icing (3)	160	4.5	27
Orange Flavored, with Icing, 1.7 oz	160	6	26
Twists, Flaky Cinnamon, with Icing	160	7	23
Grands, Refrigerated: *Per Roll*			
Cinnabon Cinnamon Roll,			
with Cream Cheese	300	8	54
Caramel Rolls, with Icing, 3.5 oz	310	9	53
Flaky Supreme Cinnabon,			
Cinnamon Roll, with Icing, 3.5 oz	360	17	48
7-Eleven: Iced Honey Bun, 6 oz	820	58	68
Glazed Honey Bun, 5 oz	620	35	70
Sara Lee, Cinnamon Roll, 2.4 oz	260	12	33

C Candy ~ Chocolate

Quick Guide

	C	F	Cb
Chocolate:			
Average All Brands			
Milk Chocolate, regular:			
Plain/Nuts/Fruit, average, 1 oz	150	9	17
1.5oz Bar	230	13	25
2 oz Bar	305	17	34
4 oz Block	610	34	68
8 oz Block	1220	68	136
1 Pound, 16 oz	2440	136	272
Dark/White Chocolate: 1 oz	155	9	17
Hershey's, Sugar Free, 5 pieces	110	13	24
Milk Chocolate-Coated:			
Almonds, 5-6, 1 oz	150	10	15
Cherry Cordial Centers, 2 pcs, 1 oz	145	6	21
Clusters, Nut, 3 pieces, 1.2 oz	210	14	20
Coffee Beans, 1.4 oz	220	13	22
Macadamias, 10 pieces, 1.4 oz	220	16	21
Mints, 1 medium, 0.5 oz	55	1	11
Nougat & Caramel, 1 oz	150	9	15
Peanuts, 12 medium, 1 oz	145	10	14
Raisins, 28 medium, 1 oz	110	4	19
Baking Chocolate:			
Baker's: Bittersweet, 1 oz	140	12	14
Semi-sweet, 1 oz	140	9	16
Nestle, Chips: Dark, 1 Tbsp. 0.5 oz	70	5	3
Semi-Sweet, 1 Tbsp. 0.5oz	70	4	9
Unsweetened, 1 oz	140	14	8
Carob, Plain, 1 oz	155	9	16

Candy ~ Brands & Generic

Per Piece/Serving

	C	F	Cb
3 Musketeers: Orig., 1 bar, 2.2 oz	260	8	46
2 To Go, 1.7 oz Bar	200	6	35
Fun Size (3), 1.6 oz	190	6	34
Minis, 7 pieces, 1.4 oz	170	5	32
100 Grand: 1.5 oz bar	190	8	30
Snack Size (1), 0.8 oz	95	4	15
Super Size, 2.8 oz	360	14	58
Abba Zabba, 2 oz bar	250	5	48
After Dinner Mints, 1 small	25	1.5	3
After Eight Mint, each	35	1.5	4
Airhead, 1 bar, 0.5 oz	60	1	14
Almond Joy: 2 bars, 1.6 oz	220	13	26
King Size, 4 bars, 3.3 oz	460	26	54
Snack Size, 0.6 oz bar	80	4.5	9
Pieces (46), 1.4 oz	200	10	27

Per Piece/Serving

	C	F	Cb
Almond Roca, 3 pieces, 1.3 oz	200	15	17
Almond: Sugar-coated (15), 1.4 oz	190	7	27
Jordan, 15 pieces, 1.4 oz	180	8	28
Almond Clusters:			
True North, 1 oz	170	12	9
Trader Joe's, 1.2 oz	190	14	13
Altoids, 3 pieces	10	0	2
Andes, Thins (8), av. all var., 1.4 oz	205	13	22
Anthon Berg:			
Creamy Mint (4), 1.4 oz	180	6	31
Marzipan with Plum, in Madeira	120	6	14
Atomic Fireball, 1 piece, 0.3 oz	35	0	9
Baby Ruth: King Size, 3.5 oz bar	500	24	66
2 oz bar	280	14	39
Fun size, 2 bars	170	8	24
Minis, 4 bars	210	11	28
Baci (Perugina),			
1 piece, 0.5 oz	75	6	7
Baskin-Robbins: Sugar Candy, 3 pcs	60	1	12
Sugar Free, 4 pieces, average, 0.6 oz	40	1	16
Carbs include 16g sugar alcohol			
Big Hunk, 2 oz Bar	230	3	47
Bit-O-Honey:			
1.7 oz bar	180	3.5	39
Chews, 6 pieces, 1.4 oz	150	3	32
Bliss (Hershey's):			
Milk/Dark Choc./Caramel, 6 pieces	120	14	25
Meltaway Centers:			
Milk Chocolate, 6 pieces	220	15	24
Raspberry, 6 pieces	220	14	24
Blow Pops, each, 0.6 oz	60	0	17
Bon Bons, 3 pieces	65	0	15
Boston Baked Beans, (11), 0.5 oz	70	2	11
Brach's:			
Almond Supremes (10)	200	14	20
Bridge Mix (15), 1.4 oz	190	10	26
Double Dippers (15), 1.4 oz	210	14	22
Gummi Bears (14), 1.4 oz	130	0	30
Lemon Drops, Sugar Free, 4 pieces	35	0	17
Carbs include 17g Sugar Alcohol			
Mandarin/Orange Slices (3), 1.6 oz	150	0	37
Maple Nut Goodies (8), 1.5 oz	190	9	27
Milk Maid Crmls (4), 1.3 oz	150	4	25
Peanut Cluster (3), 1.4 oz	210	15	20
Breath Savers, all varieties, each	5	0	2
Bubble Gum ~ *See Page 75*			
Bulls Eyes, 3 pieces, 1.2 oz	130	3	23
Buncha Crunch: ½ cup, 1.4 oz	180	9	25
Movie Box, 3.2 oz	450	20	65
Burnt Peanuts, (31), 1.4 oz	170	6	29

Candy ~ Brands & Generic (Cont)

Per Piece/Serving	C	F	Cb
Butterfinger: 2 oz bar	270	11	43
King Size (3 bars), 3.5 oz	480	18	75
Fun Size, (1), 0.8 oz	100	4	15
Giant, (Pieces in Chocolate), ¼ bar, 1 oz	150	8	21
Miniatures:			
1 piece, 0.4 oz	45	2	8
4 pieces, 1.4 oz	180	8	32
Snack Pack, 4 pcs, 1.4 oz	180	7	29
Crisp Bar: Original, 2 oz bar	270	11	44
King Size, 3 pieces, 2 oz	310	17	38
Minis, 2 bars, 1.4 oz	210	11	25
Snackerz:			
Single, 1.3 oz	170	8	23
Fun Size, 2 pcs, 1.2 oz	150	7	21
King Size, 10 pcs, 1.4 oz	190	8	25
Butter Mints, 7 pieces, 0.5 oz	50	0	12
Butterscotch: 3 pieces	60	0	15
Discs (Walgreens), 3 pieces, 0.6 oz	70	0	17
Cadbury: Caramello Bar, 1.6 oz	220	10	29
Caramel Egg, 1.2 oz	170	8	22
Dairy Milk Bar, 7 pieces, 1.4 oz	200	11	23
Mini Eggs (Candy), 12 pcs, 1.4 oz	190	8	28
Candy Apple, medium, 6.5 oz	280	0	60
Candy Cane, medium, 5", 0.5 oz	40	0	14
Candy Corn, 20 pieces, 1.4 oz	150	0	38
Candy Jar Mix (Jewel), 3 pcs, 0.6 oz	60	0	14
Candy Necklace (Smarties), (1), 0.8 oz	90	0.5	20
Caramels: Each, 0.4 oz	40	1	8
Chocolate, each, 0.3 oz	25	0.3	6
Creams (3), 1.3 oz	130	3	23
Caramel Popcorn, ⅔ cup	150	6	23
Cella's,			
Milk Choc. Cherries, 3 pieces, 1.5 oz	160	6	27
Certs, Breath Mints, 1 piece	5	0	2
Charleston Chew:			
Chocolate Bar (1), 1.4 oz	160	4.5	30
Mini Bars, 13 pieces	190	6	34
Charms: Blow Pop	60	0	17
Flat Pop, 0.5 oz	50	0	14
Chew-ets, Peanut Chews, Original (4), 1.6 oz	230	12	29
Chewz, 1 roll, 1 oz	120	1	28
Chick O Stick, 2 oz	240	9	42

Per Piece/Serving	C	F	Cb
Chunky Bar (Nestlé), King Size, 2.5 oz	340	19	44
Chupa Chups, 1 Pop	50	0	12
Cinn. Buttons (Walgreens), 3 pieces	60	0	16
Cinnamon Disks (Walmart), 3 pieces	70	0	18
Circus Peanuts (Spangler), 6 pieces, 1.3 oz	165	0	41
CocoaVia, Orig., 0.8 oz	100	6	12
Coconut Stacks, (8)	320	16	46
Coffee Go, Candy, (4)	60	1	12
Conversation Hearts (Necco):			
Small (40), 1.4 oz	160	0	39
1 large	10	0	3
Cookie Dough Bites, 1.4 oz	200	10	27
Cote d'Or: Dark 86% Coca, 4 pcs	270	22	14
Dark, 70%, Orange, 3.5 oz	575	46	34
Dark, Raspberry, 3.5 oz	580	46	34
Milk, Intense, 3.5 oz	575	40	45
Cotton Candy, 1 oz	110	0	28
Cough Drops ~ See Page 75			
Cracker Jack, ½ cup, 1 oz	120	2	23
Creme Savers: 3 pieces, 0.5 oz	60	1	11
Sugar-Free, 3 pieces	30	1	8
Crisped Rice, Choc Chip, 1 bar, 1 oz	115	4	20
Crows, 11 pieces, 1.4 oz	130	0	33
Crunch Bar ~ See Nestle			
Dots, 11 dots, 1.4 oz	130	0	33
Double Dip Stick, 1 stick	15	0.5	3
Dove:			
Milk Choc: Singles Bar, 1.4 oz	220	13	24
Large Tablet Bar, 9 pieces, 1.5 oz	230	13	25
Choc. Covered Almonds, 13 pcs, 1.4 oz	220	15	19
Promises: Milk Choc., 1 piece, 0.3 oz	45	2.5	5
With Caramel, 1 piece, 0.3 oz	40	2	5
With Peanut Butter, 1 piece, 0.3 oz	45	3	4
Swirls, all varieties, 9 pieces 1.5 oz	230	14	25
Dark Choc: Singles Bar, 1.3 oz	220	13	24
Large Tablet Bar, 9 pieces, 1.5 oz	220	14	25
Choc. Covered. Almds, 13 pcs, 1.4 oz	210	15	19
Promises, Almond, 1 piece, 0.3 oz	40	3	4
Swirls, Raspberry, 9 pieces, 1.4 oz	220	14	24
Sugar Free, all varieties, 5 pcs, 1.4 oz	195	15	21
Dum Dum Pops (Spangler), 1 pop	25	0	7
Drops (Hershey's):			
Cookies 'n' Creme, 14 pieces, 1.5 oz	210	11	26
Milk Chocolate, 15 pieces, 1.4 oz	200	12	25

Candy ~ Brands & Generic (Cont)

Per Piece/Serving

	C	F	Cb
English Toffee, 1 piece, 0.4 oz	70	4	6
5th Avenue: 2 oz bar	260	12	38
King Size, 3.5 oz	440	20	64
Fannie May:			
Mint Meltaway (1)	230	15	24
Pixie (1), 1.5 oz	210	12	24
Trinidad (1), 1.5 oz	200	12	23
Fast Break (Reese's): 2 oz bar	260	12	35
3.5 oz bar	460	22	62
Ferrero Rocher: 1 piece	75	5	5
3 pieces, 1.3 oz	220	16	16
Rondnoir, 3 pieces, 1.4 oz	180	13	14
Fifty 50 Snack Bars:			
Milk Chocolate: 5 pieces, 1 oz	135	11	14
Almond, 5 pieces, 1 oz	135	11	14
Crunch Bar, 7 pcs, 1 oz	140	12	16
Dark Chocolate, 5 pieces, 1 oz	120	11	15
Carb figures include 9-12g Sugar Alcohol			
Fluffy Stuff (Charms),			
Cotton Candy, 1.4 oz	150	0	40
Fondant: Choc-coated, 1.2 oz	125	3	27
Mint, 1 oz	105	0	25
Fran's:			
Gold Bar, Almond (1)	250	14	27
GoldBite, Almond (1)	120	7	13
Fruit Drops (Sunkist), (1), ¼ oz	20	0	4
Fruit Gems (Sunkist), (4), 1.4 oz	130	0	33
Fruit Leathers, average, 0.5 oz	50	0.5	12
Fruit Pastilles (Rowntree), 1 roll	185	0	45
Fruit Roll-Ups (Betty Crocker/Sunkist),			
1 roll, 0.5 oz	50	1	12
Fruit Runts (Walgreens),			
12 pieces	60	0	14
Fruit Flavored Shapes (Betty Crocker),			
all varieties, 0.8 oz	80	0	19
Fudge:			
Chocolate; Mint, 1 oz	130	8	14
Peanut Butter & Choc., 1 oz	130	8	13
Brevin's: Cashew, 1 oz	195	9	28
Triple Decker, 1 oz	165	7	25
Ghirardelli:			
3 oz Bars: Dark Chocolate, 4 squares	220	17	23
Filled, Peanut Butter, 4 squares	250	17	22
Intense Dark Bars, Ev'ng Dream, 3 pcs	190	15	20
Squares:			
Dark Chocolate (4), 1.5 oz	210	16	23
Milk & Caramel (3), 1.5 oz	220	12	27
Sea Salt Escape (4), 1.5 oz	210	15	24

Per Piece/Serving

	C	F	Cb
Godiva:			
Bars: Milk/Dark, av., 1.5 oz	230	14	26
Extra Dark: 75%, 1.5 oz	230	17	18
85%, 1.4 oz	260	21	14
Chocoiste:			
Dark Chocolate Cherries (12)	190	7	30
Milk Chocolate Cashews (14)	230	15	19
Hearts: Dark Ganache (4)	200	12	23
Milk Praline (4)	220	13	23
Go Lightly:			
Assorted Toffee, 5 pieces, 1 oz	85	2	24
Fruit Chews, 5 pieces, 1 oz	95	2	26
Hard Candy, Assorted (4), 0.5 oz	45	0	15
Carb figures include 15-25g sugar alcohol			
Goobers Peanuts, 1 package, 1.4 oz	200	13	21
Good & Plenty (Hershey's), (33), 1.4 oz	140	0	35
GooGoo Clusters, 1 piece, 1.8 oz	240	12	30
Gum ~ *See Page 75*			
Gum Drops: 1 small, 0.1 oz	15	0	3
5 pieces, 0.5 oz	75	0	15
Gummi (Shur Fine):			
Bears (15), 1.4 oz	130	0	29
Chewy Sweet Tarts (4)	160	0	36
Worms (9), 1.5 oz	140	0	31
Guylian:			
Bars: Dark Chocolate (3), 1 oz	150	12	11
Milk Choc. with Hazelnuts (3),1 oz	170	11	15
No Sugar Added Bars:			
Milk Chocolate, 3 squares	150	11	16
54% Cocoa, Dark Choc., 3 squares	140	11	16
Seashells:			
Bar, 1.4 oz	210	13	21
Boxed, Originals (1), 0.4 oz	60	4	6
Truffles (1), 0.4 oz	70	5.5	5
Heath: Original (1), 1.4 oz	210	13	24
King Size, 2.8 oz	410	22	49
Snack Size, 3 pieces, 1.5 oz	230	14	27
Hershey's:			
Cookies 'n' Creme, 1.6 oz Bar	220	12	26
Milk Chocolate:			
Bars: 1.6 oz	210	13	26
With Almonds, 1 bar, 1.4 oz	210	14	21
King Size, 1 Bar, 2.5 oz	370	22	44
Kisses, 9 pieces, av., 1.4 oz	200	12	25
Nuggets: 4 pieces, 1.4 oz	200	13	20
W/Toffee & Alm., 4 pcs, 1.3 oz	200	13	21
Sugar Free Choc., 5 pieces, 1.4 oz	160	13	24
Extra Dark Choc., 4 pieces, 1.4 oz	180	14	21
Simple Pleasures, 6 pieces, av.	180	8	29
Special Dark Choc., 1.5 oz bar	190	12	25

Candy ~ Brands & Generic (Cont)

Per Piece/Serving **C F Cb**

Hershey's, (Cont):

Pot of Gold Chocolate Asstd:

	C	F	Cb
Carmel, 4 pieces, 1.4 oz	190	10	26
Average other var., 4 pieces, 1.4 oz	210	12	24

Candy-Coated Eggs:

Milk Chocolate: (8) 1.2 oz	170	8	27
With Almonds (8) 1.2 oz	200	12	18

Honeycomb: Plain, 1 oz	115	0	27
Choc-coated, 2 pieces	180	7	31

Hot Tamales,

20 pieces, 1.4 oz	150	0	36

Hugs ~ See Kisses

Jawbreakers (Sathers), (15), 0.6 oz	60	0	16
Jells (Joyva), Raspb., 3 pieces, 1.6 oz	160	0	38

Jelly Beans, average all brands

Small Size (Jelly Belly): 1 bean	5	0	1
12 beans, 0.5 oz	50	0	13
Regular Size: 1 bean	10	0	2
10 beans, 1 oz	105	0	26
Large Size: 1 bean	15	0	38
10 beans, 1.5 oz	150	0	38

Sugar Free,

average all brands, 25 beans, 1 oz	60	0	26

Carb figures include 26g sugar alcohol

Jelly Belly: 25 beans, 1 oz

25 beans, 1 oz	105	0	26
3.5 oz package	360	0	90

Sugar Free,

25 beans, 1 oz	60	0	26

Carb figures include 26 sugar alcohol

Chocolate Dips:

All flavors: 1 bean	4	0	1
10 beans	40	1	8
2.8 oz bag	300	8	62

Jelly Rings (Jewel), 5 pieces, 1.4 oz	110	0	26

Jolly Rancher:

Bites: Soft, 15 pieces	150	1.5	32
Sours, 16 pieces	130	0	34
Crunch 'N Chew, 1 oz pkg	160	0.5	40
Filled Fruity Bites, 22 pieces	140	1	31
Gummies, 9 pieces	120	0	28
Hard Candy, 3 pieces	70	0	17
Jelly Beans/Sours, 1.4 oz	140	0	34
Lollipops (1), 0.55 oz	60	0	15
Jujubes, all varieties (52), 1.4 oz	110	0	28
Juju Bears, 5 pieces	130	0	34
Juju Mix (Sathers), 11 pieces, 1.5 oz	150	0	36
Jujyfruits, 16 pieces, 1.4 oz	120	0	32
Junior Caramels: 13 pieces, 1.5 oz	190	6	33
Mini, 2 boxes, 1 oz	130	4	23

Per Piece/Serving **C F Cb**

Junior Mints: 1.8 oz

1.8 oz	220	4	45
16 pieces, 1.4 oz	170	3	35

Justin's, Peanut Butter Cups,

Milk Choc, 2 cups, 1.4 oz pkg	200	14	18

Kisses (Hershey's):

Air Delights (11), 1.4 oz	200	12	24
Cookies 'n' Creme (9), 1.5 oz	220	12	26
Hugs (9), 1.4 oz	210	12	24
Milk Chocolate: (1), 0.16 oz	25	1.5	3
(9), 1.4oz	200	12	25
With Almonds (9), 1.4 oz	200	13	22
Caramel Filled (9), 1.5 oz	190	9	27
Special Dark (9), 1.4 oz	180	12	25

Kit Kat (Nestle):

Milk Chocolate:

4 piece bar, 1.5 oz	210	11	28
Extra Crispy, 1.6 oz bar	220	12	29
King Size, 8 pcs, 3 oz bar	420	22	56
Minis, 5 pieces	210	11	28
Snack Size, 6 pcs, 1.5 oz	210	11	28

White Chocolate, 4 pieces, 1.5 oz	220	12	26
Peanut Bar (Lance), 2.2 oz package	340	19	29
Lemon Drops: (4), 0.6 oz	60	0	16
Walgreens, Sugar Free (3), 0.6 oz	50	0	17
Lemonhead, (26), 1.4 oz	140	0	36

Licorice:

Avearage all varieties, 1oz	100	0	25
Chews (Panda), (1)	10	0	3
Tid Bits (1)	10	0	2
Twists: Black/Red, av., 1 pc	35	0	8
Sugar Free, 1 piece	15	0	2.5

American Licorice Co.:

Natural Vines: Black (9), 1.4 oz	140	1	33
Strawberry (9), 1.4 oz	150	1	34
Red Vines (4), 1.4 oz	140	0	34
Sip-n-Chew, 1 oz package	100	1	23
Snaps (31), 1.4 oz	140	0.5	33
Sour Punch (6), 1.4 oz	150	0.5	34
Super Ropes (1), 2 oz	200	0	46

Lifesavers: Large size, 1 candy

Large size, 1 candy	15	0	3
Regular: All flavors, 1 candy	10	0	3
1 Roll (14 candies), 1.2 oz	140	0	35
Creme Savers: 3 pieces, 0.5 oz	60	1	11
Sugar Free (3)	45	1.5	13
Pep-o-mint (3), 0.2 oz	20	0	5
Fruit Splosion (10), 1.4 oz	130	0	31
Sugar-Free Delites,			
Orchard Fruits; Summer Blend (1)	5	0	2
Butter Toffee; European Collection	10	1	3

Candy ~ Brands & Generic (Cont)

Per Piece/Serving	C	F	Cb
Lik-m-aid (Nestle), Fun Dip, 1 package	50	0	13
Lindt: Lindor Truffles (1), average	75	6	5
Swiss Milk Chocolate Bars:			
70% Cocoa, 4 pieces	220	17	13
Classic, with Hazelnuts, 10 pieces	230	16	20
Raspberry filled, 7 pieces	200	10	25
Dark Choc. Truffles,			
with filling, 7 pieces	240	18	18
Lollipops: Mini, 0.3 oz	25	0	6
Small, 0.5 oz	50	0	12
Medium, 1 oz	100	0	25
Giant (4" diam), 7 oz	790	0	198
M & M's:			
Dark Chocolate: 1.5 oz package	210	10	29
Peanuts, 1.5 oz	220	12	25
Milk Chocolate: 28 piece, 1 oz	145	6.5	21
1.5 oz package	210	9	30
1.7 oz package	240	10	34
Almond Choc., 1.5 oz	220	12	25
Minis, 1 tube, 1 oz	150	7	21
Peanut: 28 pieces, 1 oz	155	8	17
1.75 oz pkg	250	13	30
Peanut Butter, 1.6 oz package	240	14	26
Premiums: Chocolate Trio, 1.5 oz	230	14	25
Mint Thrills, 1.5 oz	240	14	25
Pretzels, ½ pkg, 1.4 oz	180	6	29
Snack Mix, av. all var., ⅓ cup, 1.5 oz	200	9	25
Mamba Sours, Fruit Chews,			
6 pieces, 1 oz	100	1	22
Marshmallow Egg, 1 egg, 1 oz	120	3	22
Mary Jane (Necco), 5 pieces, 1.4 oz	160	3.5	32
Marshmallows: Firm/Soft, 1 oz	90	0	23
Regular size, 4 pieces, 1 oz	100	0	24
Mini-Marshmallow, ⅔ cup, 1 oz	95	0	24
Joyva, Choc-coated Twists	95	2	10
Fluff, 2 Tbsp, 0.6 oz	60	0	15
Kraft: Creme, 0.5 oz	45	0	11
Funmallows, ⅔ cup, 1 oz	100	0	24
Jet-Puffed, 5 pieces, 1 oz	100	0	24
Mini, 1 oz	90	0	23
Marzipan, 2 Tbsp, 1.4 oz	160	4	29
Mauna Loa, Mountains, 4 pcs	230	17	21
Mexican Hats, (7), 1.4 oz	120	0	30
Mentos: Regular	10	0	3
Sugar Free	5	0	2
Mike & Ike:			
Original: 2.1 oz package	220	0	55
23 pieces, 1.4 oz	140	0	36
Milk Duds, 1 box, 1.8 oz	230	8	38

Per Piece/Serving	C	F	Cb
Milky Way (Mars):			
Bars: Single, 2 oz	240	9	37
Fun Size, 2 bars, 1.2 oz	160	6	24
To Go, 1.8 oz	230	9	36
Minis, 5 pieces, 1.5 oz	190	7	30
Midnight Bars: 1.8 oz	230	8	36
Minis, 5 pieces, 1.4 oz	190	7	30
Simply Caramel, 1.9 oz	250	11	37
Mints: Uncoated, 3 pieces	70	0	17
1 mint , medium	7	0	1
1 large mint	15	0	3
Mon Cheri (Ferrero), 4 pieces, 2 oz	260	18	20
Mounds: 1.75 oz bar	230	13	29
King Size, 4 pieces, 3.5 oz	460	26	58
Snack Size, 1 piece, 0.6 oz	80	4.5	10
Mr Goodbar: 1.8 oz bar	250	17	26
King Size, 2.6 oz bar	380	26	38
Munch Bar, 1.4 oz	220	15	18
Necco, Candy Wafers (40), 2 oz	220	0	56
Nestle Crunch: Orig.,1.6 oz bar	220	11	30
Fun Size, 3 bars, 1.4 oz	180	9	26
Miniatures, 4 bars, 1.4 oz	200	10	27
Buncha Crunch, ⅓ cup, 1.2 oz	180	9	25
Crunch Crisp, 1.8 oz	240	13	32
Newman's Own:			
Milk Chocolate: Caramel Cups (3)	160	8	21
Peanut Butter Cups (3)	180	12	17
Dark Chocolate: Caramel Cups (3)	160	9	20
Peanut Butter Cups (3)	180	13	16
Nips, all varieties, 2 pieces, 0.5 oz	60	2	11
Nougat: 3 pieces, 1.5 oz	170	1	39
Chocolate Covered, 1 oz	125	4	22
Nuggets ~ See Hershey's			
Nutrageous Bar (Reese's), 1.8 oz	260	16	28
Oh Henry!: Fun Size, 0.9 oz	120	5	16
1.8 oz bar	230	11	33
Orange Slices:			
Jewel, 3 pieces, 1.5 oz	140	0	35
Walgreens, 4 pieces, 1.6 oz	160	0	39
Pastel Mints (Walgreens), 20 pieces	60	0	14
PayDay Bar: 1.8 oz bar	240	13	27
King Size, 3.5 oz bar	440	24	50
Snack Size, 0.7 oz	90	5	10
Avalanche, 1.4 oz	250	13	29
Peanut Bar (Planter's), 1.6 oz	240	14	21
Peanut Butter Cups ~ See Reese's; Newman's Own			
Peanut Brittle: 1 piece, 1.5 oz	190	5	32
Sugar Free (Russell Stover),			
4 pieces, 1.3 oz	140	10	24

Candy ~ Brands & Generic (Cont)

Per Piece/Serving

	C	F	Cb
Peanuts, choc-covered, 14 pieces	230	14	23
Pearson's, Mint Patties, (5), 1.3 oz	150	2.5	31
Peppermints: 7 small, 0.5 oz	60	0	15
Brach's, Star Brites (3)	60	0	16
Pez, 1 roll	35	0	9
Planters:			
Double Peanut Bar, 1.6 oz	240	14	21
Pop Rocks, 0.4 oz package	35	0	9
Pot of Gold (Hershey's):			
Assortment: Caramel, 4 pieces	190	10	25
Nut, 4 pieces	210	13	23
Pretzels: Choc-covered, Mini (6)	200	9	25
White Choc Bites (23), 1.4 oz	200	9	25
Pretzel Flipz (Nestlé), 8 pieces, 1 oz	130	5	20
Raisinets: Milk Choc:			
1.58 oz package	190	8	32
Movie Pack, 3.5 oz	380	16	64
Dark Chocolate, ¼ cup, 1.6 oz	180	8	32
Reese's:			
Clusters, 3 pieces, 1.5 oz	220	12	24
Crispy Crunchy Bar: 1.7 oz	260	18	22
2 pieces, 1.2 oz	170	10	19
King Size, 3 oz	480	32	40
Fast Break, 2 oz bar	260	12	35
Peanut Butter Chips, 1 Tbsp, 0.5 oz	80	4	8
Peanut Butter Cups, Milk Chocolate:			
(2), 1.5 oz	210	13	24
Miniatures (5), 1.5 oz	220	13	26
Minis (11)	200	12	23
Big Cup, 1 cup, 1.4 oz	220	12	24
Sugar Free, Minis (5), 1.4 oz	180	13	27
Dark Chocolate (2), 1.5 oz	210	14	23
Pieces, Peanut Butter (51)	200	9	25
Sticks: 1.5 oz package	220	13	23
King Size, 3 oz package	440	26	46
Snack Size (1), 0.6 oz	90	5	9
Snacksters, 1 package, 0.8 oz	100	4	14
Whipps, 1.5 oz	230	9	37
Rice Krispies Treats (Kellogg's),			
1 bar, average all varieties, 0.8 oz	95	2.5	17
Riesen, Choc. Chew, 4 pieces, 1.3 oz	170	6	28
Rocky Road, Milk/Dark, 1.8 oz bar	240	11	34
Roca Thins, 3 pieces, av. all varieties	210	14	24
Rolo: Regular, all varieties, 1.7 oz roll	220	10	33
Mini Chews, Caramel in milk choc. (11)	190	9	26
Root Beer Barrels, (3), 0.6 oz	60	0	17

Per Piece/Serving

	C	F	Cb
Russell Stover Candy:			
Boxed Chocolates: Chocolate Coated			
Assorted (2), 1.2 oz	150	7	22
Cherry Cordials (3), 0.4 oz	150	5	25
Dairy Cream Caramels (2), 1.2 oz	160	7	22
Elegant Collection (3), 1.6 oz	210	10	25
French Choc. Mints (4), 1.4 oz	220	13	22
Nut, Chewy & Crisp Centers (2)	160	8	21
Sugar Free:			
Assorted Hard Candies (3), 1.6 oz	210	16	24
Bags: Caramel (3), 1.3 oz	180	8	25
Coconut (3), 1.5 oz	160	10	28
Mint Patty (3), 1.5 oz	180	12	26
Peanut Butter Cups (2), 1.2 oz	160	12	17
Pecan Delight (3), 1.2 oz	160	12	19
Note: Carbohydrates include sugar alcohol			
Salt Water Taffy (Brach's), (5)	170	2.5	36
Seashells (Guylian), (4), 1.6 oz	260	17	24
See's Candies:			
Almond Royal (5), 1.3 oz	190	13	18
Butterscotch Chews (5), 1.5 oz	210	12	27
Krispy's: Caffe Latte (5),1.3 oz	180	8	27
Mint (5), 1.3 oz	170	8	27
Little Pops:			
Butterscotch (4), 0.5 oz	60	2	12
Chocolate (4), 0.5 oz	60	3	10
Vanilla (4), 0.5 oz	50	2	9
Lollypops, average, 0.7 oz	90	3	17
Milk Molasses Chips, 6 pieces, 1.4 oz	180	12	20
Milk Peppermints, 2 pieces, 1.3 oz	150	4	28
Peanut Brittle Bar, 1 oz	150	10	15
Peanut Butter Patties, 2 pieces, 1.2 oz	170	10	16
Peppermint Twists (3), 0.5 oz	60	0	15
Toffee-ettes, 3 pieces, 1.6 oz	270	21	17
Sugar Free: Dark Bar, 1.5 oz	180	16	24
Dark Walnut Clusters (4), 1.5 oz	230	21	17
Peanut Brittle, 1.5 oz	170	14	17
Skinny Cow:			
Dreamy Clusters, all var., 1 pouch	120	6	20
Heavenly Crips, all varieties, 1 bar	110	6	14
Skittles: Original, 2 oz	230	2.5	52
Sour, 1.8 oz	200	2	44
Tropical; Wild Berry, 2.2 oz	250	2.5	56
Fun Size, 1 bag, 0.5 oz	60	1	14
Tear & Share, 4 oz bag	420	4.5	93
Skor, Toffee Bar (1), 1.4 oz	200	12	25
Smarties: Candy Rolls (1), 0.3 oz	25	0	6
Giant, 1 roll, 1 oz	100	0	25

C Candy ~ Chocolate

Candy ~ Brands & Generic (Cont)

Per Piece/Serving

	C	F	Cb
Snickers:			
Milk Chocolate:			
1.9 oz bar	250	12	33
Fun Size, 2 bars, 1.2 oz	160	8	21
To Go Bar, 1.6 oz	220	10	29
Miniatures: (4)	170	8	22
Sugar Free, 5 pcs	180	13	27
Almond Bar, 1.8 oz	230	11	32
P'nut Butter Squared, 2 bars, 1.8 oz	250	13	30
Dark Chocolate Bar, 1.8 oz	250	12	31
Sno Caps, ¼ cup, 1.4 oz	180	8	30
Soft 'N Chewy, Butter Toffee, 1 piece	30	0.5	5
Sorbee, Crystal Light Hard Candy, 4 pieces	25	0	13
Note: Carb figures include Isomalt which has fewer calories than sugar.			
Sour Patch: Kids, average, 2 oz	210	0	52
Extreme, 1.8 oz	190	0	47
Spearmint Leaves:			
Jewel, 5 pieces, 1.4 oz	140	0	35
Walgreens, 4 pieces, 1.6 oz	160	0	39
Spree Candies: Original, 15 pieces	50	0	13
Chewy, 8 pieces	60	0	13
Starburst:			
Candy Canes, 0.5 oz	70	0	18
Fruit Chews: Original, 1 piece	20	0.5	4
8 pieces, 1.4 oz	160	3.5	33
Gummibursts, 9 pieces, 1.4 oz	130	0	31
Jellybeans, 1.5 oz	150	0	37
Starlight Mints, 3 pieces, 0.5 oz	60	0	15
Suckers (Walgreens), 1 piece, 0.4 oz	45	0	11
Sugar Babies, Original, 1.4 oz	160	1.5	37
Sugar Coated Peanuts, 1 oz	120	8	10
Sunbursts Sunflowers (Kimmie):			
Choco Rocks Milk, 1.4 oz	210	10	27
Kettle Corn Nuggets, 1.4 oz	200	9	29
Sunburst Milk, 1.4 oz	210	11	23
Swedish Fish, 7 pieces, 1.5 oz	150	0	38
SweeTARTS:			
Orig., 8 pieces, 0.5 oz	50	0	13
Mini Chewy, 23 pieces, 0.5 oz	50	0.5	12
Symphony (Hershey's):			
Milk Choc: 1.5 oz bar	220	14	23
Large Block: 5 pieces, 1.4 oz	200	12	22
W/ Alm. & Toffee, 5 pcs, 1.3 oz	200	13	21

Per Piece/Serving

	C	F	Cb
Taffy,			
Fruit Chews, 1 piece	20	0.5	4
Take 5 (Hershey's): Orig., 1.5oz	200	11	25
King Size, 2.3 oz	300	16	37
Snack Size, 2 pcs, 1 oz	150	8	19
3 Musketeers:			
Original, 1.9 oz	240	7	42
2 To Go, 1 bar, 1.6 oz	200	6	35
Fun Size, 3 bars, 1.6 oz	190	6	34
Minis, 7 pieces, 1.4 oz	170	5	32
Tang-a-Roos, 1 roll	25	0	6
Terry's: Chocolate Orange (5), 1.5 oz	230	12	27
Dark Chocolate Orange (5), 1.5 oz	240	13	28
Tic Tac, all varieties, 1 piece	2	0	0
Toblerone: 1.3 oz bar	190	10	22
1.8 oz bar	270	15	31
3.5 oz bar	540	30	63
5.3 oz Package, 5 pieces, 1.5 oz	230	13	27
Toffees, Regular, 1 oz	160	9	18
Tootsie Pops, (1), 0.6 oz	60	0	15
Tootsie Roll: 2.3 oz roll	245	2	55
Midgees, 1.4 oz	140	3	28
Truffles: Reg., 1 piece, 0.4 oz	60	4	6
Large (Godiva), 1 piece	110	6.5	12
Extra Large (J.Schmidt), 1.5 oz	220	13	24
Turtles: Original, 1 piece, 0.6 oz	85	5	10
Sugar Free, 1 piece, 0.4 oz	50	3.5	7
Twists, Licorice; Strawb., sugar free, 7 pieces, 1.4 oz	90	0	25
Twix:			
Caramel: 2 cookies, 1.8 oz	250	12	34
Fun Size, 2 cookies, 1.7 oz	250	14	27
4 To Go, 1 cookie, 0.8 oz	110	5	15
6 To Go, 1 cookie, 0.5 oz	80	4	11
Minis, 3 pieces, 1 oz	150	7	20
Peanut Butter:			
Single, 2 cookies, 1.7 oz	250	14	27
4 to Go, 1 cookie, 0.8 oz	250	12	34
Twizzlers: Cherry Bites (17), 1.4 oz	140	0.5	32
Cherry Nibs, 29 pieces, 1.4 oz	140	1	32
Pull 'n' Peel, Cherry, 1 piece, 1.2 oz	110	0.5	26
Twists Strawb., 1.3 oz	120	0.5	29
U-No Bar, 1.5 oz	250	17	22
Weight Watchers (Whitman's):			
Caramel Medallions (3)	160	9	24
Coconut (3)	150	9	23
English Toffee Squares (3)	150	9	21
Mint Patties (3)	150	9	23
Peanut Butter Cups (4)	180	8	31
Pecan Crowns (3)	160	10	24

Candy ~ Brands & Generic (Cont)

Per Piece/Serving

	C	F	Cb
Werther's:			
Hard Candy: Original (3), 0.5 oz	70	1.5	14
Sugar-Free Original (5)	40	1.5	15
Note: Carb figure includes 14g sugar alcohol			
Soft, Chocolate Caramel (4), 1.4 oz	190	8	28
Whatchamacallit: 1.5 oz Bar	230	12	28
King Size Bar, 2.5 oz	370	20	45
Whitman's, Boxed Chocolates:			
Sampler (4), 1.6 oz	220	12	27
12 oz Box, 3 pieces, 1.2 oz	170	9	21
Reserve, 7 oz Box, 2 pieces, 1.2 oz	160	9	21
Sugar Free, 10 oz Box, 3 pcs, 1.5 oz	190	13	25
Whoppers, av. all varieties, 18 pcs	190	7	31
Wonka:			
Bar (1), 2.5 oz	360	19	49
Exceptional Bars, average, 4 pieces	200	13	23
Gobstopper, 9 pieces, 0.5 oz	60	0	14
Laffy Taffy: Ropes, all var., 0.8 oz	80	1.5	18
Stretchy & Tangy, all var., 1.5 oz	150	3.5	29
Nerds, Giant, Chewy, 1.8 oz package	180	0	42
Yogurt Candy,			
Coated Raisins, 27 pieces, 1.4 oz	180	8	28
York: Mints, (3)	10	0	3
Peppermint Pattie, reg, 1.4 oz	140	2.5	31
Pieces (50)	170	6	34
Zagnut, 1.75 oz bar	220	9	35
Zero Bar: 1.8 oz bar	230	8	37
King Size, 3.5 oz	400	14	68

Gum

Per Piece

	C	F	Cb
Bazooka	15	0	4
Beechies	6	0	2
Big League Chews	10	0	2
Bubble Yum: Original	25	0	6
Sugarless	10	0	2
Candilicious	30	0	7
Carefree, Sugarless/Regular	5	0	2
Chiclet	5	0	1
Dentyne	5	0	0.5
Double Bubble Ball	20	0	5
Estee, Bubble/Regular	5	0	2
Extra (Wrigley's), Sugar-Free	5	0	2
Freshen-Up	10	0	2
Hubba Bubba: Regular	25	0	6
Sugar-free, average	14	0	0.5
Ice Breakers	5	0	2
Jolt Gum	5	0	2
Super Bubble	15	0	4
Trident, Orig.; White	5	0	0
Wrigley's, all flavors	10	0	2

Carob Candy

Per Piece/Serving

	C	F	Cb
Carob, Plain/Natural, 1 oz	155	9	15
Carob Coated: Raisins, 1 oz	130	8	15
Almonds/Peanuts, 1 oz	150	10	14
Caramels, 1 oz	110	4	18
Dates, 1 oz	125	5	20
Malt Balls, 1 oz	135	8	15
Soybeans	145	9	16
Trail/Party Mix, 1 oz	150	9	15

Cough Drops

Per Drop/Piece

	C	F	Cb
Beech Nut, 1 drop	10	0	4
CVS, Honey Lemon Cough Drops	15	0	4
Diabetic Tussin	0	0	4
Halls, Defense Vitamin C: Regular	15	0	4
Sugar Free	5	0	3
Fruit Breezers	15	0	4
Menthol Drops: Regular	15	0	4
Sugar Free	5	0	4
Plus	20	0	5
Listerine (Amer. Chicle), Lozenge	10	0	2
Luden's, Throat Drops: Reg., all var.	10	0	2
Sugar Free	0	0	2
Pine Bros, Cough Drops	10	0	2
Ricola, Cough Drops:			
Natural Herbs	10	0	3
Sugar-Free Lemon Mint	0	0	1
Rolaids, Sodium Free	5	0	1
Sathers, Peppermint Lozenges	15	0	3
Sucrets (Beecham), Lozenges	10	0	2.5
Wintergreen, Lozenges	15	0	3

Eat at least 5 servings of fruit and vegetables every day . . . and Enjoy Better Health!

C Cheese

Quick Guide · C · F · Cb

Firm/Hard Cheeses
American, Cheddar, Jack, Swiss:
Average All Brands
Regular Cheese:

	C	F	Cb
Thin Deli slice, 0.8 oz	80	6	0.5
1 oz slice/piece	110	9	0.5
8 oz package	880	72	3
Cubes: 1" cube, 0.6 oz	70	5.5	0.5
1¼" cube, 1 oz	115	9	0.5
Diced, 1 cup, 4.5 oz	510	41	3
Melted, ¼ cup, 2 oz	245	20	1
Shredded: ¼ cup, 1 oz	110	9	0.5
1 cup, 4 oz	440	36	2

Cheese & Cheese Products

Per 1 oz Unless Indicated

	C	F	Cb
Almond (Lisanatti), Chunks, average	50	1	3
American:			
Regular: 1 slice, 1 oz	105	9	0.5
Kraft, Regular, 0.67 oz slice	60	4.5	1
Land O'Lakes, 1 oz slice	100	9	2
Reduced Fat:			
Alpine Lace, Yellow/White, 0.8 oz	90	6	1
Borden, 1 slice, 0.8 oz	50	3	2
Kraft, 2% Milk, Deli Deluxe, 0.67 oz	60	4	1
Land O Lakes, 2% Milk, 1 oz	90	6	1
Babybel (Laughing Cow), Mini:			
Original (1), 0.8 oz	70	6	0
Light (1), 0.8 oz	50	3	0
Bonbel (1), 0.8 oz	70	6	0
Light Original (1), 0.8 oz	50	3	0
Gouda (1), 0.8 oz	80	6	0
Blue/Bleu: *Average all Brands*			
Crumbled, ¼ cup, 1 oz	100	8	1
Light, 0.8 oz	35	1.5	2
Brie: Average, 1 oz	95	8	0
Alouette,			
Baby Brie Wedge, 1 oz	110	10	1
Camembert, 1 oz	85	7	0
Caraway, 1 oz	105	8	1
Castello, 1 oz	120	12	0
Cheddar:			
Regular: Medium/Sharp, av., 1 oz	110	9	1
Shredded, ¼ cup, 1 oz	110	9	1
Cracker Barrel: Extra Sharp, 1 oz	120	10	0
Sharp, Shreds, 1 oz	110	9	1

Cheese & Cheese Products (Cont)

Per 1 oz Unless Indicated · C · F · Cb

	C	F	Cb
Cheddar (Cont):			
Reduced Fat,			
2% Milk, Shredded:			
Borden, ¼ cup, 1 oz	80	6	0
Cracker Barrell, 1 oz	80	6	1
Cheese Curds:			
Fresh: ¼ cup, 1 oz	110	9	0
1 cup, 4 oz	440	36	0
Breaded & Fried:			
A&W, 5 oz	570	40	27
Culver's, Wisconsin, 6.7 oz	670	38	54
Cheese Logs (Kaukana), average	90	6	4
Cheese Whiz:			
Original, 2 Tbsp, 1 oz	90	7	4
Light, 2 Tbsp, 1 oz	80	3.5	6
Salsa Con Queso,			
2 Tbsp, 1 oz	90	7	4
Cheshire, 1 oz	110	9	1.5
Colby, Regular, 1 oz	110	8	1
Colby-Jack:			
Regular, 1 oz	110	9	1
Kraft, 2% Milk, 1 oz	60	4	0
Cottage Cheese: *Average All Brands*			
Creamed (4% milk fat):			
2 Tbsp, 1 oz	30	1	1.5
½ cup, 4 oz	110	5	4
With fruit, ½ cup, 4 oz	115	4	5
Reduced-Fat (2%): 2 Tbsp, 1 oz	25	0.5	1
½ cup, 4 oz	100	3	4
Low-Fat (1%): 2 Tbsp, 1 oz	20	0.5	1
½ cup, 4 oz	80	1	3
Fat-Free/Non-Fat: 2 T., 1 oz	20	0	1
½ cup, 4 oz	80	0	5
Cottage Cheese: *Brands*			
Fiber One, 1% Fat, ½ c., 4 oz	80	2	8
Friendship:			
1% Low-Fat with Pineapple, 4 oz	120	1	16
Nonfat with Pineapple, ½ cup, 4 oz	110	0	17
Pot Style, 2%, ½ cup, 4 oz	90	2.5	3
Hood, with Chive/Onion, 4 oz	90	1	5
Knudsen/Breakstone's:			
Free, Non-Fat, ½ cup, 4 oz	70	0	7
2% Milk Fat, ½ cup, 4 oz	100	2.5	6
On the Go!,			
Low-Fat, 4 oz carton	90	2.5	6
Lactaid, Low-Fat, ½ cup, 4 oz	80	1	7
Light n' Lively:			
Fat-Free, ½ cup, 4.4 oz	80	0	8
Low-Fat, ½ cup, 4.4 oz	80	1.5	6

Cheese & Cheese Products (Cont)

Per 1 oz Unless Indicated **C · F · Cb**

Item	C	F	Cb
Cream Cheese: *Average All Brands*			
Regular/Soft:			
2 Tbsp, 1 oz	95	10	1
3 oz package	290	29	3.5
8 oz package	780	78	9
Light, Plain, 1 oz	60	4.5	2.5
Fat-Free, Plain, 1 oz	30	0	2
Easy Cheese (Kraft),			
American, 2 Tbsp, 1.2 oz	90	6	2
Edam, 1 oz	100	8	0.5
Farmer, Low-Fat, 1 oz	40	2.5	0
Feta: Regular, 1 oz	75	6	1
Crumbled, ½ cup, 2.5 oz	190	15	3
Athenos, Reduced-Fat,			
1 oz	60	4	1
Fontina, 2 Tbsp, 1 oz	110	9	0.5
Galaxy, *Cheese Substitute:*			
Grated Parmesan Flavor, 2 tsp, 0.2 oz	15	0	1
Rice, Mozzarella flavor, 1 sl., 0.6 oz	40	2.5	0.5
Veggy, all varieties, 1 slice, 0.5 oz	40	2.5	0.5
Goat's Milk Cheese:			
Chevre: Original, 2 Tbsp	75	6	0.5
Semi-Soft, 1 oz	100	8.5	1
Hard, 1 oz	130	10	0.5
Chavrie: Regular, 2 Tbsp, 1 oz	50	3.5	1
Caramelized Onion, 2 Tbsp	50	3	4
Logs, average all varieties, 1 oz	80	7	3
Gjetost, fresh, 1 oz	130	8	12
Myzithra, grated, 1 oz	80	4	2
Gorgonzola, 1 oz	100	8	0.5
Galbani, Dolcelatte, 1 oz	95	8	1
Gouda, 1 oz slice	100	8	0.5
Gruyere, 1 oz	115	9	1
Handi-Snacks (Kraft):			
Breadsticks 'n Cheez Single, 1 oz	110	4.5	14
Ritz Crackers 'n Cheez Dip, 1 oz	100	6	11
Havarti (Land O'Lakes), 0.8 oz	80	7	0
Italian Pasta Blend (Sargento), 1 oz	90	6	3
Jarlsberg: Average, 1 oz	100	8	0
Reduced Fat, shredded, 1 oz	70	3.5	0
Labneh, (Lebanese Cream Chse) 1.8 oz	70	4	4

Cheese & Cheese Products (Cont)

Per 1 oz Unless Indicated **C · F · Cb**

Item	C	F	Cb
Laughing Cow, Wedges:			
Original Creamy Swiss (1)	50	4	1
Light Varieties, av., (1)	35	2	2
Lifetime, Cholesterol Reducing,			
Low Fat, all varieties, 1 Slice, 1 oz	45	1.5	1
Limburger, 1 oz	95	8	0
Mascarpone, av., 1 oz	125	13	0.5
Mexican:			
Cacique: Asadero, sliced	70	5	1
Cotija	100	8	0
Enchilado; Manchego	90	7	0
Panela	80	6	0
Queso Fresco	80	6	0
Queso Quesadilla	90	7	0
Ranchero	80	6	0
Chi-Chi's, Salsa Con Quéso, Mild	45	3	4
El Mexicano: Asadero, Regular	90	7	0
Cotija, Regular	110	9	0
Kraft, Mexican Four Cheese; Taco,			
Shredded,	100	8	1
Sargento, 4 Cheese Mexican	110	9	1
Supremo: Quéso Chihuaha, 1 oz	100	8	0
Quéso Oaxaca	80	5	1
Monterey Jack:			
Regular, shredded, 1 oz	100	8	1
Alpine Lace, Co-Jack, 1 oz	70	5	0
Kraft, 1 oz	100	8	1
Mozzarella:			
Regular: Average 1 oz	85	6.5	0.5
Land O'Lakes/Polly-O:			
Slice, average, 1 oz	90	6	1
Shredded, 1 oz	90	6	1
Fat-Free:			
Kraft, Shredded, 1 oz	45	0	2
Light:			
Kraft, 2% Milk Fat, Reduced Fat	70	4	1
Polly-O Lite, Shredded, 1 oz	60	2.5	1
Part Skim:			
Alpine Lace, 25% Reduced Fat	60	4	1
Borden/Kraft, Shredded	80	5	2
Kraft, String	80	6	0
Muenster:			
Regular, 1 oz	105	9	0.5
Low-Fat, 1 oz	85	5	1

Cheese & Cheese Products (Cont)

Per 1 oz Unless Indicated

	C	F	Cb
Parmesan:			
Fresh/Block, Dry, 1 oz	110	7.5	1
Grated (Packaged): 1 Tbsp	20	1.5	0
1 oz	120	8	1
½ cup, 1.8 oz	215	14	2
Kraft, Reduced-Fat Topping, 1 Tbsp	20	1	2
Philadelphia:			
Cream Cheese: Original, 2 T. 1 oz	100	9	1
3 oz package	300	27	3
Regular, 1 oz	90	9	2
Creme, Cooking, av. all var., ¼ cup	110	9	4
Flavored:			
Blueberry, 1 oz	80	6	5
Honey Nut; Strawberry, av., 1 oz	80	7	5
Garden Vegetable, 1 oz	80	7	2
Salmon, 1 oz	70	7	1
Light, Plain, 1 oz	70	5	2
⅓ Less Fat: Plain, 2 T., 1 oz	70	6	2
Garden Veggie; Chive & On., 1 oz	70	5	2
Neufchatel, 2 T., 1 oz	70	6	1
Fat-Free, Plain, 1 oz	30	0	2
Indulgence:			
Milk/White Chocolate:			
1 Tbsp, 0.6 oz	60	3.5	6
Mini Tub, 1.3 oz	125	7	13
8 oz container	800	47	80
Dark Chocolate, 1 T., 0.6 oz	55	3.5	6
Spread: Regular, 1 oz	80	7	2
Flavors, average, 1.2 oz	80	6	5
Whipped:			
Regular, 0.8 oz	60	5	2
Mixed Berry, 0.7 oz	70	5	3
Pizza Four Cheese, shredded,			
Kraft/Sargento, Regular, av., 1 oz	90	7	1
Port de Salut, 1 oz	100	8	0
Port Wine *(Kaukauna/WisPride):*			
8 oz Tub: Average, 1 oz	85	7	3
Lite, 2 Tbsp, average, 1 oz	60	3	5
Ball, 1 oz	100	6	4
Log, 1 oz	100	7	4
Provolone: Regular, 1 oz	100	7.5	0.5
Alpine Lace, Reduced-Fat, 0.8 oz	60	4.5	0
Sargento, Deli Style 1 slice, 0.67 oz	50	3	0
Pub *(Rondele)*, average all varieties	75	7	1
Quark: 40% fat	45	3	1
20% fat	30	1.5	1
Skim/Non-Fat	20	0	1.5
Queso:			
Anejo/Asadero/Blanco, 1 oz	105	9	1
Chichuahua/De Papa, 1 oz	110	9	2
Rice Cheese Chunks *(Lisanatti)*,			
average, 1 oz	60	3	2
Swiss *(Lifetime)*, Fat Free, 1 oz	40	0	1

Cheese & Cheese Products (Cont)

Per 1 oz Unless Indicated

	C	F	Cb
Ricotta Cheese:			
Whole Milk: 1 oz	50	3.5	1
½ cup, 4.5 oz	215	16	4
Part Skim: 1 oz	40	2	1.5
½ cup, 4.5 oz	170	10	6
Light/Low-Fat: 1 oz	25	1	1.5
½ cup, 4.5 oz	125	5	6
Fat-Free, ½ cup, 4.5 oz	100	0	10
Baked Ricotta, 2 oz	130	9	3
Romano: Block/Loaf	110	8	1
Grated: 1 oz	120	9	1
1 Tbsp, 0.2 oz	20	1.5	0
Roquefort, 1 oz	105	9	0.5
Sheep's Milk, (Manchego),			
Trader Joes/Wegman's, 1 oz	120	10	0
Soy Cheese:			
Trader Joe's, Cheddar flavor, 0.7 oz	45	2	3
Soy Kaas: Cheddar, 1 oz	50	2	8
Monterey Jack, 1 oz	60	4	0
Soy Sation, Chunks,			
all varieties, 1 oz	60	3	2
Smoked Cheddar, average, 1 oz	110	10	0
Stilton, average, 1 oz	110	10	0
String:			
Regular, average all brands	80	6	0.5
Kraft, Twist-Ums & String-ums,			
Super Long, 1 stick, 1.1 oz	90	6	1
Light/Lite:			
Frigo, String	60	2.5	0.5
Polly-O, String,			
2% Red-Fat, 0.8 oz	60	2.5	0
Sargento: 1 piece, 0.8 oz	50	2.5	1
Part Skim, 0.9 oz	70	4.5	1
Swiss: Regular, 1 oz	110	8	1.5
Alpine Lace, Reduced-Fat, 0.8 oz	70	4.5	1
Kraft Singles, 2% Milk, 0.67 oz	45	2.5	2
Tilsit, 1 oz	100	7.5	0.5
Tybo, 1 oz	100	7	0.5
Tofutti, Better Than Cream Cheese,			
all varieties, 1 oz	85	5	9
Velveeta *(Kraft):*			
Original, 1 oz	80	5	3
Reduced Fat, 2% Milk, 1 oz	60	3	4
Extra Thick, 1 oz	100	7	3
Mexican: Hot, 1 oz	90	6	3
Mild, 1 oz	80	6	3

Dips/Spreads　C　F　Cb

Per 2 Tbsp, 1 oz, Unless Indicated
Average All Brands

	C	F	Cb
Avocado/Guacamole	45	4	2
Baba Ghanoush (Eggplant/Sesame)	70	6	2
Cheese Fondue, ½ cup, 4 oz	260	15	4
French Onion Dip	60	4.5	3
Hummus: 2 Tbsp	50	1	5
½ cup, 4.5 oz	220	4.5	23
Tzatziki (Cucumber/Yogurt)	30	2.5	2
Clearman's, Original Spread	150	16	0
De La Casa, 5 Layer Party Dip	45	2.5	4

Fritos: *Per 2 Tbsp*
Dips:

	C	F	Cb
Chili Cheese	45	3	3
Bean; Hot Bean w/ Jalap.	35	1	5
Jalapeno Cheddar Cheese	50	3.5	3

Guiltless Gourmet,

	C	F	Cb
Black Bean/Spicy Black Bean Dip	40	0	7

Heluva Good Cheese,

	C	F	Cb
French Onion Dip, 2 Tbsp	50	4.5	2

Hidden Valley,

	C	F	Cb
For Everything Topping, av.	130	14	3

Kaukauna *(Wisconsin)*:
Spreadable Cheddar:

	C	F	Cb
Sharp/Smokey Cheddar	90	7	3
Cheese Balls, all varieties	100	6	4
Cheese Logs, all varieties	100	7	4

Kemps: *Per 2 Tbsp*
Dips:

	C	F	Cb
French Onion	60	5	2
Ranch Style	60	5	2
Top The Tater,			
Taco Fiesta; Veggie Ranch	60	5	3
Kroger, Dips, all varieties	60	5	2

Kraft: *Per 2 Tbsp*
Dips:

	C	F	Cb
Average all varieties	60	5	3
Cheez Whiz: Original	90	7	4
Light	80	3.5	6
Salsa Con Queso	90	7	4

Spreads:

	C	F	Cb
Olive & Pimento, 1.2 oz	70	6	3
Old English Sharp; Roka Blue, av	85	8	2

Marzetti: *Per 2 Tbsp*
Dips:

	C	F	Cb
Choc Fruit, 1.4 oz	110	1	25
Caramel Apple, fat free, 1.4 oz	100	1	25
Veggie: Dill, Light, 1 oz	60	5	2
Ranch, Singles, 1.5 oz	180	18	2.5
Ranch, Fat-Free, 1 oz	30	0	6

Dips/Spreads (Cont)　C　F　Cb

Per 2 Tbsp, 1 oz, Unless Indicated
Marie's:

	C	F	Cb
Dips: Buttermilk Ranch; Crmy Dill. av.	100	10	2
Guacamole	40	3	3
Nalley's, Ranch Chip Dip	100	10	2

Naturally Fresh: *Per 2 Tbsp*
Dips:

	C	F	Cb
Chocolate	70	0	12
Cream Cheese Strawb.	90	3.5	14
Caramel	100	4	16

Old Dutch:
Dips:

	C	F	Cb
French Onion, 1 oz	50	3	5
Mild Cheddar, 1 oz	40	3	4
Nacho Cheese, 1 oz	35	2.5	2

Old El Paso: *Per 2 Tbsp*
Dips:

	C	F	Cb
Cheese & Red Pepper	35	2	3.5
Thick N' Chunky Salsa	10	0	2.5

Price's: *Per 2 Tbsp*
Dips:

	C	F	Cb
Pimiento Cheese	85	7	3
Light Pimiento	55	3	3
Zesty Jalapeno	75	6	2.5

Stop & Shop: *Per 2 Tbsp*
Dips:

	C	F	Cb
Veggie	100	10	3
Sour Cream French Onion	60	4.5	3

TGI Fridays,

	C	F	Cb
Spinach, Cheese & Artichoke Dip	30	1.5	3
Toby's, Tofu Pate, 2 Tbsp	80	7	2

Tostitos: *Per 2 Tbsp*
Dips:

	C	F	Cb
Creamy Spinach, 1 oz	50	4	2
Salsa Con Quéso	40	2.5	5
Smooth & Cheesy, 1 oz	50	3.5	4

Wise: *Per 2 Tbsp*
Dips:

	C	F	Cb
French Onion, 1.2 oz	60	5	3
Ranch, 1.2 oz	50	4	3

New Diet Aid
- The Refrigerator Air Bag!

POOF!

Condiments, Sauces | C | F | Cb

Average of Brands & Homemade

Apple Sauce:

	C	F	Cb
Sweetened, ¼ cup, 2.5 oz	55	0	13
Unsweetened, ¼ cup, 2 oz	25	0	7

Barbecue Sauce:

	C	F	Cb
Regular, all flavors, 2 Tbsp, 1 oz	40	0	10
Bull's Eye, Original, 1 oz	60	0	14
Bearnaise Sauce, ¼ cup, 2.5 oz	190	19	5
Buffalo Wing Sce: Hon. Mustard, 1 T.	40	3	3
Average other varieties, 1 Tbsp	25	2	2
Cheese, h/made, ¼ cup, 2.5 oz	150	10	12
Chef-Mate, Hot Dog, ¼ cup	70	2.5	9
Chili Sauce (Heinz), 1 Tbsp	20	0	5
Cocktail Sauce, ¼ cup	110	0	15
Walden Farms, Fat-Free, 1 Tbsp	0	0	0
Cranberry Sauce, av. all varieties: 2 T.	45	0	11
¼ cup, 2.5 oz	110	0	27
Demi Glaze Gold, 2 tsp	30	0.5	3
Honey Mustard (French's), 2 Tbsp	60	0.5	12
Horseradish: 1 tsp	2	0	0
Kraft, 1 tsp	15	1.5	1

Ketchup:

	C	F	Cb
Regular, 1 Tbsp	15	0	4
Heinz, Reduced Sugar, 1 Tbsp	5	0	1
Simply Heinz, 1 Tbsp	20	0	5

Mole:

	C	F	Cb
Dona Maria, av. all varieties., 2 T.	150	10	10
Rogelio Bueno, 2 Tbsp, 1 oz	160	11	12
Mushroom Sce, ½ cup, 2 oz	50	2	5
Mustard, average, 1 tsp	5	0	0.5
Pesto Sauce, ¼ cup, 2 oz	270	28	2
Pizza Sauce, ¼ cup, 2 oz	30	0	6
Seafood Cocktail Sce, ¼ cup	60	0	15
Soy Sauce: Average all, 1 Tbsp	10	0	1
Kikkoman, Lite Soy, 1 Tbsp	10	0	1
Spaghetti Sce, ½ cup, 4.5 oz	135	6	19

Steak Sauce:

	C	F	Cb
Kraft, A1, 1 Tbsp, 0.5 oz	15	0	3
Lea & Perrins, 1 Tbsp, 0.5 oz	20	0	5
Strawb. Puree Sauce, Unsweet., 2 T.	10	0	2

Sweet & Sour Sauce:

	C	F	Cb
Contadina, 1.2 oz	40	1	8
Kraft, 1 Tbsp	60	0	13
Tabasco Sauce, 1 tsp	2	0	0
Taco Sauce, average all, 2 Tbsp, 1 oz	10	0	1

Tartar Sauce: (Heinz), 2 Tbsp, 1 oz

	C	F	Cb
(Heinz), 2 Tbsp, 1 oz	120	11	4
Hellmann's, Regular, 2 Tbsp, 1 oz	80	7	4
McCormick, Fat-Free, 2 Tbsp, 1 oz	30	0	7
Teriyaki Sauce (Kikkoman), 1 T., 0.5 oz	15	0	2
Vinegar, White or Wine, 2 T.	4	0	1
White Sauce, ½ cup, 5 oz	130	7	10
Worcestershire Sauce, 1 tsp	5	0	1

Pickles & Relish | C | F | Cb

Average All Brands

	C	F	Cb
Bread & Butter Pickles, 4 sl.,1 oz	25	0	6
Chutney, 2 Tbsp, 1.25 oz	50	0.5	11

Dill Pickles:

	C	F	Cb
Slices, 4 slices, 1 oz	4	0	1
1 large, (3¾"x 1¼" diam.), 2.25 oz	12	0	3
Extra large (4"x 1¾" diam.), 5 oz	30	0	6
Halves: Small, 1 oz	3	0	0.5
Large, 2.5 oz	8	0	2
Gherkins, sweet, 1 medium, 1 oz	30	0	7
Green Chiles, chopped, 2 Tbsp	5	0	1
Horseradish, 1 Tbsp	10	0	2
Jalapenos, pickled (2), 2 oz	10	0.5	2
Jalapeno Relish, 1 Tbsp, 0.5 oz	5	0	1
Mustard, av. all brands, 1 tsp	5	0	0.5
Peppers, Hot/Mild (1), 1.5 oz	20	0	4
Pickled: Beets, ½ cup, 4 oz	75	0	19
Cocktail Onion, 1 onion	2	0	0
Red Cabbage, ½ cup, 3 oz	65	0	15
Pickles: Sweet, 2 Tbsp, 1 oz	35	0	8
Large (3" x ¾ diam.),1.25 oz	40	0	10
Pickle in a Pouch, 1 large	12	0	3

Relishes:

	C	F	Cb
Cranberry-Orange, 1 Tbsp	30	0	7
Hot Dog (Heinz), 1 T., 0.5 oz	17	0	3
S'wich Spread, 1 tsp	20	1	5
Sweet Pickle, 1 Tbsp, 0.5 oz	20	0	5
Sweet Cauliflower, 1 tsp	35	0	8
Sugar Free Relish, 1 tsp	5	0	1
Sweet Gherkins (2), 1 oz	5	0	1
Sauerkraut, Drained, 1 cup, 5 oz	25	0	6

Salsa

Average all Types:

	C	F	Cb
Regular, w/out oil, 2 T., 1 oz	15	0	3.5
Made with oil, 2 Tbsp, 1 oz	40	3	8
La Victoria, 2 Tbsp, 1 oz	10	0	2
Old El Paso, 1 Tbsp, 1 oz	10	0	3
TGI Friday's, 1.2 oz	15	0	4

Quick Guide

C **F** **Cb**

Cookies:
Average All Brands: Per Cookie

	C	F	Cb
Biscotti: Small, 0.5 oz	70	3	10
Regular, 1 oz	140	6.5	18
Chocolate Chip:			
Small/Thin, 0.5 oz	70	3.5	9
Regular, 1 oz	140	7	18
Large (*Mrs Fields*), 3 oz	350	17	45
Extra Large, 4 oz	555	28	73
Oatmeal/Oatmeal Raisin:			
Small/Thin, 0.5 oz	65	2.5	10
Regular, 1 oz	130	5	20
Large (*Mrs Fields*), 2.5 oz	330	14	44
Extra Large, 4 oz	510	20	78
Peanut Butter:			
Small/Thin, 0.5 oz	70	3.5	9
Regular, 1 oz	135	7	17
Large (*Mrs Fields*), 2.5 oz	330	17	41
Extra Large, 4 oz	540	27	67
Low-Fat Cookies:			
Choc Chip (Low-Fat), (1), 0.5 oz	65	2	10
Oatmeal Raisin (Fat-Free), (1), 1 oz	95	0.5	22
Peanut Butter (Low-Fat), (1), 1 oz	105	5	15

Quick Guide

Crackers
Average All Brands: Per Cracker Unless Indicated

	C	F	Cb
Cheese Crackers:			
Plain: 1" square	5	0	0.5
Bag, single serving, 1 oz	140	7	16
Cheese/P'nut Butter filled	30	1.5	4
Crispbread, Rye	35	0	8
Grahams, 2½" square	30	0.5	5
Melba Toast, Plain, 1 piece	20	0	4
Matzo, Plain, 1 oz	110	0.5	23
Oyster/Soup, ½ cup	95	2	17
Rice: 1 crackers	70	1.5	11
Oriental Style, 1 oz	130	3.5	23
Saltines, 5 crackers	65	2	11
Snack-type, 1 round cracker	15	1	2
Soda Crackers (*Saltine*), 2	25	1	4.5
Water Cracker (*Carr's*), Original	15	0.5	2.5
Wheat:			
Wheat Thins	10	0.5	1.5
Cheese/Peanut Butter filled	35	2	4

Cookies & Crackers ~ Brands

Per Cookie/Cracker, Unless indicated **C** **F** **Cb**

	C	F	Cb
Albertsons:			
Animal Crackers (6), 1 oz	130	3.5	22
Chocolate Chip:			
Original (3), 1 oz	150	7	20
Chewy (2), 1 oz	130	6	18
Chunky (1), 0.5 oz	80	3.5	10
Chocolate S'wich Cremes: (3) 1 oz	150	6	25
Double Filled (2), 1 oz	140	6	22
Fudge Graham (3), 1 oz	140	7	18
Fudge Wafer (3), 1 oz	140	8	18
Fudge Marshmallow Ring	120	5	19
Pinwheels, Chocolate Marshmallow	120	5	20
Vanilla Wafers (9), 1 oz	140	4	25
Graham: Cinnamon (2)	150	3	28
Honey (2), 1 oz	140	2	28
Annie's:			
Bunny Grahams:			
Chocolate; Choc Chip, 1 oz	130	4.5	21
Cinnamon, 1 oz	140	4.5	23
Friends, 1 oz	120	4	20
Honey, 1 oz	140	4.5	23
Gluten Free: Cocoa & Vanilla, 1 oz	120	3.5	22
Ginger Snaps; SnickerDoodles, 1 oz	130	4	21
Cheddar Bunnies:			
Regular: 1 oz Snack Pack	140	6	19
7.5 oz Box	1050	45	145
Sour Cream & Onion, 1 oz	150	7	19
White Cheddar, 1 oz	140	6	19
Whole Wheat, 1 oz	140	6	19
Austin:			
Sandwich Crackers: *Per Package*			
Cheese: With Cheddar Cheese	190	10	23
With Peanut Butter	190	10	23
Chocolate Peanut Butter	190	8	26
Toasty, with Peanut Butter	190	9	23
Barbara's Bakery:			
Fig Bars: Raspberry, 1.4 oz	120	0	27
Wheat/Multigrain	110	0.5	26
Snackimals:			
Choc Chip, 1 oz	120	4	19
Double Choc.; P'nut Butter, av., 1 oz	145	6	22
Bear Naked:			
Soft-Baked Granola,			
Double Choc.; Fruit & Nut, av.	130	6	19

Cookies & Crackers ~ Brands (Cont)

Per Cookie/Cracker, Unless Indicated **C** **F** **Cb**

BelVita *(Nabisco):*
Breakfast Biscuits:

	C	F	Cb
Crunchy, 1 pack (4 biscuits), average	230	8	36
Soft Baked, 1 biscuit, average	190	7	32

Blue Diamond:
Nut Thins, (17), average all varieties	130	3	23
Artisan Nut Thins, (13), av. all var.	130	3.5	22

Brent & Sam's: *Per 2 Cookies*
Natural: Choc. Chip Pecan	130	7	14
Key Lime White Chocolate	120	6	16
Triple Chocolate Bliss, 1 oz	120	6	16

Carr's: Ginger Lemon Cremes (2)
	140	6	21
Poppy & Sesame Crackers(4)	80	4	10
Rosemary Crackers(4)	70	2.5	11
Whole Wheat Crackers (2)	80	4	10

Cheez-It ~ *See Sunshine, Page 87*
Chips Ahoy! ~ *See Nabisco, Page 85*
Country Choice:
Sandwich Cremes (2),
all varieties	130	5	19

Snacking:
Ginger Snaps (5); Vanilla Wafers (7)	140	4	22
Iced Oatmeal (4)	120	4	21

Dr. Kracker:
Crispbread:
100% Whole Wheat (1)	80	1	16
Average other varieties (1)	100	4	12
Snackers, average all varieties (8)	125	5	15

Erin Baker's:
Original Breakfast: *Per 3 oz*
Banana Walnut	300	8	53
Peanut Butter	320	11	49

Minis: *Per 1 oz Cookie*
Peanut Butter	110	3.5	16
Dble Chocolate; Oatmeal Raisin, av.	100	2	18

Famous Amos:
Bite Size: Choc. Chip,
4 Cookies, 1 oz	150	7	20
Choc. Chip & Pecans (4)	150	8	18
Sandwich, Creme Filled:			
Chocolate (3), 1 oz	160	7	25
Vanilla (3), 1 oz	170	7	25

Per Cookie/Cracker, Unless Indicated **C** **F** **Cb**

Fig Newtons ~ *See Nabisco, Page 85*
Fifty50:
Butter (4)	190	9	24
Average other varieties (4)	165	9	22
Wafers, average all varieties, (6)	165	9	22

Gamesa:
Animalitos, 14 cookies, 1 oz	110	1	25
Arcoiris Marshmallow,			
2 oz pkg, 6 cookies	220	5	38
Chocolatines Marshmallow,			
2 cookies, 1 oz	130	5	18
Chokis, Chocolate Chip, 1.4 oz pkg	190	9	27
Emperador: Cream Cookie Sandwich			
Lemon Creme, 1 pkg, 6 cookies	270	8	45
Av. other flavors, 1 pkg, 6 cookies	360	12	57
Fruitbars, average, 1 cookie, 1 oz	110	4.5	18
Giro, 3 cookies, 1 oz	140	6	20
Mamut, Choc Marshmallow,			
1 cookie, 1 oz	130	5	19
Marias, 8 cookies, 1 oz	120	2	24
Sugar Wafers, average, 3 wafers, 1.2 oz	160	7	25

Girl Scouts Cookies:
Caramel DeLites/Samoas (2)	130	6	19
Do-si-dos (3)	160	7	22
Peanut Butter Patties (2)	130	7	15
Savannah Smiles (5)	140	5	23

Goya:
Lady Fingers, 3 cookies	65	0.5	13
Maria, 5 cookies, 1 oz	130	3	24
Wafers, average all flavors,			
4 wafers, 1 oz	150	7	20

Grandma's:
Frosted,
average all flavors (1)	230	9	34

Homestyle: *Per Cookie*
Chocolate Brownie	190	8	21
Chocolate Chip	170	9	22
Oatmeal Raisin	150	6	23
Peanut Butter	170	9	19
Peanut Butter Chocolate Chunks	200	10	22

Sandwich Cremes:
Peanut Butter (5)	200	9	25
Vanilla (5)	190	9	27
Mini's, Vanilla (9)	150	7	22

Cookies & Crackers ~ Brands (Cont)

Per Cookie/Cracker, Unless Indicated

	C	F	Cb
Great American Cookies:			
Chewy Chocolate Supreme	180	7	27
Chewy Pecan Supreme	230	12	31
Double Fudge with Reese's	230	11	33
Original, w/ Reese's M&M's	240	12	31
Peanut Butter w/ M&M's	250	14	29
White Chunk Macadamia	250	14	30
Double Doozies:			
Original, 5.3 oz	690	34	94
M&M Big Bite, 2.5 oz	340	17	46
Cookie Cakes: 16", 3.5 oz	460	22	67
16" M&M, 4 oz	500	24	73
Heart Shaped, 3.5 oz	440	21	64
Great Value *(Walmart):*			
Chocolate Chip, all varieties (1)	160	7	23
Soft Cookies, Fudge & Cream (1)	150	6	22
Twist & Shout, all varieties (1)	140	6	22
Buttery Rounds, Baked (5)	80	4.5	10
Reduced Fat (5)	70	2	11
Cheese, 1 oz	150	8	18
Joseph's:			
Sugar Free: *Per 4 Cookies*			
Almond; Chocolate Walnut, average	95	3.5	14
Chocolate Chip; Pecan Choc. Chip, av.	95	5	14
Average other varieties	95	4	15
Carb figures include 6 grams Maltitol			
Kashi:			
Chocolate Almond Butter	130	5	19
Happy Trail Mix, Chewy	140	5	21
Oatmeal: Dark Chocolate	130	5	20
Raisin Flax	120	4.5	19
Crackers:			
Country Cheddar (18)	130	4.5	20
Fire Roasted Veggie (15)	120	3.5	19
Honey Sesame (15)	120	3	22
Original 7 Grain (15)	120	3.5	19
Toasted Asiago (15)	130	4.5	21
Heart To Heart Whole Grain, Original; Roasted Garlic (7)	120	3.5	22
Pita Crisps:			
Original 7 Grain with Salt (11)	120	3	22
Zesty Salsa (11)	120	3	24

Per Cookie/Cracker, Unless Indicated

	C	F	Cb
Keebler:			
Animals: Frosted (8)	160	7	22
Iced (6)	140	4.5	22
Cinnamon Roll (2), all varieties	150	6	23
Chips Deluxe: Original (2)	160	8	19
Soft & Chewy (2)	160	6	21
Chocolate Lovers (2)	170	9	20
Coconut (2)	160	9	18
Peanut Butter Cups (2)	170	9	19
Rainbow: Choc. Chip (2)	160	8	20
Minis, 1.4 oz package	200	10	27
Danish Wedding, (4)	140	7	19
E.L. Fudge: Original (2)	170	7	25
Double Stuffed (2)	180	9	24
Fudge Shoppe:			
Cheesecake Middles, Orig. Grahams (3)	130	7	17
Deluxe Grahams (3)	140	7	18
Fudge Sticks: Original (3)	150	8	20
Jumbo (1)	160	8	21
Fudge Stripes: Original (2)	140	6	19
Dark Chocolate (3)	150	7	22
Filled Pretzel Bites, Peanut Butter & Fudge, average, 1 pkg	170	9	21
Grasshopper (4)	140	7	20
Mint Creme Middles, Choc. Graham (3)	130	7	17
Gripz, Chips Deluxe, 0.9 oz pouch	120	5	18
Oatmeal (2), average all varieties	140	6	20
Sandies Cookies:			
Dark Choc. Almond; Pecan Shtbrd, av.	170	10	19
Average other varieites	160	9	19
Vienna Fingers:			
Creme Filled (2)	150	6	23
Reduced Fat (2)	140	4.5	24
Wafers: Vanilla (8)	140	5	22
Mini Vanilla (18)	140	5	22
Crackers:			
Club: Original (4)	70	3	9
Reduced Fat (5)	70	2	12
Grahams: Original (8)	120	3.5	22
Honey (8)	140	4.5	23
Town House: Original (5)	90	5	9
Reduced Fat (6)	60	1.5	12

C Cookies ◆ Crackers

Cookies & Crackers ~ Brands (Cont)

Per Cookie/Cracker, Unless Indicated

	C	F	Cb
Kraft, Macaroni & Cheese Crackers,			
av. all varieties, 1. oz	150	7	18
Kroger:			
Chip Mates: Orig. (3), 1.5 oz	150	7	22
Chunky (2), 1 oz	120	6	17
Peanut Butter (2), 1 oz	120	7	15
White Chip (2), 1 oz	120	6	16
Chocolate Sandwich:			
Original (3), 1.2 oz	150	6	24
Chocolate Sandwich (2), 1 oz	150	6	23
Double Filled (2), 1 oz	140	6	22
Olde Southern Pecan Shortbread (2)	150	9	16
Vanilla Wafers (7)	130	3.5	23
Crackers:			
Grahams, Original; Honey, (4)	120	3	20
Saltines, Original (5), 0.5oz	60	1.5	10
Lance:			
Cookies:			
6 Pack: *Per Pack of 6 Cookies*			
Choc-O-Lunch/Van-O-Lunch, av.	225	9	34
Nekot, Peanut Butter	240	11	32
Crackers:			
Cracker Creations: *Per 2 Crackers*			
Five Grain,			
Peanut Butter Filling (2), 1 oz	140	7	16
Granola, all flavors (2), 1.3 oz	190	9	24
Cracker Sandwiches: *Per 6 Crackers*			
Malt, with Peanut Butter Filling	180	8	20
Nip Chee, Cheddar Cheese	190	9	24
Toastchee:			
Peanut Butter	210	10	25
Toasty, Peanut Butter	180	8	21
Wholegrain, Cheddar Cheese	200	9	26
Little Debbie:			
Apple Oatmeal Pies (1)	140	4.5	24
Chocolate Chip Cream Pie (1)	150	6	23
Cookie Wreaths (1)	100	5	12
Marshmallow Puffs (1)	150	5	25
Oatmeal Creme Pie (1)	170	7	26
Star Crunch(1)	150	6	22
Lu:			
Petit Beurre (1), 1.2 oz	140	4	24
Petit Ecolier, av. all var., (1), 0.9 oz	130	6	17
Pim's, Raspberry (1), 0.9 oz	100	3	16
Manischewitz:			
Crackers:			
Tam Tams: Original (10)	110	4	16
Everything; Garlic (1), av.	140	5	20

Mary's Gone Crackers:	C	F	Cb
Cookies:			
Chocolate Chip; Double Choc (2)	130	6	19
Ginger Snaps (3)	140	5	23
"N'Oatmeal" Raisin without Oats (2)	120	4	20
Crackers,			
all varieties (13), 1 oz	140	5	21
Miss Meringue:			
Madeleines:			
Traditional (2), 1.2 oz	160	9	19
Traditional & Dipped (2), 1.2 oz	160	9	18
Meringue Classiques:			
Cappuccino (4), 1 oz	110	0	26
Mint Choc. Chip (4), 1 oz	120	1.5	25
Triple Chocolate (4), 1 oz	120	1.5	25
Vanilla Rainbow/Van. (4), 1 oz	110	0	27
Meringue Minis, Low Fat:			
Mini: Choc. Chip (12), 1 oz	130	1.5	27
Mint Choc. Chip (12), 1 oz	120	1.5	26
Meringue Minis, Fat Free:			
Chocolate (12), 1 oz	110	0	26
Vanilla; Rainbow Vanilla (13), 1 oz	110	0	27
Mother's:			
Chocolate Chip (4), 1 oz	150	7	20
Circus Animal (7), 1 oz	150	7	21
Coconut Cocadas (5), 1.2 oz	160	8	21
Double Fudge (2), 1.3 oz	170	7	27
Iced: Lemonade (4), 1 oz	150	7	19
Oatmeal (4), 1.2 oz	150	6	23
Macaroons (2), 1 oz	170	11	17
Peanut Butter Gauchos (2), 1.3 oz	180	8	25
Taffy; Vanilla Cream (2), av., 1.3 oz	185	8	27
Mrs Fields Cookies ~ *See Page 219*			
Murray:			
Cookies, Sugar Free:			
Fudge-Dipped:			
Grahams (4)	140	8	19
Mint Cookies (4)	130	7	17
Vanilla Wafers (4)	150	10	19
Oatmeal (3)	140	7	21
Peanut Butter (3)	150	9	16
Sandwiches, Lemon Creme (3)	130	7	19
Shortbread (8)	130	5	21
Shortbread Pecan (3)	160	11	18
Vanilla Creme Wafers (4)	130	8	19
Carb figures include 3-9g sugar alcohol			

Cookies & Crackers ~ Brands (Cont)

Per Cookie/Cracker, Unless Indicated **C** **F** **Cb**

Nabisco:

Cookies:

100 Calorie Packs:

	C	F	Cb
Chips A'hoy!, Thin Crisps, Baked, 0.8 oz	100	3	18
Lorna Doone, Shortbread Cookie Crisps, 0.7 oz	100	3	16

Chips Ahoy!, Chocolate Chip:

	C	F	Cb
Original: (2), 1.1 oz	160	8	22
Single Serve, 1.4 oz	190	9	27
Reduced Fat (2), 1.2 oz	150	6	24
Candy Blasts (2),1.2 oz	180	9	22
Chewy (2), 1.1 oz	140	6	21
Chunky, Choc. Chunk (2), 1.2 oz	160	8	20
Mini Choc. Chips:			
3 oz Package	410	19	60
Go-Pak, 3.5 oz	525	25	70

	C	F	Cb
Mallomars, (1), 1 oz	120	5	18

Newtons:

100% Whole Grain:

	C	F	Cb
Fig (2), 1 oz	110	2	23
Other varieties (2), 1 oz	100	1.5	21
Original Fig: 2 cookies, 1 oz	100	2	20
Single Serve, 2 oz package	200	4	40
Fat-Free: 2 cookies, 1 oz	100	0	23
Single Serve, 2 oz package	200	0	46
Strawberry, (2), 1 oz	100	1.5	21
Fruit Thins, Crispy (3), all var., 1 oz	140	5	21

Nilla Wafers:

	C	F	Cb
8 wafers, 1 oz	140	6	21
Reduced-Fat (8), 1 oz	120	2	24

Nutter Butter, Peanut Butter Sandwich:

	C	F	Cb
16 oz package, 1 cookie 1 oz	130	5	20
4.8 oz package, 2 cookies, 0.9 oz	120	5	17
1.9 oz package, 4 cookies	250	10	37
Bites:			
Big Bag, 3 oz pkg	420	18	63
Go-Paks!, 1 oz	140	6	21

Per Cookie/Cracker, Unless Indicated **C** **F** **Cb**

Nabisco (Cont):

Oreo Cookies, Chocolate/Golden:

Average all Creme Fillings:

	C	F	Cb
1 cookie	55	2.5	8
3 cookies	160	7	25
Single Serve package (6), 2 oz	270	11	41
5.25 oz package, 15 cookies	800	35	125
Sugar Free, 1 cookie	50	2.5	5
Mini Bite, Single Sve pkg, 1.25 oz	170	7	25
Double Stuf:			
(2), 1 oz	140	7	21
King Size			

Fudge Cremes, average all varieties:

	C	F	Cb
1 cookie	60	3	8
3 cookies	180	9	24

Snackwell's:

	C	F	Cb
Creme Sandwich:			
7.8 oz Package, 1 cookie, 0.9 oz	110	3	20
1.7 oz Package, 4 cookies	210	5	38

Teddy Grahams:

	C	F	Cb
Snacks: Honey; Cinnamon (24), 1 oz	130	4	23
Chocolate (24), av. all var., 1 oz	130	4.5	22

Crackers:

Barnum's Animals:

	C	F	Cb
8 crackers, 1 oz	120	3.5	21
Snack Saks (17), 1 oz	140	4	24

Honey Maid:

	C	F	Cb
Grahamfuls, av. all var., 0.9 oz pkg	115	5	18
Grahams (8), average all var., 1 oz	130	3	24

Premium:

	C	F	Cb
Saltine: Original, 5 crackers, 0.5 oz	70	1.5	12
Round, 6 crackers, 0.5 oz	60	1.5	12
Unsalted Tops (5), 0.5 oz	70	1.5	13

Triscuit:

	C	F	Cb
Original, 6 crackers, 1 oz	120	4	20
Reduced Fat (7), 1.1 oz	120	2.5	23
Brown Rice (6), av. all varieties, 1 oz	130	4.5	21
Thin Crisps (10), all varieties, 1 oz	130	3	23

Wheat Thins: *Per 9 oz Box*

	C	F	Cb
Original (14), 1.1 oz	140	5	22
Av. other flavors (14), 1.1 oz	140	5	21
Multigrain (14), 1.1 oz	130	4	22
Flatbread, Garlic & Parsley, 0.5 oz serving	60	1.5	11

Wheatsworth,

	C	F	Cb
Stone Ground Wheat (5)	80	4	10

C Cookies ◇ Crackers

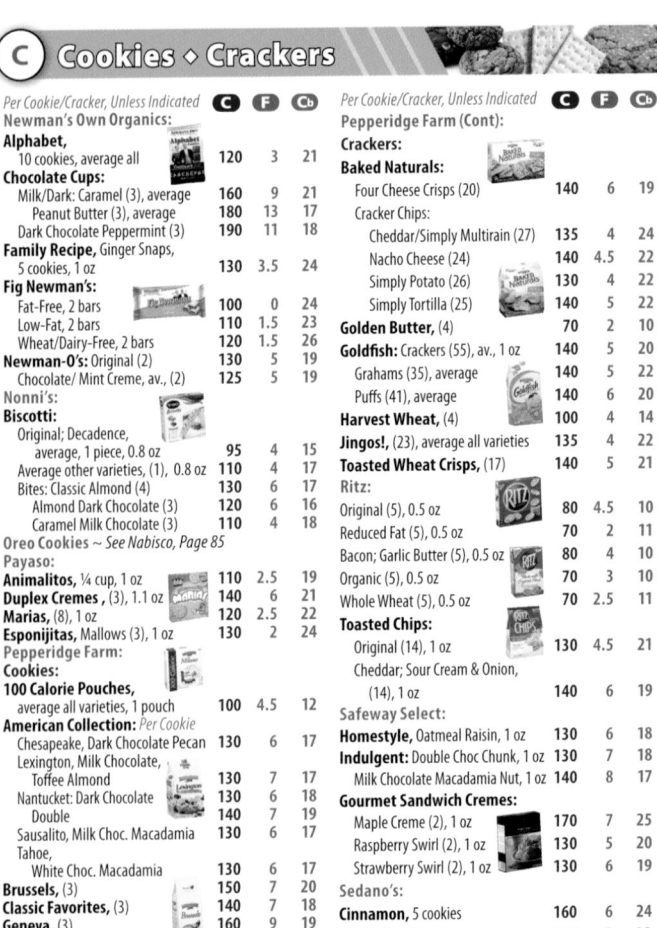

Per Cookie/Cracker, Unless Indicated **C** **F** **Cb**

Newman's Own Organics:

Alphabet,
10 cookies, average all	120	3	21

Chocolate Cups:
Milk/Dark: Caramel (3), average	160	9	21
Peanut Butter (3), average	180	13	17
Dark Chocolate Peppermint (3)	190	11	18

Family Recipe, Ginger Snaps,
5 cookies, 1 oz	130	3.5	24

Fig Newman's:
Fat-Free, 2 bars	100	0	24
Low-Fat, 2 bars	110	1.5	23
Wheat/Dairy-Free, 2 bars	120	1.5	26

Newman-O's: Original (2) | 130 | 5 | 19

Chocolate/ Mint Creme, av., (2)	125	5	19

Nonni's:

Biscotti:
Original; Decadence,			
average, 1 piece, 0.8 oz	95	4	15
Average other varieties, (1), 0.8 oz	110	4	17
Bites: Classic Almond (4)	130	6	17
Almond Dark Chocolate (3)	120	6	16
Caramel Milk Chocolate (3)	110	4	18

Oreo Cookies ~ See Nabisco, Page 85

Payaso:
Animalitos, ¼ cup, 1 oz	110	2.5	19
Duplex Cremes , (3), 1.1 oz	140	6	21
Marias, (8), 1 oz	120	2.5	22
Esponijitas, Mallows (3), 1 oz	130	2	24

Pepperidge Farm:

Cookies:

100 Calorie Pouches,
average all varieties, 1 pouch	100	4.5	12

American Collection: Per Cookie
Chesapeake, Dark Chocolate Pecan	130	6	17
Lexington, Milk Chocolate,			
Toffee Almond	130	7	17
Nantucket: Dark Chocolate			
Double	140	7	19
Sausalito, Milk Choc. Macadamia	130	6	17
Tahoe,			
White Choc. Macadamia	130	6	17

Brussels, (3) | 150 | 7 | 20

Classic Favorites, (3) | 140 | 7 | 18

Geneva, (3) | 160 | 9 | 19

Milano: Milk Chocolate (3) | 170 | 9 | 21
Double Chocolate (3)	140	8	17
Mint; Orange; Raspb. (2), av.	130	7	16
Melts (2), av. all varieties	140	7	18
Slices (3), av. all var.	150	8	18

Pirouettes, (2), av. all var. | 120 | 5 | 19

Tahiti, Coconut (2) | 170 | 10 | 17

Per Cookie/Cracker, Unless Indicated **C** **F** **Cb**

Pepperidge Farm (Cont):

Crackers:

Baked Naturals:
Four Cheese Crisps (20)	140	6	19
Cracker Chips:			
Cheddar/Simply Multirain (27)	135	4	24
Nacho Cheese (24)	140	4.5	23
Simply Potato (26)	130	4	22
Simply Tortilla (25)	140	5	22

Golden Butter, (4) | 70 | 2 | 10

Goldfish: Crackers (55), av., 1 oz | 140 | 5 | 19
Grahams (35), average	140	5	20
Puffs (41), average	140	6	20

Harvest Wheat, (4) | 100 | 4 | 14

Jingos!, (23), average all varieties | 135 | 4 | 22

Toasted Wheat Crisps, (17) | 140 | 5 | 21

Ritz:
Original (5), 0.5 oz	80	4.5	10
Reduced Fat (5), 0.5 oz	70	2	11
Bacon; Garlic Butter (5), 0.5 oz	80	4	10
Organic (5), 0.5 oz	70	3	10
Whole Wheat (5), 0.5 oz	70	2.5	11

Toasted Chips:
Original (14), 1 oz	130	4.5	21
Cheddar; Sour Cream & Onion,			
(14), 1 oz	140	6	19

Safeway Select:

Homestyle, Oatmeal Raisin, 1 oz | 130 | 6 | 18

Indulgent: Double Choc Chunk, 1 oz | 130 | 7 | 18
Milk Chocolate Macadamia Nut, 1 oz	140	8	17

Gourmet Sandwich Cremes:
Maple Creme (2), 1 oz	170	7	25
Raspberry Swirl (2), 1 oz	130	5	20
Strawberry Swirl (2), 1 oz	130	6	19

Sedano's:
Cinnamon, 5 cookies	160	6	24
Maria, 5 cookies, 1 oz	120	3	22

Shar Gluten Free ~ See CalorieKing.com

Special K: Per 1 oz Serving
Crackers, Multigrain (24)	120	3	23
Cracker Chips, av. all varieties	110	3	22
Popcorn Chips, av. all varieties	120	2.5	23

Cookies & Crackers ~ Brands (Cont)

Per Cookie/Cracker, Unless Indicated **C F Cb**

Stella D'Oro:

	C	F	Cb
Biscotti, av. all varieties, 0.8 oz	100	4.5	13
Breakfast Treats (1), av. all var.	90	3	15
Margherite: Chocolate (2)	130	6	19
Vanilla (2)	120	4	20
Roman Egg Biscuits, 1 oz	130	4.5	19
Swiss Fudge (3)	170	9	22

Toast & Sponge:

Almond Toast (2)	100	2	20
Anisette Sponge (3)	90	1	18
Anisette Toast (3), 1 oz	130	1	27

Streit's:

Flavored Wafers:

Chocolate (3)	160	9	19
Lemon (3)	170	10	19
Rolls, Chocolate Cream filled (3)	105	6	12

Sunshine:

Cheez-It Snack:

Original (27), 1 oz	150	8	17
1.25 oz bag	180	9	20
Colby, 0.8 oz pouch	110	6	12
Average other varieties (25), 1 oz	145	8	18
Big: Original,(13)	150	8	17
Monterey Jack (14), 1 oz	150	8	17
Reduced Fat: Original (29), 1 oz	130	4.5	20
White Cheddar (25), 1 oz	130	4	22

Trader Joe's:

100 Calorie Packs, average	100	2.5	18
Almond Windmill (2), 1 oz	140	6	19
Charmingly Chewy Choc Chip (2), 1 oz	130	5	20
Cherry Granola (2), 1 oz	110	4	18
Chocolate Chip: Small (4), 1 oz	140	7	18
Large, singles, 1.7 oz	280	14	35
Vegan (1), 1 oz	130	6	18
Caramel Cashew (3), 1 oz	140	7	16
Crispy Crunchy Choc Chip (12)	150	9	19
Crispy Oatmeal Choc Chip (12)	150	9	19
Dark Choc Chunks with almonds (3)	140	7	17
Dunkers: Chocolate Chip (2), 1.2 oz	160	7	21
Choc. Coated Choc. Chip (2), 1.3 oz	190	9	25

Per Cookie/Cracker, Unless Indicated **C F Cb**

Trader Joe's: (Cont)

Ginger Snaps, Gluten Free (5), 1 oz	140	6	21
Highbrow Chocolate (2)	140	7	17
Joe Joe's S'wich Cremes, Choc./ Vanilla (2), 1 oz	130	6	19
Macarons A La Parisienne (2)	90	3	10
Meringues, Vanilla (4)	110	0	27
Oatmeal Raisin, 1.8 oz	270	12	35
Pecan S'thrn Style (4), 1 oz	150	9	15
Thins: Meyer Lemon (9)	130	4.5	22
Toasted Coconut (8)	130	4.5	22
Triple Choc Chunk, 1 oz	140	7	20
Ultimate Vanilla Wafers (5)	120	6	15
Way More Chocolate Chip (3)	160	11	14
Crackers, Water (4)	60	1	12

Triscuits ~ *See Page 85*

Voortman:

Classics: Almond Krunch (2), 1 oz	140	6	20
Chunky Chip (1), 0.8 oz	100	4.5	14
Wafers, all varieties (3), 1 oz	140	6	20
Sugar Free: Chocolate Chip (1), 0.7 oz	80	5	13
Peanut Butter Wafer (4), 1 oz	150	7	17

Note: Carb figures include 6g of sugar alcohols

Whole Foods (365 Organic):

Choc Chip (2), 1 oz	150	7	21
Classic Fig Bars (2), 1.3 oz	140	2.5	27
Lemon Wafers (7), 1 oz	110	3	19
Oatmeal (2), 1 oz	130	4.5	20
S'wich Cremes; Sugar (2), average	130	5	20

WhoNu?:

Original Cookie (3), 1.3 oz	160	7	22
2X Chocolate (2), 1.1 oz	140	6	21
Chocolate/Vanilla S'wich (3), 1.3 oz	150	6	24
Soft & Chewy, Chocolate Chip Cookie, (3) 1.5 oz	150	6	24

Cookie ~ Mixes

Prepared as Directed

Betty Crocker:

Pouch Mix: *Per 2 Cookies*

Double Choc. Chunk; P'nut Butter, av.	140	6	20
Walnut Chocolate Chip	170	9	20
Average other varieties	145	6	20
Duncan Hines, Chocolate Chip, 2 cookies, 1 oz	180	9	23

Thaw, Bake & Serve **C** **F** **Cb**

Per Cookie/Cracker Unless Indicated

Pillsbury Cookies:

Refrigerated Cookie Dough: *Per Cookie*

	C	F	Cb
Chocolate Chip Cookie	130	6	18
Create N Bake, Peppermint, 0.77 oz	100	4.5	14
Peanut Butter	120	5	17
Sugar, Regular	120	5	18

Ready To Bake:

Chocolate Chip (2)	170	8	23
Chocolate Chunk & Chip (2)	170	8	23
Holiday Cookies, Sugar, average all varieties, (2)	120	6	15
Oatmeal Chocolate Chip (2)	160	7	24

Big Deluxe Classics:

Chocolate Chip (1)	170	8	23
Oatmeal Raisin (1)	150	6	24
Peanut Butter Cup (1)	160	7	22
White Chunk Macadamia (1)	170	9	22
Simply Cookies: Choc. Chip (1)	150	7	20
Peanut Butter (1)	140	6	19

Refrigerated Sweet Buns/Rolls~ *See Page 67*

Toll House (Nestle):

Refrigerated Dough Bars: *Per Cookie*

Chocolate Chip	90	4	11
Oatmeal Raisin	80	3	12
P'B Chocolate Chip	80	4.5	10
Sugar Cookie	80	3.5	12
Walnut Chocolate Chip	90	4.5	11

Ultimates Refrigerated Dough: *Per Cookie*

Chocolate Chip Lovers	180	9	23
Chocolate Pecan Deluxe	190	10	22
Choc. P'nut Butter Deluxe	180	9	23
Dark Chocolate Delight	160	8	21
Pecan Turtle Delight	160	7	23

Crispbreads **C** **F** **Cb**

Per Crispbread Unless Indicated

Finn Crisp:

	C	F	Cb
Classic: Traditional Rye	40	0.5	7
Hi-Fibre	40	0.5	6.5
Round: Original	45	0.5	7.5
Sesame	50	1	8
Thin Crisps, Original	20	0	4

Kavli Norwegian:

Crispy Thin (3)	60	0	13
Golden Rye (2)	60	0.5	12
Hearty Thick (2)	60	0	12
Malsovit, Meal Wafers	75	4	7

New York Flatbread Crisps,

Everything, 0.4 oz	50	1.5	7
Ry-Krisp: Natural (2)	50	0	11
Seasoned (2)	60	1	11
Sesame (2)	60	1.5	10

Ryvita:

Crackerbreads, Original; Wholegrain	20	0	4
Crispbreads, Original; Dark	35	0	6.5

WASA:

Crisp'n Light 7 Grain (3)	60	0	13
Fiber, 0.35 oz	35	0.5	8
Hearty; Multi Grain, 0.5 oz	45	0	11
Light Rye (2), 0.5 oz	60	0	14
Whole Wheat, 0.5 oz	50	1	10

Matzos

Manischewitz:

	C	F	Cb
Matzos: Egg 'n Onion, 1 oz	80	0.5	17
Thin Salted/Tea, average, 0.9 oz	95	0	20
Whole Wheat, 1 oz	110	1	21
Yolk Free, 1.2 oz	100	0	20

Crackers:

Tam Tam: Original (10), 1 oz	110	4	16
Everything (10), 1 oz	140	5	19
Sesame (10), 1 oz	140	6	19

Streit's:

Mediterranean Matzos, 1 Matzo, 1 oz	90	0.5	18
Unsalted Matzos, 1 Matzo, 1 oz	100	0	23

Quick Guide	**C**	**F**	**Cb**

Cream

Average All Brands

Half & Half Cream:

1 Tbsp, 0.5 oz	20	1.5	0.5
2 Tbsp, 1 oz	40	3	1
¼ cup, 2 oz	80	6	2

Light: Coffee/table (20% fat): 1 Tbsp | 30 | 3 | 0.5

2 Tbsp, 1 oz	60	6	0.5

Sour Cream:

Regular: 1 Tbsp, 0.5 oz | 25 | 2.5 | 1

1 cup, 8 oz	445	45	7

Low-Fat/Light: 1 Tbsp, 0.5 oz | 20 | 1.5 | 1

2 Tbsp, 1 oz	40	3	2

Fat-Free: Av., 2 Tbsp, 1 oz | 20 | 0 | 4.5

Hood, 2 Tbsp, 1 oz	25	0	4
Knudsen, 2 Tbsp, 1 oz	30	0	5
Kroger, 2 Tbsp, 1 oz	20	0	3
Naturally Yours; Oak Farm, 2 Tbsp	20	0	3

Sour Cream Substitute:

Albertson's, 2 Tbsp, 1 oz	60	5	2
Tofutti, Sour Supreme, 2 Tbsp, 1 oz	85	5	9

Whipping Cream:

Heavy, (37% fat):

1 Tbsp fluid/2 Tbsp whipped	50	5.5	0.5
¼ cup whipped	105	11	1
½ cup fluid/1 cup whipped	410	44	3.5

Light, (30% fat):

1 Tbsp fluid/2 Tbsp whipped	45	4.5	0.5
½ cup fluid/1 cup whipped	350	37	3.5

Coconut Cream/Milk

Coconut Cream, (Canned):

Plain/unsweetened: 2 Tbsp, 1 oz | 75 | 6.5 | 3

½ cup, 4 oz	285	26	12

Sweetened:

Coco Lopez: 1 oz	130	5	21
½ cup, 4 oz	520	20	84

Coconut Milk: (Canned):

Thai Kitchen: Lite, ⅓ cup, 2 fl.oz	50	4.5	1
Premium/Organic, 2 fl.oz	115	10	4
Unsweetened, ⅓ cup	140	14	3

Coconut Water, (Center), 1 cup | 45 | 0.5 | 9

Whipped Toppings	**C**	**F**	**Cb**

Average All Brands

Cream (Pressurized): 2 Tbsp | 20 | 1.5 | 1

¼ cup	40	3.5	2

Cream Topping, Lite, 2 Tbsp | 20 | 1 | 3

Kraft:

Cool Whip: Regular, Original, ⅓ oz | 25 | 1.5 | 2

Extra Creamy, 2 Tbsp	25	2	2
Lite, 2 Tbsp, ¼ oz	20	1	3
Free, 2 Tbsp, 0.3 oz	15	0	3
Chocolate; Vanilla, 0.7 oz	60	3.5	8

Dream Whip, 2 Tbsp | 10 | 0 | 2

Reddi wip:

Original, 2 Tbsp, 0.3 oz	15	1	1
Extra Creamy, 2 Tbsp, 0.3 oz	15	1	1
Fat-Free, 2 Tbsp, 0.3 oz	5	0	1
Chocolate, 2 Tbsp, 0.3 oz	15	1	1

Creamers (Non-Dairy)

Powder:

Coffee-Mate/Cremora/N-Rich:

Original: Unsweetened, 1 tsp | 10 | 0.5 | 1

1 heaping tsp	25	2	2
Lite, 1 tsp	10	0	2
Sweetened, 4 tsp	60	2.5	9
Flavors: Av., 4 tsp	60	3	9
Fat-Free, average, 4 tsp	50	0	11

Liquid/Refrigerated:

Per Tablespoon

Bailey's: Average all flavors | 35 | 1.5 | 5

Fat Free, all flavors	25	0	5

Coffee-Mate: *Per Tablespoon*

Flavors: Average all flavors	35	1.5	5
Fat-Free, all flavors	25	0	5
Sugar free, all flavors	15	1	2
Unflavored: Original	20	1	2
Fat-Free	10	0	1
Low-Fat	10	0.5	1
Natural Bliss: All flavors	35	1.5	5
Vanilla, Low-fat	20	1	3

Hood, Country Creamer, 1 Tbsp | 20 | 1.5 | 2

International Delight: *Per Tbsp*

American/Classic/Coffee House:

Regular, all flavors	35	1.5	6
Fat-Free, all flavors	30	0	7

Kroger: *Per Tbsp*

Coffee Creamers: Original | 20 | 1 | 3

Caramel Vanilla; Hazelnut	35	1.5	6
Fat-free, Hazelnut	30	0	6

Silk: Original | 15 | 1 | 1

French Vanilla; Hazelnut	20	1	3

Ready-To-Serve | C | F | Cb

	C	F	Cb
Hunt's:			
Snack Pack Puddings: *Per 3.3oz Cup*			
Regular: Butterscotch; Tapioca	110	2.5	21
Chocolate/ Chocolate Fudge	120	3	21
Vanilla	100	2.5	20
Fat Free: Chocolate	90	0	20
Tapioca	80	0	19
Sugar Free: Chocolate	70	3	14
Caramel; Vanilla	60	3	10
Fruit Blasts: Lemon Pudding	120	2.5	24
Juicy Gels: Regular, all flavors	100	0	24
Sugar Free, Cherry	10	0	2
Jell-O *(Kraft)*:			
Ready To Eat Puddings:			
Banana Split, 3.9 oz	110	2	23
Butterscotch, 3.9 oz	110	1.5	23
Cinnamon Rice, 3.7 oz	110	3	20
Vanilla Rice, 3.7 oz	110	3	20
Kozy Shack:			
Puddings:			
Bread, average all flavors, 3.5 oz	155	3.5	27
Butterscotch, 4 oz	120	2	23
Chocolate, 4.6 oz	140	2.5	27
Rice:			
Original, ½ cup, 4.6 oz	130	2.5	24
Av. other varieties, ½ cup, 4.6 oz	145	3	26
No Sugar Added:			
Chocolate, 4 oz	90	2.5	13
Rice; Tapioca, 4 oz	90	1.5	14
Flan, Creme Caramel, 1 cup, 4 oz	160	4	28
Lactose Free: *Per 4 oz Cup*			
Chocolate	130	3.5	21
Rice; Tapioca, average	125	3	21
Kroger: *Per Container*			
Puddings: *Per 3.5 oz*			
Butterscotch	110	2	22
Chocolate	110	2.5	21
Swiss Miss: *Per 4 oz Cup*			
Puddings:			
Classic Butterscotch	130	3.5	22
Creamy : Milk Chocolate	150	3.5	27
Vanilla	140	3.5	24
Old Fashioned Tapioca	140	3.5	24
Sugar Free: Chocolate	70	3.5	15
Vanilla	60	3	11

Homemade Puddings | C | F | Cb

	C	F	Cb
Apple Tapioca, ½ cup	150	0	32
Bread Pudding, ½ cup	250	8	40
Blancmange, ½ cup	140	5	19
Chocolate, ½ cup	190	6	30
Crème Brûlée, ½ cup	400	35	16
Plum Pudding, 2 oz	170	3	32
Rice with Raisins, ½ cup	200	4	38
Sponge Pudding, 3.5 oz	340	16	45
Tapioca Cream, ½ cup	110	4	15
Trifle, ½ cup	180	7	26

Custards

	C	F	Cb
Custard Mix *(Jello/Royal Flan)*, average:			
Dry, ¼ of 2.9 oz package, 0.7 oz	80	0	19
Prepared: Whole milk, ½ cup	155	4	25
2% milk, ½ cup	140	2.5	25
Non-Fat milk, ½ cup	125	0	25
Home Made Egg Custard:			
With Whole Milk, ½ cup	170	8	18
With 2% Milk, ½ cup	155	6.5	18

Gelatin • Parfait • Jell-O

Prepared As Directed

	C	F	Cb
Jell-O:			
No Bake: Oreo, ⅑ package	370	17	51
Peanut Butter Cup, ⅛ package	360	21	42
Cheesecake: Real, ⅛ package	360	21	42
Strawberry, ⅑ pakage	290	10	48
Flan, Spanish Style Custard			
with Caramel Sauce, ¼ package	140	2.5	27
Gelatin Dessert Mix: All flav., ¼ pkg	80	0	19
Sugar free, all flavors, ⅛ package	10	0	0
Pudding & Pie Filling: *Prepared As Directed*			
Cook & Serve: Choc. Fudge, ⅙ pkg	150	2.5	27
Banana Crm; Vanilla, ⅙ pkg	140	2.5	27
Sugar & Fat-Free, all flav., ⅙ pkg	70	0	12
Instant Mix:			
Devil's Food, ¼ pkg	140	2.5	30
Oreo, Cookies 'N Cream, ¼ pkg	180	3.5	33
White Chocolate, ¼ pkg	150	2.5	30
Sugar free, all flavors, ¼ pkg	70	0	12
Ida Mae, Strawberry Parfait	90	2	18
Reser's, Parfaits, av. all flav., 3.9 oz	100	2	19

Meringues

	C	F	Cb
Meringue Swirl, ½ oz	50	0	8
Meringue Shell, 1 oz shell	100	0	16

Chicken Eggs

	C	F	Cb
Fresh Eggs:			
Raw:			
Small	55	4	0
Medium	65	4	0
Large	70	5	0
Extra Large	80	5.5	0
Jumbo	90	6	0
Egg Yolk, 1 extra large	55	4.5	0
Egg White, 1 extra large	17	0	0
Dried Egg Powder:			
Whole Egg, ¼ cup, 1 oz	170	12	0
1 Tbsp	30	2	0
Egg White, ¼ cup, 1 oz	105	0	0
Egg Yolk, ¼ cup, 1 oz	195	18	0

Egg Substitutes

¼ Cup (Equivalent to 1 Egg) ~ Zero Cholesterol

	C	F	Cb
All Whites (Crystal Farms), 1.6 oz	25	0	1
Better 'n Eggs (Crystal Farms):			
Regular, ¼ cup, 2 oz	30	0	1
Plus, ¼ cup, 2 oz	35	0	1
Egg Beaters (ConAgra):			
Regular, 3 Tbsp, 1.6 oz	25	0	1
Southwestern Style, 3 Tbsp, 1.6 oz	20	0	1
Egg Replacer (Ener-g), 1.5 tsp,	15	0	4
Eggs (Second Nature),			
Egg Whites, Fat-Free,			
¼ cup, 2 fl.oz	35	0	1
Egg Substitute (Albertson's), ¼ cup	30	0	1
Naturegg (Burnbrae Farms),			
Simply Egg White, ¼ cup, 2 oz	30	0	1

Other Eggs

	C	F	Cb
Duck, 1 large, 2.5 oz	130	9.5	0
Goose, 1 large, 5 oz	280	19	0
Quail, 3 eggs, 1 oz	42	3	0
Turkey, 1 large, 3 oz	135	9.5	0
Turtle, 1 egg, 1.75 oz	75	5	0

Omega-3 Fat Enriched

	C	F	Cb
Eggland's Best, 1 large	70	4	0
Horizon Organic, 1 large	70	4.5	0

Note: Cholesterol content same as regular eggs, but Omega-3 fats inhibit blood cholesterol increase.

Cooked Eggs

	C	F	Cb
Boiled Egg: *Same as Raw Egg*			
Hard-Cooked, Small, peeled	65	4	0
Fried Egg:			
With fat: 1 large egg	105	9	0.5
2 small eggs	175	13	1
No fat/nonstick pan, 1 large	75	5	0.5
Deviled Egg, 2 halves	145	13	0.5
Eggs Benedict, (2),			
on Toast or English Muffin	860	56	25
Eggs Florentine, (2),			
on Toast or English Muffin	890	59	25
Pickled Egg, 1 large	80	5.5	0
Poached Egg, 1 large	65	4	0
Quiche (Homemade):			
Egg & Bacon, 1 slice, 5.3 oz	580	43	27
Ham & Cheese, 1 slice, 5.3 oz	475	33	29
Scotch Egg, 1 egg	300	21	16
Scrambled Eggs:			
1 large egg:			
With 1 Tbsp milk + 1 tsp fat	120	9	0.5
With 1 Tbsp skim milk/no fat	85	5.5	1
2 large eggs:			
With 2 Tbsp milk + 2 tsp fat	260	20	2
With 2 Tbsp skim milk, w/o fat	180	11	2

Omelets

	C	F	Cb
1 Egg:			
Plain (with 1 tsp fat)	125	10	0.5
With: ½ oz cheese	175	15	0.5
½ oz cheese + ½ oz ham	200	16	0.5
2 Eggs:			
Plain (with 2 tsp fat)	250	20	1
With: 1 oz cheese	360	29	2
1 oz cheese + 1 oz ham	410	32	2
3 Eggs:			
Plain (with 1 Tbsp fat)	360	29	1.5
With: 2 oz cheese	580	47	2.5
2 oz cheese + 2 oz ham	680	53	2.5
Extras, Tomato/Onion/Veggies, 2 oz	20	0	4.5
Egg Substitute (EggBeaters):			
2 eggs (½ cup) + 1 tsp fat	100	4	2
3 eggs (¾ cup) + 2 tsp fat	160	8	3
Extras: 1 oz Cheese	110	9	1
1 oz Ham	50	3	1

Egg Nog

Average all Brands,

	C	F	Cb
½ cup, 4 oz	170	9.5	17
Borden, Regular, 4 fl.oz	160	8	18
Hood, Golden, ½ cup, 4 fl.oz	180	9	22
Horizon/Hood, Light/Low-Fat,	140	4	22

Breakfast Sides

	C	F	Cb
Toast:			
Plain, 1 thick slice	85	1	13
With: 2 tsp butter/marg.	155	9	13
3 tsp/1 Tbsp fat	190	13	13
English Muffin:			
Plain, 2 oz	130	1	26
With 3 tsp fat	230	12	26
Bacon, 2 strips	70	5	0
Ham, lean, 2 oz	100	3	0
Hash Brown:			
½ cup, 3 oz	125	6.5	14
1 cup serving, 6 oz	250	13	28
Sausages, 2 oz link	180	16	1.5

Frozen Egg Breakfasts

	C	F	Cb
Aunt Jemima:			
Breakfast Sandwich: *Per Sandwich*			
Croissant, Sausage, Egg & Cheese	350	23	23
Griddlecake, Ham, Egg & Cheese	240	8	33
Jimmy Dean:			
Breakfast Sandwich: *Per Sandwich*			
Biscuit, Bacon, Egg & Cheese	310	19	26
Croissant, Sausage, Egg & Cheese	410	28	27
Muffin, Sausage, Egg & Cheese	350	21	26
Omelets: *Per Omelet*			
Three Cheese	290	23	4
Ham & Cheese	250	19	4
MorningStar Farms:			
Breakfast Sandwich: *Each*			
Sausage, Egg & Cheese	220	10	20
Veggie Scramble with Cheese	140	4.5	18
Pillsbury,			
Egg Scrambles, Bacon & Veggies	290	15	22
Red Baron:			
Scrambles: *Each*			
Bacon, 5 oz	390	19	38
Sausage; Western, 5 oz	360	17	38
Frozen Pancake/Waffles ~ *See Page 132*			
Toaster Pastries ~ *See Page 64*			

Frozen Egg Rolls

	C	F	Cb
Kahiki: *Each, without sauce*			
Chicken,; Pork, av., 3.3 oz	145	3.5	22
Vegetable, 3.3 oz	130	3	22
Lotus Restaurant:			
Imperial, Chicken/Pork (1)	160	7	25
Vegetarian (1)	120	4.5	21
Pagoda Express: *Each, without sauce*			
Chicken	140	4.5	20
Pork	180	9	19
Pork & Shrimp	170	7	19
Vegetable	130	4.5	20

Fast-Foods/Restaurants

	C	F	Cb
Arby's,			
Bacon, Egg & Cheese Croissant	400	26	25
Au Bon Pain, 2 Egg on Plain Bagel	430	12	58
Bob Evans:			
Omelets:			
Border Scramble	630	45	15
Western	495	35	7
Bojangles: Egg & Cheese Biscuit	515	34	35
Bacon, Egg & Cheese Biscuit	550	37	35
Bruegger's:			
Bagel: With Egg & Cheese, 6.8 oz	430	18	63
With Egg, Cheese & Sausage, 8.3 oz	590	34	63
Burger King:			
Breakfast Burrito: Sausage	310	19	22
Southwestern	600	38	43
Croissan'wich:			
Bacon, Egg & Cheese	370	21	31
Ham, Egg & Cheese	390	20	33
Double, Sausage, Egg & Cheese	790	57	35
Carl's Jr:			
Burrito: Bacon & Egg	570	34	38
Big Country	720	43	55
Loaded Breakfast	770	48	53
Steak & Egg	640	36	43
Chick-fil-A, Chicken, Egg & Cheese,			
on Sunflower Multigrain Bagel	480	20	48
Del Taco, Egg & Cheese Burrito	400	17	38
Denny's: *With Hashbrowns, Without Bread*			
Omelette:			
Ultimate	870	63	37
Veggie-Cheese	650	44	37
Dunkin Donuts:			
Bagel, Ham, Egg & Cheese	440	8	67
Croissant, Bacon, Egg & Cheese	480	27	40
Eat 'N Park:			
Omelette:			
Ham & Cheese	535	35	5
Meat Lovers	725	55	4
Hardee's:			
Biscuit: Loaded Omelet	490	28	40
Sausage & Egg	560	37	39
IHOP: T-Bone Steak & Eggs, 12 oz	1270	70	76
Omelette, Spinach & Mushroom	1000	82	22
Jack in the Box:			
Biscuit: Bacon, Egg & Cheese	410	25	26
Sausage, Egg & Cheese	535	38	27
McDonald's:			
Biscuit, Bacon, Egg & Cheese, regular	460	26	38
McMuffin, Egg	290	12	31
Whataburger, Breakfast Platter,			
with Bacon	640	41	34

Quick Guide C F Cb

Butter
Average All Brands

		C	F	Cb
Regular: 1 tsp, 0.2 oz		35	4	0
1 Tbsp, 0.5 oz		100	11	0
2 Tbsp, 1 oz		205	23	0
1 Stick, ½ cup, 4 oz		810	92	0
1 Pound, 2 cups, 16 oz		3255	368	0
Light: Regular, 40% Fat				
1 tsp, 0.2 oz		30	3	0
1 Tbsp, 0.5 oz		70	7.5	0
2 Tbsp, 1 oz		140	15	0
Whipped Butter: Regular				
1 tsp, 0.1 oz		20	2.5	0
1 Tbsp, 0.3 oz		65	7.5	0
1 Stick, 2.7 oz		545	62	0
Whipped Light Butter (Land O Lakes):				
1 tsp, 0.15 oz		15	1.5	0
1 Tbsp, 0.4 oz		45	5	0
2 Tbsp, 0.8 oz		90	10	0
Unsalted ~ *Same as Salted*				

Flavored Butter/Spreads
Average All Brands

		C	F	Cb
Honey Butter, (60% Fat):				
1 Tbsp, 0.5 oz		90	8	4
Downey's, 2% Fat,				
1 Tbsp, 0.5 oz		60	1	11
Garlic Butter, (80% Fat):				
1 Tbsp, 0.5 oz		100	11	0
Sweet Cream Butter:				
Land O Lakes: Regular, 1 Tbsp		100	11	0
Honey Butter Spread, 1 Tbsp		70	6	4

Butter & Butter Blends
Per 1 Tablespoon

		C	F	Cb
Challenge: Stick, 0.5 oz		100	11	0
Tub, Whipped, 0.3 oz		70	7	0
Brummel & Brown,				
Spread Made with Yogurt, 0.5oz		45	5	0
Land O'Lakes:				
Sticks: Original, 0.5oz		100	11	0
Light, 0.5 oz		50	6	0
Tubs: Butter With Olive Oil, 0.5 oz		90	10	0
Light, with Canola Oil, 0.5 oz		50	5	0
Smart Balance:				
Original Buttery Spread, 0.5 oz		80	9	0
Butter & Canola, 0.5 oz		100	11	0

Ghee (Clarified Butter) C F Cb
(Example ~ *Purity Farms*)
Note: Ghee is 100% fat compared to
regular butter (80% fat + 20% water)

		C	F	Cb
1 tsp, 0.2 oz		45	5	0
1 Tbsp, 0.5 oz		120	14	0

Light & Reduced Fat Spreads
Per Tablespoon

		C	F	Cb
bestlife, Buttery Spread, 0.5 oz		60	6	0
Benecol: Regular, 0.5 oz		70	8	0
Light, 0.5 oz		50	5	0
Blue Bonnet:				
Stick, Light Spread, 0.5 oz		50	5	1
Tub, Original Soft Spread, 0.5 oz		60	6	0
Country Crock (*Shedd's*):				
Tubs: Regular Spread, 0.5 oz		70	7	0
Light Spread, 0.5 oz		50	5	0
Churn Style, 0.5 oz		60	7	0
Fleischmann's:				
Original: Soft Spread, 0.4 oz		70	7	0
Spread, 0.5 oz		80	9	0
Light Spread, 0.5 oz		40	4.5	0
I Can't Believe It's Not Butter!:				
Tubs: Original Spread, 0.5 oz		70	8	0
Light, 0.5 oz		45	5	0
Olive Oil Spread, 1 Tbsp		70	8	0
Parkay:				
Original Spread, 0.4 oz		70	7	0
Spray, 5 sprays		0	0	0
Squeeze Bottle, 0.5 oz		70	8	0
Promise:				
Activ, Light Spread, 0.5 oz		45	5	0
Buttery Spread, 0.5 oz		80	8	0
Light Spread, 0.5 oz		45	5	0
Smart Balance:				
Tubs, Buttery Spread:				
Original, 0.5 oz		80	9	0
Light Original, 0.5 oz		50	5	0
HeartRight, Light, 0.5 oz		50	5	0
Omega 3: Reg., 0.5 oz		80	8	0
Light, 0.5 oz		50	5	0

Butter Substitutes

		C	F	Cb
Butter Buds:				
Butter Flavored: Mix, 1 tsp		5	0	2
Sprinkles, 1 tsp		5	0	2
Earth Balance,				
Original, 1 Tbsp		100	11	0
Molly McButter, 1 tsp		5	0	1
Sunsweet, (Butter/Oil Replacement),				
Lighter Bake, 1 Tbsp, 0.7 oz		35	0	9

Animal Fats/Lards   **C** **F** **Cb**

Average All Types
Beef Tallow/Drippings, Lard (Pork), Chicken, Duck, Goose, Turkey:

	C	F	Cb
1 Tbsp, 0.5 oz	115	13	0
2.25 Tbsp, 1 oz	255	28	0
1 cup, 7.3 oz	1850	205	0
½ pound, 8 oz	2040	227	0

Ghee/Butter/ Oil ~ *See Page 93*

Vegetable Shortening

Average All Types

	C	F	Cb
1 Tbsp, 0.5 oz	115	13	0
2.25 Tbsp, 1 oz	250	28	0
1 cup, 7.3 oz	1810	205	0

Vegetable Oils

Includes almond, avocado, canola, corn, coconut, flaxseed, grapeseed, linseed, mustard, olive, palm, peanut, rice bran, safflower, sesame, sunflower, soybean, wheat germ. Note: Oil is 100% fat.

	C	F	Cb
1 tsp, 0.2 oz	45	5	0
1 Tbsp, 0.5 oz	120	14	0
2 Tbsp, 1 oz	240	28	0
1 cup, 7.3 oz	1930	205	0

Fish Oils

Average All Types
(Includes Cod Liver, Herring, Salmon, Sardines): 1 Tbsp, 0.5 oz   125   14   0

Cooking Sprays/Squeezes

Cooking Sprays: (PAM, Mazola, I Can't Believe It's Not Butter, Weight Watchers, Wesson):

	C	F	Cb
Pam: ¼ second spray	2	0	0
1-3 second spray	6	1	0
I Can't Believe It's Not Butter, Original Spray	0	0	0
Parkay, Buttery Spray	0	0	0

Olestra (Olean)   **C** **F** **Cb**

Olestra *(Olean)*   0   0   0
Note: Olean is Proctor & Gamble's brand name for Olestra – a no-calorie cooking oil that gives snacks (like potato chips, tortilla chips and crackers) taste and texture without adding fat or calories.
Examples:
• *Frito-Lay,* Light Products (Lays, Ruffles, Tostitos, Doritos)
• *Pringles,* Fat-Free Potato Crisps

Quick Guide   **C** **F** **Cb**

Mayonnaise:
Regular: *Per 1 Tbsp, 0.5 oz Unless Indicated*

	C	F	Cb
Average All Brands	90	10	0
Best Foods; Hellman's; Kraft:			
Original/Real	90	10	0
½ cup, 4 oz	720	80	0
Hain, Safflower Mayonnaise	100	11	0
Spectrum, Canola Mayo	100	11	0
Light/Reduced Fat: *Per 1 Tbsp, 0.5 oz*			
Best Foods/Hellman's	35	3.5	1
Kraft, Light/Olive Oil	35	3	2
Smart Balance, Omega	50	5	1
Spectrum, Light Canola Mayo, Eggless	35	3.5	0
Fat Free:			
Kraft: Original, 1 Tbsp	10	0	2
½ cup, 4 oz	80	0	16
Sugar Free:			
Dukes Mayo, 1 Tbsp	100	12	0

Mayonnaise Style Dressing:
Per 1 Tbsp, 0.5 oz

	C	F	Cb
Best Foods, Sandwich Spread	60	5	2
Kraft:			
Miracle Whip Dressing:			
Original	40	3.5	2
Light	20	1.5	2
Fat Free	15	0	3
Sandwich Shop Mayo:			
Chipotle	40	4	2
Horseradish-Dijon	40	3.5	2
Hot & Spicy	100	11	0
Nasoya, Egg & Dairy Free:			
Nayonaise: Regular/Whipped	40	3.5	1
Light	20	1.5	1

Quick Guide C F Cb

Fresh Fish

Low Oil: *Less than 2.5% fat*
White/Lightly-colored flesh. Examples:
Cod, Flounder, Haddock, Halibut, Mahi Mahi, Perch, Pike,
Pollock, Snapper, Sole, Whiting.

	C	F	Cb
Raw, without bones, 4 oz	100	1	0
Steamed, Broiled, Baked, 4 oz	140	1.5	0
Fried: Lightly Floured, 4 oz	210	8	3.5
Breaded, 4 oz	260	12	8
In Batter, 4 oz	320	16	27

Medium Oil: *2.5-5% fat*
Lightly-colored flesh. Examples:
Bluefin Tuna, Catfish, Kingfish, Orange Roughy, Salmon
(Pink), Swordfish, Rainbow Trout, Yellowtail.

Raw, without bones, 4 oz	145	7	0
Baked/Broiled, 4 oz	195	8	0
Fried, 4 oz	230	11	8

High Oil: *Over 5% fat*
Darker-colored flesh. Examples:
Albacore Tuna, Mackerel,
Salmon (Atlantic/Chinook/Sockeye), Sardines, Trout.

Raw, without bones, 4 oz	220	14	0
Baked, Broiled, 4 oz	275	17	0
Fried, 4 oz	340	23	12

Cooking Yields (Fin Fish):

4 oz Raw wt. = 3.5 oz Cooked weight
4 oz Cooked wt = 5 oz Raw weight

Calorie & Fat Variations:

The amount of fat/oil in fish varies with the species, season
and locality. Within the same fish, fat/oil content is generally
higher towards the head.

Fish & Shellfish

Edible Weights: (no bones/shell)

	C	F	Cb
Abalone: Raw, 3 oz	90	0.5	5
Fried, 3 oz	160	6	9.5
Ahi Tuna, grilled, 6 oz fillet (w/o fat)	235	2	0
Anchovy: Paste, 1 Tbsp, 0.5 oz	45	3	0
Canned in oil, drained, (5), 0.7 oz	40	2	0
Barracuda (Pacific), raw, 4 oz	130	3	0
Basa/Swai, raw, 4 oz fillet	70	2	0
Bass:			
Sea: Raw, 4.6 oz fillet	125	2.5	0
Baked, 3 oz	105	2	0
Striped: Raw, 1 fillet, 5.5 oz	150	3.5	0
Baked, 3 oz	105	3	0
Freshwater: Raw, 3 oz	95	3	0
Baked, 3 oz	125	4	0

Fish & Shellfish (Cont) C F Cb

Edible Weights: (no bones/shell)

	C	F	Cb
Calamari/Squid:			
Raw, 4 oz	100	1.5	3.5
Baked, 1 cup	190	6.5	5.5
Fried, 3 oz	150	6	7
Catfish:			
Farmed: Raw, 1 fillet 5.6 oz	190	9.5	0
Baked, 1 fillet 5 oz	205	10	0
Wild: Raw, 1 fillet, 5.6 oz	150	4.5	0
Baked, 1 fillet, 5 oz	150	4	0
Breaded, fried, 1 fillet, 3 oz	200	12	0
Caviar, black/red, 1 Tbsp, 16g	40	3	0.5
Clams: Raw (4 large/9 small), 3 oz	70	1	3
Breaded, Fried (20 small), 6.6 oz	380	21	20
Canned, drained, ½ cup, 2.8 oz	115	1	0
Steamed (10 small), 3.3 oz	140	2	5
Clam Juice *(Snow's),* 1 Tbsp	0	0	0
Cod:			
Atlantic: Raw, 4 oz	95	1	0
Baked, 3 oz	90	1	0
Canned, solids & liquid	90	0.5	0
Pacific: Raw, 4 oz	80	0.5	0
Baked, 3 oz	70	0.5	0
Crab:			
Alaska King,			
1 leg, cooked, 4.7 oz	130	2	0
Blue: Raw, 1 crab, 6 oz	150	1	0
Steamed, 3 oz	70	0.5	0
Canned, drained, 6.5 oz can	105	0.5	0
Dungeness: Raw, 1 crab, 5.8 oz	140	1.5	0
Steamed, 4.45 oz	140	1.5	0
Crab Cakes *(Capt. D's),* (1), 2.8 oz	250	16	16
Crayfish:			
Farmed: Raw, 3 oz	60	1	0
Steamed, 3 oz	75	1	0
Wild: Raw 3 oz	65	1	0
Steamed, 3 oz	70	1	0
Cuttlefish, raw, 3 oz	70	1	1
Dolphinfish *~ See Mahi-Mahi*			
Eel: Raw, 3 oz	155	10	0
Baked, 3 oz	200	13	0
Fish & Chips *(Red Lobster),*			
battered, without condiments	630	26	54
Fish Sandwich *(Burger King),*			
without Tartar Sauce	410	12	53
Fish Oil, 1 Tbsp, 0.5 oz	125	14	0
Flounder/Sole:			
Raw, 4 oz	80	2	0
Baked, 3 oz	75	2	0
Frozen Fish *~ See Pages 114-122*			

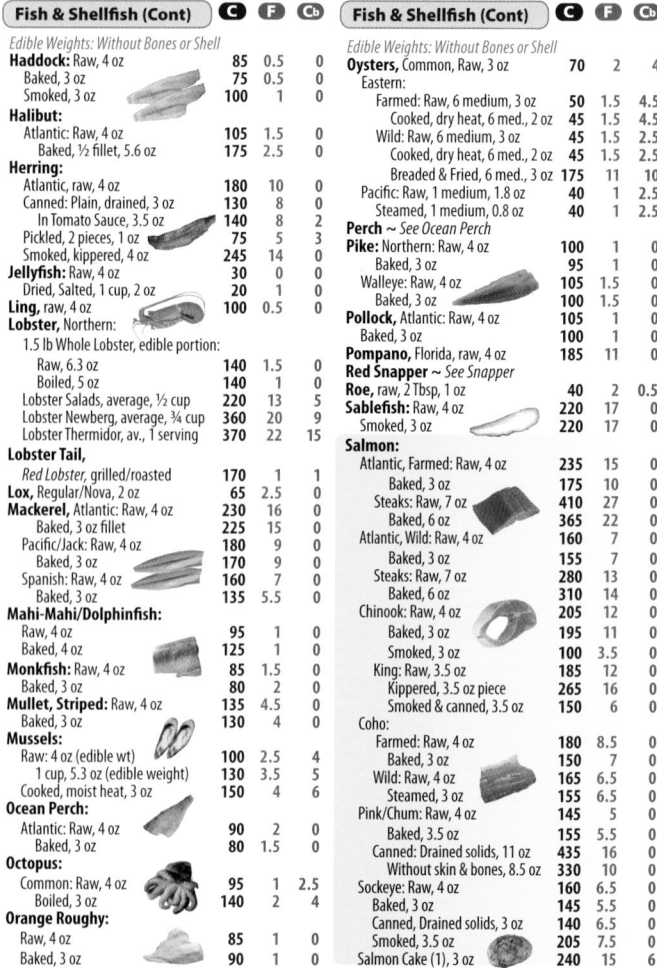

Fish & Shellfish (Cont)	C	F	Cb
Edible Weights: Without Bones or Shell			
Haddock: Raw, 4 oz	85	0.5	0
Baked, 3 oz	75	0.5	0
Smoked, 3 oz	100	1	0
Halibut:			
Atlantic: Raw, 4 oz	105	1.5	0
Baked, ½ fillet, 5.6 oz	175	2.5	0
Herring:			
Atlantic, raw, 4 oz	180	10	0
Canned: Plain, drained, 3 oz	130	8	0
In Tomato Sauce, 3.5 oz	140	8	2
Pickled, 2 pieces, 1 oz	75	5	3
Smoked, kippered, 4 oz	245	14	0
Jellyfish: Raw, 4 oz	30	0	0
Dried, Salted, 1 cup, 2 oz	20	1	0
Ling, raw, 4 oz	100	0.5	0
Lobster, Northern:			
1.5 lb Whole Lobster, edible portion:			
Raw, 6.3 oz	140	1.5	0
Boiled, 5 oz	140	1	0
Lobster Salads, average, ½ cup	220	13	5
Lobster Newberg, average, ¾ cup	360	20	9
Lobster Thermidor, av., 1 serving	370	22	15
Lobster Tail,			
Red Lobster, grilled/roasted	170	1	1
Lox, Regular/Nova, 2 oz	65	2.5	0
Mackerel, Atlantic: Raw, 4 oz	230	16	0
Baked, 3 oz fillet	225	15	0
Pacific/Jack: Raw, 4 oz	180	9	0
Baked, 3 oz	170	9	0
Spanish: Raw, 4 oz	160	7	0
Baked, 3 oz	135	5.5	0
Mahi-Mahi/Dolphinfish:			
Raw, 4 oz	95	1	0
Baked, 4 oz	125	1	0
Monkfish: Raw, 4 oz	85	1.5	0
Baked, 3 oz	80	2	0
Mullet, Striped: Raw, 4 oz	135	4.5	0
Baked, 3 oz	130	4	0
Mussels:			
Raw, 4 oz (edible wt)	100	2.5	4
1 cup, 5.3 oz (edible weight)	130	3.5	5
Cooked, moist heat, 3 oz	150	4	6
Ocean Perch:			
Atlantic: Raw, 4 oz	90	2	0
Baked, 3 oz	80	1.5	0
Octopus:			
Common: Raw, 4 oz	95	1	2.5
Boiled, 3 oz	140	2	4
Orange Roughy:			
Raw, 4 oz	85	1	0
Baked, 3 oz	90	1	0

Fish & Shellfish (Cont)	C	F	Cb
Edible Weights: Without Bones or Shell			
Oysters, Common, Raw, 3 oz	70	2	4
Eastern:			
Farmed: Raw, 6 medium, 3 oz	50	1.5	4.5
Cooked, dry heat, 6 med., 2 oz	45	1.5	4.5
Wild: Raw, 6 medium, 3 oz	45	1.5	2.5
Cooked, dry heat 6 med., 2 oz	45	1.5	2.5
Breaded & Fried, 6 med., 3 oz	175	11	10
Pacific: Raw, 1 medium, 1.8 oz	40	1	2.5
Steamed, 1 medium, 0.8 oz	40	1	2.5
Perch ~ *See Ocean Perch*			
Pike: Northern: Raw, 4 oz	100	1	0
Baked, 3 oz	95	1	0
Walleye: Raw, 4 oz	105	1.5	0
Baked, 3 oz	100	1.5	0
Pollock, Atlantic: Raw, 4 oz	105	1	0
Baked, 3 oz	100	1	0
Pompano, Florida, raw, 4 oz	185	11	0
Red Snapper ~ *See Snapper*			
Roe, raw, 2 Tbsp, 1 oz	40	2	0.5
Sablefish: Raw, 4 oz	220	17	0
Smoked, 3 oz	220	17	0
Salmon:			
Atlantic, Farmed: Raw, 4 oz	235	15	0
Baked, 3 oz	175	10	0
Steaks: Raw, 7 oz	410	27	0
Baked, 6 oz	365	22	0
Atlantic, Wild: Raw, 4 oz	160	7	0
Baked, 3 oz	155	7	0
Steaks: Raw, 7 oz	280	13	0
Baked, 6 oz	310	14	0
Chinook: Raw, 4 oz	205	12	0
Baked, 3 oz	195	11	0
Smoked, 3 oz	100	3.5	0
King: Raw, 3.5 oz	185	12	0
Kippered, 3.5 oz piece	265	16	0
Smoked & canned, 3.5 oz	150	6	0
Coho:			
Farmed: Raw, 4 oz	180	8.5	0
Baked, 3 oz	150	7	0
Wild: Raw, 4 oz	165	6.5	0
Steamed, 3 oz	155	6.5	0
Pink/Chum: Raw, 4 oz	145	5	0
Baked, 3.5 oz	155	5.5	0
Canned: Drained solids, 11 oz	435	16	0
Without skin & bones, 8.5 oz	330	10	0
Sockeye: Raw, 4 oz	160	6.5	0
Baked, 3 oz	145	6.5	0
Canned, Drained solids, 3 oz	140	6.5	0
Smoked, 3.5 oz	205	7.5	0
Salmon Cake (1), 3 oz	240	15	6

Fish ~ Fresh ◆ Shellfish (F)

Fish & Shellfish (Cont)

	C	F	Cb
Sardines: *Canned, Average all Brands*			
Drained of Oil:			
¼ cup drained, 2.2 oz	130	9	0
3.75 oz can, drained, 3.3 oz	190	11	0
1 large/2 medium, ⅓", 0.8 oz	50	3	0
In Tomato Sauce, 3.8 oz	190	8	3
Sashimi ~ *See Japanese Foods, Page 171*			
Scallops: Raw, 6 lge/15 small, 3 oz	65	0.5	3
Breaded, Fried (6), 5 oz	385	20	39
Steamed, 3 oz	95	0.5	0
Sea Bass ~ *See Bass*			
Seafood Salad, Deli Style,			
½ cup, 3.5 oz	250	21	11
Shark: Raw, 4 oz	145	5	0
Baked, 4 oz	185	7	0
Batter-dipped, fried, 4 oz	260	16	7
Shrimp:			
Raw: Small/Medium (4), 0.8 oz	15	0	0
Large (4), 1 oz	20	0	0
Breaded & Fried, 4.8 oz	395	24	27
Steamed, in shell, 3 oz	100	1.5	0
Canned, 1 can, 4.5 oz	130	2	0
Snapper: Raw, 4 oz	115	1.5	0
Baked: 3 oz	110	1.5	0
6 oz fillet	220	3	0
Sole: Raw, 4 oz	80	2	0
Baked, 3 oz	75	2	0
Squid ~ *see Calamari*			
Surimi, (Imitation Crab), 4 oz	110	0.5	17
Swai/Basa, raw, 4 oz	70	2	0
Swordfish: Raw, 4 oz	165	7.5	0
Medium Steak, 6 oz	250	11	0
Baked: Small Steak, 4 oz	205	7	0
Medium Steak, 6 oz	290	13	0
Tilapia: Raw, 4 oz	110	2	0
Baked: 3 oz	110	2	0
Trout, Rainbow:			
Farmed: Raw, 4 oz	160	7	0
Baked, 3 oz	145	6.5	0
Wild: Raw, 4 oz	135	4	0
Baked, 3 oz	130	5	0
Tuna:			
Raw: Bluefin, 4 oz	165	5.5	0
Skipjack, Yellowfin, av., 4 oz	120	1	0
Baked: Bluefin, 3 oz	155	5.5	0
Skipjack, Yellowfin, av., 3 oz	110	1	0
Canned: In Water, drained			
Chunk Light: 2 oz	50	1	0
3 oz can	75	1.5	1
5 oz can	125	2.5	1.5

	C	F	Cb
Tuna (Cont):			
In Water, drained (Cont):			
Solid White: 2 oz	60	0.5	0
5 oz can	150	1.5	0
7 oz can	210	2	0
In Oil, drained:			
Chunk Light: 2 oz can	80	4	0
5 oz can	200	10	0
Solid White: 2 oz can	90	4	0
6 oz can	270	12	0
Tuna Salad, Deli Style, ½ cup, 4oz	280	20	8
Whitefish: Raw, 4 oz	150	6.5	0
Baked, 3 oz	145	6.5	1
Smoked, 3 oz	90	1	0
Whiting: Raw, 4 oz	100	1.5	0
Baked, 3 oz	100	1.5	0
Yellowtail: Raw, 4 oz	165	6	0
Grilled, 3 oz	160	6	0

Other Canned/Packaged Fish

	C	F	Cb
Bumble Bee:			
Ready To Eat Tuna Salad: *With Crackers*			
Original: 3.5 oz package	300	22	18
Fat-Free, 3.5 oz	150	2	24
Kit, with reduced fat mayo,			
4.8 oz	410	21	25
Lunch on the Run Kit, 8.2 oz	500	26	52
Seafood Salad,			
with Crackers, 3.3 oz pkg	150	5	24
Chicken of the Sea:			
Albacore White Tuna in Water,			
2.5 oz pouch	80	1.5	0
Pink Salmon, skinless/boneless,			
2.5 oz pouch	70	2	0
Shrimp, medium, 4 oz can	90	1	2
Gorton's ~ *Page 114*			
Kroger ~ *Page 116*			
Starkist:			
Autentico, average all, 2 oz drained	85	5	3.5
Pouch: *Per 2.6 oz Pouch*			
Albacore White Tuna in water	80	1.5	0
Chunk, Light, Tuna in water	70	0.5	0
Lunch-To-Go Kit: Chunk Light Tuna			
With Mayonnaise & Crackers, 4 oz	230	9	20
Tuna Creations: *Per 2.6 oz*			
Herb & Garlic	110	4	2
Lemon Pepper	80	0.5	0
Van De Kamp's *(Frozen)* **~** *Page 122*			

Restaurant Chains

Captain D's Seafood ~ *Page 187*
Long John Silver's ~ *Page 213*
Southern Tsunami ~ *Page 242*

Updated Nutrition Data ~ www.CalorieKing.com
Persons with Diabetes ~ See Disclaimer (Page 22)

97

Flours & Grains	C	F	Cb
Amaranth Flour, ½ cup, 3.5 oz	365	6.5	65
Arrowroot Flour, ½ cup, 2.3 oz	230	0	56
Barley: Grain, regular, ½ cup, 2.6 oz	255	1	55
Pearled, raw, 3.5 oz	350	1	78
Buckwheat: Grain, ½ cup, 3 oz	290	3	61
Flour, whole-groat, ½ cup, 2 oz	200	2	42
Groats: Rstd, dry, ½ cup, 3 oz	285	2	62
Roasted, cooked, 3.5 oz	80	0.5	17
Bulgur: Dry, ½ cup, 2.5 oz	240	1	53
Cooked, ½ cup, 3.2 oz	75	0.5	17
Carob Flour, ½ cup, 1.8 oz	115	0.5	46
Corn Kernels, cooked, av., ½ cup	80	0.5	18
Corn Bran, ½ cup, 1.3 oz	85	0.5	33
Corn Flour/Masa, ½ cup, 2 oz	215	2.5	43
Corn Grits:			
Dry, ½ cup, 2.8oz	290	1	62
Cooked, ½ cup, 4.3 oz	70	0.5	15
Corn Germ, toasted, ½ cup, 4 oz	100	1.5	22
Cornmeal, average all varieties:			
3 Tbsp, 1 oz	105	0.5	22
½ cup, 2.5 oz	255	1	54
Mixes, same as above	230	1	48
Cornstarch: 1 Tbsp, 0.3 oz	30	0	8
½ cup, 2.3oz	245	0	58
Couscous: Dry, 1 oz	110	0	22
1 cup cooked, 5.5 oz	175	0.5	37
Farina: Dry, ½ cup, 3 oz	325	0.5	69
Cooked, ½ cup, 4 oz	55	0	12
Flaxseed: Whole, 1 T., 0.3 oz	45	3.5	2
Ground, 2 Tbsp, 0.3 oz	60	4.5	4
Garbanzo, (Chick Pea), ½ cup, 1.6 oz	180	3	27
Gluten Free Flour, 3 Tbsp	100	0	24
Matzo Meal, ½ cup, 2.2 oz	230	0.5	48
Millet: Raw, ½ cup, 3.5 oz	380	4	73
Cooked, ½ cup, 3 oz	105	1	21
Oat Bran: Raw, ⅓ cup, 1 oz	75	2	21
Cooked, ½ cup, 3.8 oz	45	1	13
Oats, Rolled/Oatmeal:			
Dry/Groats, ½ cup, 1.5 oz	160	3	28
Cooked, ½ cup, 4.2 oz	75	1	13
Polenta ~ See Cornmeal			
Potato Flour, ½ cup, 2.8 oz	285	0.5	66
Psyllium Husks, 1 Tbsp, 0.2 oz	10	0	4
Quinoa: Dry ½ cup, 3 oz	320	5	59
Cooked, ½ cup, 3.8 oz	130	2	24
Rice Bran, ½ cup, 2 oz	180	12	28
Rice Flour, ½ cup, 2.8 oz	290	1	63

Flours & Grains (Cont)	C	F	Cb
Rice Polish, ½ cup, 3.5 oz	360	0.5	80
Rye Flour:			
Dark, ½ cup, 2.3 oz	210	2	44
Light, ½ cup, 1.8 oz	190	1	41
Medium, ½ cup, 1.8 oz	180	1	40
Rye Grain: ½ cup, 3 oz	280	2	59
Flakes, ¼ cup, 1 oz	100	0.5	21
Semolina Flour, ½ cup, 3 oz	300	1	61
Sorghum, ½ cup, 3.4 oz	325	3	72
Soy Flour:			
Defatted, 1 cup, 3.5 oz	330	1	38
Low-Fat, 1 cup, 3 oz	325	6	33
Full-Fat, 1 cup, 3 oz	365	17	29
Soy Meal, defatted, 1 cup, 4.3 oz	415	3	49
Spelt Flour, ½ cup, 2 oz	190	1	41
Tapioca Pearl:			
Dry, ½ cup, 2.7 oz	270	0	67
3 Tbsp, 1 oz	100	0	25
Teff Seed Flour, 2 oz	215	2	42
Tortilla Flour Mix,			
½ cup, 2 oz	220	6	37
Triticale:			
½ cup, 3.4 oz	325	2	70
Flour, wholegrain, ½ cup, 2.3 oz	220	1	48
Wheat Bran, unprocessed, ½ cup, 1 oz	65	1	19
Wheat Flakes, ½ cup, 1.5 oz	160	1	35
Wheat Germ:			
Raw, ¼ cup, 1 oz	105	3	15
Toasted, ¼ cup, 1 oz	110	3	14
Wheat Flour:			
White, All Purpose/Self-Rising:			
1 level Tbsp, 0.3 oz	30	0	6
½ cup, 2.2 oz	230	0.5	48
1 cup, 4.4 oz	455	1.5	95
Whole Wheat, 1 cup, 4.2 oz	405	2	87

FRUIT TIME

Fruit ~ Fresh

	C	F	Cb

Weights As Purchased

Apples, all varieties, average:
Whole, with skin:			
1 small, 4 oz	55	0	14
1 medium, 5.5 oz	75	0	19
1 large, 8 oz	110	0	28
1 extra large, 11 oz	145	0	36
Flesh only, no skin or core: 1 oz	15	0	3.5
Slices, 1 cup, 4 oz	55	0	14
Candy/Caramel Apple, 1 med., 6.5 oz	245	4	54
Chiquita, Apple Bites, 14 slices, 5 oz	80	0	20

Apricots: 1 small, 1.5 oz
1 small, 1.5 oz	20	0	4
1 medium, 2 oz	25	0	6
1 large, 3 oz	40	0	10
1 extra large, 4 oz	50	0	12

Asian Pear, (Nashi Fruit), 1 med., 7 oz — 85 | 0 | 21

Avocado:
Fuerte (Florida) variety:			
¼ medium, 2.7 oz pulp	90	7.5	6
½ medium, 5.4 oz pulp	180	15	12
Mashed, 2 Tbsp, 1 oz	35	3	2
Hass variety (Californian/Mexican):			
Cubes, ½ cup, 2.5 oz	120	11	6
Mashed, 2 Tbsp, 1 oz	50	4	2
¼ cup, 2 oz	95	8	5
Pulp: ¼ medium, 1.5 oz	70	6.5	3
½ medium, 3 oz	140	13	7
1 medium (8.5 oz whole), 6 oz	280	26	14
Salad slices (3), 1 oz	50	4	2

Note: The fat of avocados is heart-healthy. Avocados are very low in sugars; and most of the carbohydrate is fiber. This benefits blood sugar and cholesterol levels. Use in place of butter and other high-fat spreads.

Banana:
Weight with skin:			
1 baby, 3 oz	50	0	12
1 small (5"), 4 oz	65	0	16
1 medium (7"), 5 oz	80	0	20
1 large (8"), 8 oz	120	0	30
1 extra large (9"), 9 oz	135	0	34
Flesh only, weight without skin:			
Mashed, ½ cup, 4 oz	100	0	25
Slices, ½ cup, 2.5 oz	65	0	16
Green Bananas, weight with skin:			
1 medium (7"), 5 oz	75	0	18
1 large (8"), 7 oz	110	0	27

Blackberries, 1 cup, 5 oz — 60 | 0.5 | 14

Blueberries, ¼ cup, 1 oz
¼ cup, 1 oz	15	0	4
1 cup or ½ pint container, 5 oz	80	0	20
1 pint container, 10 oz	160	0	40

Weights As Purchased

	C	F	Cb
Boysenberries, 1 cup, 4.5 oz	60	4.5	14
Breadfruit, ½ cup, 4 oz	115	0	30

Cactus Fruit:
1 small, 2 oz	15	0	4
1 medium, 5 oz	40	0	9
1 large, 7 oz	55	0	13
Pulp, no skin, 1 cup, 5.3 oz	60	0	14

Cantaloupe: Flesh, without skin, 1 oz
Flesh, without skin, 1 oz	10	0	2
Pieces/Balls, 1 cup, 5.5 oz	55	0	13
Slices, ½ cup, without rind:			
1 thin (buffet), (⅛"), 0.5 oz	5	0	1
1 medium (¼"), 1 oz	10	0	2
1 thick (½"), 2 oz	20	0	5
Wedges, length cut, without skin:			
1 thin, 1/16 medium, 2 oz	20	0	5
1 thick, ⅛ medium, 4 oz	40	0	9
Whole, weight with seeds and skin:			
½ small, 20 oz	195	1	46
½ medium, 28 oz	270	1.5	65
½ large, 2.5 lb	370	2	90

Cape Gooseberries, 1 cup, 5 oz — 70 | 1 | 15

Cherimoya: Pulp, ½ cup, 3 oz
Pulp, ½ cup, 3 oz	60	0	14
1 Fruit (11 oz), 8 oz edible	170	1	40

Cherries, (Red/White), sweet, raw:
6 medium or 4 large, 2 oz	30	0	7
1 cup, 4.5 oz	75	0	18
½ lb quantity	130	0	32
Sour, red, raw, 1 cup, 4 oz	50	0	12

Clementine, 1 medium, 2.6 oz — 35 | 0 | 9

Coconut, raw:
Young, sweet,			
Pieces (2" x 2"), 1.5 oz	35	2	4
½ cup, 3.5 oz	80	5	9
Mature, hard, 1 piece (2"x 2"), 1.5 oz	160	15	6

Crabapples, slices, ½ cup, 2 oz — 40 | 0 | 11

Cranberries, fresh, ¼ cup, 1 oz — 25 | 0 | 6.5

Custard Apple ~ See Cherimoya

Dates: Medium (1), 0.3 oz
Medium (1), 0.3 oz	20	0	5
Large Medjool (1), 0.5 oz	40	0	10
Extra Large Medjool (1), 0.9 oz	65	0	16
Chopped, ½ cup, 3 oz	240	0	58

Dragon Fruit, (Pitahaya):
1 medium, 4" long, 12 oz	60	0	12
1 large, 5" long, 16 oz	80	0	18

Durian, pulp, 4 oz — 165 | 6 | 31

Elderberries, ½ cup, 2.5 oz — 55 | 0.5 | 13

Weights As Purchased

	C	F	Cb
Feijoa, (Pineapple Guava), 1 medium, 2 oz	30	0.5	5.5
Figs, green/black:			
1 medium, 2 oz	40	0	10
1 large, 3 oz	60	0	15
Gooseberries, raw, 1 cup, 5 oz	65	1	15
Grapefruit, all varieties, average:			
½ fruit, 10 oz (6 oz flesh)	55	0	13
1 cup sections w/ juice, 8 oz	75	0	18
Grapes: Average, 1 cup, 5.5 oz	105	0	28
1 small bunch, 4 oz	80	0	20
1 medium bunch, 7 oz	140	0	36
1 large bunch, 16 oz	315	0	82
Granadilla, pulp, ½ cup, 4 oz	110	0	27
Guanabana, pulp, ½ cup, 4 oz	75	0	19
Guava, 1 medium, 4 oz	80	1	16
Honeydew:			
1 slice, ¾" thick, 3 oz	30	0	7
1 wedge, (⅛ of 7" diameter), 12 oz (with rind)	80	0	20
Cubes/Balls, 1 cup, 6 oz	60	0	14
½ small (4½ lb whole)	180	0.5	42
½ medium (6lb whole)	230	0	56
Honey Murcots, 1 only, 5 oz	45	0	11
Jaboticaba, 1 cup, 5.5 oz	55	0	14
Jackfruit, flesh, ⅛, 4 oz	105	0	27
Kiwano, ½ medium, 5 oz	35	0	8
Kiwifruit:			
1 Medium, 2.7 oz	45	0	11
1 Large, 3.2 oz	55	0	13
Langsat, Duku 1 medium, 2 oz	25	0	5
Lemons: 1 medium, 5oz	20	0	4
1 wedge, 1 oz	5	0	1
Limes, 1 medium, 2.4 oz	20	0	7
Loganberries, frozen, ½ cup, 2.5 oz	40	0	9
Longans, 5 fruit, 0.5oz	10	0	2.5
Loquats, 4 fruit, 2.3 oz	30	0	8
Lychees, 4 fruit, 2.3 oz	30	0	7
Mamey Apple, Cubes, 1 cup, 6 oz	85	1	20
Mandarin Orange:			
1 small, 3 oz	35	0	9
1 medium, 4 oz	45	0	11
1 large, 6 oz	50	0	13
Mango:			
Slices, ½ cup, 3 oz	55	0	14
1 small mango, 7 oz	90	0.5	24
1 medium: 10 oz	130	0.5	34
Side cheek, 4 oz	60	0	14
1 large, 17 oz	220	1	58
1 extra large, 24 oz	310	1.5	82
Marionberries, 1 cup, 5 oz	75	1	15

Weights As Purchased

	C	F	Cb
Melons, all varieties, average, cubes/balls, 1 cup, 6 oz	60	0	14
Mulberries, 20 fruit, 1 oz	15	0	3
Nashi Fruit/Asian Pear, 1 med. 7 oz	85	0	21
Nectarines: 1 medium, 5oz	60	0	14
1 large, 7 oz	80	0	18
Oheloberries, ½ cup, 2.5 oz	20	0	5
Olives, Pickled: Green, 10 lge, 1.5 oz	60	6.5	1.5
Ripe, Greek Style, 10 medium, 1 oz	70	6	4
Ripe (Black) Californian:			
1 small/medium	5	0	0.2
1 large/extra large	6	0.5	0.5
1 jumbo	7	0.5	0.5
1 colossal	11	1	0.5
Oranges, all varieties, average, weights with skin:			
1 small, (2.5" diam.), 5 oz	45	0	11
1 medium (3") 7 oz	75	0	18
1 large, (3.5") 10 oz	105	0	25
1 extra large, (4"), 14 oz	130	0	30
Flesh/Pulp only, 1 cup, 6 oz	85	0	21
Peel, 1 Tbsp	0	0	0
California Navel (3"), 7 oz	70	0	17
Californian Valencia, 1 medium (2¾" diam.) 6 oz	60	0	14
Florida Orange, 1 med., 7 oz	70	0	17
Sunkist Navel, large, 14 oz	130	0	30
Papaya:			
1" pieces, 1 cup, 5 oz	60	0	15
1 medium, 16 oz	120	0	30
Green (unripe), ½ cup, 3.5 oz	20	0	5
Passionfruit:			
1 small, 1.5 oz	15	0	3
1 large, 2.7 oz	30	0	6
Pulp, ½ cup, 4 oz	110	0	27
Peaches, 1 baby/donut, 3 oz	30	0	7
1 small, 5 oz	50	0	12
1 medium, 6 oz	60	0	14
1 large, 7 oz	70	0	16
1 extra large, 9 oz	90	0	21
Pears, all varieties, average:			
1 mini, 2.5 oz	35	0	8
1 small, 5 oz	75	0	18
1 medium, 7 oz	100	0	25
1 large, 9 oz	130	0	33
1 extra large, 12 oz	170	0	42
Pepino, ½ medium, 4 oz	20	0	4
Persimmons: Native, 1 oz	35	0	9
Japanese (2½"d. x 2½"h), 7 oz	120	0	30
Seedless (Maui), 1 medium, 5 oz	100	0	25

Weights As Purchased	**C**	**F**	**Cb**
Pineapple, average all varieties:		
Weights without skin:		
1 thin slice (½"), 2 oz	30	0	7
1 thick slice (¾"), 3 oz	40	0	10
1 cup, chunks, 6 oz	80	0	20
Whole fruit, wt with skin:		
Baby/Mini, 16 oz	150	0	39
Medium size, 3 lbs	450	1	118
Canned ~ *See Page 102*		
Pitanga, (Surinam-Cherry) (5), 1.2 oz	10	0	2
Plaintains:		
Fresh/Raw, weight with skin:		
1 medium, 10 oz	220	0	55
Slices, 1 cup, 5 oz	180	0	44
Cooked:		
Mashed, ½ cup, 3.5 oz	115	0	30
Slices, 1 cup, 5.5 oz	180	0	47
Fried in oil: 10 slices (¼"), 2 oz	160	6	26
1 cup, 4.2 oz	360	14	58
Plums, all varieties, average:		
1 mini/Damson, (1" diam) 0.5 oz	10	0	1.5
1 small (2"), 2.3oz	30	0	7
1 medium (2½"), 3.5 oz	45	0	10
1 large (3"), 5 oz	60	0	14
Plumcot, 1 medium, 6 oz	75	0	14
Pomegranates:		
1 small (3"), 5.5 oz	70	1	15
1 medium (3½"), 10 oz	125	2	27
1 large (4"), 16 oz	230	3	50
Seeds/Arils, ¼ cup, 2 oz	40	1	10
Pomelo, flesh, ½ cup, 3.5 oz	35	0	9
Prickly Pear ~ *See Cactus Fruit*		
Quince, 1 medium, 3.5 oz	55	0	14
Rambuta/Rambotang,		
Red/Yellow, medium, 2 oz	15	0	4
Raspberries: ½ cup, 2 oz	30	0	7
10 Raspberries, 0.8 oz	10	0	2
1 cup, 4.3 oz	65	1	15
1 Pint, 11 oz	160	2	37
Sapodilla: 1 medium, 6 oz	140	2	34
Pulp, 1 cup, 8.5 oz	200	2.5	45
Sapote:		
Black: 1 medium, 4.5 oz	60	0	14
Pulp only, ½ cup, 4 oz	100	1	22
Mamey, piece, 1 cup, 6 oz	220	1	50
Satsuma Tangerine, 1 medium, 3 oz	45	0	11
Soursop, pulp, 1 cup, 8 oz	150	0.5	38
Starfruit, (Carambola):		
1 medium, (3½" long), 3 oz	30	0	6
1 large (4½"), 4.5 oz	40	0	9
Strawberries: 1 cup, 5.5 oz	50	0.5	12
6 medium/3 large, 2 oz	20	0	4
1 pint container, heaping, 16 oz	130	0	32
Chocolate Dipped, 1 large	45	2.5	6

Weights As Purchased	**C**	**F**	**Cb**
Sugar-Apple (Sweetsop),		
pulp, ½ cup, 4 oz	120	0	28
Sugar Cane:		
Unpeeled, 1 baton (7" long), 4 oz	30	0	7
Peeled, 1 small stick (3"), 2 oz	35	0	8
Tamarillo, 1 medium, 3 oz	20	0	3
Tamarind: 1 fruit (3"x1")	5	0	1.5
Pulp, ½ cup, 2 oz	140	0.5	37
Tangelo: 1 small, 4 oz	55	0	13
1 medium, 5 oz	70	0	17
1 large, 7 oz	95	0	23
Tangerine, 1 med., (2½" diam.), 4 oz	50	0	13
Tangor, 1 medium, 4 oz	35	0	7
Tomatillos:		
3 medium, 3.5 oz	35	0.5	6
1lb (16 oz) quantity	160	2	27
Tomatoes:		
1 small (2¼" diameter), 3 oz	15	0	3
1 medium (2¾"), 5 oz	25	0	5
Sliced: 2 thin slices, 1 oz	5	0	1
2 thick (⅜"), 2 oz	10	0	2
Wedge, ¼, 1.3 oz	6	0	1
1 large (3½"), 8 oz	40	0.5	9
1 extra large (4"), 12 oz	60	0.5	14
Cherry: 4 medium, 2 oz	10	0	2
1 cup, 5 oz	25	0	6
Grape, 5 medium, 2 oz	10	0	2
Yellow Tear Drop, 3 medium, 1 oz	5	0	1
Canned Tomatoes/Products ~ *See Page 144*		
Tree Tomato/Tamarillo, 3 oz	20	0	5
Ugli Fruit, Tangelo type, 5 oz	40	0	8
Watermelon:		
Flesh only, weights without skin:		
1 thin slice (½"): ¼ circle, 3 oz	25	0	6
1 thick slice (1"): ¼ circle, 6 oz	50	0	12
½ circle, 12 oz	100	1	24
Buffet Slice, small, thin, 1 oz	8	0	2
Cubes or Balls, 1 cup, 5.5 oz	45	0	11
Round Seedless Melon, weight with skin:		
Medium size, 13 lb, (8" diam.):		
Whole melon, 13 lb	1160	5	280
Wedge, ⅛ whole, 26 oz	145	1	35
Mini size, 6 lb, (6.5" diam.):		
Whole melon, 6 lb	480	2.5	110
Wedge, ⅛ whole, 12 oz	60	0	14

Dried Fruit

	C	F	Cb
Apples, 5 rings, 1 oz	80	0	19
Apricots, 8 halves, 1 oz	65	0	16
Banana Chips, ⅓ cup, 1 oz	180	9	16
Banana Flakes, 4 Tbsp, 1 oz	80	0	20
Cranberries *(Craisins):*			
Original, ¼ cup	130	0	33
Reduced Sugar, ¼ cup	100	0	31
Chocolate Covered, ¼ cup, 2 oz	180	8	28
Dates ~ See Dates in Fresh Fruit			
Figs, 3 medium figs, 1 oz	90	0	23
Goji Berries, 3 Tbsp, 1 oz	100	1	20
Mango Slices, 5 pieces, 1.4 oz	25	0	6
Papaya Spears, 2 pieces, 1.4 oz	120	0	30
Peaches, 2 halves, 1 oz	60	0	15
Pears, 3 halves, 2 oz	140	0.5	34
Plums (Sunsweet), (5), 1.4 oz	100	0	24
Prunes/Dried Plums:			
With pits, 3 medium, 1 oz	70	0	17
Without pits, 4 medium, 1 oz	70	0	17
Cooked: With sugar, ½ cup, 5 oz	155	0	38
Without sugar, ½ cup, 4.5 oz	135	0	33
Raisins: 2 Tbsp, 1 oz pack	85	0	20
½ cup, 2.8 oz	220	0.5	56

Candied/Glazed Fruit

	C	F	Cb
Apricot, 1 medium, 1 oz	70	0	17
Cherry, Maraschino (1)	8	0	2
Citron/Fruit Peel, 1 oz	85	0	20
Ginger, 1 oz	90	0	21
Pineapple, 1 slice, 1.3 oz	120	0	29
Tamarind, dried, sweetened, 1 oz	70	0	17

Fruit Leather Rolls

	C	F	Cb
Betty Crocker: Fruit By The Foot,			
1 roll, 0.8 oz	80	0	17
Fruit Gushers, 1 oz	90	1	20
Fruit Roll-Ups, 1 roll	50	1	12
Stretch Island, Leathers, 1 pouch, 0.5 oz	45	0	12

Canned/Bottled Fruit

Solids & Liquids:
Per ½ Cup, 4½ oz Unless indicated

	C	F	Cb
Apricots/Peaches/Pears:			
In juice, light	60	0	15
In heavy syrup	105	0	28
In water/diet	35	0	8
Black/Blueberries:			
In heavy syrup	120	0	30
In light syrup	110	0	26

Canned/Bottled Fruit (Cont)

	C	F	Cb
Cherries, pitted:			
In heavy syrup	105	0	27
In light syrup	85	0	22
In water	55	0	15
Maraschino, 1 oz	50	0	12
Fruit Cocktail/Salad:			
In heavy syrup	95	0	25
In juice, light	60	0	16
In water/diet	35	0	10
Gooseberries, light syrup	90	0	24
Grapefruit, in light syrup	75	0	20
Lychees, ½ cup, 4.5 oz	105	0	26
Mixed Fruit: In fruit juices/light syrup	70	0	18
In heavy syrup	90	0	24
In water/diet	40	0	10
Pineapple, all varieties:			
In heavy syrup, 4.3 oz	110	0	26
In own juice, 4 oz	60	0	15
Prunes: With pits, 3 oz	90	0	23
Stewed in water, ½ cup	135	0	35

Fruit Snack Cups

	C	F	Cb
Deli-/Take-Out: Small, 6 oz	70	0	16
Large, 12 oz	140	0	32
Yogurt and Fruit Cup, 15 oz	380	4.5	75
Del Monte:			
Fruit Natural: All varieties, av., 7 oz	100	0	24
No Sugar Added, all varieties, 6.5 oz	55	0	12
Snack Cups: In light Syrup, av., 4 oz	70	0	18
No Added Sugar, Peaches, 4 oz	25	0	11
Dole:			
Fruit Bowls: *Per 4 oz Container*			
Pineapple; Tropical Fruit, average	60	0	15
Average other varieties	75	0	18
Fruit in Gel: *Per 4.3 oz Container*			
Mixed Fruit, in Cherry Gel	60	0	14
Average other fruits, in various Gels	90	0	23

Apple & Fruit Sauces

	C	F	Cb
Apple Sauce:			
Regular/sweetened, 2 Tbsp, 1 oz	20	0	6
4 oz package	90	0	22
Cranberry, Jellied, ¼ cup	110	0	25
Fruit Sauces & Purees:			
All fruit types, average: 2 Tbsp, 1 oz	25	0	6
½ cup, 4 oz	100	0	24
Mott's:			
Apple Sauce: Original, 4 oz	90	0	24
Fruit Flavored, average, 4 oz	90	0	23
Healthy Harvest, all flavors, 4 oz	50	0	13
Ocean Spray,			
Cranberry varieties, ¼ cup	110	0	25

Ice Cream ◇ Frozen Yogurt I

Quick Guide   C F Cb

Ice Cream
Average all Flavors:
Regular (10% fat):
Examples: Dreyer's Grand, Hood, Friendly's

	C	F	Cb
½ cup, 4 fl.oz	140	7	16
1 cup, 8 fl.oz	280	14	32
1 pint, 16 fl.oz	560	28	64

Rich/Premium (16-17% fat):
Examples: Baskin Robbins, Ben & Jerry's, Haagen-Dazs

½ cup, 4 fl.oz	250	16	24
1 cup, 8 fl.oz	500	32	48
1 pint, 16 fl.oz	1000	64	96

Reduced-Fat/Light (5% fat):
Examples: Breyers ½ The Fat, Friendly's Light, Hood Light

½ cup, 4 fl.oz	140	5	21
1 cup, 8 fl.oz	280	10	42
1 pint, 16 fl.oz	560	20	84

Fat-Free:
Example: Breyers

½ cup, 4 fl.oz	90	0	21
1 cup, 8 fl.oz	180	0	42
1 pint, 16 fl.oz	360	0	84

Scoop Shops:
Average all Brands
Add extra for cone (see next column)

Kids, 3 fl.oz	125	8	12
Regular, 6 fl.oz	250	16	24
Large, 9 fl.oz	375	24	36

Soft Serve:
Average all Brands

Regular: ½ cup, 4 fl.oz	255	15	25
1 cup, 8 fl.oz	510	30	50
Light: ½ cup, 4 fl.oz	145	3	25
1 cup, 8 fl.oz	290	6	50

Quick Guide

Frozen Yogurt
Average all Brands

Hard: Low-Fat, ½ cup	110	3	19
Non-Fat, ½ cup	110	0	24
Soft: Low-Fat, ½ cup	120	4	17
Non-Fat, ½ cup	100	0	30

Brands ~ See Ice Cream & Novelties Section

Quick Guide   C F Cb

Gelato/Ices/Frozen Custard
Gelato: *Per ½ Cup*

	C	F	Cb
Milk base: Vanilla	160	6	25
Chocolate Hazelnut	230	15	21
Water base, ½ cup	100	0	26

Frozen Custard, Choc./Vanilla, av:

½ cup	210	11	23
Single Scoop, 5 oz wt	300	15	38
Double Scoop, 10 oz wt	600	30	76

Ice (Milk base:) *Average all flavors*

Hard (4% fat), ½ cup	100	3	15
Soft Serve (3% fat), ½ cup	110	2	19
Shaved Ice, 12 fl.oz	160	0	40
Sherbet, average, ½ cup	110	1.5	22
Sorbet, Fruit, fat free, ½ cup	70	0	19
Fruit Ice Pops	80	0	20

Sundaes

Baskin Robbins:

Classic: Banana Royale	620	28	87
Banana Split	1010	34	173
Brownie	920	47	119
Denny's, Banana Split, 15 oz	810	31	125

Toppings ~ See Page 195
McDonald's:

Sundaes: Hot Caramel, 6.4 oz	340	8	60
Hot Fudge, 6.3 oz	330	9	53
Strawberry, 6.4 oz	280	6	49
Toppings, Peanuts, 0.3 oz	40	3.5	1

Ice Cream Cones & Cups

Average all Brands

Wafer Cone/Cup, average	20	0	4
Sugar Cone, average	50	0	14
Waffle Cone: Small	50	1	10
Large	90	0.5	19
Brands: *Comet,* Sugar Cone	50	0	11
Keebler, Sugar Cone	50	0	10
Oreo, Chocolate Cone	50	1	10

Ice Cream ~ Brands

C   **F**   **Cb**

Baskin-Robbins ~ *See Fast-Foods Section*

Ben & Jerry's:

Scoop Shop Ice Cream: *Hand Scooped, per ½ Cup*

	C	F	Cb
Americone Dream	250	13	29
Butter Pecan	270	19	19
Choc. Chip Cookie Dough	250	13	28
Chocolate Fudge Brownie	230	12	28
Chocolate Nougat Crunch	250	13	28
Chocolate Therapy	240	13	26
Chunky Monkey	260	16	26
Coconut Seven Layer Bar	270	17	27
Mint Chocolate Chunk	240	15	24
NY Super Fudge Chunk	270	18	25
Strawberry Cheesecake	220	13	24
Sweet Cream & Cookies	240	13	26
Vanilla Toffee Bar Crunch	120	4	27

Ice Cream, 1 Pint Tubs: *Per ½ Cup*

	C	F	Cb
Banana Split	260	14	28
Boston Cream Pie	250	13	29
Cake Batter	260	14	29
Cherry Garcia	240	13	28
Chocolate Chip Cookie Dough	280	16	32
Chubby Hubby	340	21	32
Everything But The....	310	19	29
Imagine Whirled Peace	270	16	27
Milk & Cookies	280	17	28
Peanut Brittle	260	15	29
Peanut Butter Cup	360	26	27
Phish Food	290	14	37
Red Velvet Cake	250	13	30
S'mores	290	15	36
Triple Caramel Chunk	280	16	32
What a Cluster	320	19	31

Frozen Yogurt: *Per ½ Cup*

Fro Yo: Cherry Garcia

	C	F	Cb
Cherry Garcia	200	3	37
Chocolate Fudge Brownie	180	2.5	35
Half Baked	200	3	38
Phish Food, 3.6 oz	240	6	41

Greek: Raspberry Fudge Chunk

	C	F	Cb
Raspberry Fudge Chunk	200	7	29
Strawberry Shortcake	180	5	28
Vanilla Honey Caramel	190	5	30

Sorbet, average all flavors | 95 | 0 | 23 |

Blue Bunny:

C   **F**   **Cb**

Premium Ice Cream (Pint Ctn): *Per ½ Cup*

	C	F	Cb
Banana Split	160	7	21
Bunny Tracks	190	11	21
Chocolate	130	6	16
Cookies 'n Cream	150	7	20

Fat Free, No Sugar Added: *Per ½ Cup*

	C	F	Cb
Brownie Sundae	80	0	23
Caramel Toffee Crunch	90	0	23
Vanilla	80	0	20

Carb figures include 4-8 g sugar alcohols

Hi Lite: *Per ½ Cup*

	C	F	Cb
Homemade Vanilla	110	3.5	18
Vanilla, 2.3 oz	100	2.5	17

Frozen Yogurt, Personals: *Per Container*

	C	F	Cb
Bordeaux Cherry Chocolate	170	4	31
Caramel Praline Crunch	180	5	30

Bars/Pops ~ *See Page 108*

Breyers:

Original Ice Cream: *Per ½ Cup*

	C	F	Cb
Butter Pecan	140	6	18
Cherry Vanilla	120	3	21
Cookies & Cream	140	4.5	23
Mint Chocolate Chip	150	8	17
Natural Strawberry	110	5	14
Vanilla, Chocolate	130	7	16

Fat Free, average all flavors | 90 | 0 | 21 |

Half The Fat: *Per ½ Cup*

	C	F	Cb
Cookies & Cream	120	4	20
Creamy, Chocolate or Vanilla, av.	105	3	18

No Added Sugar:

	C	F	Cb
Butter Pecan	100	6	13
Vanilla; Vanilla, Choc., Strawberry	80	4	13

Carb figures include 5g sugar alcohol and 4g fiber

Blasts!: *Per ½ Cup*

	C	F	Cb
Chips Ahoy	140	5	23
Mrs Field's Choc Fudge Brownie	140	4	25
Oreo Cookies and Cream Mint	120	4	20
Snickers	150	5	23
Strawberry Waffle Cone	130	4	22

CarbSmart, average all flavors, ½ cup | 115 | 6 | 14 |

Carb figures includes 5g sugar alcohol and 4g fiber

Ice Cream ~ Brands (Cont)

Bruster's:

	C	F	Cb
Ice Cream, Choc./Vanilla, av., ½ cup	210	12	24

Fat Free, No Added Sugar: *Per ½ Cup*

Chocolate	100	0	26
Chocolate Caramel Swirl	120	0	31
Cinnamon; Coffee; Vanilla	100	0	23
Fudge Ripple	110	0	30

Frozen Yogurt,

Chocolate; Vanilla, average, ½ cup	150	4.5	24

Carvel Ice Cream ~ See Fast-Foods Section

Clemmy's: *Per ½ Cup*

Butter Pecan	200	15	20
Chocolate; Chocolate Chip, average	175	13	22
Coffee; Vanilla Bean, average	160	11	21
Orange Cream	120	6	23
P'B Chocolate Chip	220	16	22
Toasted Almond	170	11	26

Carb figures include 13-15g sugar alcohol

Coldstone Creamery ~ See Fast-Foods Section
Dairy Queen/Brazier ~ See Fast-Foods Section

Dippin' Dots:

Original Dots: *Per ½ Cup*

Banana Split	160	8	20
Caramel Brownie Sundae	190	9	23
Cookies 'n Cream	200	11	22
Mint Chocolate	170	8	21
Rocky Road	200	10	22
Strawberry	160	8	18
Vanilla	160	8	18

Dove:

Ice Cream: *Per ½ Cup*

Mint/Vanilla Choc. Chunk	180	11	17
Unconditional Chocolate	200	12	23
Vanilla Chocolate Chunk	180	11	17

Dreyer's/Edy's:

Ice Cream: *Per ½ Cup*

Grand: Chocolate

Grand: Chocolate	140	7	17
Mint Chocolate Chip	150	8	18
Neapolitan	130	6	16
Real Strawberry	120	5	16
Vanilla	140	7	16

Slow Churned, ½ The Fat: *Per ½ Cup*

Chocolate	100	3.5	15
Double Fudge Brownie	120	3	19
Fudge Tracks	120	3.5	18
Mint Chocolate Chip	120	4.5	17
Peanut Butter Cup	130	4	17

Friendly's:

Rich & Creamy Ice Cream: *Per ½ Cup*

	C	F	Cb
Butter Crunch	150	7	19
Chocolate Almond Chip	160	9	17
Classic Chocolate	150	8	16
Coffee	130	7	15
Strawberry	140	6	18
Vanilla	140	8	15
Vienna Mocha Chunk	170	9	18

Smooth Churned Ice Cream: *Per ½ Cup*

Light: Black Raspberry	110	3	18
Chocolate Chip Cookie Dough	140	5	21
Fudge Swirl	130	4	21
Mint Chocolate Chip	120	4.5	19
Purely Pistachio	120	4.5	18
Vanilla	110	3.5	17

Sundae Cup: *Per Container*

Original Fudge	300	14	39
Choc. Chip Cookie Dough	330	15	46
Reese's P'nut Butter Cup	430	25	42
Sherbet, all flavors, ½ cup	130	1.5	28

Yogurt Frozen: *Per ½ Cup*

Regular, average all flavors	145	5	24
Fat Free, all flavors	110	0	23

Gelati-da:

Gelato: *Per ½ Cup*

Amaretto Chocolate	150	4.5	23
Choc Mint Milano	120	2.5	22
Coffee Fudge Latte	130	2	22
Limoncello; Vanilla Marsala, average	120	3	23
Red Raspberry	130	1.5	25

Great Value (Walmart):

Ice Cream: *Per ½ cup*

Chocolate Chip Cookie Dough	150	8	19
Peanut Butter Lovers	300	16	34
Sherbet, all flavors	110	0	26

Haagen-Dazs:

Regular: *Tubs, Per ½ Cup*

Butter Pecan	300	22	20
Chocolate Peanut Butter	340	23	26
Cookies & Cream	250	16	22
White Chocolate Raspberry Truffle	280	16	31

Gelato: *Per ½ Cup*

Black Cherry Amaretto	240	9	35
Sea Salt Caramel	270	11	38

Healthy Choice,

Greek Frozen Yogurt,

average all varieties,	100	2	18

Bars ~*See Page 109*

Ice Cream ~ Brands (Cont)

Hood:

	C	F	Cb
Ice Cream: *Per ½ Cup*			
Chocolate	140	6	18
Classic Trio	140	7	17
Cookie Dough	160	8	19
Cookies 'N Cream	150	8	19
Creamy Coffee	140	7	16
Fudge Twister	140	6	20
Golden/Natural Vanilla; Patchwork	140	7	17
Maple Walnut	150	9	17
Churned, Light: *Per ½ Cup*			
Chocolate Chip	120	4.5	18
Coffee	100	3	16
Moosehead Lake Fudge	160	7	21
Under The Stars	160	8	18
Vanilla	110	3	16
Frozen Fat-Free Yogurt: *Per ½ Cup*			
Maine Blueberry & Sweet Cream	90	0	19
Mocha Fudge	100	0	22
Strawberry	80	0	18
Strawberry Banana	90	0	20

New England Creamery ~ www.CalorieKing.com

Jerseymaid *(Vons): Per ½ Cup*

	C	F	Cb
Ice Cream:			
Cookies & Cream	160	8	18
Choc Chip; Mint Choc Chip	150	9	16
Heavenly Hash	165	9	19
Mocha Almond Fudge; Chocolate	150	9	16
Neapolitan; Real Vanilla	140	8	15
Strawberry	130	6	17

Oberweis:

Super Premium Ice Cream: *Per 6 oz Scoop*

	C	F	Cb
Chocolate	480	31	43
Chocolate Peanut Butter	550	39	42
Cookie Dough	500	28	56
Vanilla	460	31	40

Pinkberry:

Frozen Yogurt: *Without Toppings*

	C	F	Cb
Original: Mini, 3.2 oz wt	90	0	19
Small, 5 oz wt	140	0	29
Medium, 8 oz wt	230	0	48
Large: Original, 13 oz wt	370	0	78
Chocolate Hazelnut	370	9	60
Cookies & Cream	320	4.5	60
Mango; Passionfruit, av.	255	0	53

Purely Decadent:

Soy Based: *Per ½ Cup*

	C	F	Cb
Chocolate Obsession	210	7	27
Peanut Butter Zig Zag	230	12	24
Gluten Free, Cookie Dough	230	8	36

Red Mango:

Frozen Yogurt: *No Toppings Included*

	C	F	Cb
Original: 3.3 oz wt	80	0	19
Small, 4.7 oz wt	120	0	27
Regular, 7.5 oz wt	190	0	43
Large, 11.4 oz wt	290	0	65
Pomegranate: 3.3 oz wt	90	0	21
Small, 4.6 oz wt	130	0	30
Regular, 7.5 oz wt	210	0	48
Large, 11.4 oz wt	320	0	73

Rice Dream:

Frozen Dessert: *Per ½ Cup*

	C	F	Cb
Carob Chip	180	7	28
Cocoa Marble Fudge	170	6	31
Cookies n' Dream	180	7	28
Neapolitan	160	6	26
Strawberry	170	6	30
Vanilla	160	6	26

Bars ~ *See Page 110*

Skinny Cow:

Bars/Sandwiches/Cones ~ *See Page 110*

So Delicious:

Coconut Based: *Per ½ Cup*

	C	F	Cb
Cherry Amaretto	130	6	22
Chocolate	150	9	20
Coconut Almond Chip	180	12	20
Turtle Trails	160	8	26

Soy Based: *Per ½ Cup*

	C	F	Cb
Chocolate Peanut Butter	140	4.5	23
Chocolate Velvet	130	3.5	23
Creamy Vanilla	130	3	24
Mint Marble Fudge	140	3	27
Mocha Fudge	130	3	26
Neapolitan	120	3.5	23

Ice Cream ~ Brands (Cont)

	C	F	Cb
Soy Dream:			
Frozen Dessert: *Per ½ Cup*			
Butter Pecan	190	11	23
Choc. Fudge Brownie	170	9	21
French Vanilla; Vanilla	170	9	21
Vanilla Fudge	170	9	23
Stonyfield Farm:			
Frozen Yogurt: *Per ½ Cup*			
After Dark Chocolate	100	0	21
Creme Caramel	130	1.5	26
Gotta Have Vanilla	100	0	20
Stop & Shop:			
Ice Cream: *Per ½ Cup*			
Chocolate	150	8	18
Neapolitan; Vanilla, average	140	7.5	17
Vanilla Fudge Swirl	140	7	18
Light: Moose Tracks	130	5	18
Vanilla	100	3	17
Premium:			
Cookies & Cream	170	9	21
Mint Chocolate Chip	160	9	18
Simply Enjoy:			
Chocolate	210	12	22
Strawberry; Vanilla, average	225	13	25
Tasti D-Lite:			
Soft Serve: *Per ½ Cup*			
Calories will vary with density (air in product) and serving size. Best to weigh product and calculate on 25 cals per 1 oz weight.			
Banana	70	1	13
Blueberry Cheesecake	80	1.5	15
Brownie Batter	70	1.5	13
Buttercrunch Mania	90	3.5	13
Chocolate Cookie Dough	80	1.5	14
Marshmallow	80	1	14
Tofutti:			
Premium Pints: *Per ½ Cup*			
Better Pecan	250	15	27
Chocolate	210	13	20
Vanilla	210	13	21
Vanilla Almond Bark	240	15	24
Vanilla Fudge; Wild Berry Supreme	190	9	25
TCBY ~ See Page 250			

	C	F	Cb
Turkey Hill:			
All Natural, average all flavors, ½ cup	160	9	17
Light: *Per ½ Cup*			
Moose Tracks	140	6	20
Vanilla Bean	100	2	17
Average other flavors	130	4	19
No Sugar Added: *Per ½ Cup*			
Cherry Fudge Ripple	80	0	22
Dutch Chocolate; Vanilla Bean, av.	70	0	20
Moose Tracks	120	5	22
Premium Ice Cream: *Per ½ Cup*			
Black Cherry	130	6	18
Butter Pecan; Choco Mint Chip, av.	160	10	16
Chocolate Peanut Butter Cup	180	11	18
Cookies 'n Cream; Tin Roof Sundae	150	8	19
Rocky Road	170	8	23
Vanilla Bean	140	7	16
Frozen Yogurt: *Per ½ Cup*			
Chocolate Chip Cookie Dough	120	2.5	22
Fat-Free: Chocolate Marshmallow	110	0	24
Average other flavors	95	0	19
Sherbet, av. all flavors	120	1	27
Wawa:			
Premium Ice Cream: *Per ½ Cup*			
Butter Pecan; Mint Choc. Chip, av.	180	10	20
Chocolate; Vanilla Bean, average	160	8	20
Cookies & Cream	180	9	21
Strawberry Shortcake	160	7	22
Wegmans: *Per ½ Cup*			
Chocolate	130	7	15
Cookies & Cream	160	8	21
French Vanilla; Vanilla, av.	145	7	19
Neapolitan	130	7	17
Peanut Butter Sundae	220	14	20
Premium, Vanilla	270	18	22
Yoplait:			
Go-Gurt!, Frozen Yogurt, tube, 2.3 oz wt	60	0.5	12
Frozen Yogurt: *Per ½ Cup*			
Original Fruit flavors, average	115	2	21
Vanilla	110	2.5	19
Greek:			
Fruit Flavors, average	130	2	21
Honey Caramel	140	2.5	22
Vanilla	120	2.5	17

Ice Cream Bars & Pops ~ Brands

Per Bar/Serving Unless Indicated **C** **F** **Cb**

Ben & Jerry's:

	C	F	Cb
Bars: Cherry Garcia	270	17	26
Half Baked	340	20	34

Big Bear – *See Klondike*

Blue Bunny:

Bars:

	C	F	Cb
Caramel Crunch, 1.4 oz	120	8	12
Chocolate Sundae Crunch, 2.2. oz	170	7	24
Cookies 'n Cream, 2.4 oz	180	9	25
English Toffee, 1.4 oz	130	8	13
Fudge Bar, 2.2 oz	80	1	16
Orange Dream: 1.7 oz Bar	70	1	13
2.5 oz Bar	90	1.5	19
Root Beer Float, 1.9 oz	60	1	12
Star Bar, 1.5 oz	110	7	12
King Size: Chocolate Eclair, 2.8 oz	210	9	30
Crunch with Candy Center, 3 oz	350	28	25
Strawberry Shortcake, 2.8 oz	200	10	27
Bomb Pops, Banana Fudge, 4 oz	160	2	31

Champ Cones:

	C	F	Cb
6 Pack: Caramel Lovers, 3.4 oz	310	16	37
Chocolate Lovers, 3.2 oz	270	13	35
Cookies 'n Cream, 3.2 oz	270	13	37
Single, Caramel Lovers, 3.8 oz	350	19	40
King Size:			
Bunny Tracks, 5.9 oz	490	27	57
Vanilla Brownie, 5.8 oz	460	22	60

FrozFruit:

	C	F	Cb
Chunky: Mango	140	0	35
Pineapple	120	0	30
Strawberry	130	0	33
Creamy Coconut	210	5	39
Double Lime	120	0	32
Jolly Rancher, Cool Tubes, 3 oz	110	1	23

Ice Cream Sandwiches:

	C	F	Cb
Birthday Party, 2.6 oz	180	5	30
Cookies-N-Cream, 3 oz	250	10	36
Simply Vanilla, 2.5 oz	160	5	27
Big: Bopper, 5 oz	470	23	61
Double Strawberry, 3.9 oz	250	7	42
Mississippi Mud, 4 oz	280	9	46
Neapolitan, 3.7 oz	240	7	40

Per Bar/Serving Unless Indicated **C** **F** **Cb**

Breyers:

Carb Smart:

	C	F	Cb
Fudge Bar	100	7	9
Carb figure includes 3g sugar alcohol			
Vanilla Ice Cream Bar	180	14	9
Vanilla Almond Ice Cream Bar	190	15	11
Carb figures include 2 sugar alcohol			

Butterfinger *(Nestle):*

Ice Cream Bar:

	C	F	Cb
King Size	280	18	27
Loaded	270	17	28

Clemmy's,

	C	F	Cb
Bars, average all flavors, 2 oz	70	3	16

Cool Classics:

Arctic Blasters:

	C	F	Cb
Crispy Bar	160	11	15
Fudge Bar	100	1	21
Ice Cream Bar	150	10	13
Orange Cream	100	2.5	18
Strawberry Shortcake	150	8	20
Toffee Bar	160	11	14
Icepix: Grape; Cherry; Orange	35	0	8
Honeydew; Watermelon; Cantelope	35	0	9
Swirl Pops, Mango-Cherry	80	0	20
Creamsicles: 100 Calorie Bar	100	2	20
Sugar-Free, all flavors	40	0.5	12
Carb figures include 5g sugar alcohol			

Diana's Bananas:

Banana Babies:

	C	F	Cb
Milk/Dark Chocolate (1)	130	6	18
Milk Chocolate & Peanuts (1)	215	13	21
Banana Bites, (5), 2 oz	130	8	16

Dove:

Bars: *Per 2.6 oz Bar*

	C	F	Cb
Vanilla: With Milk Chocolate	250	16	24
And Almonds	250	17	21
Caramel Swirl & Cashews	250	16	23
Vanilla, with Dark Chocolate	250	17	24
Miniatures, Variety Pack, with Milk Chocolate, 5 pieces, 3.2 oz	340	22	32

Dreyer's/Edy's:

Outshine Fruit Bars:

	C	F	Cb
Coconut Waters, average all flavors	60	0	15
Creamy Coconut	120	3	20
Grape	60	0	16
Mango; Pineapple	80	0	20
Average other varieties	70	0	20

Ice Cream Bars/Pops ~ Brands (Cont)

Per Bar/Serving	C	F	Cb
Drumstick (Nestlé):			
Classic Cones: Vanilla	290	16	33
Vanilla Caramel	310	16	38
Super Nugget	310	18	34
Lil' Drums, av. all flavors	120	6	16
Simply Dipped: Mint	270	13	37
Vanilla	270	13	37
Edy's ~ See Dreyer's			
Eskimo Pie (Nestlé):			
Crunch	200	13	19
Dark Chocolate, No Sugar Added	150	10	13
Fat Boy:			
Sundae On A Stick:			
Nut Sundae	270	20	23
Toffee Crunch	280	20	26
Vanilla Dipped	260	19	22
Sandwiches: Chocolate, 3 oz	210	9	31
Cookies n' Cream 3 oz	220	8	34
Mint Chocolate Chip 3 oz	220	9	33
Premium Vanilla, 3 oz	210	8	31
Rasp. Cheesecake, 3 oz	210	7	35
Strawberry, 3 oz	210	7	35
Fresh & Easy, Vanilla Sundae Cone	260	15	29
Fudge Bar (Nestlé),			
Regular, 2.8 oz	110	2	21
Fudgesicle,			
Orig. Fudge Bar, 2.3 oz	100	2	17
Good Humor:			
Bars, Single:			
Original Vanilla, 2.8 oz	250	15	27
Candy Center Crunch	300	21	27
Chocolate Eclair	210	9	30
Oreo Bar, 2.8 oz	240	13	31
Toasted Almond, 2.7 oz	210	10	27
Cones:			
Sundae, Vanilla, 2.6 oz	240	12	29
King:			
Giant:			
Triple Choc. Brownie, 5.5 oz	380	14	57
Vanilla Chocolate, 5 oz	360	17	48
Vanilla, 3 oz	240	12	32
Sandwiches: Choc. Chip Cookie	270	10	44
Giant Neapolitan, 3.3 oz	220	5	40
Giant Vanilla, 3.3 oz	220	5	40

Per Bar/Serving	C	F	Cb
Haagen-Dazs:			
Dark Chocolate Bar, Chocolate	280	20	22
Milk Chocolate Bars:			
Peanut Butter	310	23	21
Salted Caramel	290	19	27
Vanilla & Almonds	300	22	21
Vanilla	280	20	21
Snack Size:			
Coffee & Almond Crunch	190	14	15
Vanilla & Almonds	195	15	13
Healthy Choice: Fudge Bar	80	1.5	13
Mocha Swirl	90	1	17
Frozen Yogurt Bars, av.	85	1	16
Hershey's:			
Cones: Candy Bar Overload	320	12	48
Incredible	250	13	28
Moose Tracks	430	27	43
P-Nutty	210	13	20
Low fat, Cookies & Cream; Crazy, av.	120	2	25
Pops, all flavors	35	0	10
Sandwiches:			
99 Cent Vanilla Ice Cream	210	9	30
Giant: Andes Creme de Menthe	350	16	48
Neopolitan	320	14	43
Vanilla, 6 oz	300	12	43
Signature Bars: Chocolate Eclair	230	10	34
Cookies & Cream	290	15	33
Cotton Candy	280	15	33
Strawb. Shortcake	230	9	34
Hood:			
Bars: Ice Cream Bar	150	11	12
Fudge Stix	60	0	14
Harvey: Cookies 'n Cream, 2.8 oz	240	14	28
Toffee Crunch, 2.8 oz	240	14	25
Vanilla, 2.8 oz	220	13	25
Hoodsie:			
Cups, Chocolate; Vanilla, 3 oz	100	5	12
Sundae Cups, 3 oz	120	5	19
Sandwich, av., 2.2 oz	175	6	29
Klondike:			
Bars: Multipacks, Per Bar			
Original Vanilla	250	14	29
Dark Chocolate	240	14	29
Double Chocolate	250	14	29
Heath; Rocky Road, average	230	13	28
Krunch	250	14	29
Neapolitan	250	14	29
Oreo Cookies & Cream	250	15	29
Reese's	260	16	26
Slim-A-Bear	170	9	21
Sandwiches: Each			
Chocolate; Classic Vanilla	180	4.5	31
Oreo	200	7	34

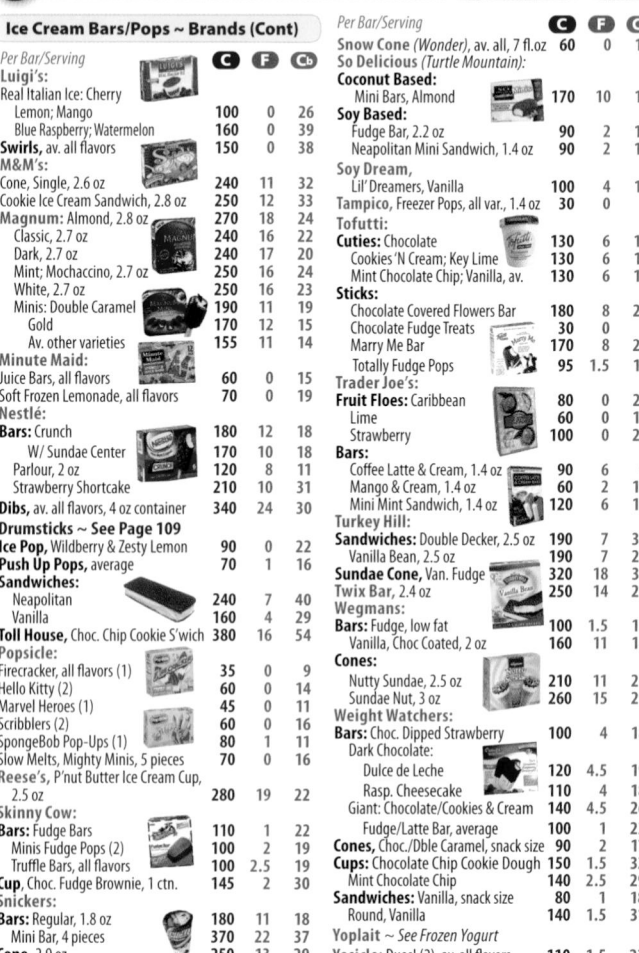

Ice Cream Bars/Pops ~ Brands (Cont)

Per Bar/Serving

	C	F	Cb
Luigi's:			
Real Italian Ice: Cherry			
Lemon; Mango	100	0	26
Blue Raspberry; Watermelon	160	0	39
Swirls, av. all flavors	150	0	38
M&M's:			
Cone, Single, 2.6 oz	240	11	32
Cookie Ice Cream Sandwich, 2.8 oz	250	12	33
Magnum: Almond, 2.8 oz	270	18	24
Classic, 2.7 oz	240	16	22
Dark, 2.7 oz	240	17	20
Mint; Mochaccino, 2.7 oz	250	16	24
White, 2.7 oz	250	16	23
Minis: Double Caramel	190	11	19
Gold	170	12	15
Av. other varieties	155	11	14
Minute Maid:			
Juice Bars, all flavors	60	0	15
Soft Frozen Lemonade, all flavors	70	0	19
Nestlé:			
Bars: Crunch	180	12	18
W/ Sundae Center	170	10	18
Parlour, 2 oz	120	8	11
Strawberry Shortcake	210	10	31
Dibs, av. all flavors, 4 oz container	340	24	30
Drumsticks ~ See Page 109			
Ice Pop, Wildberry & Zesty Lemon	90	0	22
Push Up Pops, average	70	1	16
Sandwiches:			
Neapolitan	240	7	40
Vanilla	160	4	29
Toll House, Choc. Chip Cookie S'wich	380	16	54
Popsicle:			
Firecracker, all flavors (1)	35	0	9
Hello Kitty (2)	60	0	14
Marvel Heroes (1)	45	0	11
Scribblers (2)	60	0	16
SpongeBob Pop-Ups (1)	80	1	11
Slow Melts, Mighty Minis, 5 pieces	70	0	16
Reese's, P'nut Butter Ice Cream Cup, 2.5 oz	280	19	22
Skinny Cow:			
Bars: Fudge Bars	110	1	22
Minis Fudge Pops (2)	100	2	19
Truffle Bars, all flavors	100	2.5	19
Cup, Choc. Fudge Brownie, 1 ctn.	145	2	30
Snickers:			
Bars: Regular, 1.8 oz	180	11	18
Mini Bar, 4 pieces	370	22	37
Cone, 2.9 oz	250	13	29
Ice Cream Brownie, 3.3 oz	300	13	41

Per Bar/Serving

	C	F	Cb
Snow Cone (Wonder), av. all, 7 fl.oz	60	0	15
So Delicious (Turtle Mountain):			
Coconut Based:			
Mini Bars, Almond	170	10	15
Soy Based:			
Fudge Bar, 2.2 oz	90	2	18
Neapolitan Mini Sandwich, 1.4 oz	90	2	18
Soy Dream,			
Lil'Dreamers, Vanilla	100	4	15
Tampico, Freezer Pops, all var., 1.4 oz	30	0	7
Tofutti:			
Cuties: Chocolate	130	6	16
Cookies 'N Cream; Key Lime	130	6	17
Mint Chocolate Chip; Vanilla, av.	130	6	18
Sticks:			
Chocolate Covered Flowers Bar	180	8	23
Chocolate Fudge Treats	30	0	6
Marry Me Bar	170	8	22
Totally Fudge Pops	95	1.5	19
Trader Joe's:			
Fruit Floes: Caribbean	80	0	21
Lime	60	0	16
Strawberry	100	0	24
Bars:			
Coffee Latte & Cream, 1.4 oz	90	6	9
Mango & Cream, 1.4 oz	60	2	10
Mini Mint Sandwich, 1.4 oz	120	6	18
Turkey Hill:			
Sandwiches: Double Decker, 2.5 oz	190	7	30
Vanilla Bean, 2.5 oz	190	7	29
Sundae Cone, Van. Fudge	320	18	33
Twix Bar, 2.4 oz	250	14	28
Wegmans:			
Bars: Fudge, low fat	100	1.5	19
Vanilla, Choc Coated, 2 oz	160	11	14
Cones:			
Nutty Sundae, 2.5 oz	210	11	25
Sundae Nut, 3 oz	260	15	29
Weight Watchers:			
Bars: Choc. Dipped Strawberry	100	4	18
Dark Chocolate:			
Dulce de Leche	120	4.5	19
Rasp. Cheesecake	110	4	18
Giant: Chocolate/Cookies & Cream	140	4.5	26
Fudge/Latte Bar, average	100	1	22
Cones, Choc./Dble Caramel, snack size	90	2	17
Cups: Chocolate Chip Cookie Dough	150	1.5	32
Mint Chocolate Chip	140	2.5	19
Sandwiches: Vanilla, snack size	80	1	18
Round, Vanilla	140	1.5	31
Yoplait ~ See Frozen Yogurt			
Yosicle: Duos! (2), av. all flavors	110	1.5	22
Torpedoes! (2), 2 oz	90	2	16

Canned & Packaged Meals ~ Brands

	C	**F**	**Cb**
Amy's: *Per Serve*			
Frozen:			
Asian Meals:			
Stir-Fry: Asian Noodle,10 oz	300	7	50
Thai, 9.5 oz	310	11	45
Bowls: Baked Ziti, 9.5 oz	390	12	62
Broccoli & Cheddar Bake, 9.5 oz	430	20	44
Pesto Tortellini, 9.5 oz	440	20	50
Burritos: Bean & Cheese, 6 oz	310	9	46
Bean & Rice, 6 oz	320	8	52
Breakfast Burrito, 6 oz	270	8	38
Entrees: Cheese Enchilada, 4.5 oz	240	14	18
Cheese Lasagna, 10.3 oz	410	16	46
Macaroni & Cheese, 9 oz	400	16	47
Roasted Vegetable Lasagna, 9.8 oz	350	11	47
Light & Lean: *Per 8 oz Serve*			
Black Bean & Cheese Enchilada	250	5	44
Mattar Paner	260	6	42
Soft Taco Fiesta	220	4.5	40
Pot Pies:			
Broccoli, 7.5 oz	460	24	50
Mex. Tamale; Shephd's Pie, av., 8 oz	165	3.5	27
Vegetable, 7.5 oz	430	20	54
Snacks: Nacho, Chse & Bean, 5-6 pcs	220	9	25
Cheese Pizza, 5-6 pieces	210	9	25
Whole Meals:			
Black Bean Enchil., 10 oz	330	8	53
Southern Dinner, 9 oz	310	7	51
Veggie Loaf, 10 oz	290	8	47
Veggie, Steak & Gravy, 11 oz	380	16	49
Wraps:			
Indian Samosa, 5 oz	250	9	35
Indian Spinach Tofu, 5.5 oz	270	13	28
Teriyaki, 5.5 oz	310	7	51
Atkins: *Per 9 oz Tray/Bowl*			
Frozen:			
Beef Merlot	310	21	9
Chicken & Broccoli Alfredo	330	20	9
Chili Con Carne	320	21	8
Crustless Chicken Pot Pie	330	22	8
Italian Sausage Primavera	330	25	10
Meatloaf with Portob. Mshrm Gravy	340	23	11

	C	**F**	**Cb**
Bagel Bites:			
Frozen:			
Cheese, Ssge & Pepp., 4 pcs	200	6	28
Supreme; Three Cheese, av., 4 pcs, 3 oz	190	4.5	31
B & M:			
Baked Beans: *Per 16 oz Can, ½ cup, 4.6 oz*			
Original; Vegetarian, av.	160	1	31
Barbeque	190	0.5	39
Raisin Brown Bread,			
½" slice, 2 oz	130	0.5	29
Banquet:			
Homestyle Bakes: *Includes Topping*			
Asian Style Fried Rice,			
½ filling & ¼ cup rice	240	1.5	47
Cheesy Ham & Hashbrowns,			
½ cup filling & ⅓ cup potato	270	15	27
Frozen:			
Dinners: Boneless Pork Rib, 10 oz	310	11	37
Cheesy Smothered Meat Patty, 7 oz	280	16	20
Chicken Fingers, 7 oz	480	21	56
Chicken Nuggets, 6.7 oz	320	15	31
Chicken Pasta Marinara, 6.5 oz	290	14	30
Fettuccine Alfredo, 8 oz	290	11	39
Fish Sticks, 7.5 oz	310	9	47
Fried Beef Steak, 10 oz	360	17	41
Lasagna, with Meat Sauce, 8 oz	270	7	38
Meatloaf, 9.5 oz	250	11	26
Pepperoni Pizza, 5.8	330	11	48
Salisbury Steak, 9.5 oz	230	9	26
Spaghetti & Meatballs, 9 oz	360	16	38
Turkey, 9.3 oz	230	6	31
Family:			
Broccoli Chicken & Cheese,			
with Rice, 7.7 oz	210	7	26
Chicken Alfredo,			
with Broccoli & Noodles, 8 oz	210	6	29
Salisbury Steak & Gravy, 4.5 oz	180	12	11
Pot Pies:			
Breakfast Ham & Potato, 7 oz	410	22	44
Breakfast Sausage Gravy, 7 oz	450	28	39
Chicken; Turkey, average, 7 oz	400	24	37
Chicken with Broccoli, 7 oz	380	23	34
Select Recipe Dinners:			
Chicken Parmigiana, 10 oz	350	15	37
Original Fried Chicken, 10 oz	340	17	36
Slow Cooker: Beef Pot Roast, 8.8 oz	240	6	28
Chicken Dumplings, 8.3 oz	300	12	32

	C	F	Cb
Barilla:			
Microwaveables: *Per 9 oz Container*			
Ital. Ssg; Meat Sauce Gemelli, av	350	7	60
Marinara/tomato & Basil Penne, av.	310	4	60
Betty Crocker:			
Bowl Appetit:			
Cheddar Broccoli Rice	290	6	52
Homestyle Chicken Flavored Pasta	250	5	44
Pasta Alfredo	350	9	55
Three-Cheese Rotini	340	7	59
Hamburger Helper: *Per 1 Cup, Prepared*			
Beef Pasta	280	12	24
Cheeseburger Macaroni	320	13	30
Cheesy Baked Potatoes	310	12	30
Cheesy Italian Shells	310	12	27
Crunchy Taco	330	14	33
Salisbury	280	11	27
Helper Complete Meals: *Per 1 Cup, Prepared*			
Cheesy Beef Taco	220	5	35
Chicken & Buttermilk Biscuits	260	9	39
Chicken with Cheesy Rice & Broccoli	230	6	36
Stroganoff	230	8	33
Potatoes: *Per Serving, Prepared*			
Casserole: Au Gratin, ½ cup	150	5	24
Cheddar & Bacon, ½ c.	150	5	24
Roasted Garlic, ½ cup	120	3	21
Scalloped, ⅔ cup	130	3	23
Sour Cream and Chives, ⅔ cup	130	3	24
Flavored Potatoes, prepared,			
average all varieties, ⅔ cup	145	6	18
Seasoned Skillet:			
Hash Brown, ½ cup	120	4	18
Rstd Garlic & Herb Potatoes, ⅔ c.	170	9	21
Trad'nl Recipe Potatoes, ½ cup	180	9	22
Tuna Helper: *Per 1 Cup, Prepared*			
Creamy Parmesan	270	10	30
Average other varieties	260	10	30
Biggest Loser:			
Refrigerated:			
Simply Sensible: *Per ½ Package*			
Beef Pot Roast & Gravy	220	5	16
Beef Tips & Gravy	200	3.5	21
Lasagna	200	5	28
Mediterranean-Style Chicken	250	6	36
Zing Chicken	230	1.5	38

	C	F	Cb
Birds Eye:			
Frozen:			
Voila!: *Per 1 Cup Prepared Unless Indicated*			
Alfredo Chicken, 1½ cups	280	12	37
Beef & Broccoli Stir Fry	160	6	13
Chicken Florentine	230	6	27
Chicken Parmesan	360	11	50
Garlic Shrimp	230	9	30
Shrimp Scampi	190	2.5	31
Sweet & Sour Chicken	200	1	38
Boca:			
Frozen:			
Burger:			
All American Flame Grilled, 2.5 oz	120	5	6
Cheeseburger, 2.5 oz	100	4.5	6
Grilled Vegetables, 2.5 oz	80	1	7
Original Vegan, 3.5 oz	100	0.5	6
Chik'n: Orig. Nuggets, 3 oz	180	7	17
Patties (1), 2.5 oz	160	6	15
Veggie Patties, Bruschetta	90	1.5	9
Boston Market:			
Frozen:			
Dinners: Beef Steak & Pasta, 14 oz	470	15	52
Chicken Parmesan, 13 oz	500	13	70
Oven Roasted Chicken, 13 oz	280	7	32
Salisbury Steak, 14.5 oz	530	32	38
Swedish M'balls, 13 oz	570	26	55
Buitoni: *Per ½ Package Unless Indicated*			
Refrigerated:			
Ravioli: Chicken Marsala, 1 c., 3.9 oz	280	8	36
Crab, 1 cup, 3.8 oz	300	11	36
Four Cheese, 1¼ cups, 3.7 oz	330	12	42
Tortellini: Herb Chicken, 1 c., 3.8 oz	330	8	52
Spinach Cheese, 1 cup, 3.7 oz	320	7	49
Other Varieties ~ See Page 133			
Bush's Best: *Per ½ Cup, 4.6 oz*			
Baked Beans: Original	140	1	29
Vegetarian	130	0	29
Average other varieties	150	1	32
Black Beans	105	0.5	23
Chili Pinto Beans, with sauce	110	1	20
Dark Red Kidney Beans	100	0	22
Garbanzo Beans	105	2	20
Grillin' Beans:			
Black Bean Fiesta	110	1	21
Sweet Mesquite	160	1	32
Texas Ranchero	120	2	20
Average other varieties	165	0.5	35
Refried Beans: Traditional	150	3	24
Fat Free	130	0	24

Campbell's:

	C	**F**	**Cb**
Pork & Beans, 28 oz can, 4.6 oz	140	1.5	25

Chunky Microwaveable Bowls: *Per 15.25 oz Can*

Firehouse; Roadhouse, Beef & Beans Chili	440	12	56

Spaghetti O's: *Per Can*

Original, 15 oz	285	1.5	59
With Meatballs, 14.8 oz	350	10	50
With Sliced Franks, 14.8 oz	365	10	53

Chef Boyardee: *Per 1 Cup*

Canned (14.5 oz can):

Beefaroni, 8.8 oz	250	10	30
Lasagna, with Tomato & Meat Sce, 8.8 oz	250	9	32
Ravioli			
Beef, in Tomato & Meat Sauce:			
Regular, 8.7 oz	220	7	31
99% Fat Free, 8.6 oz	170	2	31
Overstuffed, 9.2 oz	230	5	37
Cheese Ravioli, in Meat & Tomato Sce, 8.7 oz	230	6	34
Pepperoni Pizza Ravioli, in Zesty Sauce, 9.1 oz	210	4	36
Spaghetti & Meatballs, in Tomato Sauce, 9 oz	260	11	31

Microwaveable: *Per 7.5 oz Bowl*

Beef Ravioli, in Tomato & Meat Sauce	190	5	29
Mini Beef Ravioli, in Tomato & Meat Sauce	240	9	32

Boxed Pizza Maker Kits: *Single Kits*

Cheese, ¼ package, 4 oz	260	4.5	47
Pepperoni, ¼ package, 4 oz	280	8	42
Pizza Sauce, ¼ cup, 2 oz	35	1.5	4

Country Crock (Hormel):

Side Dishes:

Cheddar Broccoli Rice, 7 oz	260	11	33
Elbow Mac. & Cheese, 8 oz	330	14	38
Garlic Mashed Potato, 5 oz	120	4	19
Loaded Mashed Potatoes, 5 oz	190	11	18

Dennison's Chili: *Per Cup*

	C	**F**	**Cb**
Chili Con Carne:			
Original: W/- Beans, 9 oz	350	15	31
Without Beans, 8.8 oz	310	16	20
Chili: Original, with Beans, 9 oz	360	14	38
Chunky, with Beans, 8.8 oz	300	10	32
Hot, with Beans, 9 oz	350	14	36
Vegetarian, 99% fat free, 9 oz	190	1.5	34

Dinty Moore:

Big Bowl (Microwave): *Per ½ of 15 oz Bowl*

Beef Stew, 8.3 oz	200	10	17
Chicken & Dumplings, 8.5 oz	220	7	29
Scalloped Potatoes & Ham, 8.7 oz	280	16	23

Hearty Meals: *Per ½ of 20 oz Can*

Beef Stew, 9 oz	190	7	21
Chicken & Dumplings, 8.5 oz	230	8	28
Chicken Pot Pie, 8.6 oz	240	11	24
Noodles & Chicken, 8.3 oz	170	6	22

Dr. McDougall's: *Per 2 oz Package*

Asian Noodle Entree Cups, average all varieties	200	1.5	41
Quinoa Cups: Black Bean	280	3	51
Curry Almond and Rice	260	3	51
Tomato Pine Nut	260	5	44

Eden Organics: *Per ½ Cup, 4.6 oz*

Baked Navy Beans, w/ Sorghum, Mstrd	150	0	27
Chili Beans, w/- Jalap. & Chili Peppers	130	0	21
Lentils, with Onions & Bay Leaf	90	0	13
Refried: Black Beans	110	1.5	18
Pinto; Kidney Beans, average	85	1	17

Farmhouse:

Rice: *Per 1 Cup, Prepared*

Long Grain & Wild Herb & Butter	250	7	43
Mexican, 6 oz	230	5	42
Roasted Chicken Flavor, 6 oz	230	5	44

French's:

French Fried Onions:

Original; Cheddar:			
2 Tbsp, 0.3 oz	45	3.5	3
¼ cup, 0.5 oz	90	7	6
1 cup, 2 oz	360	28	24

	C	F	Cb
GardenBurger:			
Veggie Burger:			
Original, 3 oz	110	3	16
Black Bean Chipotle, 2.5 oz	90	3	16
Garden Lites: *Per 7 oz Serving*			
Meals: Veggie & Cheese	180	7	21
Veggie Chili & Cornbread Melt	200	4.5	33
Zucchini Marinara/Portabella	110	4	18
Souffle: Broccoli	140	1.5	23
Butternut Squash; S'thwestern, av.	180	2.5	32
Loaded Potato	200	5.5	27
Roasted Veggie; Zucchini	140	1.5	25
Muffins, average all varieties (1), 2 oz	120	3	23
Gorton's:			
Battered Pollock Fillets:			
Beer Battered (2), 3.6 oz	230	14	20
Crispy Battered (2), 3.8 oz	240	14	20
Breaded Pollock Fillets:			
Crunchy (2), 3.8 oz	250	13	23
Lemon Herb Crunchy (2), 3.7 oz	240	13	21
(Grilled Fillets):			
Garlic Butter Pollock (1), 3.5 oz	80	3	0
Lemon Butter Pollock (1), 3.5 oz	90	3	0
Signature Tilapia (1), 3.2 oz	80	2	2
Shrimp:			
Crispy Beer Battered (9), 3.5 oz	240	12	25
Crunchy Butterfly Shrimp (5), 3.5 oz	220	8	27
Garl. Butter Shrimp Scampi (6), 4 oz	120	5	8
Great Value (Walmart):			
Breakfast Bowls: *Per 8 oz*			
Sausage	390	25	22
Sausage & Gravy	360	24	21
Complete Skillet Meals: *Per ½ Package*			
Chicken Florentine & Farfalle	575	32	40
Shrimp Scampi & Linguini, 12 oz	550	23	58
Meals: Cheese Manicotti, 8 oz	320	16	24
Lasagna, 7.6 oz	280	9	36
Party Size: Lasagna, 7.5 oz	270	9	32
Mexican Style Lasagna, 8 oz	380	17	38
Health Valley:			
Vegetarian Chili: *Per 8.7 oz*			
3 Bean Chipotle	200	3	37
Black Bean Mango	210	3	41
Average other varieties	200	3	37

	C	F	Cb
Healthy Choice:			
100% Natural Cafe Steamers:			
Asian Potstickers, 9.8 oz	330	3.5	67
Portabella Spin. Parmesan, 9.8 oz	230	5	38
Pumpkin Squash Ravioli, 9.5 oz	260	6	44
Tortellini Primavera Parm., 9.5 oz	250	4.5	42
Asian/Mediterranean Cafe Steamers:			
Balsamic Garlic Chicken, 9.5 oz	250	5	34
Beef Teriyaki, 9.5 oz	270	5	39
Grilled Basil Chicken, 10 oz	250	6	32
Baked: 4 Cheese Ziti Marin., 9.2 oz	310	5	46
Italian Sausage Pasta, 8.5 oz	270	6	40
Roasted Chicken & Potatoes, 9.7 oz	180	3.5	21
Complete Meals:			
Beef Pot Roast, 11 oz	250	6	32
Chicken Parmigiana, 11.5 oz	340	9	49
Lemon Pepper Fish, 10.7 oz	330	5	58
Extra Product Listings ~ www.CalorieKing.com			
Heinz, Vegetarian Beans, ½ cup, 4 oz	140	0.5	27
Hormel:			
Compleats: *Per 10 oz Container*			
Balanced Selection:			
Beef Steak & Peppers	220	3.5	29
Chicken Marinara	230	4	30
Chicken Pasta Primavera	230	4	32
Spaghetti & Turkey Meatballs	250	7	29
Cafe Creations:			
Cheese Manicotti w/ Meat Sauce	290	9	42
Cheesy Ravioli	410	20	38
Italian Herb & Cheese Rigatoni	440	25	33
Homesyle: Beef Pot Roast	230	6	22
Beef Stew	250	11	22
Chicken Alfredo	340	18	28
Chicken Breast & Msh'd Potatoes	210	3.5	26
Meatloaf & Mashed Potatoes	300	11	34
Salisbury Steak	280	11	30
Swedish Meatballs	350	18	32
Chili with Beans: *Per 8.7 oz Serving*			
Regular; Hot; Chunky	260	7	33
Turkey	210	3	28
Vegetarian	190	1	35

continued next page...

Hormel (Cont):	C	F	Cb
Chili without Beans: Per 8.3 oz Serving			
Chunky/Hot Chili , average	215	9	19
Turkey	190	3	16
Kid's Kitchen: Per 7.5 oz Microwave Cup			
Cheezy Mac 'n Cheese	270	14	24
Noodle Rings & Chicken	140	4	18
Spaghetti Rings & Franks	240	8	32
Hot Pockets:			
Sandwiches: Per Sandwich			
Crispy Buttery Crust: BBQ Rcpe Beef	330	13	44
Cheeseburger	310	12	39
Ham & Cheese	300	12	37
Crispy Crust:			
Five Cheese Pizza	350	17	37
Pepperoni Pizza	350	19	33
Croissant Crust:			
Chicken, Broccoli & Cheddar	300	14	35
Ham & Cheese	320	15	35
Garlic Buttery Crust:			
Four Cheese Pizza	320	13	39
Four Meat & Four Cheese	320	14	36
Meatballs & Mozz.	330	15	34
Pepperoni Pizza	320	15	34
Pepperoni & Sausage	330	15	34
Pretzel Bread:			
Bacon Cheddar Cheese Melt	320	14	36
Queso Chicken	280	10	34
Seasoned Crust:			
Beef Taco	300	13	36
Philly Steak & Chse	310	12	38
Spicy Nacho	260	10	34
Hungry Jack:			
Easy Mash'd Cheesy: Per ⅔ Cup, Prepared			
Creamy Butter; Homestyle	110	1.5	21
Hearty Baked; Roasted Garlic	110	1	22
Hungry Man:			
Dinners: Boneless Fried Chicken	800	38	85
Boneless Pork Ribs	810	36	98
Classic Fried Chicken	1030	62	63
Country Fried Chicken	560	26	53
Home-Style Meatloaf	660	35	61
Pub Favorites: Beer Battered Chkn	760	34	74
Bourbon Steak Strips	500	14	73
Grilled Beef Patty	530	32	36
Grilled Bourbon Steak Strips	480	11	71
Honey Bourbon Chicken Strips	620	24	69

Hungry Man (Cont):	C	F	Cb
XXL Sandwiches: Per Box			
Angus Beef Charbroil	740	47	52
BBQ Pork Ribs	690	39	62
Buffalo Fried Chicken	650	27	73
Chicken Parmesan	610	29	63
Crispy Fried Chicken	670	32	64
Hunt's, Manwich Sloppy Joe,			
Canned, Original, ¼ cup, 2.3 oz	35	0	7
José Olé:			
Breakfast Burritos:			
Egg & Bacon, 4 oz	260	9	33
Egg & Sausage, 4 oz	270	10	34
Premium Burritos:			
Chicken Monterey (1)	270	6	41
Steak & Cheese (1)	300	10	40
Premium Chimichangas:			
Chicken & Cheese (1), 5 oz	330	11	45
Steak & Cheese (1), 5 oz	350	14	41
Snacks:			
Mini: Chimichangas,			
Steak & Cheddar (3)	370	20	37
Quesadillas,			
Grilled Chicken & 3 Cheese (4)	210	8	25
Tacos, Beef & Cheese (4)	230	12	23
Taquitos: Chicken, Corn Tortillas, (3)	200	8	26
Steak & Cheese, Flour Tortillas, (2)	250	12	26
Kashi:			
Entrees: Per Package			
Chicken Florentine, 10 oz	290	9	31
Chicken Pasta Pomodoro, 10 oz	280	6	38
Pesto Pasta Primav., 10 oz	290	11	37
S'west Style Chicken, 10 oz	310	5	49
Kid Cuisine: Per Meal			
Cheese Stuffed Crust Pizza	330	7	54
Chicken Breast Nuggets, 8 oz	430	18	54
Fish Sticks, 7.6 oz	320	11	45
Fried Chicken, 10 oz	530	22	53
Hot Dog, 7.2 oz	320	5	55
Mac. & Cheese, 10.6 oz	420	11	69
Pancakes, 7.2 oz	400	15	59
Popcorn Chicken, 8.6 oz	370	12	53
Spaghetti & Mini Meatballs, 10.2 oz	290	6	45

Knorr: Sides, Prepared as Directed	C	F	Cb
Asian: Chicken Fried Rice	290	7	48
Teriyaki Noodles	280	9	45
Teriyaki Rice	280	7	48
Cajun, Garlic Butter Rice	260	4	48
Fiesta: Mexican Rice	280	6	48
Spanish Rice	280	6	49
Taco Rice	270	6	46
Pasta: Alfredo	290	10	39
Alfredo Broccoli	300	10	39
Butter	260	8	39
Butter & Herb	260	7	39
Cheesy Cheddar	270	7	39
Parmesan	290	10	39
Stroganoff	260	7	39
Rice: Cheddar Broccoli	280	6	48
Chicken Flavor Broccoli	270	5	48
Chicken Flavor	280	6	48

Kraft:

Macaroni & Cheese Dinner: Per Cup, Prepared

	C	F	Cb
Original flavor, 2.5 oz	400	19	47
Cheesy Alfredo, 2.5 oz	400	17	50
White Cheddar, 2.5 oz	380	15	48
Thick 'N Creamy, 2.5 oz	410	17	50
Deluxe: Four Cheese, 3.5 oz	320	10	46
Sharp Cheddar, 3.5 oz	320	9	46

Velveeta Potatoes: Per ½ Cup, Prepared

	C	F	Cb
Cheesy: Au Gratin	190	7	24
Bacon Scalloped	200	7	27
Mashed, Twin Pack	180	9	21
Shells & Cheese, Original, 4 oz	360	12	49

Kroger:

Kitchen Creation Skillet Dinners: Per Cup, Prepared

	C	F	Cb
Creamy Broccoli	300	12	33
Creamy Pasta	300	13	33
Double Cheeseburger	320	13	30
Lasagna	280	12	26
Stroganoff	320	14	27

Frozen:

Healthy Meals Made Simple: Refrigerated, Per Cup

	C	F	Cb
Braised Beef Pot Roast & Gravy	220	5	15
Lean Beef Tips & Gravy	210	4	20
Lem. Herb Chkn w/ Rice	170	1.5	23
Sweet & Spicy Chicken	270	1.5	48

Kroger (Cont):	C	F	Cb
Frozen (Cont):			
Meals Made Simple:			
Beef Stir Fry, 1¾ cups	180	4	26
Chicken Florentine, 2¼ cups, 6.9 oz	320	18	22
Chicken Stir Fry, 1½ cups	180	2	25
Shrimp Fried Rice, 1¼ cups, 8 oz	240	0	44
Oven Ready:			
Breaded Calamari Rings (10), 3 oz	200	10	21
Coconut Shrimp (5), with 1 oz sweet chili sauce	350	20	34

La Choy:

Family Meals, Canned: Per 1 Cup

	C	F	Cb
Beef Pepper Oriental, 8.9 oz	80	1	11
Beef Chow Mein, 8.7 oz	80	0	11
Chicken Chow Mein, 8.8 oz	100	4	11
Sweet & Sour Chicken, 8.9 oz	180	1.5	35

Lean Cuisine:

Culinary Collection: Per Complete Meal

	C	F	Cb
Baked Chicken	240	7	30
Beef & Broccoli	270	5	43
Beef Chow Fun	320	5	54
Beef Portabello	200	6	24
Beef Pot Roast	190	4	25
Chicken with Almonds	270	4	44
Chicken Parmesan	310	9	39
Flatbread Melts:			
Chicken Ranch Club	370	9	52
Sun-Dried Tom. Basil Chicken	360	8	52
Lemon Pepper Fish	300	8	40
Paninis: Chicken Club Panini	360	9	45
Chicken, Spinach & Mushroom	300	7	40
Philly-Style Steak & Cheese	330	9	42
Roasted Turkey & Veggies	200	7	18
Salisbury Steak	260	8	23
Shrimp Alfredo	200	4	29
Spring Rolls:			
Fajita Style Chicken (2)	200	7	20
Garlic/Thai Chicken (2), average	200	8	24
Thai Style Chicken	280	6	37

	C	F	Cb
Lean Cuisine (Cont):			
Market Collections:			
Chicken Alfredo	300	7	36
Chicken Fettuccini	310	5	42
Chicken Tuscan	280	5	37
Roasted Turkey Breast	290	7	38
Shanghai Style Shrimp	250	3	41
Sweet & Spicy Ginger Chicken	290	2	45
Simple Favorites:			
Asian Style Pot Stickers	260	4	49
Cheese Ravioli	230	5	34
Macaroni and Cheese	300	6	48
Spa Collection:			
Butternut Squash Ravioli	260	7	40
Lemongrass Chicken	240	4	38
Salmon with Basil	250	2	38
Pizzas ~ See Page 136			
Extra Product Listings ~ www.CalorieKing.com			
Lean Pockets:			
Sandwiches: *Per Single Pocket*			
Garlic Buttery Crust, Pepp. Pizza	290	7	42
Pretzel Bread: BBQ Recipe Chicken	260	4	42
Chicken Japalpeno Cheddar	270	8	35
Three Cheese & Spinach	250	7	36
Seasoned Crust,			
Four Cheese Pizza	270	6	42
Whole Grain Crust:			
Bacon/Ssg, Egg & Cheese, av.	270	9	38
Garlic Chicken White Pizza	260	7	38
Ham & Cheese	270	8	39
Supreme Pizza	220	7	33
Three Cheese & Broccoli	250	6	40
Lightlife:			
Entrees:			
Amaz'n Asian Sesame Chik'n, 9.7 oz	260	4	40
Perfecto Penne Primavera,			
with Meatless Crumbles, 10 oz	240	4.5	36
Smart Cutlets:			
Original (1), 3 oz	110	1	7
Classic Marinara (1), 5 oz	150	1.5	13
Spicy Sweet & Sour (1), 5 oz	210	1.5	29
Smart Wings: Buffalo (4), 3 oz	100	2.5	6
Honey BBQ (4), 3 oz	110	0	15
Smart Tenders:			
Lemon Pepper (3), 3 oz	100	0	7
Savory Chick'n (3), 3 oz	100	0	7

	C	F	Cb
Lunchables:			
Per Package without Drink			
Crackers Stackers:			
Light Bologna & American Cheese	320	17	32
Turkey & American Cheese	330	16	37
Extra Cheesy Pizza	270	9	30
Ham & Cheddar,			
with Crackers	260	13	22
Nachos, Cheese Dip & Salsa	380	21	40
Pizza, with Pepperoni	300	13	32
Turkey & Cheddar, with Crackers	260	13	22
Lunchmakers *(Armour):* Per Package			
Bologna Cracker Crunchers	350	14	46
Cheese Pizza	340	12	51
Nachos	480	17	77
Pepperoni Pizza	330	10	55
Turkey Cracker Crunchers	350	14	45
Marie Callender's:			
Beef:			
Beef & Broccoli	370	9	50
Braised Beef Pot Roast	210	4	28
Country Fried Beef Steak & Gravy	660	31	75
Chicken: Chicken Parmigiana	530	27	47
Country Fried Chicken & Gravy	560	27	61
Fettuccini with Chicken & Broccoli	500	24	41
Sweet & Sour Chicken	560	13	93
Pot Pies: Beef	410	23	39
Cheesy chicken & Bacon	520	31	43
Chicken	380	21	38
Chicken Corn Chowder	470	27	44
Creamy: Mushroom Chicken	450	27	41
Parmesan Chicken	420	24	35
Turkey	480	28	46
Under 500 Calories:			
Chunky Chicken & Noodles	440	18	46
Country Fried Pork Chop	460	19	55
Golden Battered Filet	410	11	58
Herb Roasted Chicken	470	17	44
Meat Loaf & Gravy	450	17	43
Slow Roasted Beef	330	12	37
Spaghetti & Meatballs	420	13	52
Steak & Roasted Potatoes	350	11	40
Three Meat & Four Cheese Lasagna	280	11	30
Family size: *Per 1 Cup*			
Cheesy Chicken Lasagna, 8 oz	320	14	33
Vermont White Chedd. Mac & Chse	350	20	31

	C	F	Cb
Maruchan:			
Bowls, all varieties, 3.3 oz	380	16	50
Ramen, Noodle Soup, average all, 3 oz pkg	380	16	52
Instant Lunch, average, 1 package	290	11	39
Yakisoba: *Per 4 oz Pkg*			
Chicken/Teriyaki Beef Flavor, av.	520	21	72
Sweet & Sour Chicken	560	22	78
Michael Angelo's:			
Natural: Chicken Parmesan, 10 oz	390	8	51
Four Cheese Lasagna, 10 oz	410	13	47
Meat Lasagna, 10 oz	400	11	45
Stuffed Manicotti, w/ Sauce, 10 oz	380	15	36
Signature: Chicken Alfredo, 11 oz	410	12	47
Lasagna with Sausage, 11 oz	460	19	47
Shrimp Scampi, 10 oz	540	28	46
Minute Rice:			
Ready To Serve: *Per 4.4 oz Container, Prepared*			
Brown/Chicken Rice Mix, average	230	5	42
White/Yellow Rice	195	4	38
Morningstar Farms:			
Burgers: *Per Patty*			
Grillers Original (1)	130	6	5
Mushroom Lovers (1)	110	4	6
Spicy Black Bean (1)	110	4	13
Chik'n:			
Buffalo Wings (5)	200	9	19
Chik'n Nuggets (4)	190	9	19
Patties:			
Chik, Original (1)	140	6	15
Grillers Chik'n Veggie (1)	80	3	7
Hot & Spicy Sausage (1)	70	3	3
Pizza, Mediterranean Chickpea, 5.7 oz pizza	380	12	59
Newman's Own:			
Skillets: *Per ½ Package, 11-12 oz*			
Chicken: Fettuccini Alfredo	410	12	49
Florentine & Farfalle	370	10	42
Parmigiana & Penne	490	25	47
Garlic Chicken Lo Mein Noodles	320	7	42
Italian Ssge & Rigatoni	510	28	48
Steak Fajita	290	6	47
Sweet & Sour Chicken	330	10	46

	C	F	Cb
Nissin:			
Chow Mein: *Per 4 oz Package*			
Chicken Flavor	480	18	70
Spicy Chicken Flavor	560	30	64
Teriyaki Beef	520	20	68
With Shrimp	540	24	68
Cup Noodles,			
Beef/Chicken/Shrimp, 1 cup	300	13	38
Top Ramen, average, 3 oz pakage	380	14	52
Old El Paso:			
Dinner Kits: *Per Serving, Prepared with Chicken*			
Chicken Soft Taco	300	10	30
Enchilada	390	16	27
Frozen Meals: *Per ½ Pkg*			
Chicken Burritos (1)	480	17	59
Chicken Quesadillas (1)	620	30	57
Shredded Beef Burritos (1)	490	16	63
Pasta Roni: *Per Cup, Prepared*			
Angel Hair Pasta varieties, average	310	14	40
Butter & Herb Italiano	300	11	41
Chicken & Broccoli	360	15	49
Chicken Flavor	300	12	40
Fettuccine Alfredo	450	24	44
Four Cheese Corkscrew	370	15	49
Stroganoff	350	13	48
Tomato Parmesan	270	9	40
White Cheddar & Broccoli	300	13	39
P.F. Chang's: *Per ½ Package, 11 oz*			
Meals: Beef with Broccoli	360	17	30
General Chang's Chicken	350	14	35
Mongolian Style Chicken	310	9	40
Orange Chicken	430	18	44
Sweet & Sour Chicken	335	12	40
Noodle Meals: *Per ½ Package, 11 oz*			
Garlic Chkn with Dan Dan Noodles	370	9	53
Gr. Chkn Teriyaki w/ Lo Mein Noodle	330	6	45

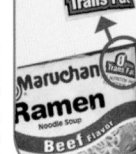

Most packaged noodle soups are high in calories and fat.

Their promotion of '0 Grams Trans Fat' does not make them heart-healthy.

They are still high in saturated fat as well as salt/sodium.

Rice-A-Roni:	**C**	**F**	**Cb**
Classic Favorites: *Per Cup, Prepared*			
Beef; Herb & Butter; Rice Pilaf, av.	310	9	52
Broccoli Au Gratin	350	16	46
Chicken Flavor	300	9	50
Chicken & Broccoli	220	5	40
Spanish Rice	260	8	44
Whole Grain Blends:			
Roasted Garlic Italiano	270	9	41
Spanish	250	8	42
Rosarita:			
Kidney Beans, ½ cup, 4.5 oz	110	0	20
Chili Beans, ½ cup, 4.5 oz	130	0.5	24
Refried Beans: *Per ½ Cup, 4.5 oz*			
Traditional	120	2	18
No Fat, Refried Beans	100	0	18
Safeway Select:			
Frozen:			
Beef Salisbury Steak, 9.4 oz	410	28	23
Chicken Cacciatore, 8.8 oz	290	10	34
Fettucini Alfredo, 11.5 oz	380	12	55
Five Vegetable Lasagna, 10.6 oz	330	8	48
Homestyle Baked Chicken, 9 oz	260	11	31
Orange Chicken, 9 oz	360	7	61
Penne Pasta, 8 oz	300	11	42
Pot Roast, 9 oz	270	11	23
Spaghetti with Meat Sauce, 12 oz	450	16	61
Swedish Meat Balls, 11.5 oz	470	24	43
Three Cheese Tortellini, 7.5 oz	350	16	38
S & W: *Per ½ Cup*			
Black Beans, 4.5 oz	110	0.5	22
Chili Beans,			
in Zesty Tomato Sauce, 4.6 oz	130	1.5	23
Kidney Beans, 4.7 oz	110	0	22
White Beans, 4.5 oz	110	0.5	21
Seapak ~ *See www.calorieking.com*			
Simply Asia:			
Noodle Bowls: *Per 8.5oz Bowl*			
Roasted Peanut	460	12	75
Sesame Teriyaki	390	13	82
Soy Ginger	420	6	84
Spicy Mongolian	430	6	86

Simply Asia (Cont):	**C**	**F**	**Cb**
Noodles & Sauce: *Per ⅓ Package*			
Sesame Teriyaki	300	3	60
Soy Ginger	320	4.5	60
Spicy Kung Pao	350	7	63
Quick Noodles: *Per 8.8 oz Tray*			
Honey Teriyaki	430	3.5	85
Pad Thai	460	3	93
Szechwan Garl. Chow Mein	460	7	83
Smart Ones *(Weight Watchers):*			
Classic Favorites: *Per Meal*			
Angel Hair Marinara	220	4	37
Chkn Enchiladas Suiza	290	5	49
Lasagna Bake with Meat Sauce	250	5	39
Lasagna Florentine	320	10	43
Lemon Herb Chicken Piccata	250	2	45
Macaroni & Cheese	260	2	51
Pasta Primavera	250	3	44
Pasta with Ricotta & Spinach	290	5	44
Ravioli Florentine	270	5	46
Salisbury Steak	260	6	28
Spaghetti with Meat Sauce	280	3.5	50
Swedish Meatballs	290	7	38
Three Cheese Macaroni	300	6	48
Traditional Lasagna w/ Meat Sauce	310	8	45
Tuna Noodle Gratin	230	3.5	39
Smart Beginnings: *Per Meal*			
Breakfast Quesadilla	230	7	29
Canadian Bacon English Muffin	210	6	27
English Muffin S'wich,			
Egg White & Cheese	210	5	28
Three Cheese Omelet	200	7	20
Smart Creations: *Per Meal*			
Chicken Fettucini	290	6	40
Chicken Parmesan	290	6	35
Homestyle Turkey Breast,			
with Stuffing	260	5	39
Meatloaf	230	6	23
Teriyaki Chicken & Vegetables	250	3	43

Stagg Chili:

	C	**F**	**Cb**
Chili with Beans: *15 oz Can, 1 cup, 8.7 oz*			
Classic	290	13	30
Chunkero	320	16	28
Dynamite Hot	320	15	30
Fiesta Grille	280	13	25
Ranch House Chicken	240	8	26
Turkey Ranchero, 1 cup	250	5	32
Vege Garden Four-Bean, 1 cup	200	1	37
White Chicken Chili	260	12	20
No Beans, Steakhouse, 1 cup	320	22	14

Stouffer's:

Satisfying Servings For One: *Per Package*			
Baked Ziti	520	18	68
Bourbon Steak Tips	490	17	61
Chicken Fettuccini Alfredo	840	38	94
Five Cheese Lasagna	330	14	33
Lasagna Italiano	290	12	30
Lasagna with Meat & Sauce	260	9	28
Macaroni & Cheese	340	16	36
Meatloaf	530	26	40
Monterey Chicken	530	21	54
Savory Beef & Vegetables	360	16	34
White Meat Chicken Pot Pie	590	34	54
Signature Classics For One: *Per Package*			
Baked Chicken Breast	240	8	17
Beef Pot Roast	320	8	41
Beef Stroganoff	380	17	34
Creamed Chipped Beef	140	7	11
Fettuccini Alfredo	630	35	63
Green Pepper Steak	240	4	32
Meatloaf	320	16	23
Spaghetti with Meatballs	360	12	45
White Meat Chicken Pot Pie	670	38	64
Simple Dishes For One: *Per ½ Package*			
Cheddar Potato Bake	270	17	21
Creamed Spinach	200	16	8
Macaroni & Cheese	340	16	33
Spinach Souffle	150	10	9

Stouffer's (Cont):

	C	**F**	**Cb**
Skillets For Family: *Per ½ Package*			
Broccoli & Beef	350	6	57
Cheesy Meatball Rigatoni	470	21	48
Chicken Alfredo	410	10	48
Chicken & Dumplings	370	13	40
Garlic Chicken	330	6	45
Garlic Shrimp	310	10	40
Grilled Chicken & Vegetables	360	9	43
Savory Chicken & Rice	330	6	50
Teriyaki Chicken	270	4	41
Yankee Pot Roast	300	8	38

Swanson:

Dinners: *Per Package*			
Chicken Nuggets	590	25	71
Rib Style Bnless Pork	540	23	71
Salisbury Steak	450	22	44
Skillets: *For Two*			
Alfredo Chicken	370	12	42
Beef Lo Mein	360	6	55
Chicken Parmesan	430	14	60
Garlic Chicken	420	15	51
Teriyaki Chicken	290	2.5	51

Tasty Bite:

Vegetarian Entrees: *Per ½ Package, 5 oz*			
Bengal Lentils	160	6	20
Bombay Potatoes	130	4	19
Jaipur Vegetables	180	11	12
Jodhpur Lentils	110	2.5	16
Madras Lentils	150	6	18
Punjab Eggplant	150	9	13

TGI Friday's:

Beer Battered Onion Rings, 3 rings	180	8	26
Cheese & Bacon Loaded Fries, 3 oz	210	11	20
Chicken Parmesan Sliders, 3 oz	260	13	27
Chicken Wings, Buffalo Style Sce, 3 oz	230	16	31
Cream Cheese Stuffed Jalap., 2.7 oz	220	18	27
Dill Pickle Chips, w/ Horseradish Sce	200	15	24
Mozzarella Sticks (1),			
w/ Marinara Sce,	100	5	10
Potato Skins, Cheddar & Bacon (3)	220	14	14

Thai Kitchen:	C	F	Cb
Take-Out Meals: *Per ½ Package*			
Original Pad Thai	250	2	54
Thai Basil & Chili	250	3	50
Thai Peanut	270	5	51
Noodle Carts: *Per 9 oz Tray*			
Pad Thai	460	2	104
Thai Peanut	510	9	96
Rice Noodle Soup Bowls,			
average all varieties, 2.5 oz	240	2	50
Stir-Fry Rice Noodles: *Per ½ Package*			
Original Pad Thai	390	3.5	84
Thai Peanut	390	2	87
Tofurky:			
Holiday Products: *Per Serving*			
Roast	350	11	19
Vegetarian Feast	555	20	50
Pies:			
Chick'N Pot Pie (1), 8 oz	520	33	45
Sausage & Veggie Quiche (1), 7.5 oz	520	28	43
Pockets: BBQ Chick'N (1), 4.5 oz	290	4	50
Broccoli Cheddar (1), 4.5 oz	240	5	40
Pepp. Pizza (1), 4.5 oz	300	5	43
Trader Joe's:			
Baked Beans, Organic,			
average all varieties, ½ cup	140	0	29
Black Beans:			
Regular, ½ cup	110	0	19
Cuban Style, ½ cup	100	0.5	19
Chicken Chili with Beans, 1 cup	290	9	32
Pasta, Shells & White Cheddar, 1 cup	280	6	47
Potatoes: Garlic Mashed, ½ cup	150	7	19
Cheddar Cheese Au Gratin, ½ cup	140	5	21
Turkey Chili w/ Beans, 1 cup	240	4.5	30
Frozen:			
Butter Chicken w/ Basmati Rice, 1 cup	270	8	33
Chicken Chow Mein, ⅓ package, 6.7 oz	210	2	35
Chicken Quesadilla (1), 6 oz	320	16	26
Citrus Glazed Chicken with Rice, 8 oz	270	5	40
Mac & Cheese: Regular, 1 cup, 7 oz	360	15	42
Reduced Guilt, 7 oz	270	6	40
Shrimp Stir Fry, 6.4 oz	70	0.5	6
Spag. & Beef Meatballs,			
1 cup, 9 oz	380	13	48
Spicy Beef & Broccoli,			
1¾ cups	430	13	64
Thai Vegetable Kao Soi, 12.6 oz	430	20	55
Vegetable Pad Thai, 10.5 oz tray	520	21	74
Pies: Chicken Pot Pie, ½ pie, 8 oz	360	22	28
Shepherd's Pie, 1 cup, 8 oz	170	3	22

Tyson:	C	F	Cb
Any'tizers Snacks:			
H'style Chicken Fries (7), 3.2 oz	230	13	14
Stuffed Chicken Cordon Bleu,			
Minis, 3 pieces, 3 oz	200	12	11
Chicken Wings: Buffalo Style Hot Wings			
bone-in, 3 oz	190	13	3
Honey BBQ, 3 oz	190	12	8
Hot & Spicy, 3 oz	190	13	1
Chicken Wyngz, Boneless:			
Buffalo Style, 3 pcs	150	7	8
Honey BBQ, 3 oz	200	8	20
Better For You: *Per 3 oz Serving*			
Grilled & Ready Chicken Breast Strips:			
100% Natural	100	2.5	1
Fajita	110	4	1
Southwestern	100	2.5	2
Breaded Chicken:			
100%: Breast Patties (1), 2.7 oz	200	13	10
Chicken Nuggets (5), 3.2 oz	270	17	15
Crispy Chicken Strips, 3 oz	190	9	12
Breast Nuggets (5), 3.1 oz	220	13	15
Buffalo Chicken Strips, 3 oz	190	9	17
Cheesy Chicken Nuggets (4), 2.8 oz	220	14	12
Fully Cooked Beef:			
Country Fried Steak, 1 pattie, 2.6 oz	250	17	13
Steak Fingers, 2 pieces, 2.5 oz	250	18	14
Grilled & Ready, Pulled Pork Loin	150	7	6
To Go Products:			
Mini Chicken Sandwich:			
Original, breaded	390	16	46
With Cheese	440	20	47
Uncle Ben's:			
Country Inn: *Per Cup, Prepared with Water Only*			
Broccoli Rice Au Gratin	200	2	41
Chicken & Vegetable Rice	200	1	43
Chicken Flavored Rice	200	1	42
Rice Pilaf	200	1	43
Flavored Grains: *1 Cup cooked As Directed*			
5 Grain Blend, French Onion	200	1.5	41
Brown & Wild Rice Mshrm Recipe	210	1	43
Brown Rice Medley,			
Roasted Garlic & Herbs, 2 oz	200	2	40
Ready Rice: *Per Package, Heat & Serve*			
Butter & Garlic Flavored	220	4	41
Garden Vegetable	200	2.5	41
Roasted Chicken Flavored	210	3	42
Teriyaki Style	220	3	42
Ready Whole Grain Medley,			
average all varieties, 1 pkt	210	3	41

	C	F	Cb
Van Camp's:			
Baked Beans, Original, ½ cup, 4.8 oz	160	1	30
Beanee Weenees, Smkd Hickory, 7.8 oz	320	9	45
Pork & Beans, 28 oz can, ½ cup, 4.6 oz	110	1	23
Van De Kamp's:			
Battered Crispy Pollock Fillets, 4 oz	210	10	21
Beer Battered Fillets, 3.8 oz	210	10	21
Breaded: Butterfly Shrimp, 4 oz	330	16	31
Crunchy: Fish Fillets, 1.8 oz	90	4	13
Fish Sticks, 3.4 oz	230	10	22
Popcorn Fish, 4.1 oz	270	13	25
Whole Foods (365):			
Chickenless Nuggets, breaded (4), 2.8 oz	180	7	16
Meatless Meatballs (4), 2 oz	110	4	9
Meatless Burgers (1), 2.5 oz	120	4.5	7
Pasta Rings in Tomato Sauce, 1 cup	150	1	31
Vegetarian Chili, 1 cup	130	2	15
Worthington/Loma Linda:			
Big Franks: 1 link, 1.8 oz	110	6	3
Low-fat, 1 link, 1.8 oz	80	2.5	3
Chili, 1 cup, 8.10 oz	280	10	25
Choplets, 2 slices, 3.2 oz	90	1	4
Diced Chik, 2 oz	50	0	2
FriChik, Original, low fat, 2 pieces, 3 oz	80	2.5	4
Linketts (1), 1.3 oz	70	4	1
Little Links (2), 1.6 oz	90	5	3
Redi-Burger, ⅝" slice, 3 oz	120	2.5	7
Super Links (1), 1.5 oz	110	8	2
Tender Rounds (6), 2.8 oz	120	4.5	6
Vegetable Skallops, ½ cup, 3 oz	90	1	4
Vegetarian Burger, ¼ cup, 1.9 oz	70	1.5	3
Veja-Links (1), 1 oz	50	3	1
Frozen:			
Chic-ketts, 2 slices	110	5	3
Dinner Roast, ¾" slice	180	11	6
FriPats, 1 pattie, 2.3 oz	130	6	5
Leanies, 1 link, 1.4 oz	100	7	2
Meatless:			
Chicken Style Roll, ⅜" slice	90	4.5	2
Smoked Turkey Roll, ⅜" slice	130	8	4
Prosage Links (2), 1.6 oz	80	3	3
Stakelets, 2.5 oz piece	150	7	3
Stripples, 2 strips, 0.6 oz	60	4.5	2

	C	F	Cb
Yves Veggie Cuisine:			
Brats: *EPer Brat*			
Veggie Classic, 3.5 oz	160	5	9
Zesty Italian, 3.5 oz	150	5	9
Burgers: Meatless Beef Burger (1)	110	4	8
Meatless Chicken (1)	100	3	5
Deli Slices:			
Meatless: Bologna, 4 slices	80	2.5	2
Ham, 4 slices	80	2.5	2
Pepperoni, 6 slices	100	2	5
Roast without the Beef, 4 slices	80	1	5
Salami, 4 slices	110	2.5	4
Smoked Chicken, 4 slices	80	0	4
Turkey, 4 slices	100	1.5	5
Ground Rounds:	100	1.5	5
Meatless: Taco Stuffers, ⅓ cup, 2 oz	90	2.5	5
Turkey, ⅓ cup, 2 oz	60	1	4
Hot Dog:			
Good Dog (1), 2 oz	70	3.5	1
Hot Dog (1), 1.5 oz	50	0.5	2
Jumbo Hot Dog (1), 2.8 oz	110	3	5
Tofu Dog (1), 1.5 oz	45	1	2
Skewers & Strips:			
Chicken Skewers (1)	100	1	7
Meatless Beef/Chicken Strips, average, 2.8 oz	115	1	7
Veggie Seafood:			
Shrimp, 3 oz	50	1.5	8
Shrimp Scampi, 3.5 oz	100	7	8
Tuna Steak, with Sesame Ginger Sce, 3.5 oz	250	20	8
Zatarain's:			
New Orleans Style: *Per Dry Mix Only*			
Black Beans & Rice, Original, 2.3 oz	230	1	47
Caribbean Rice Mix, 2.5 oz	250	2	52
Chicken Creole Rice Mix, 1.5 oz	140	1	29
Chicken Flavor Rice, 2 oz	210	0.5	45
Garlic & Herb & Rice Mix, 1.5 oz	130	0.5	29
Rice Pilaf, 2 oz	210	0.5	45
Smothered Chicken Rice Mix, 1.6 oz	160	0.5	34
Yellow Rice, 2 oz	200	0.5	43
Frozen:			
Meals: *Per Meal*			
Blackened Chicken Alfredo, 10.5 oz	500	21	56
Dirty Rice with Beef & Pork, 10 oz	430	13	64
Jambalaya Flavored w/ Ssge, 12 oz	490	10	86
Red Beans & Rice w/ Sausage, 12 oz	540	17	79
Shrimp Scampi with Pasta, 10.5 oz	350	10	49

Note: Cooking reduces weight of meat by 20-45% due to water and fat losses. Average weight loss is 30%. Actual loss depends on cooking method and cooking time.

Examples:

4 oz raw weight = approx. 3 oz cooked weight
4 oz cooked weight = approx. 5½ oz raw weight

What 3 oz Cooked Meat Looks Like:
• Rectangular piece (4" x 2½" x ½" thick)
• Deck of cards (3½" x 2½" x ⅝ " thick)

Quick Guide

C F Cb

Sirloin (Choice Grade):
External fat trimmed to ⅛"
Broiled, Edible Portion (no bone)

Small/Regular Serving, 3 oz, cooked weight:
(from 4-4½ oz raw)

	C	F	Cb
Lean + external fat (⅛"), 3 oz	220	13	0
Lean + marbling, 3 oz	185	9	0
Lean only, 3 oz	160	6	0

(No external fat or marbling)

Medium Serving, 5 oz, cooked weight:
(from approximately 7 oz raw)

	C	F	Cb
Lean + external fat (⅛"), 5 oz	365	22	0
Lean + marbling, 5 oz	310	15	0
Lean only, 5 oz	265	10	0

Large Serving, 8 oz, cooked weight:
(from approximately 11-12 oz raw)

	C	F	Cb
Lean + external fat (⅛"), 8 oz	585	36	0
Lean + marbling, 8 oz	500	24	0
Lean only, 8 oz	425	15	0

Extra Large Serving, 12 oz, cooked weight:
(from approximately 16-17 oz raw)

	C	F	Cb
Lean + external fat (⅛"), 12 oz	875	54	0
Lean + marbling, 12 oz	745	36	0
Lean only, 12 oz	640	22	0

Pan Fried:
Sirloin (Choice), medium serving,

	C	F	Cb
Lean + external fat (⅛"), 5 oz	445	30	0

Other Steaks

C F Cb

Filet Mignon (Tenderloin):
1 Medium steak, 6 oz raw weight:
Broiled, with ¼" fat trim:

	C	F	Cb
Lean + fat (¼"), 4 oz	360	27	0
Lean only, 3.5 oz	230	12	0

New York/Club Steak:
Top Loin/Short Loin:
1 steak, regular (9.25 oz raw, ¼" fat):
Broiled: Lean + fat (¼"), 6.3 oz

	C	F	Cb
Lean + fat (¼"), 6.3 oz	580	43	0
Lean + marbling, 5.5 oz	400	25	0
Lean only, 5.25 oz	360	20	0

Porterhouse Steak:
1 Medium, 6 oz raw weight, without bone, broiled:

	C	F	Cb
Lean + fat (¼"), 4.3 oz	410	33	0
Lean only, 3.5 oz	210	11	0

1 Large , 12 oz raw weight, without bone, broiled:

	C	F	Cb
Lean + fat (¼") 8.5 oz cooked	820	66	0
Lean only, 7 oz cooked	420	22	0

T-Bone Steak: *Broiled or Grilled*
Medium Size: *8 oz raw weight, without bone*
Approximately 6 oz cooked:

	C	F	Cb
Lean + fat (¼"), 5 oz	400	28	0
Lean only, 4 oz	265	12	0

Large Size: *12 oz raw weight*
Approximately 9 oz cooked:

	C	F	Cb
Lean + fat (¼"), 7 oz, without bone	560	39	0
Lean only, 6 oz, without bone	400	18	0

Extra Large Size: *20 oz raw weight*
Approximately 16 oz cooked:

	C	F	Cb
Lean + Fat (¼"), 12 oz, without bone	960	66	0
Lean Only, 10 oz, without bone	660	30	0

Also See Fast-Foods & Restaurants Section ~
Lone Star Steakhouse; Outback Steakhouse

Beef – Individual Cuts C F Cb

Average All Grades
Edible Weight, Without Bone

	C	F	Cb
Brisket, whole, braised:			
Lean + fat (¼" trim), 3 oz	330	27	0
Lean + marbling, 3 oz	250	17	0
Lean only, 3 oz	185	9	0
Chuck blade, braised:			
Lean + fat (¼"), 3 oz	310	24	0
Lean + marbling, 3 oz	295	22	0
Lean only, 3 oz	245	13	0
Flank: Raw, 4 oz	175	8	0
Braised, 3 oz	225	14	0
Broiled, 3 oz	155	6	0
Round, bottom, braised:			
Lean + marbling, 3 oz	190	7.5	0
Lean only, 3 oz	185	6.5	0
Round, eye/tip, rstd:			
Lean + fat (¼"), 3 oz	205	11	0
Lean, w/ marbling, 3 oz	150	5	0
Round, top: *Per 3 oz, Cooked Weight*			
Braised, Lean + fat	210	10	0
Lean only	170	4	0
Broiled, Lean + fat	180	8	0
Lean only	160	5	0
Pan-fried, Lean + fat	235	13	0
Lean only	195	7	0

Beef Ribs

Back Ribs: *7" long, visible fat trimmed to ¼"*
10.3 oz raw w/ bone or 3.5 oz cooked, braised, w/o bone

1 average rib	410	34	0
3 ribs	1230	102	0

Short Ribs: *2½" long, visible fat trimmed to ¼"*
6 oz raw with bone or 2.52 oz cooked, braised, w/o bone

1 average rib	320	28	0
3 ribs	960	85	0

Ground Beef

Ground Beef, Raw: *Per 4 oz*			
70% lean (30% fat)	380	34	0
75% lean (25% fat)	335	29	0
80% lean (20% fat)	290	23	0
85% lean (15% fat)	245	17	0
90% lean (10% fat)	200	12	0
95% lean (5% fat)	155	6	0
Baked/Broiled: Regular (70%), 3 oz	230	16	0
Lean (80%), 3 oz	215	14	0
Extra lean (90%), 3 oz	185	10	0
Pan-Broiled:			
Regular (70%), 3 oz	230	15	0
Lean (80%), 3 oz	210	14	0
Extra lean (90%), 3 oz	195	10	0
Ground Beef Patties: *Average, 23% Fat*			
Raw, 4 oz	330	25	0
Broiled, 3 oz (from 4 oz raw)	250	19	0

Quick Guide C F Cb

Roast Beef

Round (Eye/Tip, average): *Average All Cuts*

Small/Regular Serving: *3 oz*
(2 thin slices/1 thick slice)

	C	F	Cb
Lean + fat (⅛" fat trim)	180	9	0
Lean only	145	4	0

Medium Serving: *5 oz*
(3-4 thin slices)

Lean + fat (⅛" fat trim)	300	15	0
Lean only	245	6.5	0

Large Serving, 8 oz: *3 thick slices*

Lean + fat (⅛" fat trim)	480	24	0
Lean only	385	11	0

Roast Dinner Extras

Gravy: Thin, 2 Tbsp	20	0.5	3.5
Thick, 2 Tbsp	50	2	0.5
1 Ladle/4 Tbsp	100	4	1
Veggies: Beans, green, ½ cup	20	0	5
Cauliflower with cheese sauce, 4 oz	135	9	15
Corn, kernels, ¼ cup	35	0	9
Carrots, ¼ cup	20	0	3
Peas, ¼ cup	35	0	6
Potato:			
Baked in jacket: Plain, 1 large	280	0	63
With sour cream, 2 Tbsp	270	5	64
With whipped butter, 1 Tbsp	350	8	63
Roasted with fat, 1 small	155	8	30
Sweet Potato/Yam, 1 medium	105	1	24
Yorkshire Pudding, 1 oz	90	3.5	11

Beef Kebab: *Cooked*			
Beef & Veggies, 2 oz	160	10	4
If very lean meat	100	4	4

"347 ~ 348 ~ 349..."

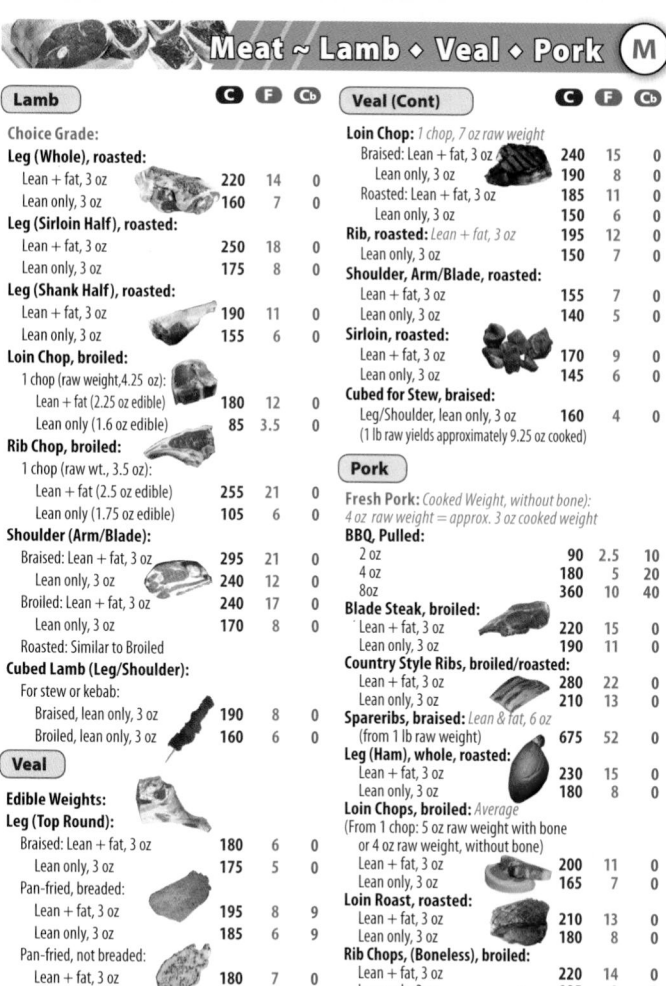

Lamb

C · F · Cb

Choice Grade:

Leg (Whole), roasted:

	C	F	Cb
Lean + fat, 3 oz	220	14	0
Lean only, 3 oz	160	7	0

Leg (Sirloin Half), roasted:

Lean + fat, 3 oz	250	18	0
Lean only, 3 oz	175	8	0

Leg (Shank Half), roasted:

Lean + fat, 3 oz	190	11	0
Lean only, 3 oz	155	6	0

Loin Chop, broiled:

1 chop (raw weight,4.25 oz):

Lean + fat (2.25 oz edible)	180	12	0
Lean only (1.6 oz edible)	85	3.5	0

Rib Chop, broiled:

1 chop (raw wt., 3.5 oz):

Lean + fat (2.5 oz edible)	255	21	0
Lean only (1.75 oz edible)	105	6	0

Shoulder (Arm/Blade):

Braised: Lean + fat, 3 oz	295	21	0
Lean only, 3 oz	240	12	0
Broiled: Lean + fat, 3 oz	240	17	0
Lean only, 3 oz	170	8	0
Roasted: Similar to Broiled			

Cubed Lamb (Leg/Shoulder):

For stew or kebab:

Braised, lean only, 3 oz	190	8	0
Broiled, lean only, 3 oz	160	6	0

Veal

Edible Weights:

Leg (Top Round):

Braised: Lean + fat, 3 oz	180	6	0
Lean only, 3 oz	175	5	0
Pan-fried, breaded:			
Lean + fat, 3 oz	195	8	9
Lean only, 3 oz	185	6	9
Pan-fried, not breaded:			
Lean + fat, 3 oz	180	7	0
Lean only, 3 oz	155	4	0
Roasted: Lean + fat, 3 oz	135	4	0
Lean only, 3 oz	130	3	0

Veal (Cont)

C · F · Cb

Loin Chop: *1 chop, 7 oz raw weight*

	C	F	Cb
Braised: Lean + fat, 3 oz	240	15	0
Lean only, 3 oz	190	8	0
Roasted: Lean + fat, 3 oz	185	11	0
Lean only, 3 oz	150	6	0

Rib, roasted: *Lean + fat, 3 oz*

	195	12	0
Lean only, 3 oz	150	7	0

Shoulder, Arm/Blade, roasted:

Lean + fat, 3 oz	155	7	0
Lean only, 3 oz	140	5	0

Sirloin, roasted:

Lean + fat, 3 oz	170	9	0
Lean only, 3 oz	145	6	0

Cubed for Stew, braised:

Leg/Shoulder, lean only, 3 oz	160	4	0
(1 lb raw yields approximately 9.25 oz cooked)			

Pork

Fresh Pork: *Cooked Weight, without bone:*
4 oz raw weight = approx. 3 oz cooked weight

BBQ, Pulled:

	C	F	Cb
2 oz	90	2.5	10
4 oz	180	5	20
8oz	360	10	40

Blade Steak, broiled:

Lean + fat, 3 oz	220	15	0
Lean only, 3 oz	190	11	0

Country Style Ribs, broiled/roasted:

Lean + fat, 3 oz	280	22	0
Lean only, 3 oz	210	13	0

Spareribs, braised: *Lean & fat, 6 oz*

(from 1 lb raw weight)	675	52	0

Leg (Ham), whole, roasted:

Lean + fat, 3 oz	230	15	0
Lean only, 3 oz	180	8	0

Loin Chops, broiled: *Average*
(From 1 chop: 5 oz raw weight with bone
or 4 oz raw weight, without bone)

Lean + fat, 3 oz	200	11	0
Lean only, 3 oz	165	7	0

Loin Roast, roasted:

Lean + fat, 3 oz	210	13	0
Lean only, 3 oz	180	8	0

Rib Chops, (Boneless), broiled:

Lean + fat, 3 oz	220	14	0
Lean only, 3 oz	185	9	0

Rib Roast:

Lean + fat, 3 oz	215	13	0
Lean only, 3 oz	180	9	0

Pork (Cont)

	C	F	Cb
Sirloin Chop, broiled:			
Lean + fat, 3 oz	180	8	0
Lean only, 3 oz	165	6	0
Sirloin Roast, roasted:			
Lean + fat, 3 oz	175	8	0
Lean only, 3 oz	170	7	0
Tenderloin (Boneless), roasted:			
Lean + fat, 3 oz	125	4	0
Lean only, 3 oz	120	3	0
Ground Pork:			
Raw, average, ¼ lb, 4 oz	300	24	0
Broiled, 3 oz	250	18	0
Pan-fried, drained, 3 oz	260	19	0

Bacon

	C	F	Cb
Raw: 1 med. slice, 0.75 oz	95	9	0
1 thick slice, 1.3 oz	175	17	0
(1 lb raw yields approximately 5 oz cooked)			
Broiled/Pan-Fried:			
1 medium slice, 0.3 oz	40	3	0
3 medium slices, 0.8	125	10	0
2 thin slices, 0.5 oz	75	6	0
1 thick slice, 0.9 oz	65	5	0
Canadian Bacon:			
Cooked 1 slice, 1 oz	45	2	0.5
2 slices, 2 oz	90	4	1
Bacon Bits, 1 Tbsp, 0.3 oz	35	2	0
Breakfast Strips, Broiled, 1 sl., 0.4 oz	50	4	0

Ham

	C	F	Cb
Boneless Ham, cooked:			
Regular, (approximately 13% fat):			
Roasted, 3 oz	150	8	0
Extra Lean (5% fat),			
Roasted, 3 oz	125	5	0
Whole Ham, cooked:			
Lean + fat (as purchased)			
Roasted, 3 oz	210	15	0
Lean only, Roasted, 3 oz	135	5	0
Canned Ham: *Similar to boneless ham*			
Chopped, canned, 3 oz	200	16	0
Ham Patties, cooked, (1), 2.3 oz	220	20	1
Ham Steak, extra lean, 2 oz	70	2.5	0
Lunch Slices ~ *See Deli Meats, Page 128*			

Game & Other Meats

	C	F	Cb
Bison Steak,			
lean, 6 oz (raw)	205	4	0
Boar (wild), roasted, 3 oz	140	4	0
Buffalo Steak,			
New West Foods, 4 oz	70	3	0
Caribou, roasted, 3 oz	140	4	0
Deer/Venison, roasted 3 oz	135	3	0
Goat (Capretto):			
Raw, 3 oz	95	2	0
Roasted, 3 oz	120	2.5	0
Ostrich:			
Blackwing Ostrich Meats:			
Sausage Patties (2) 2 oz	60	0.5	0
Sport Jerky, 0.5 oz piece	25	0	0
New West Foods:			
Ground Ostrich, 4 oz	165	7	0
Ostrich Steak, 4 oz steak	130	2.5	0
Rabbit: Roasted, 3 oz	165	7	0
Stewed, 1 cup, diced, 5 oz	290	12	0

Variety & Organ Meats

	C	F	Cb
Brain (Lamb): Braised, 3 oz	125	9	0
Pan-fried, 3 oz	230	19	0
Chitterlings, pork, simmered, 3 oz	260	25	0
Ears, pork, simmered, 1 ear, 4 oz	185	12	0
Feet, Pork: Simmered, 3 oz	200	14	0
Cured, pickled, 3 oz	170	14	0
Hormel, 2 oz	80	6	0
Head Cheese (Pork Snouts/Ears/Vinegar/Spices),			
1 oz slice	50	4	0
Heart, Beef, braised, 3 oz	140	4	0
Jowl, pork, raw, 4 oz	750	80	0
Kidneys, braised, 3 oz	140	5	0
Liver (beef): Raw, 4 oz	150	4	4
Braised, 3 oz	140	4	3
Pan-fried, 3 oz	185	7	7
Pancreas, pork, braised, 3 oz	185	8	0
Pork Cracklins, 0.5 oz	80	6	0
Pork Hocks, 1 piece, 6 oz	340	23	0
Scrapple, pork, 2 oz	120	8	8
Spleen, pork, braised, 3 oz	130	3	0
Stomach, pork, raw, 4 oz	185	12	0
Sweetbreads:			
Beef./Lamb, cooked, 3 oz	125	9	0
Tail, pork, simmered, 3 oz	340	31	0
Tongue: Raised Veal, 3 oz	170	9	0
Beef/Lamb/Pork, av., 3 oz	235	17	0
Tripe, beef, raw, 3 oz	85	3.5	0

Quick Guide | C | F | Cb |

Franks & Weiners
Average All Brands

Regular (Pork Mix): *Per Frank*

	C	F	Cb
Regular, 1.5 oz	140	13	1
Bun Length/Jumbo, 2 oz	185	17	2
Extra Long, 2.75 oz	255	24	2
Small/Cocktail, each	30	3	0.5
Beef Franks: *Per Frank*			
Regular, 1.5 oz	140	13	2
Bun Length/Jumbo, 2 oz	175	17	2.5
¼ lb Dog, 4 oz	375	33	5

Franks & Weiners

Ball Park: *Per 2 oz Frank Unless Indicated*

Angus Beef:

	C	F	Cb
Original; Bun Size, 2 oz	170	15	3
Lean, 1.8 oz	70	5	2
Beef: Original, Bun Size, 2 oz	190	16	4
Lean, 1.8 oz	80	5	2
Cheese, with Turkey, Beef & Pork	190	16	5
Deli Style: Regular, 1.8 oz	150	12	2
BunSize, 1.8 oz	150	12	2
GrillMaster,			
Hearty Beef, 2.9 oz	250	21	3
Jumbo, 2.5 oz	240	20	5
Turkey, Original, 2 oz	110	7	6
Foster Farms, Chicken; Turkey, 2 oz	140	12	1

Hebrew National: *Per Frank*

	C	F	Cb
Beef: Regular, 1.7 oz	150	14	1
¼ Pounder, 4 oz	360	33	3
Jumbo, 3 oz	270	25	2
97% Fat-Free, 1.6 oz	40	1	3
Beef Frank in a Blanket, 5 pcs, 3 oz	300	24	12

Jennie-O: *Per Frank*

	C	F	Cb
Turkey Franks: 1.2 oz	70	6	1
Jumbo, 2 oz	120	10	2

Oscar Mayer: *Per Frank*

	C	F	Cb
Beef: Classic, 1.6 oz	140	13	1
Lean, 1.8 oz	60	3.5	1
Turkey: Classic, 1.6 oz	100	8	2
Classic Bun Length, 2 oz	120	10	3

Shelton's: *Per Frank*

	C	F	Cb
Chicken, uncured, 1.2 oz	80	7	1
Turkey: Regular, 1.2 oz	60	4.5	1
Smoked, 3 oz	150	11	2
Zacky Farms, Chkn; Turkey, av, 2 oz	115	10	4

Quick Guide | C | F | Cb |

Fresh Sausages
Pork/Beef: *Average All Types*

	C	F	Cb
Small: Raw, 4"link, 1 oz	85	7.5	0
Broiled/Pan-fried	80	7	0
Medium: Raw, 2 oz	170	15	0
Broiled/Pan-fried	165	14	0
Large: Raw, 3 oz	255	22	0
Broiled/Pan-fried	245	21	0
Italian: Raw, 3.2 oz	315	28	1
Cooked, 2.4 oz	230	18	3
Chorizo: Beef Chorizo, 2.5 oz piece	250	23	5
Pork Chorizo, 2 oz piece	250	23	5

Note: Fat is lost in broiling/pan frying.
Cooked weight = approx. 60-70% raw weight

Smoked Sausages
Per Link:

	C	F	Cb
Butterball, Turkey, 2 oz	100	6	4
Eckrich:			
Grillers: Original, 2 oz	180	15	4
Cheese	190	17	1
Hillshire Farm:			
Angus Beef, 2 oz	170	15	2
Cheddar Wurst, 2 oz	180	16	2
Chicken Hardwood, 2 oz	100	7	3
Johnsonville – See CalorieKing.Com			

Breakfast Sausages/Patties

Butterball: *Fully Cooked*
Turkey:

	C	F	Cb
B'fast Sausage Links (3), 2.5 oz	110	6	2
Sausage Patties (2), 2.5 oz	110	6	2
Jennie-O,			
Turkey Breakfast Sausage, Lean, 2 oz	80	5	0

Jimmy Dean: *Fully Cooked*
Heat 'N Serve Sausage Links:

	C	F	Cb
Pork, Regular (3), 1.9 oz	210	19	2
Turkey (3), 2 oz	130	8	2
Maple Pork Sausages,(3), 2.4 oz	280	26	5

Heat 'N Serve Sausage Patties:

	C	F	Cb
Pork, Original (2), 1.8 oz	200	17	2
Turkey (2), 1.8 oz	120	8	1
Maple Pork Patties, (2), 2.4 oz	260	22	3
Breakfast Sandwiches ~ See Page 92			

Jones Dairy Farm:
All Natural Golden Brown Sausages: *Fully Cooked*

	C	F	Cb
Pork Sausage (1), 1 oz	120	12	0
Pork Patty (1),1 oz	120	11	0

Vegetarian Patties:
Boca ~ See Page 117
GardenBurger ~ See Page 114

Bagel, Corn & Hot Dogs

	C	**F**	**Cb**
Hot Dogs, Ready-To-Go:			
Includes Ketchup/Relish			
Regular, 1.5 oz frank, 1.5 oz bun	260	15	22
Bun Length, 2 oz frank, 1.5 oz bun	290	18	21
Jumbo Dog, 2 oz frank, 2 oz bun	360	20	36
¼ lb Beef Dog, 2 oz bun	480	15	36
Mile Long Dog, 2.6 oz dog, 1.5 oz bun	360	24	23

Corn Dogs
Beef/Pork Frank, average, 2.6 oz	170	10	16
Foster Farms:			
Corn Dogs:			
Chili Cheese: (1), 2.7 oz	180	9	19
Honey Crunchy:			
Regular (1), 2.7 oz	180	9	19
Jumbo (1), 4 oz	280	15	27
Mini (4), 2.7 oz	210	12	18
State Fair:			
Beef Corn Dog (1), 2.7 oz	230	11	26
Classic Corn Dog (1), 2.7 oz	190	8	23
Fiesta (1), 2.7 oz	180	9	19

Bagel Dogs:
Einstein Bros/Noah's:			
N.Y. Bagels: Asiago	530	27	56
Original	490	24	56
Vienna Beef:			
Bageldog: 5.5 oz	400	1	64
6.5 oz	470	18	56
Mini (4), 3 oz	220	13	16

Hot Dog Toppings/Extras:
American Cheese, 1 slice, 1 oz	110	9	1
Chili Con Carne, ¼ cup	50	2	5.5
Ketchup, 1 Tbsp	15	0	4
Mustard, 1 Tbsp	20	0	1
Onions, chopped, 1 Tbsp	5	0	1
Pickle Relish, 1 Tbsp	20	0	5
Sauerkraut, ½ cup	20	0	5

Deli/Lunch Meats & Sausage

Beef Jerky/Meat Snacks,			
Berliner (pork/beef), 1 oz	65	5	1
Beerwurst (Beef):			
Small (2¾"diam), ¹⁄₁₆" slice	20	2	0
Large (4" diam), ⅛" slice	75	7	0.5
Beerwurst (Pork):			
Small (2.75"diameter), ¹⁄₁₆" slice	15	1	0
Large (4"diameter), ⅛" Slice	55	4	0.5
Blood Sausage, 1 oz	100	9	0.5

Deli/Lunch Meats & Sausages (Cont)

	C	**F**	**Cb**
Bologna:			
Beef Bologna, 1 slice, 1 oz	90	8	1
Light, 1 slice, 1 oz	60	4	2
Oscar Mayer: Regular, 1 oz	90	8	1
98% Fat Free, 1 oz	25	0.5	3
Light, 1 slice, 1 oz	60	4	2
Boar's Head, Ring, 2 oz	150	13	1
Pork Bologna, 1 Slice, 1 oz	65	6	1
Fat-Free, 1 slice, 1 oz	20	0	2
Turkey Bologna, average, 1 oz	60	5	0.5
Bratwurst, average, 1 oz	80	7	1
Bob Evan's, Beer B'wurst, 2.2 oz link	170	14	0
Braunschweiger, (Pork/Liver/Sausage),			
Oscar Mayer, 2 oz slice	190	17	1
Chicken, average:			
1 thick or 2 thin slices, 1 oz	30	1	1
2 oz slice	60	2	1
Hillshire Farm,			
Rotiss. Seas'nd Chicken Breast, 2 oz	50	0.5	2
Corned Beef, average, full fat, 1 oz	60	5	0.5
Ham, Sliced:			
Baked/Broiled, 1 oz slice	35	1	1
Oscar Mayer, Baked, 1 slice	60	2	0
Honey/Brown Sugar, av., 1 oz	35	1	1
Prosciutto, average, 1 oz	70	5	0
Ham & Cheese Loaf, average, 1 oz	70	5	1
Italian Sausage, 2.6 oz	250	20	3
Kielbasa: Polish Sausage, 2 oz	65	5	1
Beef, 2 oz link	190	17	1
Hillshire Farm,			
Polska, 2 oz	180	16	3
Knockwurst, av., 1 oz	90	8	0.5
Linguica (Gaspar's), 2 oz	130	9	1
Liverwurst, 1 oz	65	5	1
Liver Pate, fresh, average, 1 oz	90	8	1
Mortadella, 1 oz	105	9	0
Olive Loaf: Average, 1 oz	70	5	3
Oscar Mayer, 1 oz	80	6	3
Pancetta ,			
Boars Head, 1 slice	50	4.5	0

Deli/Lunch Meats & Sausages (Cont)

	C	F	Cb
Pastrami (Beef):			
Boar's Head:			
1st cut Brisket, 2 oz	90	4	2
Cap-off Top Round, 2 oz	70	2.5	1
Hillshire, Deli Select,			
Ultra Thin, 7 slices., 2 oz	60	1.5	1
Peppered Beef, 1 oz slice	40	2	1
Pepperoni, 5 slices, 1 oz	140	13	0
Pickle Loaf, average, 1 oz	70	5	5
Pickle & Pepper Loaf,			
Boars Head, 2 oz	150	13	2
Proscuitto/Proscuitti, av., 1 oz	70	5	1
Roast Beef, Lean, 1 oz	40	2	0
Salami: Beef, av., 1 oz	80	7	1
Oscar Mayer, Hard, 1 slice, 1.8 oz	100	8	1
Beer Salami, average, 1 oz	50	4	0.5
Oscar Mayer, Cotto, 1 slice, 1 oz	70	6	1
Dry, Hard, average, 4 slices, 1 oz	100	8	1
Genoa: Average, 1 oz	100	8	1
Stick, 1.8 oz	175	14	2
Bridgford, Italian, 1 oz	120	11	0
SPAM (Hormel): *Per 2 oz*			
Classic: 2 oz serving	180	16	1
7 oz can	630	56	3.5
12 oz can	1080	96	6
Spam Lite: 2 oz	110	8	1
12 oz can	660	48	6
Other Spam Products: *Per 2 oz*			
Hickory Smoked	170	16	2
Hot & Spicy	180	16	2
Oven Roasted Turkey	80	4	2
Spam with Bacon	180	16	1
Spam with Cheese	170	15	2
Spam Spread	140	12	0
25% Less Sodium	180	16	1
Spam Singles: *Per 3 oz*			
Classic, 3 oz package	210	16	0
Lite, 3 oz package	160	11	2

Deli/Lunch Meats & Sausages (Cont)

	C	F	Cb
Summer Sausage:			
Armour, 2 oz	190	17	2
Hillshire Farm, 2 oz	190	16	1
Treet *(Armour),* Luncheon Loaf,			
Original, 2 oz	140	11	4
Turkey, average: 1 oz slice	30	1	0.5
0.8 oz slice	22	0.5	0.5
Turkey Breast:			
Butterball, Oven Roasted:			
Thick Slice, 1 slice 1 oz	30	0.5	2
Deli Inspirations,			
Extra Thin Slices, 4 slices, 2 oz	50	1	3
Hillshire, Deli Select,			
Oven Roasted, 6 slices, 2 oz	50	0.5	2
Turkey Ham, 1 slice, 1 oz	35	1.5	0.5
Turkey Loaf, 1 oz	30	1	0.5
Turkey Pastrami, 1 oz	35	1.5	1
Turkey Roll, 1 oz	40	2	0.5
Vegetarian Deli ~ *See Page 118*			

Meat Spreads

	C	F	Cb
Average All Brands: *Per 2 oz*			
Chicken, white meat	130	10	2
Ham, Deviled	140	11	0
Liverwurst	190	16	2
Roast Beef	130	10	2
Sandwich Spread	140	10	9
Turkey	110	7	2
Underwood: *Per 2 oz*			
Chicken, White Meat	140	11	2
Deviled Ham	180	15	1
Liverwurst	160	13	4
Roast Beef	130	10	2

Paté

	C	F	Cb
Les Trois Petit Cochons: *Per 2 oz*			
Black Peppercorn	200	19	1
Chicken & Pork Livers with Truffle	140	11	2
Country Pate	200	22	1
Smoked Salmon	110	9	2
Old Wisconsin Pate,			
Braunschweiger, 2 oz	210	18	3

Nuts **C** **F** **Cb**

Per 1 oz Unless Indicated

	C	F	Cb
Acorns, raw 1 oz	110	7	12
Almonds: Dried/Dry Roasted:			
Whole: 12 medium size, 0.5 oz	85	7.5	3
23-25 medium size, 1 oz	170	15	6
½ cup, 2.5 oz	420	37	13
Ground, 1 cup, 3.4 oz	545	47	20
Sliced, ½ cup, 1.6 oz	260	22	10
Slivered, ½ cup, 2 oz	310	27	12
Chocolate Coated (5-6), 1 oz	150	10	15
Honey Roasted, 1 oz	170	14	8
Oil Roasted (Blue Diamond), 1 oz	170	16	5
Brazil Nuts, 8 medium, 1 oz	185	19	3.5
Cashews, dry or oil roasted:			
14 large/18 med./26 small: 1 oz	165	14	9
½ cup, 2.4 oz	375	31	20
Honey Roasted, 1 oz	165	13	10
Chestnuts:			
Average, dried, 1 oz	105	1	22
Raw/Fresh, 5-6 nuts, 1 oz	60	0	13
Canned, water chestnuts,			
sliced/whole/drained, 1 oz	30	0	7
Coconut, Fresh:			
1 piece, 2"x2"x ½", 1 oz	185	18	7
Shredded, fresh, ½ cup, 1.4 oz	140	13	6
Dried (Desiccated):			
Sweetened: Shredded, 1 oz	145	10	14
Grated, ½ cup, 1.3 oz	185	13	18
Unsweetened, 1 oz	185	18	7
Cream (canned), ½ cup, 5.2 oz	285	26	12
Milk (canned), unsweetened,			
¼ cup, 2 fl.oz	100	10	3
Water (center liquid), ½ cup, 4.3 oz	25	0	4.5
Filberts or Hazelnuts:			
Shelled, 18-20 nuts	180	17	4.5
Chopped, ¼ cup, 1 oz	180	18	5
Ground, ¼ cup, 0.6 oz	120	12	3
Ginkgo Nuts, canned, 14 med., 1 oz	32	0.5	6.5
Hickory:			
30 small nuts, 1 oz	200	18	5
Macadamia Nuts, Shelled:			
Raw or Dry Roasted, avg:			
12 small or 8 med., 1 oz	200	21	4
6-7 large, 1 oz	200	21	4
½ cup, 2.3 oz	480	51	10
Mixed Nuts: Raw, 18-22 nuts, 1 oz	170	15	7
Oil Roasted, all types	170	16	6
Sweet Roasts, 26 pieces, 1 oz	160	12	10
Planters, Dry Roasted/Honey	160	12	9
Nut Toppings, chopped, 1 Tbsp, 0.3 oz	40	4	1.5

Per 1 oz Unless Indicated **C** **F** **Cb**

	C	F	Cb
Peanuts, dry or oil roasted, average:			
Small handful, 0.5 oz	85	7	3
⅓ cup, 1 oz	165	14	6
½ cup, 2.5 oz	415	35	15
3 oz bag	500	42	18
7 oz bag	1160	98	42
Planters:			
Cocktail, all varieties	170	14	5
Honey Roasted	160	13	7
Spanish Redskins	170	15	4
Sweet N' Crunchy	140	8	15
Japanese Style Peanuts,			
Coated in Crunchy Shell	150	8	13
Raw: Shelled, 1 oz	160	14	4.5
In shell, 1 oz	115	110	3
Pecans, roasted:			
10 halves, 0.5 oz	95	10	2
20 Halves, 1 oz	195	20	4
1 cup, halves, 3.5 oz	680	71	14
Pilinuts, dried, 1 oz	215	24	1
Pine Nuts,			
dried, 1 Tbsp, 0.3 oz	70	7	1.5
Pistachios, raw:			
Shelled, 45 nuts, 1 oz	160	13	8
Unshelled, 2 oz	165	14	7
Lance, Roasted, 1.5 oz	120	9	6
Sesame Nut Mix, 1 oz	160	13	9
Soy Nuts: Dry Roasted	130	6	9
½ cup, 3 oz	390	18	28
Dr Soy, Chocolate coated, 1 oz pkg	140	7	13
Trail Mix (Planters):			
Daybreak, Berry Almond, 1.5 oz	180	7	27
Energy Mix, 1.5 oz	250	20	14
Fruit & Nut	140	9	14
Nut & Chocolate, 1.3oz	150	9	14
Nuts, Seeds & Raisins, 1 oz	160	11	11
Spicy Nuts & Cajun Sticks	150	11	10
Sweet & Nutty, 1 oz	150	9	13
Walnuts: average all types:			
7-10 halves, 0.5 oz	90	9	2
15-20 halves, 1 oz	175	17	3
Chopped, ½ cup, 2.2 oz	380	36	6
Ground, ¼ cup, 0.7 oz	130	13	3

Quick Guide | C | F | Cb |

Peanut Butter: *Average All Brands*

	C	F	Cb
1 level tsp, 0.2 oz	35	3	1
1 level Tbsp, 0.6 oz	100	8.5	3.5
1 oz Quantity	165	14	6
½ cup, 5 oz	835	72	29

Peanut Butter ~ Brands

	C	F	Cb
Jif: Regular, all varieties, 2 tbsp	190	16	8
Natural, average all varieties, 2 tbsp	190	16	9
Reduced Fat, all varieties, 2 tbsp	190	12	15
To Go: Crmy/Crunch, 1.5 oz cup	250	22	11
Reduced Fat, 1.7 oz cup	250	16	20
Whipped: Creamy, 2 Tbsp	140	12	6
Chocolate flavored, 2 Tbsp	150	11	11
Laura Scudder's, Natural,			
Smooth; Nutty, 2 Tbsp	210	16	6
Peanut Wonder, Original, 2 Tbsp	100	2	13
Peter Pan:			
Natural, Creamy/Crunchy, 2 Tbsp	210	17	6
Creamy/Crunchy, Red.-Fat, 2 Tbsp	200	13	14
Creamy, Whipped, 2 Tbsp	150	12	5
Planters, Creamy/Crunchy, 2 Tbsp	180	15	8
Smucker's, Goober,			
Grape/Srawberry, 3 Tbsp. 2 oz	240	13	24
Skippy: Natural, Creamy/Chunky, 2 T.	190	16	6
Reduced Fat, all varieties, 2 Tbsp	180	12	15
Dark Chocolate Spread, 2 Tbsp	200	14	12

Peanut Butter & Jelly Sandwich

1 sandwich: *With 2 oz Bread*

	C	F	Cb
Thin Spread, 1 Tbsp Peanut Butter + 1 Tbsp Jelly	310	10	48
Thick Spread, 2 Tbsp Peanut Butter + 2 Tbsp Jelly	480	19	67

Nut & Chocolate Spread

Nutella:

	C	F	Cb
1 Tbsp, 0.7 oz	100	6	11
2 Tbsp, 1.3 oz	200	12	21

Note: Nutella contains approx. 50% sugar & 13% hazelnuts

Other Nut & Seed Butters

Per 1 Tbsp, 0.5 oz

	C	F	Cb
Almond Butter	100	10	3.5
Cashew Butter	95	8	4.5
Hazelnut Butter; Pecan Butter	110	10	2
Pistachio Butter	90	6.5	4.5
Sesame Butter (Tahini)	90	8	3
Soy Nut Butter	75	5	4

Seeds | C | F | Cb |

	C	F	Cb
Alfalfa Seeds, sprouted, ½ cup, 0.5 oz	5	0	1
Caraway/Fennel, 1 tsp	7	0.5	1
Chia Seeds: 1 Tbsp, 0.4 oz	45	3	4
3 Tbsp, 1 oz	140	8.5	12
Cottonseed Kernels, roasted, 1 Tbsp	50	3.5	2
Flax Seeds, 3 Tbsp, 1 oz	140	9	9
Lotus Seeds, dried, ½ cup, 0.5 oz	55	0.5	10
Poppy Seeds, 1 tsp	15	1	1
Pumpkin/Pepita Seeds, whole:			
Roasted/Tamari: 1 oz	150	12	4
½ cup, 4 oz	590	48	15
Dried (hulled), ¼ cup, 1 oz	155	13	5
Safflower Kernels, dried, 1 oz	150	11	10
Sesame Seeds:			
Dried, 1 Tbsp, 0.3 oz	50	4.5	2
Roasted/Toasted, 1 oz	160	14	7.5
Sunflower Kernels/Seeds:			
Dried, ¼ cup w/out hulls, 0.3 oz	200	18	7
Dry Roasted: 1 Tbsp, 0.3 oz	45	4	2
¼ cup, 1 oz	165	14	7
Oil Roasted, ⅓ cup, 1 oz	170	14	6.5
Watermelon Seeds, dried, ¼ cup, 1 oz	150	13	4

*N*ut eaters are healthier and live longer, say scientists.

Nuts are a nutritious source of protein, vitamins, minerals, fiber, healthy fats, and antioxidants.

The fat and fiber of nuts can help reduce blood cholesterol. Their protein and fiber also promotes meal satiety (fullness) and reduces hunger levels – of benefit in weight control.

Eat nuts instead of high-sugar snacks, candy and soft drinks. Add chopped nuts to breakfast cereals.

Quick Guide   C   F   Cb

Pancakes:

Plain: *Average All Types*

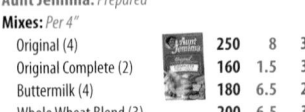

	C	F	Cb
Small (3" diameter), 0.8 oz	50	2	6
Medium (4" diameter), 1.3 oz	85	3.5	11
Large (6" diameter), 2.5 oz	175	7.5	22

Add Extra for Syrups/Butter

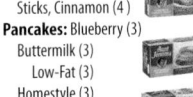

	C	F	Cb
Pancake Syrup: Regular, 1 Tbsp	50	0	12
¼ cup, 4 Tbsp	185	0	49
Lite, 1 Tbsp	25	0	6.5
¼ cup, 4 Tbsp	100	0	27

Butter/Margarine:

	C	F	Cb
Regular, 1 Tbsp	100	11	0
Whipped, 1 Tbsp	65	7.5	0

Waffles:

	C	F	Cb
Homemade, 7" waffle, 2.5 oz	220	11	25
Frozen + Toasted, (4" diam.), 1 oz	105	3	16

Pancake Brands

Prepared As Directed

Aunt Jemima: *Prepared*

Mixes: *Per 4"*

	C	F	Cb
Original (4)	250	8	36
Original Complete (2)	160	1.5	32
Buttermilk (4)	180	6.5	23
Whole Wheat Blend (3)	200	6.5	30

Bisquick: *Prepared*

Complete Pancake/Waffle Mix:

	C	F	Cb
Shake 'n Pour, Buttermilk (3)	220	3	43
Simply Buttermilk (3)	210	4	39

Hungry Jack: *Prepared*

Mixes: *Per 4"*

	C	F	Cb
Complete, Buttermilk (3)	150	1.5	32
Traditional, Original:			
With 2% Milk, Oil, Egg (3)	250	8	37
W/ Skim Milk, Oil, Egg White (3)	180	1	37
Extra Light & Fluffy (3)	150	2	31

Easy Packs:

	C	F	Cb
Blueberry Wheat	160	2.5	32
Buttermilk	150	1.5	31

Northern Pines,

	C	F	Cb
Premium Mix (3), 4", 3.5 oz, prep'd	200	3.5	38

Frozen Breakfasts   C   F   Cb

Aunt Jemima:

	C	F	Cb
French Toast: Cinnamon, 2 slices	210	4	35
Homestyle, 2 slices	210	4	34
Sticks, Cinnamon (4)	260	2.5	39
Pancakes: Blueberry (3)	260	6	45
Buttermilk (3)	250	6	41
Low-Fat (3)	210	2	42
Homestyle (3)	250	6	42
Mini Pancakes (10)	280	8	45

Eggo *(Kellogg's):*

	C	F	Cb
French Toaster Sticks, (2), average	230	6	38
Pancakes: Blueberry (3)	260	8	42
Buttermilk (3)	280	9	45

Krusteaz:

	C	F	Cb
French Toast, Cinnamon Swirl	230	5	36
Pancakes:			
Blueberry (3)	270	3	51
Buttermilk (3)	210	3	39

Pillsbury:

Pancakes:

	C	F	Cb
Buttermilk (3)	230	4	45
Mini Buttermilk (11)	240	4	45

Frozen Waffles

	C	F	Cb
Aunt Jemima: Buttermilk (2)	190	5	29
Homestyle; Blueberry, (2), average	170	5	28

Eggo *(Kellogg's):*

	C	F	Cb
Blueberry (2)	180	6	29
Chocolate Chip (2)	200	7	31
Homestyle (2)	190	7	27
Nutri-Grain:			
Blueberry (2)	180	5	31
Whole Wheat (2)	170	6	26

	C	F	Cb
Kashi, all varieties (2)	150	5	25

Nature's Path:

	C	F	Cb
Flax Plus: Fig & Flax (2)	200	9	27
Red Berry (2)	190	9	27
Homestyle (2)	210	7	34
Van's: 8 Whole Grains, Berry (2)	170	6	27
Belgian, Homestyle (2)	250	10	37
Wheat Gluten Free,			
Apple Cinnamon (2)	200	6	35
Mini, Chocolate Chip (8)	160	5	29

Spaghetti/Pasta **C F Cb**

- Pasta includes all shapes and sizes; (e.g. spaghetti, fettuccini, elbows, shells, twists, sheets, cannelloni, linguini, tubes, ziti).
- All regular pasta products have the same cals/fat/carbs on a weight basis.
- 1 oz Dry = approximately 2.5 -3 oz cooked.

Dry Spaghetti/Pasta

	C	F	Cb
1 oz quantity	105	0.5	21
1lb box/pkg, 16 oz	1685	7	339
Elbows, 1 cup, 4 oz	380	2	80
Shells, small, 1 cup, 3.3 oz	330	1.5	69
Spirals, 1 cup, 3 oz	305	1.5	64

Cooked Spaghetti/Pasta

Plain, All Types (no added fat):
	C	F	Cb
Firm/Al Dente (8-10 minutes), 1 oz	42	0.5	8.5
Medium (11-13 minutes), 1 oz	37	0.5	7.5
Tender (14-20 minutes), 1 oz	32	0.5	7

Longer cooking increases water absorbed
	C	F	Cb
Spaghetti: ½ cup, 2.5 oz	90	0.5	18
Medium serving, 1 cup, 5 oz	225	1.5	44
Large serving, 2 cups, 10 oz	450	3	88
Extra large, 3 cups, 15 oz	675	5	132
Elbows/Spirals, 1 cup, 5 oz	220	1.5	43
Small Shells, 1 cup, 4 oz	180	1	36
Protein-fortified: Dry, 1 c., 3.4 oz	350	2	61
Cooked, 1 cup, 5 oz	230	0.5	45
Spinach/Vegetable: Dry, 1 cup, 3 oz	310	1	61
Cooked, 1 cup, 5 oz	180	0.5	38
Whole-wheat: Dry, 1 cup, 3.8 oz	365	1.5	79
Cooked, 1 cup, 5 oz	175	1	37

Fresh Pasta (Refrigerated)

Average All Brands:
Plain/Spinach/Tomato:
	C	F	Cb
As purchased, 4.5 oz	370	3	70
Cooked, 1 cup, 5 oz	185	1.5	35
Home-made, w/o egg, cooked, 1 c. 5 oz	175	1	35

Buitoni:
Cut Pasta:
	C	F	Cb
Angel Hair, 3 oz	230	2	43
Fettuccine/Linguine, 3 oz	240	2	45

House Foods:
Tofu Shirataki Noodles:
	C	F	Cb
Traditional, 1.6 oz	0	0	1
Angel Hair/Fettuccini, Macaroni/Spaghetti, 4 oz	20	0.5	3

Nasoya,
Shirataki Spaghetti,
	C	F	Cb
Pasta Zero, ⅔ cup, 4 oz	20	0	4

Buitoni: *Per 1 Cup Unless Indicated* **C F Cb**
	C	F	Cb
Agnolotti: Butternut Squash, 3.7 oz	300	12	37
Wild Mushroom, 3.8 oz	280	10	34
Ravioli: Beef & Sausage, 3.8 oz	260	8	33
Chicken Marsala, 3.9 oz	280	8	36
Light 4-Cheese, 1¼ cup, 3.3 oz	260	6	39
Tortellini: Herb Chicken, 3.9 oz	330	8	52
Mixed Cheese, 3.7 oz	320	8	48
Tortellini: Italian Sausage, 4 oz	350	10	51
Spinach & Ricotta, 3.7 oz	270	7	39

Other Varieties ~ See Page 112
Pasta Sauces ~ See Page 144

Macaroni & Cheese

Packaged (Kraft) ~ See Page 116
Restaurant: *Average*
	C	F	Cb
Side Serve, 6 oz	265	13	26
Medium serve, 1 cup, 9 oz	350	17	34
Large serve, 2 cups, 18 oz	700	34	68

Noodles

Plain/Egg: Dry, 1 oz
	C	F	Cb
Dry, 1 oz	110	1.5	20
1 cup, 1.4 oz	145	1.5	27
Cooked: 1 oz	40	0.5	7
½ cup, 2.8 oz	110	1.5	20
1 cup, 5.5 oz	220	3.5	40
Stir-Fried: 1 cup, 5.5 oz	270	9	40
2 cup serving, 11 oz	540	18	80

Low Carb Noodles,
	C	F	Cb
Quest Pasta, 4 oz	10	0	3

Note: Carbs are from glucomannan fiber
Yolk Free (Cooked):
	C	F	Cb
Manischewitz, Yolk Free, 2 oz	200	1	41
Chinese: Cellophane/Rice, dry, 1 oz	100	0	25
Chow Mein/hard, dry, 1 oz	150	9	16
Japanese: Soba: Dry, 1 oz	95	0.5	21
Cooked, 1 cup, 4 oz	115	0.5	24
Somen: Dry, 1 oz	100	0.5	21
Cooked, 1 cup, 6 oz	230	0.5	49

Japanese Style Pan Fried,
	C	F	Cb
Yaki-Soba (*Maruchan's*), av., 5.6 oz	260	3	50

Ramen Noodles ~ See Page 117
	C	F	Cb
Rice Noodles: Dry, 3.5 oz	365	0.5	83
Cooked, 1 cup, 6.2 oz	190	0.5	44
Yakisoba, Stir Fry, 3.5 oz	430	6	52
House Foods, Tofu Shirataki, 4 oz	20	0.5	3
Chikara, Udon, average, 7.5 oz pkt	250	1	52

Simply Asia/Thai Kitchen ~ See Pages 119 & 121

Egg Roll/Won Ton Wrappers

	C	F	Cb
Egg/Spring Roll (1), 0.8 oz	65	0	15
Won Ton Wrapper (1), 0.3 oz	20	0	4

Quick Guide   C F Cb

Fruit Pies: *Average All Brands, 9"*
Apple; Blueberry; Cherry:

	C	F	Cb
Small Serving, ⅛ pie, 4.8 oz	350	16	49
Medium Serving, ⅙ pie, 6.5 oz	465	22	65
Large Serving ¼ pie, 9.5 oz	700	33	98
Whole Pie (9"), 38 oz	2800	131	392

Other Pies: *Per Serving, ⅙ of 8" Pie*

	C	F	Cb
Chocolate Cream Pie	345	22	38
Custard: Egg	220	12	22
Coconut	330	18	35
Lemon Meringue	305	10	53
Peach	260	12	39
Pecan	440	23	57
Pumpkin Pie	315	14	41

Fruit Pies ~ Brands

	C	F	Cb
Denny's Restaurant, Apple Pie, 7 oz	480	22	67
Hostess:			
Cherry Pie, 4.5 oz	480	20	69
Lemon Pie, 4.5 oz	490	22	69
Marie Callender's Restaurant, Banana Cream, w/out whip, 8.2 oz	470	24	59
Mrs Smith's:			
Classsic Pies: *Per ⅙ Pie, 4.5 oz*			
Apple	320	14	47
Coconut Custard	330	18	35
Cherry	320	14	44
Dutch Apple	340	14	52
Original Flaky Crust: *Per ⅛ Pie, 4.6 oz*			
Cherry	360	18	46
Peach	340	19	41
Sara Lee:			
Creme Pies:			
Chocolate, ⅓ pie, 3.9 oz	450	27	50
Coconut, ⅙ pie, 4.5 oz	370	20	44
Key Lime, ⅓ pie	410	17	60
Lemon Meringue, ⅓ pie, 4.6 oz	390	13	64
Oven Fresh Pies: *Per 9" Pie, 4.6 oz Slice*			
Apple	340	16	43
Cherry	340	17	44
Peach	320	15	42
Seasonal: Pumpkin, 4.6 oz	270	10	41
Sthrn Sweet Potato, 4.6 oz	280	9	46
Tastykake: Apple	270	11	41
Coconut Cream	360	20	41
Lemon	300	14	44

Croissants   C F Cb

Average all Brands

	C	F	Cb
Plain/Butter/Cheese: Mini, 1 oz	115	6	13
Small, 1.5 oz	170	9	19
Medium, 2 oz	230	12	26
Large, 2.5 oz	290	15	32
Sweet Croissants:			
Almond Filled, 3 oz	330	18	39
Chocolate Filled, 3 oz	360	19	43
Dunkin' Donuts, Plain Croissant	330	13	37
Sara Lee:			
French Style: Original, 1.8 oz	185	9	21
Mini, 1 oz	230	11	26

Croissant Sandwiches ~ *See Page 165*

Pastry & Pie Crust

	C	F	Cb
Pie Crust, Baked, 9" diameter shell:			
1 Pie Shell, 6.5 oz	970	64	87
2-crust Pie, 9", 11.3 oz	1660	109	150
Filo Pastry: 4 sheets, 2.5 oz	210	2.5	40
Athens, Filo Dough, 5 sheets, 2 oz	170	1	36
Puff:			
Pepperidge Farm, ½ sheet	480	30	48
Bake & Fill Shell (1)	180	11	18
Arrowhead Mills, Graham Cracker Pie Crust, ⅛ of 9"	110	5	14
Keebler:			
Ready Crust: *Per ⅛ of 9" Crust*			
Chocolate	100	4.5	14
Graham: Regular	110	5	14
Reduced Fat	100	3.5	15
Shortbread Crust	100	5	14
Marie Callenders, Deep Dish Pie Crust, ⅛ pie, 1 oz	140	10	11
Mrs Smith's, Deep Dish, ⅛ pie, 1 oz	130	7	14
Nabisco:			
Honey Maid, Graham Crackers, ⅛ pie, 0.75 oz	110	5	14
Nilla, Pie Crust, ⅙ of 9", 1 oz	140	8	18
Pillsbury, Rolled, ⅛, 0.9 oz	100	6	12
Trader Joe's, Pie Crust, ⅛ pie, 1.2 oz	190	13	17

Pie Fillings ~ Canned

	C	F	Cb
Apple/Blueb./Cherry/Strawb., average:			
Sweetened: ⅓ cup, 3.2oz	90	0	22
1 cup, 9.5 oz	270	0	66
1 can, 21 oz	600	0	150
Light/Lite, ⅓ cup, 3.2 oz	60	0	15
Unsweetened, ⅓ cup, 3.2 oz	35	0	8
Lemon Crm/Creme, ⅓ cup, 3.2 oz	130	1.5	28

Pizzas ~ Ready To Eat **C** **F** **Cb**

Figures Based On Pizza Hut

Chicken Supreme:
Medium Size (12"):

Hand Tossed/Classic Crust:

	C	F	Cb
⅛ Pizza (1 slice)	210	8	26
½ Pizza (4 slices)	840	32	104
Whole Pizza (8 slices)	1680	64	208

Pan/Deep Dish:

	C	F	Cb
⅛ Pizza (1 slice)	230	9	27
½ Pizza (4 slices)	920	36	108
Whole Pizza (8 slices)	1840	72	216

Thin 'N Crispy Crust:

	C	F	Cb
⅛ Pizza (1 slice)	190	6	23
½ Pizza (4 slices)	760	24	92
Whole Pizza (8 slices)	1520	48	184

Meat Lovers:
Medium Size (12"):

Hand Tossed/Classic:

	C	F	Cb
⅛ Pizza (1 slice)	300	16	26
½ Pizza (4 slices)	1200	64	104
Whole Pizza (8 slices)	2400	128	208

Pan/Deep Dish:

	C	F	Cb
⅛ Pizza (1 slice)	320	18	26
½ Pizza (4 slices)	1280	72	104
Whole Pizza (8 slices)	2560	144	208

Thin Crust:

	C	F	Cb
⅛ Pizza (1 slice)	280	16	22
½ Pizza (4 slices)	1120	64	88
Whole Pizza (8 slices)	2240	128	176

Pepperoni:
Medium Size (12"):

Hand Tossed/Classic Crust:

	C	F	Cb
⅛ Pizza (1 slice)	230	10	25
½ Pizza (4 slices)	920	40	100
Whole Pizza (8 slices)	1840	80	200

Pan/Deep Dish:

	C	F	Cb
⅛ Pizza (1 slice)	260	13	26
½ Pizza (4 slices)	1040	52	104
Whole Pizza (8 slices)	2080	104	208

Thin Crust:

	C	F	Cb
⅛ Pizza (1 slice)	210	10	21
½ Pizza (4 slices)	840	40	84
Whole Pizza (8 slices)	1680	80	168

Supreme: **C** **F** **Cb**
Medium Size (12"):

Hand Tossed/Classic Crust:

	C	F	Cb
⅛ Pizza (1 slice)	260	12	27
½ Pizza (4 slices)	1040	48	108
Whole Pizza (8 slices)	2080	96	216

Pan/Deep Dish:

	C	F	Cb
⅛ Pizza (1 slice)	280	14	27
½ Pizza (4 slices)	1120	56	108
Whole Pizza (8 slices)	2240	112	216

Thin Crust:

	C	F	Cb
⅛ Pizza (1 slice)	230	12	23
½ Pizza (4 slices)	920	48	92
Whole Pizza (8 slices)	1840	96	184

Large (14"):

Hand Tossed:

	C	F	Cb
Cheese: ⅛ Pizza (1 slice)	300	12	35
½ Pizza (4 slices)	1200	48	140
Chicken Supreme: ⅛ Pizza (1 sl.)	290	9	36
½ Pizza (4 slices)	1160	36	144
Meat Lover's: ⅛ Pizza (1 slice)	410	23	35
½ Pizza (4 slices)	1640	92	140
Pepperoni: ⅛ Pizza (1 slice)	310	13	35
½ Pizza (4 slices)	1240	52	140
Supreme: ⅛ Pizza (1 slice)	350	17	36
½ Pizza (4 slices)	1400	68	144
Veggie Lover's: ⅛ Pizza (1 slice)	270	9	36
½ Pizza (4 slices)	1080	36	144

Individual Personal Pizzas (6"):

Pan/Deep Dish:

	C	F	Cb
Cheese	590	25	68
Chkn Supreme	590	21	69
Pepperoni	620	28	68
Supreme	730	38	69
Veggie Lovers	540	20	69

Extra Large, Single Slices:
Figures Based On Sbarro's

Pan: Cheese	590	8	69
Meat Delight	700	10	69
Pepperoni	650	10	69
Supreme	650	9	70

Frozen Pizzas	C	F	Cb
Amy's: *Per ⅓ Pizza*			
Cheese Pizza	290	12	33
Mushroom & Olive	260	10	33
Pesto	310	12	39
Roasted Vegetable	280	9	42
Vegan, Roasted Vegetables, no Cheese	260	4.5	50
California Pizza Kitchen:			
Crispy Thin Crust: *Per ⅓ Pizza*			
Margherita	320	16	31
Sicilian Recipe	360	18	30
Signature Pepperoni	350	19	29
White	320	17	30
Small Crispy Thin Crust: *Per Whole Pizza:*			
BBQ Recipe Chicken; Margh., av	400	16	43
Four Cheese	400	18	40
Hawaiian	350	12	43
Sicilian	430	21	40
Original Restaurant Style Crust:			
BBQ Recipe Chicken, ⅓ Pizza	390	13	46
Hawaiian Recipe, ¼ Pizza	290	11	33
Signature Pepperoni, ¼ Pizza	330	15	32
Thai Style Chicken, ⅓ Pizza	360	13	41
Celeste:			
Pizza For One: Original, 1 pizza	320	14	42
Deluxe	340	15	41
Four Cheese	330	15	38
Pepperoni	340	13	43
Sausage & Pepperoni	380	19	41
Zesty Four Cheese	350	16	43
DiGiorno: *Per Slice, Unless Indicated*			
Cheese Stuffed Crust:			
Bacon Cheeseburger, ⅙ pizza, 4.5 oz	310	13	34
Five Cheese, ⅕ Pizza, 5.3 oz	380	16	40
Pepperoni, ⅕ pizza, 5.3 oz	380	16	40
Three Meat, ⅙ pizza 4.8 oz	340	16	34
Supreme, ⅙ pizza, 5 oz	350	16	34
Classic Thin Crust, Supreme, ⅕ pizza, 5 oz	310	14	32
Garlic Bread: *Per ⅙ Pizza*			
Pepperoni, 5 oz	380	17	40
Supreme, 4.3 oz	300	12	36

DiGiorno (Cont):	C	F	Cb
Original Rising Crust: *Per ⅙ Pizza*			
Four Cheese, 4.7 oz	310	10	38
Italian Sausage, 5 oz	340	14	39
Spicy Chicken Supreme, 5.3 oz	310	9	39
Small Pizzas, Cheese Stuffed Crust: *Per ½ Pizza*			
Four Cheese, 4.2 oz	320	15	34
Pepperoni, 4.2 oz	330	16	34
Three Meat, 4.6 oz	360	18	34
Ultimate Toppings: *Per ⅕ Pizza*			
Pepperoni, 4.8 oz	360	17	35
Supreme, 5.3 oz	360	17	35
Freschetta:			
Brick Oven: *Per ⅕ Pizza Unless Indicated*			
5 Italian Cheese, ¼ Pizza, 5.2 oz	380	19	40
Chicken Club, ¼ Pizza, 5.5 oz	360	15	41
Pepp. & Italian Style Cheese, 4.6 oz	350	18	33
Rstd Portab. M'shrms & Spin., 4.6 oz	270	11	35
Three Meat Medley, 4.6 oz	350	19	32
Zesty Italian Supreme, 4.6 oz	330	16	33
Naturally Rising: *Per ⅙ of Large Pizza Unless Indicated*			
4 Cheese Medley, ⅛ Pizza, 5 oz	380	14	46
Canada Style Bacon P'apple, 4.5 oz	280	8	39
Classic Supreme, 5 oz	350	15	39
Ssg & Pepperoni, 4.9 oz	370	16	40
Signat. Pepperoni, 4.5 oz	340	14	39
Jeno's: *Per Pizza*			
Crispy 'N Tasty: Cheese, 6.8 oz	460	22	50
Pepperoni, 6.8 oz	490	26	48
Kashi:			
Thin Crust: *Per ⅓ Pizza*			
Four Cheese, 4 oz	260	8	36
Mediterranean, 4.2 oz	290	9	37
Mushroom Trio & Spinach, 4 oz	250	9	28
Kroger:			
3 Minute Microwave: *Per 8 oz Pizza*			
3-Meat	500	17	64
Cheese	490	16	66
Combination	520	20	65
Pepperoni	530	20	65
Supreme	490	18	63
French Bread, Pepperoni, 5 oz	380	17	42

Frozen Pizzas (Cont)

	C	F	Cb
Lean Cuisine (Cont):			
Culinary Collection: *Per 6 oz Pizza*			
Deep Dish:			
Spinach & Mushroom	340	7	52
Three Meat	380	9	55
Traditional:			
Four Cheese	350	6	57
Mushroom	300	5	50
Pepperoni	380	9	56
Simple Favorites: *Per Pizza*			
French Bread Pizzas: Pepperoni	310	8	48
Cheese; Deluxe, av.	340	7	53
Red Baron:			
Classic Crust: *Per ¼ Pizza*			
4 Cheese, 5.2 oz	380	16	41
Pepperoni, 5 oz	370	16	41
Sausage & Pepp., 5.3 oz	390	18	42
Fire Baked: *Per ¼ Pizza*			
4 Cheese, 4.9 oz	360	15	40
Pepperoni, 5.3 oz	370	17	40
Spicy Pepperoni, 4.9 oz	350	15	39
Rising Crust: *Per ¼ Pizza*			
Cheese; Pepperoni, average, 4.8 oz	335	12	44
Sausage & Pepperoni, 5 oz	360	14	45
Thin & Crispy Crust: *Per ⅓ Pizza*			
5 Cheese, 5 oz	360	16	40
Pepperoni, 5.3 oz	400	19	40
Singles: *Per Pizza*			
Deep Dish: Hawaiian, 5.3 oz	350	13	47
Meat-Trio, 5.6 oz	400	18	46
Sausage, 5.8 oz	430	20	46
French Bread:			
5 Cheese & Garlic (1)	430	23	41
Pepperoni (1)	380	15	43
Personal Pan: Meat-Trio, 5 oz	370	17	42
Pepperoni, 4.8 oz	340	14	41
Supreme, 5.3 oz	360	16	42
Safeway Select:			
Pizzeria Crust:			
Cheese Trio, ¼ pizza	340	15	34
Fajita Chicken Ole, ⅕ pizza	250	10	29
Pepperoni & Sausage, ⅓ pizza	320	17	30
Self Rising: *Per ⅙ Pizza*			
Four Cheese	300	9	41
Pepperoni	350	14	41
Sausage & Pepperoni	340	13	41

	C	F	Cb
Smart Ones *(Weight Watchers):*			
Classic Favorites, Thin Crust, Cheese Pizza, 6 oz	290	6	42
Smart Anytime, Brick Oven Style, Pepperoni Pizza, 6 oz	430	13	57
Stouffer's:			
French Bread Pizzas:			
Two Per Box:			
Deluxe, 1 piece, 6 .2 oz	430	21	44
Sausage & Pepperoni, 1 piece, 6.3 oz	460	24	43
Nine Per Box:			
Cheese, 1 piece, 5.9 oz	380	16	43
Pepperoni, 1 piece, 5.7 oz	430	21	44
Tombstone:			
Original: *Per ¼ Pizza*			
Canadian Style Bacon	320	12	37
Extra Cheese	350	15	36
Pepperoni	390	20	36
Pepperoni & Sausage	360	17	37
Thin Crust: *Per ¼ Pizza*			
Three Cheese	310	15	28
Pepperoni; Sausage, average	315	16	28
Brick Oven Style: Cheese, ⅓ pizza	350	15	37
Pepperoni; Supreme, av., ¼ pizza	315	16	29
Tony's:			
Pizzeria Style Crust: *Per ⅓ Pizza*			
Cheese, 4.8 oz	330	12	43
Pepperoni, 4.7 oz	330	13	42
Supreme, 5.3 oz	350	14	43
Singles: *Per Pizza*			
French Bread: Pepperoni, 5 oz	360	16	43
Supreme, 5.2 oz	350	15	43
Totino's:			
Crisp Crust Party Pizza: *Per ½ Pizza*			
Cheese	320	15	35
Combination	360	19	36
Hamburger	350	18	36
Pepperoni	360	19	35
Pizza Rolls:			
Cheese (6), 3 oz	210	8	28
Pepperoni (6), 3 oz	220	9	26
Trader Joe's:			
3 Cheese, ⅓ pizza	310	9	42
Parlanno, ¼ pizza	340	16	34
Pizza 4 Formaggi, ⅓ pizza	310	9	42
Spinach, ⅓ pizza	300	12	38

Quick Guide

	C	**F**	**Cb**
Chicken			
From 3lb ready-to-cook chicken			
Breast/Wing Quarter:			
Roasted: With skin	300	15	0
Without skin	185	5	0
Fried, batter dipped	530	30	17
Leg Quarter:			
Thigh & Drumstick:			
Roasted: With skin	270	16	0
Without skin	185	8	0
Fried, batter dipped	435	25	15
KFC ~ See Fast-Foods Section			

Per 4 oz Edible Portion

	C	**F**	**Cb**
Average of Light Meat: *Per 4 oz Without Bone*			
Roasted: With skin	250	12	0
Without skin	175	4.5	0
Stewed: With skin	230	12	0
Without skin	180	4.5	0
Fried: Batter-dipped, with skin, 4 oz	315	17	11
Flour-coated, with skin, 4 oz	280	14	2
Average of Dark Meat: *Per 4 oz Without Bone*			
Roasted: With skin	290	18	0
Without skin	235	11	0
Stewed: With skin	265	17	0
Without skin	220	10	0
Fried: Batter-dipped, with skin, 4 oz	340	21	11
Flour-coated, with skin, 4 oz	325	19	5

Chicken Parts

	C	**F**	**Cb**
Broilers or Fryers: *Edible Weights (no bone)*			
Breast: *Per ½ Breast*			
Raw: With skin, 5 oz	250	14	0
Without skin, 4.25 oz	140	3	0
Roasted: With skin, 3.5 oz	195	8	0
Without skin, 3 oz	140	3	0
Stewed: With skin, 4 oz	200	8	0
Without skin, 3.3 oz	145	3	0
Fried: Batter-dipped, w/ skin, 5 oz	365	19	13
Flour-coated, with skin, 3.5 oz	220	9	2
Drumstick: *Per Drumstick*			
Roasted: With skin, 2 oz	115	6	0
Without skin, 1.5 oz	75	2.5	0
Stewed: With skin, 2 oz	115	6	0
Without skin, 1.5 oz	80	3	0
Fried: Batter-dipped, w/ skin, 2.5 oz	195	11	6
Flour-coated, with skin, 1.8 oz	120	7	1

Chicken Parts (Cont)

	C	**F**	**Cb**
Broilers or Fryers (Cont): *Edible Weights (no bone)*			
Thigh Portion:			
Raw: With skin, 3.3 oz			
(4¼ oz with bone)	200	14	0
Without skin, 2.4 oz	80	3	0
Roasted: With skin, 2.3 oz	155	10	0
Without skin, 2 oz	110	6	0
Stewed: With skin, 2.5 oz	160	10	0
Without skin, 2 oz	105	5	0
Fried: Batter-dipped, with skin 3 oz	240	14	8
Flour-coated, with skin, 2.3 oz	165	9	2
Wing: *Per Wing, Bone In*			
Raw Weight, 3.2 oz			
Raw: With skin	110	8	0
Without skin	35	1	0
Roasted: With skin	100	7	0
Without skin	45	2	0
Fried: Batter-dipped, with skin	160	11	5
Flour-coated, with skin	105	7	1
Stewed, with skin, 4 oz	100	7	0
Buffalo Wings ~ *See Fast-Foods Section*			
Neck: Simmered, with skin	95	7	0
Without skin	30	2	0
Skin Only: *Skin from ½ Chicken*			
Raw skin, 3 oz	275	26	0
Roasted skin, 2 oz	255	23	0
Stewed skin, 2.5 oz	260	24	0
Fried, flour-coated, 2 oz	280	24	5
Fried, batter-dipped, 6.8 oz	750	55	44
Roasters: *Average of Light & Dark Meat*			
Roasted: With skin, 4 oz	250	15	0
Without skin, 4 oz	190	8	0
Light Meat, without skin, roasted	175	5	0
Dark Meat, without skin, roasted	200	10	0
Stewing Chicken: *Per 4 oz, average of Light & Dark Meat*			
Stewed: With skin	325	22	0
Without skin	270	14	0
Light Meat, without skin	240	9	0
Dark Meat, without skin	290	17	0
Capon Chicken:			
Roasted: With skin, 4 oz	260	13	0
½ Chicken, with skin, 22.5 oz	1460	74	0
Chicken Offal & Stuffing:			
Giblets: Simmered, 1 cup	230	7	0.5
Fried, flour-coated, 1 cup	400	20	6
Gizzard, simmered, 1 cup	210	4	0
Heart, simmered, 1 cup	270	12	0.2
Liver: Raw, 4 oz	130	5.5	0
Simmered, 1 cup	215	8.5	1
Liver Pate, Fresh, 1 Tbsp, 0.5 oz	30	2	1
Stuffing, average, ½ cup	180	9	22

Chicken Products	C	F	Cb

Bumble Bee:
Chicken In Water: *Per 2 oz Drained*

Premium White	70	1.5	0
Premium Breast	70	1	0

Foster Farms:

Chicken Breast Strips, grilled, 3 oz	100	2	0
Wings: Chipotle, 3 wings, 3 oz	190	13	4
Honey BBQ Glazed, 3 wings, 3 oz	190	11	7
Hot 'n' Spicy, 3 wings, 3 oz	190	14	1

Tyson:
Anytizers, Frozen:
Wings:

Hot Wings, Buffalo Style (3)	190	13	1
Honey BBQ Seasoned (3)	190	12	8

Wyngz, Boneless:

Buffalo Style, 3 pieces, 3 oz	150	7	8
Sweet Garlic Glazed, 3 pcs, 2.8 oz	130	5	10

Duck, Goose, Quail			

Duck: Roasted,

With skin, 3 oz	290	24	0
Without skin, 3 oz	170	10	0
½ duck, with skin, 13.5 oz	1290	108	0
Goose: Roasted with skin, 3 oz	260	19	0
Without skin, 3 oz	200	11	0
Pheasant, cooked, 3 oz	210	10	0
Quail, cooked, 1 whole, 6 oz	385	24	0

Turkey			

Fryer-Roasters: *Per 3 oz Serving*
Roasted:

Light Meat: With skin	140	4	0
Without skin	120	1	0
Dark Meat: With skin	155	6	0
Without skin	140	4	0

½ of Whole Turkey: (Approx. 3.3 lbs raw weight without neck and giblets; 1.8 lbs cooked weight)

Roasted: With skin	1650	74	0
Without skin	1125	31	0

Ground Turkey, raw: (4 oz raw wt. = 3 oz ckd wt.)

85% lean, regular, 4 oz	170	10	0
93% lean: Average, 4 oz	160	8	0
Jennie-O, 4 oz	170	8	0
Trader Joe's, 4 oz	150	8	0
94% lean,			
Foster Farms, 4 oz	150	7	0
Breast, no skin, 4 oz	115	1	0
Patties: Small, 3 oz	130	7	0
Medium, 4 oz	170	10	0

Turkey Parts	C	F	Cb

Roasted, Edible Weights, without bone:
Breast, (½), (from 17.3 oz raw weight with bone):

With skin, 12 oz (no bone)	525	11	0
Without skin, 10.8 oz	415	2	0
Back (½): With skin, 4.5 oz	265	13	0
Without skin, 3.5 oz	165	6	0

Leg (Thigh & Drumstick):
(from 1 lb raw weight with bone)

With skin, 8.5 oz (without bone)	410	13	0
Without skin, 7.8 oz	355	8.5	0

Wing: (From 7.3 oz raw weight)

With skin, 3 oz (without bone)	185	9	0
Without skin, 2 oz (with bone)	100	2	0
Neck: Simmered, 1 neck, 9 oz (with bone)	275	11	0
Giblets, simmered, 1 cup, 5 oz	240	7	3

Young Hens (Roasted)			

Light Meat:

With skin, 3 oz	175	8	0
Without skin, 3 oz	135	3	0
Dark Meat: With skin, 3 oz	200	11	0
Without skin, 3 oz	165	7	0

Young Toms ~ *Similar to Young Hens*

Turkey Products			

Foster Farms: *Cooked & Frozen*
Meatballs, cooked:

Homestyle (3)	160	9	3
Italian Style (3)	160	8	5
Hormel, Canned Turkey Breast, in water, 2 oz	50	1	0

Jennie-O:

Bacon, cured, 1 sl., 0.5 oz	30	2.5	1
Bratwurst, lean, 1 link, 3.85 oz	170	10	2
Burgers, uncooked,			
All Natural, White Meat, 5.3 oz	200	10	0
Meatballs, Fully Cooked: Italian, 3 oz	180	13	2
Home Style, 3 oz	180	13	3
Spam, Oven Roasted Turkey, 2 oz	80	4	2

Trader Joe's,

Italian Turkey Meatloaf, 3 oz	140	8	5

Valley Fresh,
Canned Prem. White Turkey Breast,

in water, 97% Fat-Free, 2 oz	45	1	0

White Rice

	C	F	Cb
Raw:			
Glutinous, 1 cup, 6.5 oz	685	1	151
Long Grain, 1 cup, 6.5 oz	675	1	148
Short Grain, 1 cup, 7 oz	715	1	158
Wild Rice, 1 cup, 5.5 oz	570	2	120
Cooked Rice: *Boiled/Steamed*			
Short/Medium Grain:			
½ cup, 3.3 oz	140	0	30
1 cup (½ Pint), 7.2 oz	265	0.5	59
2 cups (1 Pint), 13 oz	480	1	106
Long Grain: ½ cup, 2.8 oz	100	0	22
1 cup, 5.5 oz	205	0.5	44
Glutinous/Sticky, 1 cup, 6 oz	170	0.5	37
Parboiled, ½ cup, 3 oz	105	0.5	22
Precooked/Instant:			
Dry, ½ cup, 3.5 oz	380	1	82
Cooked, ½ cup, 3 oz	95	0.5	21
Wild Rice,			
Cooked, 1 cup, 5.8 oz	165	0.5	35

Brown Rice

Average of Short or Long Grain

	C	F	Cb
Raw/Dry: ½ cup, 3.3 oz	340	2.5	71
1 cup, 6.5 oz	685	5.5	143
Cooked: ½ cup, 3.5 oz	110	1	22
1 cup, 7 oz	220	2	46

Rice Dishes

	C	F	Cb
Chinese Fried Rice:			
½ cup, 2.5 oz	140	4.5	21
1 cup, (½ Pint), 5 oz	280	9	42
2 cups, (1 Pint), 10 oz	565	18	84
Mexican Style Rice:			
Taco John's, Cilantro Lime, 6 oz	220	3	39
Taco Time, Mexi, 3.5 oz	80	0.5	17
Rice-A-Roni ~ *See Page 119*			
Rice with Raisins/Pinenuts, 1 cup	400	11	60
Rice Pilaf: Restaurant, 1 cup	275	7.5	46
O'Charley's, A La Carte, 1 order	220	6	36
Rice Pudding,			
Kozy Shack, Original, 1 pudding cup	130	2.5	24
Risotto, 1 cup	420	12	70
Saffron Rice, 4 oz	175	7	25
Spanish Rice: 1 cup, 5 oz	390	9	72
El Pollo Loco, Small, 4.5 oz	170	2.5	33
Taco Cababa, 3.6 oz	120	0.5	25
Sticky Rice, 1 cup, 5 oz	155	0.5	34
Sushi Rice: 1 Tbsp	25	0	5
1 cup, 5.2 oz	390	0	77
Other Packaged Rice Products:			
Uncle Ben's / Zatarain's ~ *See Page 121*			

CalorieKing.com Recipes

See the CalorieKing website for a salubrious selection of healthy recipes – all analyzed for calories, fat, protein, carbohydrate, fiber and sodium.

Choose from:
- Starters/Appetizers
- Salads
- Entrees: Meat, Fish and Chicken
- Vegetarian
- Desserts
- Cakes, Cookies
- Drinks

www.CalorieKing.com/recipes

HEALTHY RECIPE TIPS

- **Use non-fat milk** in place of whole or 2% milk
- **Use low-fat yogurt** in place of sour cream
- **Skim fat** from surface of soups and casseroles after cooling
- **Add extra vegetables** to soups and hot entrées
- **Cakes/cookies/muffins:** Replace most or all the fat/oil with applesauce and/or prune puree (Example, *Sunsweet Lighter Bake*)
- **Drinks:** Replace sugar with no-calorie sweeteners such as *Equal, Stevia, Splenda* and *Sweet 'N Low*

Deli Salads

C F Cb

Average All Outlets

	C	F	Cb
Antipasto Salad, ½ cup	135	8	13
3-Bean Salad, ½ cup	90	4.5	12
Bulgur Salad, ½ cup	70	2	12
Caesar Salad, Classic, 1 cup	200	14	15
Side Salad, without Dressing	25	0	6
Carrot Raisin: With Dressing, ½ cup	135	12	6
Without Dressing, ½ cup	20	0	5
Chef's Salad: Regular, w/o Dressing	620	37	8
With 2 oz Thousand Island Drssng	860	61	8
Chicken Salad, ½ cup/scoop, 4 oz	280	21	2
Coleslaw: Traditional, ½ cup	150	8	18
W/ Low Cal Dressing, ½ c.	50	2	8
Corn, Mexican, ½ cup	240	12	33
Cucumber: Non-Oil Dressing, ½ cup	60	0	14
With Oil Dressing, ½ cup	140	12	8
Eggplant Salad, ½ cup	75	5	7
Fettucini, with veges, ½ cup	135	6	16
Garden Salad, without Dressing, 1 cup	10	0	2
Greek Salad, 1 cup	105	8	7
Greek Vegetables, 1 cup	110	8	6
Lobster Salad, ½ cup, 4 oz	250	21	11
Macaroni Salad, ½ cup, 5 oz	360	26	26
Nicoise, 1 cup	450	32	18
Pasta Salad, ½ cup	200	11	19
Potato Salad: Dijon, 3 oz	120	7	13
With Mayonnaise, ½ cup, 4 oz	215	15	17
Lowfat, ½ cup	110	1.5	21
Rice Salad, ½ cup	150	10	13
Saffron Rice, 4 oz	175	7	25
Spinach Salad, 1 cup	180	13	13
Tabouli, ½ cup	125	7	13
Three Bean Salad, ½ cup	90	4.5	12
Tomato & Mozzarella, ½ cup	180	14	10
Tortellini, with Basil Pesto, ½ cup	150	9	15
Waldorf, with Mayo, ½ cup	110	7	12

Signature Salads: Per 6 oz Serving
(Supplied to Deli's and Institutions)

	C	F	Cb
Antipasto Salad	510	50	4
Artichoke Salad, marinated	400	41	8
California Medley	120	7	15
Cheese Agnolotti	250	8	23
Chicken Salad	420	33	11
Crabmeat Flavored	450	38	20
Egg Salad	300	23	14
Fresh Button Mushroom	190	16	6

Signature Salads (Cont): Per 6 oz

	C	F	Cb
Fresh Button Mushroom	190	16	6
Ham Salad	400	32	14
Prima Pasta Salad	360	30	18
Seafood Pasta Del Mar	170	10	21
Seafood, Crab & Shrimp	420	34	20
Shrimp Salad	360	32	8
Tuna Salad	450	36	14

~ Also See Fast-Foods & Restaurants Section

Fresh Salad Packs

Pre-Packaged (Supermarkets):
Dole:
Kits: Per 3.5 oz, With Dressing

	C	F	Cb
Caesar	150	12	8
Chopped: Chipotle & Cheddar	120	8	10
Sesame Asian	160	16	13
Southwest	140	10	10

Salad Blends: Without Dressing

	C	F	Cb
American; Mediterranean, 3 oz	15	0	3
Arugula; Baby Spinach, average, 3 oz	20	0.5	3

Fresh Express:
Complete Salad Kits: Per 3½ oz, Prepared

	C	F	Cb
Asian	120	5	17
Caesar: Regular	150	12	7
Lite	90	6	7
Supreme	160	14	6
Pear Gorganzola	130	6	17

Gourmet Cafe: Per Package

	C	F	Cb
Chopped Santa Fe	290	19	18
Tuscan	330	28	9

Ready Pac:
Complete Salad Kits: Per 3.5 oz

	C	F	Cb
Baby Spinach, 2 cups	140	3	24
Caesar: Classic, 2 cups	170	13	10
Lite, 2 cups	110	6	9
Santa Fe, 1¾ cups	150	12	7

Salad Toppings

	C	F	Cb
Bac'n Pieces, McCormick, 1Tbsp, 0.3 oz	30	1	2
Bacon Bits, Hormel, 1Tbsp	25	1	0
Bac-Os, Bits, Betty Crocker, 1 Tbsp	30	1	2
Chow Mein Noodles, dry, ½ cup	120	7	13
Croutons, 2 Tbsp, 0.3 oz	40	1	7
Olives, 5 medium	25	2	0
Salad Toppins, McCormick, 4 tsp	35	1.5	3
Sunflower Seeds, 1 Tbsp, 0.3 oz	45	4	1.5
Toasted Sliced Almonds, 2 T., 0.5 oz	85	7	3

Quick Guide Ⓒ Ⓕ Ⓒb

Salad Dressings
Average All Brands: *Per 2 Tbsp, Approx 1 fl.oz*

	C	F	Cb
Balsamic Vinaigrette:			
Regular	90	9	3
Light, 2 Tbsp	45	4	2
Fat Free, 2 Tbsp	25	0	6
Blue Cheese: Regular, 2 Tbsp	145	15	1.5
Regular, ¼ cup, 2 oz	280	30	3
Light, 2 Tbsp	30	1	4
Caesar: Regular, 2 Tbsp	165	17	1
Regular, ¼ cup, 2 oz	310	34	2
Light, 2 Tbsp	35	1.5	5.5
Coleslaw: Regular, 2 Tbsp	125	11	8
Regular, ¼ cup, 2 oz	245	21	15
Light, 2 Tbsp	110	7	14
French: Regular	145	14	5
Regular, ¼ cup, 2 oz	260	25	9
Light, 2 Tbsp	65	4	9
Fat/Oil-Free, 2 Tbsp	40	0	10
Italian: Regular, 2 Tbsp	85	8.5	3
Regular, ¼ cup, 2 oz	165	16	6
Light, 2 Tbsp	55	5.5	2
Fat/Oil-Free, 2 Tbas	15	0	2.5
Ranch: Regular, 2 Tbsp	145	16	2
Regular, ¼ cup, 2 oz	290	30	4
Light, 2 Tbsp	60	4	6.5
Fat-Free, 2 Tbsp	35	0.5	8
Thousand Island: Reg., 2 T.	115	11	4.5
Regular, ¼ cup, 2 oz	210	20	9
Light, 2 Tbsp	60	3.5	7
Fat-Free, 2 Tbsp	40	0.5	10

Enjoy a healthy salad but don't drown it in high-fat salad dressings.

Use 'light' dressings to halve the fat and calories.

Brands ~ Salad Dressings

	C	F	Cb
Annie's Naturals: *Per 2 Tbsp*			
Organic: Buttermilk	70	6	1
French	110	11	3
Papaya Poppy Seed	90	8	5
Thousand Island	90	8	5
Vinaigrettes: Pomegranate	70	7	2
Red Wine & Olive Oil	140	15	0
Sesame Ginger	90	8	4
Shitake & Sesame	120	13	1
Bernstein's: *Per 2 Tbsp*			
Creamy Caesar	120	13	1
Herb Garden French	130	12	6
Italian	110	12	1
Restaurant Recipe Italian	120	12	1
Sweet Herb Italian	130	11	8
Fat-Free, Cheese & Garlic Italian	10	0	2
Light Fantastic: Cheese Fantastico	25	1.5	3
Roasted Garlic Balsamic	45	3.5	3
Best Foods: *Per 1 Tbsp Unless Indicated*			
Dijonnaise, 1 tsp	5	0	1
Mayonnaise: Real	90	10	0
Light	35	3.5	1
Low-Fat	15	1	2
Canola	40	4	1
Creamy Balsmic	50	6	1
Olive Oil	60	6	1
Mayonesa, Lemom-Lime	90	10	0
Cardini's: *Per 2 Tbsp*			
Aged Parmesan Ranch	150	16	1
Caesar: Original	160	17	1
Fat-Free Caesar	40	0	9
Light Caesar	80	7	5
Honey Mustard	120	11	6
Roasted Asian Sesame	120	10	6
Vinaigrette, Balsamic:			
Regular	100	8	5
Lite	50	3	5
Great Value *(Walmart): Per 2 Tbsp*			
Caesar	120	12	2
Ranch: Bacon	140	14	1
Buttermilk	110	11	2
Chipotle	120	13	2
Classic	130	14	1
Zesty Italian	70	6	3
Hidden Valley: *Per 2 Tbsp*			
Cole Slaw	150	15	5
Ranch Originals: Regular	140	14	2
Light Original	80	7	3
Buttermilk	130	14	2

Brands ~ Salad Dressings (Cont)

	C	F	Cb
Hidden Valley (Cont):			
Ranch, Bacon; Spicy, average	145	15	2
Farmhouse Originals,			
Dijon Mustard Vinaigrette	100	9	4
Homestyle Italian	100	10	3
Southwest Chipotle	100	10	2
Kraft: *Per 2 Tbsp*			
Regular Dressings:			
Caesar Vinaigrette, with Parmesan	70	6	3
Catalina	90	6	9
Classic Caesar	120	12	2
Creamy Ranch	110	11	2
Creamy Italian	100	10	2
Greek Vinaigrette	110	11	2
Roka Blue Cheese	120	13	1
Sweet Honey Catalina	100	8	8
Thousand Island	130	12	4
Tuscan House, Italian	130	13	3
Fat Free: Catalina; Classic Ranch	50	0	11
French Style	45	0	11
Italian	15	0	3
Thousand Island	45	0	10
Lite: Asian Toasted Sesame	50	2.5	7
Balsamic Vinaigrette	30	1	4
Creamy Caesar	35	2	4
Zesty Italian	25	1.5	3
Seven Seas:			
Green Goddess	130	13	2
Viva Robust Italian	90	9	2
Reduced Fat: Viva Italian	45	4	2
Red Wine Vinaigrette	45	4	3
Marie's: *Per 2 Tbsp*			
Blue Cheese, Premium Super	160	17	1
Caesar	170	19	1
Ranch, all varieties	170	19	1
Classics:			
Chunky Blue Cheese	160	17	0
Coleslaw	140	13	7
Creamy Italian Garlic	170	19	1
Creamy Ranch	170	19	1
Thousand Island	150	15	4
Specialty: Honey Dijon	130	12	5
Jalapeno Ranch	160	17	1

	C	F	Cb
Marzetti's:			
Organic: Blue Cheese	130	14	1
Caesar	140	15	1
Parmesan Ranch	130	14	2
Chunky Blue Cheese	150	15	1
Classic Ranch	160	17	1
Honey Dijon	130	12	6
Newman's Own: *Per 2 Tbsp*			
Regular: Balsamic Vinaigrette	90	9	3
Creamy Caesar	170	18	1
Family Recipe Italian	130	13	1
Olive Oil & Vinegar	150	16	1
Parmesan & Rstd Garlic	110	11	2
Ranch	150	16	2
Lite: Italian	60	6	1
Raspberry & Walnut	70	5	7
Organic:			
Light Balsamic Vinaigrette	45	4	3
Tuscan Italian	100	11	2
Wish-Bone: *Per 2 Tbsp*			
Creamy: Chunky Blue Cheese	150	14	1
Caesar	180	18	1
Deluxe French	120	11	5
Italian	110	10	4
Ranch	130	13	2
Russian	110	6	14
Sweet 'n Spicy French	140	12	7
Thousand Island	130	12	5
Light: Blue Cheese	70	6	2
Creamy Caesar	70	6	2
Honey Dijon	70	5	6
Italian	35	2.5	3
Parmesan Peppercorn Ranch	60	5	2
Ranch	70	5	4
Thousand Island	60	5	4
Vinaigrette: Balsamic & Basil	50	4	3
Asian with Sesame & Ginger	70	5	5
Raspberry Walnut	70	4	7
Fat-Free:			
Chunky Blue Cheese	30	0	7
Ranch	30	0	6
Oil & Vinegar:			
Balsamic Vinaigrette	60	5	3
House Italian	110	10	3
Red Wine Vinaigrette	70	5	6
Robusto Italian	80	7	4

C F Cb

Gravy

Homemade Gravy, average:

	C	F	Cb
Thin, little fat, 2 Tbsp, 1 oz	20	1	3
Thick: 2 Tbsp, 1.3 oz	50	2	9
¼ cup, 2.5 oz	100	4	18

McCormick:

	C	F	Cb
Brown, 1 Tbsp	25	0.5	3
Turkey, 1 Tbsp	20	0.5	4

Gravy-In-Jars

Boston Market,

	C	F	Cb
Classic Beef, ¼ cup, 2 oz	30	1	4

Campbell's, Slow Roast,

	C	F	Cb
Beef/Chicken/Turkey, ¼ cup, 2 oz	25	1	3

Heinz: *Per ¼ Cup, 2 oz*

	C	F	Cb
Homestyle: Classic Chicken	30	2	3
Savory Beef	30	1	4
Sausage	45	1.5	6
Other varieties, average	20	0.5	3
Fat-Free, all varieties	20	0	4
Safeway, all varieties, ¼ cup, 2 oz	20	0.5	4

Tomato Products

Whole/Chopped/Crushed/Diced:

	C	F	Cb
Regular: 1 cup, 8.5 oz	50	0	10
In Aspic, ½ cup	50	0	12
With Green Chili 1 c., 8.5 oz	60	0	16
Stewed, ½ cup, 1.7 oz	40	1.5	9
Wedges in Tomato Juice, 1 cup	70	0.5	18
Salsa, average, 2 Tbsp, 1 oz	25	0	6

Tomato Ketchup:

	C	F	Cb
Regular: 1 Tbsp, 0.5 oz	15	0	4
Single Serve, 1 packet	10	0	3
Heinz, One-Carb, 1 Tbsp, 0.5 oz	5	0	1

Tomato Paste:

	C	F	Cb
Regular: 2 Tbsp, 1 oz	25	0	6
¾ cup, 6 oz	140	1	32

Tomato Puree, ½ cup, 4.5 oz | 50 | 0 | 10 |

Tomato Sauce:

	C	F	Cb
Regular, ½ cup, 4.4 oz	50	0	11
Spanish Style, ½ cup, 4.3 oz	40	0	9
With Mushr., ½ cup, 4.3 oz	45	0	10
With Onions, ½ cup, 4.3 oz	50	0	12
Tomato Seasoning, 3 tsp	20	0	4

Sundried Tomatoes:

	C	F	Cb
Natural, 5-6 pieces, 0.4 oz	20	0	5
In Oil, drained, 6 pieces, 0.5 oz	40	2.5	4

Sauces ~ Brands

C F Cb

A-1:
Marinades: *Per Tablespoon, ½ oz*

	C	F	Cb
Chicago Steakhouse	20	1	3
Classic	15	0	4
New Orleans Cajun	25	0	5
New York Steakhouse	20	0	5
Steak Sauce: Original	15	0	3
Bold & Spicy	20	0	4
Cracked Peppercorn	15	0	0
Thick & Hearty	25	0	6

Barilla:
Pasta Sauces: *Per ½ Cup*

	C	F	Cb
Marinara; Tom. & Basil, av.	70	1	15
Mushroom	80	2.5	12
Rstd Garlic; Traditional, av.	70	1	14
Spicy Marinara	60	0.5	13
Sweet Peppers; Three Cheese, av.	70	1	13
Tuscan Herb	70	0.5	14

Bertolli:
Alfredo Sauces: *Per ¼ Cup*

	C	F	Cb
Four Cheese Rosa; Regular, average	110	10	3
Garlic	100	10	2
Mushroom	80	7	2

Traditional: *Per ½ Cup*

	C	F	Cb
Italian Sausage	90	3	14
Olive Oil & Garlic	80	3	14
Tomato & Basil	70	2	13

Best Foods/Hellmann's,

	C	F	Cb
Tartar Sauce, 2 Tbsp	80	7	4

Buitoni:
Pasta Sauces:

	C	F	Cb
Alfredo: Regular, ¼ cup	140	12	4
Light, ¼ cup	90	6	4
Marinara: Regular ½ cup	70	3	10
With Roasted Garlic, ½ cup	60	1	10
Pesto: With Basil, ¼ cup	270	26	4
Reduced Fat, ¼ cup	230	17	8

Bull's-Eye: *Per 2 Tbsp*

	C	F	Cb
Original BBQ Sauce	60	0	14
Regional: Carolina/Memphis/Kansas	50	0	11
Texas Style	45	0	11

Catelli: *Per ½ Cup*

	C	F	Cb
Pasta, Garden Select Six Vegetable:			
Country Mushroom	70	1.5	11
Diced Tomato & Basil	70	1	12
Meat Sauce	80	2.5	11
Pizza Sauce, Tomato & Basil	60	1.5	11

Sauces ~ Brands (Cont)

	C	F	Cb
Cento: Per ½ Cup			
Clam, Red, 4.4 oz	60	2	6
San Marzano Pasta:			
Arrabbiata, 4 oz	50	3	6
Marinara, 4.4 oz	60	3.5	6
Passata, crushed or pureed	25	0	8
Classico:			
Alfredo: Per ¼ Cup			
Creamy	80	7	3
Roasted Red Pepper	60	4	4
Pesto: Per ¼ Cup			
Basil Pesto	240	23	5
Sun-Dried Tomato Pesto	100	6	9
Red Sauces: Per ½ Cup			
Signature Recipes Sauce:			
Caramelized Onion & Rstd Garlic	70	1.5	12
Fire Roasted Tomato & Garlic	60	1.5	10
Florentine Spinach & Cheese	60	3	7
Mushrooms & Ripe Olives	60	1	10
Spicy Red Pepper	50	1.5	8
Sun-Dried Tomato	80	4	9
Traditional Favorites: Four Cheese	60	1.5	10
Italian Sausage, w/ Peppers & Onions	70	2.5	10
Roasted Garlic	50	1	8
Tomato & Basil	45	0.5	8
Colgin, Liquid Smoke, 1 tsp	0	0	0
Contadina:			
Pizza Sauce: Per 2.2 oz			
Flavored with Pepperoni	35	1	5
Original; Four Cheese	30	0.5	6
Tomato Sauce, average	20	0.5	4
Crosse & Blackwell:			
Meat: Ham Glaze, 1 Tbsp	25	0	7
Mint Meat Sauce, 1 tsp	5	0	2
Seafood:			
Cocktail, ¼ cup, 2.5 oz	80	0	20
Shrimp, ¼ cup, 2.5 oz	80	0	21
Dave's Gourmet: Per ½ Cup			
Pasta Sauce:			
Butternut Squash	100	4	17
Organic: Red Heirloom	45	1.5	7
Rstd Garlic & Sweet Basil	70	4.5	8
Del Monte:			
Pasta Sauces: Per ½ Cup			
With Four Cheeses	70	1	12
Mushrooms; Traditional	60	1	12
Average other varieties	70	1	13
Sloppy Joe Sauce, Orig., ¼ cup	30	0	13

	C	F	Cb
Emeril's:			
Pasta Sauces: Per ½ Cup			
Homestyle Marinara	90	3	14
Kicked Up Tomato	80	3.5	11
Roasted Garlic	80	3.5	12
Roasted Red Pepper	70	3.5	9
Vodka Sauce	110	7	12
Francesco Rinaldi: Per ½ Cup			
Hearty: Super Mushroom	110	4.5	13
Three Cheese	90	2	16
Traditional: Original	80	3	14
Meat Flavored	90	3.5	14
Mushroom	80	3	13
French's,			
Worcestershire Sce, 1 Tbsp	5	0	1
Heinz: Per 1 Tbsp			
57	20	0	5
Barbecue Sauces, all flavors	35	0	9
Chili Sauce	20	0	5
Cocktail Sauce, Original, ¼ cup, 2.2 oz	60	0	15
Horseradish Sauce	75	6	3
Tomato Ketchup: Regular	20	0	5
Reduced Sugar	5	0	1
Worcestershire Sauce, 1 Tbsp	5	0	1
House of Tsang: Per 1 Tbsp			
Bangkok Peanut Sauce	40	2	4
Ginger Flavored Soy	20	0	4
General Tsao	45	0.5	10
Hibachi Grill: Kobe Steak	50	4	3
Sweet Ginger Sesame	40	1	8
Tokyo Teriyaki	40	0	10
Hoisin, 1 tsp	15	0	4
Oyster Flavored	30	0	7
Saigon Sizzle Stir-Fry	45	2	7
Sweet & Sour Stir-Fry	35	0	9
Hunt's:			
BBQ Sauce, Original, 2 Tbsp	60	0	15
Hickory & Brown Sugar BBQ Sce, 2 Tbsp	70	0	18
Manwich, Sloppy Joe Sauce, Original, ¼ cup, 2.3 oz	35	0	7
Pasta Sauce: Per ½ Cup			
Four Cheese	60	1	10
Garlic & Herb	40	1	8
Meat Flavor	60	1	10
Mushroom	50	0.5	9
Traditional	60	1	11

Brands (Cont)   **C** **F** **Cb**

Kikkoman:

Asian Authentic:

	C	F	Cb
Black Bean Sauce, with Garlic, 2 Tbsp	50	1	6
Hoisin Sauce, 2 Tbsp	80	0	19

Marinades: *Honey Mustard, 1 Tbsp*   30   0   6

	C	F	Cb
Roasted Garlic	20	0	4
Soy Sauce	10	0	0
Teriyaki Marinade & Sauce	15	0	2

Knorr:

Classic Sauce: *Per Whole Package*

	C	F	Cb
Bernaise, dry mix only	100	0	20
Hollandaise, dry mix only	100	0	20

Kraft:

Barbecue Sauces, av., 2 Tbsp   65   0   15

Specialty Sauce: Cocktail, 2 Tbsp   60   0.5   11

	C	F	Cb
Coleslaw Dressing, 1.2 oz	110	8	9
Horseradish, 1 oz	100	9	4
Sandwich Spread, 1 Tbsp	35	2.5	3
Sweet 'n Sour, 2 Tbsp	60	0	13
Tartar, Original, 1 Tbsp	60	4.5	4

Las Palmas:

	C	F	Cb
Green Enchilada Sauce, all varieties, 2 oz	25	1.5	3
Red Chili Sauce, 2 oz	15	0.5	2

La Victoria,

Red/Green Enchilada Sauce, av., 2 oz   15   0.5   3

Lawry's:

30 Minute Marinade: *Per Tbsp*

	C	F	Cb
Caribbean Jerk	20	0	5
Herb & Garlic; Lemon Pepper	10	0	2
Mesquite, w/ Lime Juice	5	0	1
Steak & Chop, w/ Garl. Pepp.	5	0	1
Sesame Ginger, w/ Mandarin	30	0	7

Packet Seasonings: *Dry*

	C	F	Cb
Fajitas; Taco, average, 2 tsp	15	0	3
Other varieties, average, 2 tsp	20	0	4

Lea & Perrins:

	C	F	Cb
Marinade In-A-Bag, all varieties, 0.5 oz	15	0	4
Marinade for Chicken, 1 Tbsp	10	0	3
Steak Sauce, Bold, 1 Tbsp	20	0	5
Worcestershire Sauce, Original 1 tsp, 5 ml	5	0	1

McCormicks:

Seafood Sauces: *Per 2 Tbsp*

	C	F	Cb
Asian	50	1.5	7
Cajun Style	15	0	3
Mediterranean; Santa Fe Style	20	0	4
Lemon Butter Dill	100	9	4
Lemon Herb	140	15	1
Scampi	160	17	2

Mrs. Dash: **C** **F** **Cb**

Marinades: *Per 1 Tbsp*

	C	F	Cb
Garlic Herb	15	0	3
Lemon Pepper	10	0	2
Lime Garlic	15	0	3
Sweet Teriyaki	35	0	9

Newman's Own: *Per ½ Cup*

	C	F	Cb
Five Cheese	80	3	10
Fra Diavolo	70	3	10
Marinara; Sockarooni	70	2	12
Roasted Garlic & Peppers	70	2.5	11
Tomato & Basil Bombolina	90	4.5	13
Vodka	110	5	11

O Organics (Von's): *Per ½ Cup*

	C	F	Cb
Marinara; Roasted Garlic, av.	60	1.5	9
Mushroom; Tomato Basil	50	1.5	8

Old El Paso:

Enchilada Sauce:

	C	F	Cb
Green Chile, ¼ cup	25	1.5	4
Other varieties, ¼ cup	20	0	4
Salsa, Thick & Chunky, all var., 2 Tbsp	10	0	2
Taco Sauce, all varieties, 1 Tbsp	5	0	1

Pace: *Per 2 Tbsp*

	C	F	Cb
Picante Sauce	10	0	3

Salsa: Chunky   10   0   3

Fire, Mango & Habanero   10   0   2

Prego: *Per ½ Cup*

Classic Italian:

	C	F	Cb
Flavored with Meat	80	2.5	13
Fresh Mushroom; Traditional	70	1.5	13
Italian Sausage & Garlic	90	3	13
Marinara	80	3	10
Roasted Garlic & Herb	80	2	13
Three Cheese; Tom. Basil & Garlic, av.	80	2	13

Chunky Garden:

	C	F	Cb
Combo	70	2	12
Mushroom Supreme	90	3	13

Heart Smart: Ricotta Parmesan   90   2.5   13

Other varieties   70   1.5   13

Pizza Sauce, Pizzeria Style   70   2   12

Premier Japan,

Hoisin; Teriyaki, 1 Tbsp   15   0   3

Progresso: *Per ½ Cup*

Recipe Starters:

	C	F	Cb
Creamy Roasted Garlic	70	5	4
Fire Roasted Tomato	60	2	10
Average other varieties	90	7	5

Brands (Cont)

	C	F	Cb

Ragu:

Cheesy: Per ¼ Cup

	C	F	Cb
Classic Alfredo	90	8	2
Light Parmesan Alfredo	60	4	2
Roasted Garlic Parmesan	100	9	3

Chunky: Per ½ Cup

Mushroom & Green Pepper	80	2	13
Average other varieties	90	2.5	14

Light, Tomato Basil | 50 | 0 | 10 |

Old World Style: Per ½ Cup

Flavored with Meat	70	2.5	10
Marinara	80	2.5	11
Mushroom	70	2	11
Traditional	80	2	11

Pizza: Homemade Style, ¼ cup | 30 | 1 | 5 |

| Quick Sauce, Traditional, ¼ cup | 45 | 1.5 | 6 |

Robusto!: Per ½ Cup

7-Herb Tomato	90	3	13
Chopped Tomato, Olive Oil & Garlic	100	4	13
Roasted Garlic	80	2.5	13
Sauteed Onion & Garlic	90	3.5	13
Six Cheese	90	3	13

Safeway Select:

Salsa, all varieties, average, 2 Tbsp	15	0	3

Select Sauces: Per ½ Cup

Arrabbiata	110	8	10
Artichoke Pesto	60	2	9
Four Cheese	80	3.5	4
Marinara	60	2	10
Spicy Red Bell Pepper	50	1	9
Sundried Tomato & Olive	60	1.5	11
Tomato Alfredo; Vodka	130	10	9

Taco Bell, Jalapeno Sauce, 2 T., 1 oz | 110 | 11 | 3 |

Tony Roma's:

Bold & Spicy BBQ Sauce, 2 Tbsp	50	0	12
Carolina Honeys BBQ Sauce, 1.2 oz	60	0	17

Trader Joe's:

BBQ Sauce,

Kansas City Style, 2 Tbsp	60	0	15
Tomato Basil Marinara, ½ cup	80	4.5	10

Walnut Acres,

Organic Pasta Sauces,

all varieties, average, ½ cup, 4.5 oz	50	1	9

Seasonings & Flavorings

	C	F	Cb
Auromatic Bitters (Angostua), 1 tsp	15	0	4
Bacon Bits, average, 1 Tbsp	35	2	2
Bacon Chips (Durkee), 1 Tbsp	30	1	0
Bac-Os (Betty Crocker), 1Tbsp	30	1.5	2
Blends (Mrs Dash), 1 tsp	0	0	0
Butter Buds, 1 tsp	5	0	2
Flavor Enhancer (Accent), 1 tsp	0	0	0
Flavor Sprinkles (Molly McButter), Natural/Cheese, 1 tsp	5	0	1
Garlic Bread Sprinkle, 1 tsp	8	0.5	1
Garlic Salt, 1 tsp	2	0	0
Italian Seasoning, 1 tsp	4	0	1
Lemon Pepper Seasoning, 1 tsp	7	0	1
Meat Tenderizer, av., 1 tsp	7	0	1
Salad Crunchies (McCormick), 1 tsp	10	0.5	1
Salt, Reg., Sea Salt, Lite Salt	0	0	0
Seasoning (Old Bay), ¼ tsp	0	0	0
Seasoning Mix (Vegit), ¼ tsp	0	0	0
Seasoning Mixes, av., ¼ pkg	70	1	9
Taco Seasoning, av., ¼ pkg	30	0.5	4
Bragg's, Liquid Aminos	0	0	0
Old El Paso: Chili Season. Mix, 1 Tbsp	8	0.5	1.5
Cheesy Taco Season Mix, 1 Tbsp	10	0.5	2
Taco/Burrito Seasoning Mix, 2 tsp	15	0	4
Fajita Seasoning Mix, 1 tsp	5	0	1.5

Spices & Herbs

	C	F	Cb
Average all types, 1 tsp	5	0	1
All Purpose, 1 tsp	0	0	0
Allspice, ground	5	0	1
Chili Powder	8	0	1
Cinnamon, ground	6	0	2
Curry Powder	6	0	1
Garlic Powder	9	0	2
Nutmeg, ground	12	0	1
Onion Powder	7	0	2
Parsley, dried	4	0	1
Pepper, average	6	0	1
Saffron	2	0	0
Salt-Free Blends, 1 tsp	0	0	0
Tumeric, ground	8	0	1
Seeds: Fenugreek	12	1	2
Mustard, Poppyseed	15	1	1
Other varieties, average	7	0	1

Home-Popped Popcorn   C   F   Cb

	C	F	Cb
Popping Corn Kernels, 2 Tbsp, 1 oz (makes approximately 5 cups)	110	1	26
Air-popped, without oil: Plain, 1 oz	110	1	22
1 cup, 0.2 oz	20	0	5
Oil-popped: Plain, 1 oz	145	8	16
1 cup, 0.4 oz	55	3	6
Popcorn Oil, 1 Tbsp	120	14	0

Microwave Popcorn

Average all Brands: Per 1 Cup Popped, Unless Indicated

	C	F	Cb
Butter: Regular, 1 cup	35	2	4
Light, 1 cup	25	1	4
Act II Popcorn:			
Butter: 1 cup	25	1	4
4½ cups, 1 oz	120	5	19
94% Fat-Free Butter: 1 cup	20	0.5	4
6½ cups, 1 oz	130	2	27
Butter Lovers: 1 cup	25	1	4
4½ cups, 1 oz	120	4	19
Xreme Butter: 1 cup	25	1	4
4½ cups	120	4	19
Jolly Time:			
Blast O Butter, 1 cup	45	3	4
Light Butter, 1 cup	25	1	4
Xtra Butter: 1 cup	40	2.5	4
4 cups	160	10	16
Newman's Own:			
Butter Flavor, Microwave:			
Regular, 3½ cups	130	5	18
Light, 3½ cups	120	4	19
Butter Boom, 3½ cups	130	5	18
Orville Redenbacher's:			
Family Favorites:			
Butter: 4 cups	170	12	17
Light, 5½ cups	120	5	19
Movie Theater Butter, 4 cups	160	9	19
Ultimate Butter, 5 cups	170	12	16
Sweet & Savory:			
Cheddar Cheese, 4½ cups	180	14	16
Sea Salt & Vinegar, 5 cups	150	7	21
Pop Secret: *Per Cup*			
94% Fat-Free, Butter	15	0	3
Average other flavors	30	2	3

Bagged Popcorn   C   F   Cb

Average All Brands (Ready-to-Eat)

	C	F	Cb
Regular/Plain: ½ oz package	80	5	8
1 oz package	160	10	16
4 oz package	640	40	64
2 oz Box (store/airport)	320	16	32
3 oz Bag (9" high x 5" wide)	480	24	48
Caramel Popcorn, with nuts, 1 cup, 1.5 oz	230	12	39

Bagged Popcorn ~ Brands

	C	F	Cb
Boston's, Lite, 3½ cups, 1 oz	130	4.5	20
Cracker Jack: Original, 1 cup, 2 oz	240	4	46
Butter Toffee Flavored, 1 cup, 2 oz	220	2	50
Crunch 'N Munch:			
Buttery Toffee: ⅔ cup, 1 oz	150	6	22
1 cup, 1.6 oz	220	9	32
Caramel: ⅔ cup, 1 oz	160	8	20
1 cup, 1.6 oz	230	12	29
12 oz box	1745	87	218
Fiddle Faddle:			
Average all varieties: 1 oz	120	2	24
1 cup, 2 oz	240	4	48
6 oz box	720	12	144
PopCorners, Butter/Kettle, 1 oz	125	3.5	25
Popcorn Indiana:			
Kettlecorn:			
Original, 2 cups, 1 oz	130	5	21
Cinn. Sugar, 2½ cups, 1 oz	130	4.5	21
Popcorn:			
Aged White Cheddar, 1 oz	150	9	14
Caramel, ½ cup, 1 oz	110	0	26
Movie Theater, 1 oz	160	12	13
Seasalt, 3 cups, 1 oz	130	6	18
Poppycock:			
Original/Pecan Delight, av:			
½ cup, 1 oz	155	8	20
1 cup, 2 oz	310	16	40
Cashew Lovers, ½ cup, 1 oz	150	6	20
Chocolate Lovers, 1 oz, 1.2 oz	160	7	22

Movie Theater Popcorn

	C	F	Cb
Small, (7 cups): Plain	385	21	44
With Butter (3 pumps, 0.8 oz)	570	42	44
Medium, (15 cups): Plain	825	45	94
With Butter (4 pumps, 1 oz)	1075	73	94
Large, (20 cups): Plain	1100	60	124
With Butter (6 pumps, 1.5 oz)	1485	102	124
Butter: 1 Pump, 0.3 oz	65	7	0
4 Pumps (2 Tbsp), 1 oz	250	28	0

Corn & Tortilla Chips	C	F	Cb
Average All Brands			
Corn Chips:			
Average all types: 1 oz	150	8	18
8 oz bag	1200	64	144
Fritos, Original, 32 chips, 1 oz	160	10	15
Tortilla Chips: Average, 1 oz	140	7	18
(1 oz = approx. 12 chips or 13 strips)			
Doritos: Original, 1 oz	140	7	18
Nacho Cheese; Salsa Verde, av., 1 oz	140	8	18
Popchips: Chili Limon, 1 oz	120	4	19
Nacho Cheese, 1 oz	130	5	18
Snyder's:			
El Restaurante, all flavors, 1 oz	150	8	17
Yellow Corn/White, av., 1 oz	135	5	21
Tostitos:			
Average all flavors, 1 oz	145	7	19
Baked! Scoops, 1 oz	120	3	24
Utz: Multigrain, 1 oz	150	8	16
Other flavors, 1 oz	140	8	18

Potato Chips/Crisps			
Average All Brands			
Regular:			
Plain or flavored, (4 chips)	30	2	3
1 oz package (20 chips)	150	10	15
4 oz quantity	600	40	60
14 oz package	2100	140	210

Chips/Crisps ~ Brands			
Lay's *(Fritolay):*			
Regular, average all flavors, 1 oz	160	10	15
40% Less Fat, Kettle, 1 oz	135	6	19
Air Popped, av. all flavors, 1 oz	125	4	21
Oven Baked, Original, 1 oz	120	2	23
Pringles:			
Original, 1 oz	150	9	15
Large can, 6 oz	900	54	90
Snack Stacks: Original, 1 tub	110	7	11
Other flavors, 1 tub	110	7	11
Reduced Fat, all flavors, 1 oz	140	7	17
Fat Free, all flavors, 15 crisps, 1 oz	70	0	15
Multi Grain, all flavors, 1 oz	140	8	16
Cheez Ummms, all flavors, 1 oz	150	9	15
Ruffles: Regular, av. all flavors, 1 oz	160	11	15
Baked!, average all flavors, 1 oz	120	3.5	22
Sun Chips, Original, 16 crisps, 1 oz	140	6	18

Pretzels	C	F	Cb
Average All Brands			
Hard-Baked Pretzels: *Each*			
1 oz quantity	110	1	23
Sticks, thin, 2¼" (9/oz)	12	0	3
Twists, thin, ¼" thick, (5/oz)	25	0	5
Dutch (2¾"x 2⅝"), 0.5 oz	55	1	11
Snyders, Sourdough, 0.8oz	100	0	22
Soft Pretzel Twists, average: *Each*			
Plain: Small, 2 oz	210	2	43
Medium, 4 oz	390	3.5	80
Large, 5 oz	485	4.5	100
Big Cheese, 1.8 oz	130	3	22
New York Street Vendors, 7 oz	660	6	135
Trader Joe's, Peanut Butter filled, 1 oz	140	8	14
Snyder's: Milk Chocolate Dips, 1 oz	140	6	19
White Creme Dips, 1 oz	130	6	19

Pretzels ~ Brands			
Flipz: Milk Choc, 8 pieces, 1 oz	130	5	20
White Fudge, 7 pcs, 1 oz	130	5	20
Rold Gold *(Frito-Lay):*			
Braided Twists,			
Honey Wheat (8), 1 oz	110	1	24
Pretzel Sticks, 1 oz	110	0	23
Rods/Tiny Twists, av., 1 oz	110	1	23
Sourdough, 1 pretzel	90	1	19
Tiny Twists, Fat-Free, 1 oz	110	1	23
Snyder's of Hanover:			
Gluten Free Pretzel Sticks (30)	110	1.5	25
Homestyle (4), 1 oz	120	1	25
Pieces, Bacon Cheddar , 1 oz	140	7	17
Rods (3), 1 oz	120	1	24
Sticks (28), 1 oz	110	1	23
Thins (11), 1 oz	110	0	23
SuperPretzel:			
Soft: Original (1), 2.3 oz	160	1	34
Sweet Cinnamon (1),			
with topping, 2.5 oz	200	2	42
Bites (5), 1.9 oz	140	0.5	32
Softstix (2), 1.8 oz	130	3	22
Pretzelfils: Pizza (2), 1.9 oz	120	2	20
Pepperjack; Mozzarella, (2), average	130	4.5	20
Utz: Sourdough, Hard (1)	90	0	18
Cinnamon, 1 oz	120	1.5	24

Snacks   C F Cb

Note: Actual weight of packaged snacks is usually 5-10% more than label Net Wt. For accuracy, weigh snack and allow extra calories, fat and carbs for any extra weight.

	C	F	Cb
Apple Chips (Seneca), av., 1 oz	140	7	20
Bagel Crisps (N.Y. Style), 6 crisps, 1 oz	130	6	17
Baguette Chips (Pillsbury), av., (21)	130	5	20
Banana Chips (T.Joe's), 13 chips, 1 oz	160	11	13
Beef Jerky (Jack Link's), av., 1 oz	80	1	4
Beef Sticks: (Slim Jim), Orig., 2 oz	150	3	10
Jack Links, Original, 1.5 oz	160	13	2
Bugles, Original, Nacho Cheese, 1 oz	160	9	18
Cheese Balls (Utz), 1 oz serving	150	9	15
Cheese Nips, 1.3 oz package	170	7	22
Cheese Puffs, average, 1 oz	160	10	15
Cheese Twists, 1 oz	140	8	15
Cheerios, Snack Mix, average, ⅔ cup, 1 oz	120	3	21
Cheetos:			
Crunchy: Av. all flavors, 1 oz	155	11	13
4 oz package	640	40	60
Baked!; Fantastix, all varieties, av., 1 oz	130	5	19
Simply Puffs, White Cheddar, 1 oz	150	9	16
Cheez-It Crackers (Sunshine):			
Original, 1.3 oz package	180	9	20
Original Big (13), 1 oz	150	8	17
Colby, 0.8 oz pouch	110	6	12
Mozzarella (25), 1 oz	150	7	19
Reduced Fat: Original, 1 oz	130	4.5	20
White Cheddar, 1 oz	130	4	22
Chester's: Fries, Flamin' Hot, 1 pkg	140	8	16
Puffcorn, Cheese, 1 oz	160	11	14
Chex Mix, (General Mills), Traditional, 1 oz	120	3.5	21
Chips Ahoy!, Choc Chip Cookies:			
1.4 oz Single Serve Pack	190	9	27
Minis: Go-Pak!, 1 package, 3.5 oz	525	25	70
Snak Sak, 1 package, 8 oz	1050	49	147
Chicharrones ~ See Pork Skins			
Churros (Rubio's), 9", 1.6 oz	170	8	22
Combos,			
Crackers, av. all flavors, ⅓ cup, 1 oz	140	6	18
Pretzels, average all flavors, 1 oz	135	5	19
Cool Cuts, Carrot & Ranch, 2.3 oz	70	5	5
Corn Chips ~ See Page 149			
Corn Nuts: Av all flav., 1 oz	130	4.5	20
1.7 oz bag	210	8	34
Corn Puffs/Twists, (32 approx), 1 oz	160	11	15
Dunkin Stix (Dolly Madison), (3)	490	25	63

Snacks (Cont)   C F Cb

	C	F	Cb
Edamame,			
Seapointe, Dry Roasted, 1 oz	130	4	10
Fritos: Corn Chips, all varieties, av., 1oz	150	10	15
Flavor Twists, Honey BBQ, 1 oz	150	9	16
Funyuns, Onion Flavored, 1 oz	140	7	18
Goldfish, av. all flavors 1 oz	140	5	20
Gold-n-Chees (Lance):			
Snack Mix, 1 oz	150	8	17
Tube, 1 oz	130	6	18
Gripz, (Sunshine), Mighty Tiny, 0.9 oz	120	6	15
Hot Peanuts (Munchies), 1.7 oz	310	25	10
Lance:			
Cracker Creations, Granola, av. all ,(2)	190	9	24
Sandwich Crackers, av. all, 6 crackers	200	9	25
Munchies (Frito-Lay),			
Snack Mix, all flavors, 1 oz	140	7	18
Munchos, all flavors, 16 pieces, 1 oz	160	10	16
Newtons:			
Single Serve: 2 oz pkg	200	4	40
Fat-Free, 2 oz package	200	0	46
Nutter Butter, Sandwich Cookies:			
Singles, 1.9 oz pkg	250	10	37
Bites, Go-Pak, 3.5 oz	490	21	74
Onion Rings (T.G.I. Friday), 1 oz	140	7	16
Oreo Cookies, all Creme Fillings:			
Double Stuf (2), 1 oz	140	7	21
Mini Bite Size:			
1.3 oz pkg	170	7	25
Go-Pak, 3.5 oz	455	21	74
Oreo Cakesters, soft, 2 oz	250	12	36
Oriental Mix Rice Snacks, 1 oz	125	3.5	21
Peanut Butter Nuggets, (10), 1 oz	140	6	15
Pepitas, dried or roasted, ¼ cup, 1 oz	155	14	3
Pirate's Booty:			
Aged White Cheddar, 4 oz bag	520	20	76
Fruity Booty, 4 oz bag	520	20	68
Pita Chips, (9), average, 1 oz	130	4	18
Plaintain Chips,			
Goya, 34 chips, 1 oz	150	8	19
PopCorners, Butter/Kettle, 1 oz	125	3.5	19
Popcorn ~ See Page 148			
Pork Cracklins, 1 oz	160	12	0
Pork Skins/Rinds: 1 oz	160	10	0
Baken-ets, Traditional, 0.5 oz	80	5	0
Mission, Chiccarones, 4 oz package	640	40	0
Potato Chips ~ See Page 149			
Potato Skins (TGI Friday), all flavors, 16 chips, 1 oz	140	8	15
Puffed Wheat,			
Sabritones, Chili & Lime, 1 oz	150	10	13
Pretzels ~ See Page 149			

Snacks (Cont) | C | F | Cb

	C	F	Cb
Rice Cakes:			
Lundberg, (1), average, 0.7 oz	75	0.5	16
Quaker, Plain, lightly salted, 0.3 oz	35	0	7
Chocolate (1), 0.5 oz	60	1	12
Rice Chips:			
Lundberg, average, 1 oz	140	7	18
Quaker, Popped White Cheddar & Herb, 16 chips, 1 oz	130	5	19
Sandwich Crackers:			
Austin, Cheese Crackers:			
With Cheddar, 1.4 oz	190	10	23
With Peanut Butter, 1.3 oz	190	10	23
PB & J Flavored, 1.4 oz	190	8	26
Lance:			
Nip Chee, 6 pieces	190	9	24
Toasty, 6 pieces	180	8	21
Toast Chee, 6 pieces	210	10	25
Ritz Bits:			
Cheese: 1.5 oz package	220	12	23
Go-Pak: 13 crackers, 1 oz	150	8	16
3.5 oz Pak	520	29	58
P'nut Butter: 1.3 oz pkg	170	10	20
Big Bag, 3 oz	450	25	50
Sesame Sticks,			
SunRidge Farm, 1 oz	170	12	14
Smart Puffs,			
Pirates Booty, 1 oz	140	7	16
Snack Mix,			
Quaker, Baked Cheddar, 1 package	230	8	34
Soy Crisps, average, 1 oz	120	3	17
Soy Nuts: Dry Roasted, ¼ cup, 1 oz	130	6	9
Choc-coated, 1 oz	140	7	13
Sun Chips,			
Fritolay, average, 1 oz	140	6	19
Takis: Fajitas, 1 oz	140	7	17
4 oz package	560	28	68
Tings,			
Robert's, 2 oz bag	300	16	36
Toasted Chips (Ritz), av. all, 1 oz	130	5.5	20
Tortilla Chips/Tostitos ~ Page 149			
Trail Mix (Nuts/Seeds/Dried Fruit):			
Regular, 3 Tbsp, 1 oz	140	9	13
Tropical, 3 Tbsp, 1 oz	130	7	16
Turkey Jerky: Teriyaki, 1 oz	80	1	8
Trader Joe's, Original, 1 oz	60	0.5	6
Veggie Crisps,			
Snyder's, 1 oz	140	7	18
Wasabi Peas, ¼ cup, 1 oz	120	3	19
Wheat Thins (Nabisco), av. all, 1 oz	135	5	19
Yogurt Pretzels, 1.5 oz	190	8	28
Yogurt Raisins,			
Sun-Maid, 1 oz	120	4.5	20

Fruit Snacks | C | F | Cb

	C	F	Cb
Betty Crocker: Fruit Gushers, 0.9 oz	90	1	20
Fruit by the Foot, 1 roll, 0.8 oz	80	1	17
Fruit Roll Ups, 1 roll, 0.5 oz	50	1	12
Fruit Flavored Shapes, all varieties, 0.9 oz	80	0	19
Sunkist: Fruit Snacks, 1 pouch	80	0	19
Fruit Smoothie Blitz, 1.3 oz	140	1	32

Vending Machines | C | F | Cb

	C	F	Cb
Bugles, Nacho Cheese, 1 oz	160	9	18
Cheese Balls (Utz), 1 oz	150	9	16
Cheetos, Crunchy, 1 oz	150	10	13
Cheeze-It, Snack Mix, 1.5 oz	195	6.5	30
Chex Mix, Cheddar, 1 oz	120	3.5	22
Chester's, Flamin' Hot Fries, 1 oz	140	8	16
Choc Chip Cookies:			
Chips Ahoy, 1.4 oz	190	9	27
Famous Amos, (4), 1 oz	150	8	18
Grandma's, (2), 2.5 oz	340	28	55
Chocolate Bars:			
Hershey's, Milk Choc.,1.6 oz	210	13	26
Kit Kat, 1.5 oz	210	11	27
Snickers, 1.9 oz bar	250	12	33
Donut, plain cake, 1.4 oz	160	9	18
Doritos, av. all flavors, 1 oz	145	8	18
Fritos, Corn Chips, Orig., 1.8 oz	280	17	26
Fruit Pie,			
Hostess, 4.5 oz	480	20	68
Granola/Cereal Bars, av., 1 oz	140	3	26
M & M's:			
Milk Chocolate, 1.7 oz	240	10	34
Peanuts, 1.8 oz	250	13	30
Oreo Cookies, 2 oz	270	11	41
Peanut Butter Cups,			
Reese's, 1.5 oz	210	13	24
Popcorn, plain, 1 oz	160	10	16
Pop Chips, 0.8 oz	100	3	16
Pork Skins, 1.5 oz	240	15	0
Potato Chips: 1 oz	150	10	15
Baked! (Ruffles), Orig.,1 oz	160	10	15
Potato Skins (TGI Friday's), all flavors, 1 oz	140	8	15
Pretzels (Snyder's), Old Time, 1 oz	120	1	24
Raisins, 0.5 oz package	45	0	11
Rice Krispies Treat	90	2	17
Skittles, 2 oz	230	2.5	52
Starburst, Fruit Chews, Orig., 1.4 oz	160	3.5	33
Tortilla Chips, 1 oz	140	7	18

Homemade & Restaurant

Restaurant & Take-Out:	C	F	Cb
Average All Preparations: Per 8 fl.oz			
Bean Medley	200	3	34
Beef Consomme	30	0	2
Borscht, with Sour Cream	130	8	14
Bouillabaisse	400	15	10
Chicken & Corn	290	14	20
Chicken & Wild Rice	80	4	9
Chicken Consomme	50	0	2
Chicken Curry	180	8	18
Chicken Jambalaya	160	7	8
Chicken Noodle	80	2	12
With Chicken	160	4	12
Chicken Soup	80	2	6
Chili with Beans	250	12	25
Clam Chowder	240	15	17
Corn & Crab	120	3	18
Corn Chowder	150	8	16
Cream of Broccoli	200	12	20
Cream of Potato	150	6.5	17
Cream of Mushroom	200	13	15
Fish Chowder	220	15	6
French Onion	420	15	15
Gazpacho	50	0	5
Lentil Soup	250	9	28
Lobster Bisque	320	15	10
Matzo Ball, with 1 large ball	180	7	24
Minestrone	125	2.5	20
Mulligatawny	300	15	8
Pea & Ham	240	10	25
Potato & Bacon	170	7	19
Pumpkin, Creamy	210	10	26
Shark Fin Soup	100	4	8
Spicy Shrimp Soup, 1 bowl	160	7	10
Split Pea Soup	180	2.5	30
Vegetable (Fat Free)	75	0	18
Vegetable Beef	80	2	10
Vichyssoise	200	9	15
Watercress	90	4	13

Other Soups ~ *See International & Fast-Foods Sections (Arby's, Au Bon Pain, Boston Market, Dunkin' Donuts, Denny's, Schlotzsky's, Sizzler, Souplantation, Sweet Tomatoes, Zoup!)*

Homemade Soups: *Calculate calories, fat and carbohydrates from recipe ingredients.*

Bouillon Cubes & Powders

Bouillon Cubes: *Average all types*	C	F	Cb
Regular, 1 cube	5	0	1
Extra Large, 1 cube	20	1	1
Powders, average, 1 tsp	10	0	1

Herb-Ox:

Instant Broth & Seasoning,			
Beef, 1 envelope, 0.14 oz	5	0	1
Chicken, 1 envelope, 0.14 oz	5	0	1

Soup ~ Brands

Amy's:

Heat & Serve (Organic): *Per 1 Cup, Unless Indicated*

	C	F	Cb
Alphabet	80	0	16
Chunky Vegetable	60	0	13
Cream of M'shrm, ¾ cup	150	9	13
Curried Lentil	230	8	30
Fire Roasted Southwestern Veggie	140	3	21
Lentil	180	5	25
Lentil Vegetable	160	4	24
Rustic Italian Vegetable	140	6	18
Split Pea	100	0	19
Thai Coconut	140	10	9
Tuscan Bean & Rice	160	4.5	25

Andersen's: *Per 1 Cup*

	C	F	Cb
Split Pea	130	0	24
Split Pea flavored with Bacon	140	1	23

Bertoli: *Per ½ Package, 12 oz*

Meal Soups: Chicken Minestrone	370	18	32
Roasted Chicken & Rotini Pasta	290	12	28
Ricotta & Lobster Ravioli,			
in Seafood Bisque	380	16	41
Tomato Florentine			
& Tortellini with Chicken	410	19	36

Campbell's:

Chunky: *Per 8 fl.oz Cup*

	C	F	Cb
Baked Potato w/ Ched. & Bacon Bits	190	9	23
Chicken Corn Chowder	190	10	20
Classic Chicken Noodle	120	3	15
Hearty: Beef Noodle	120	2	17
Italian Style Wedding,			
with Meatballs & Spinach	120	3	15
Tomato with Pasta	150	1	30

Campbell's (Cont):

	C	F	Cb
Condensed Soup: *Per ½ Cup, 4 fl.oz*			
Bean with Bacon	160	3	26
Beef with Veggies & Barley	80	1	15
Chicken Noodle	60	2	8
Cream of Broccoli	90	5	9
Cream of Celery/Mushroom	100	7	9
Cream of Potato	90	2	16
Homestyle Chicken Noodle	70	2	10
Old Fashioned Tomato Rice	130	1.5	26
Split Pea with Ham & Bacon	180	2	29
Tomato	90	0	20
Gourmet Bisques: *Per 8 fl.oz Cup*			
Golden Butternut Squash	110	2	21
Sweet Potato Tomatillo	160	8	19
Thai Tomato Coconut	170	5	27
Tomato Roasted Garlic Bacon	210	8	31
Homestyle: *Per 8 fl.oz Cup*			
Butternut Squash Bisque	110	3	19
Chicken Noodle	90	2.5	10
Creamy Chicken & Herb Dumplings	160	8	16
Creamy Gouda Bisque with Chicken	140	6	15
Harvest Tomato with Basil	110	1	23
Italian-Style Wedding	120	3.5	15
Maryland-Style Crab Soup	80	0.5	14
Mexican-Style Chicken Tortilla	130	2	20
Minestrone	100	1	18
New England Clam Chowder	170	10	15
Potato Broccoli	160	9	17
Southwest-Style Chicken Chili	130	2.5	20
Vegetable	90	0.5	18
Zesty Tomato Bisque	110	2	19
Light: Chicken Noodle	70	1	9
New England Clam Chowder	120	4	15
Italian-Style Wedding	80	1.5	11
Southwestern-Style Vegetable	60	0	12
Healthy Request, Chunky: *Per 8 fl.oz Cup*			
Beef with Country Vegetables	110	1.5	14
Chicken Corn Chowder	140	3	22
Chicken Noodle	110	2.5	14
New England Clam Chowder	130	3	20
Split Pea & Ham, Smoke Flavor	160	2.5	22
Microwaveable Soup On The Go: *Per 10.75 oz*			
Chicken & Stars	70	1.5	10
Chicken with Mini Noodles	70	2	11
Creamy Chicken	130	9	10
Creamy Broccoli	160	11	13
Creamy Tomato Parmesan Bisque	220	7	35
New England Clam Chowder	160	11	13
Vegetable Beef	70	1	11

Campbell's (Cont):

	C	F	Cb
Slow Kettle Style: *Per 8 fl.oz*			
Braised Beef Stew, with Vegetables & Wine	150	3	19
Portobello Mushroom & Madeira Bisque	250	18	16
Sthwest Style Chkn Chili	190	2	28
Tomato & Sweet Basil Bisque	260	14	30
Tuscan Style Chicken	140	2.5	17
Health Valley:			
Fat Free, 40% Less Sodium: *Per 8 fl.oz Cup*			
Organic: Black Bean Vegetable	110	0	25
Corn & Vegetable	100	0	22
Lentil & Carrot	110	0	24
Split Pea & Carrots	120	0	26
Tomato Vegetable	70	0	17
Creamed: *Per 8 fl.oz Cup*			
Organic: Cream of Chicken	110	3	15
Cream of Celery	90	5	11
Cream of Mushroom	90	2	14
Healthy Choice:			
Canned: *Per 8 fl.oz Cup*			
Bean & Ham	180	2.5	28
Chicken & Dumplings	150	3	22
Chicken Tortilla	140	1.5	23
Chicken with Rice	110	2	17
Country Vegetable	100	0	19
New England Clam Chowder	110	1.5	20
Split Pea & Ham	160	2.5	27
Tomato Basil	100	0	22
Microwaveable Bowls: *Per 8 fl.oz Cup*			
Beef Pot Roast	110	1.5	17
Chicken Tortilla	140	1.5	23
Chicken with Rice	90	2	13
Country Vegetable	100	0	20
Hearty Vegetable Barley, 8.8 oz	140	1	30
Imagine:			
Broths:			
Organic: Beef	20	1	2
Free Range Chicken	20	0.5	2
Vegetable	20	0	4
Vegetarian, No-Chicken	15	0	2
Chunky Style:			
Chicken & Dumplings	130	4.5	18
Cream of Mushroom	100	3.5	15
Italian Vegetables & Beans	120	1.5	24

S Soups

Imagine (Cont):	C	F	Cb
Creamy: *Per 8 fl.oz Cup*			
Acorn Squash & Mango	70	1	15
Portobello Mushroom	70	2.5	12
Potato Leek	80	2.5	13
Sweet Pea	80	1.5	14
Tomato Basil	110	2	21
Kettle Cuisine: *Per 8 oz*			
Aztec Chili with Ancient Grains	190	4	32
Caribbean Jerk Chicken	220	6	31
Carrot Ginger	110	4	18
Cream of Crab	330	26	15
Manhattan Clam Chowder	130	3	17
North Atlantic Haddock Chowder	290	19	14
Gluten Free: Broccoli Cheddar	340	26	15
Angus Steak Chili with Beans	230	7	23
Chicken Enchilada	290	16	19
Chipotle Sweet Potato	150	7	20
Coconut Curry Chicken	300	10	40
Manhattan Clam Chowder	130	3	17
Knorr:			
Cubes: *Per ½ Cube, 1 Cup, Prepared*			
Beef; Chicken, average	15	1.5	1
Vegetable	20	1	1
Homestyle Stock: *Per 1 Tsp*			
Beef	10	1	0
Chicken	10	2	0
Lipton:			
Cup-a-Soup: *Per Envelope*			
Chicken Noodle, Original	50	1	8
Cream of Chicken	60	1.5	12
Hearty Chicken Noodle	60	0	10
Recipe Secrets: *Per 1 Tbsp Dry Mix*			
Onion	20	0	4
Onion Mushroom	25	0	7
Savory Herb with Garlic	25	0	6
Manischewitz:			
Cans: *Per ½ Cup Soup*			
Chicken Consomme, Clear	15	0	2
Chicken Noodle	60	1.5	7
Quart Jars: *Per 6 fl.oz*			
Borscht with Beets	50	0	13
Borscht, Low Calorie	15	0	4
Ready To Serve,			
Matzo Ball Chicken, 1 cup, 8 fl.oz	120	4.5	12
Maruchan:			
Instant Lunch,			
average all flavors, 1 pkg	290	12	38
Ramen, all flavors, 1 pkg, 3 oz	380	14	52

Nissin:	C	F	Cb
Souper Meal: *Per ½ of 4.3 oz Ctn*			
Chicken Flavor, with Vege Medley	280	13	37
Picante Shrimp Flavor, Hot & Spicy	290	13	37
Top Ramen, all flavors, 3 oz pkg	380	14	53
Pacific Foods:			
Condensed: Cream of Chicken, ½ cup	90	3.5	10
Cream of Mushroom, ½ cup	100	2.5	18
Organic: *Per ¼ of 32 fl.oz Container*			
French Onion	30	1	5
Cashew Carrot Ginger Bisque	120	5	19
Curried Red Lentil	140	5	20
Rst Pepper & Tomato	110	2	16
Progresso:			
Broths: Beef, 1 cup	20	0	3
Chicken, 1 cup	20	0	1
Chili: Pork/Beef with Beans, 1 cup	320	20	24
White Chicken with Beans, 1 cup	210	6	24
Heart Healthy: *Per Cup*			
Creamy Tomato with Basil	120	3	22
Creole Style Chkn Gumbo	110	2	18
Homestyle Vegetable Beef	120	2	19
Italian Wedding with Meatballs	80	2.5	11
Savory Garden Vegetable	90	0	21
S'West Style Black Bean & Vegetable	110	2	21
Rich & Hearty: *Per 1 Cup*			
Chkn & Homestyle Noodles	110	3	14
Chicken Corn Chowder	200	9	23
New Engl. Clam Chowder	180	8	22
Savory Beef Barley Vegetables	110	1.5	17
Traditional: *Per ½ Can, 1 Cup*			
Chicken Noodle	100	2.5	12
Chicken & Sausage Gumbo	130	3.5	18
Italian-Style Wedding	120	4	15
Split Pea with Ham	140	1	24
Vegetable Classic: *Per 1 Cup*			
French Onion	50	1	9
Green Split Pea with Bacon	160	2.5	29
Garden Vegetable	90	0	20
Minestrone	100	2	20
Tomato Rotini	130	0.5	28
Light: *Per 1 cup*			
Beef Pot Roast	80	2	10
Chicken Pot Pie Syle	100	3	16
Italian Style Vegetable	70	0	16
Vegetable & Noodle	60	0.5	13

Safeway (Vons):	C	F	Cb
Signature Soups: *Per Cup*			
Broccoli & Cheesy Cheddar	250	18	12
Chunky Chicken Noodle	160	5	14
Fiesta Chicken Tortilla	110	2	15
Italian-Style Wedding	120	4	14
Pacific Coast Clam Chowder	320	20	27
Tuscan Tomato & Basil Bisque	290	22	20
Swanson:			
Broth: *Per 8 fl.oz Cup*			
Beef	15	0	1
Chicken	10	0.5	1
Organic Chicken	15	0.5	1
Vegetable	15	0	3
Flavor Boost: *Per Pouch*			
Beef	10	0	2
Chicken	35	2	3
Vegetable	20	0	4
Tabatchnick:			
Frozen:			
Dairy: *Per 7.5 oz Pouch*			
Corn Chowder	130	4.5	21
New England Potato	130	4.5	20
Gluten Free: *Per 7.5 oz Pouch*			
Southwest Bean	220	5	36
Split Pea	140	0	34
Vegetarian Chili	200	3.5	32
Low Sodium: *Per 7 .5oz Pouch*			
Barley Mushroom	80	1	17
Split Pea	140	0	34
Vegetable	90	1.5	17
Meat: *Per 7.5 oz Pouch*			
Frenchman's Onion	60	1.5	11
Wilderness Wild Rice	90	0.5	19
Parve: *Per 7.5 oz Pouch*			
Barley Mushroom	80	1	17
Black Bean	220	2.5	39
Minestrone	110	1.5	20
Shelf Stable: *Per ⅔ Cup, 5.3 fl.oz*			
Broth: Classic Chicken	5	0	0
Kosher Chicken	10	0	1
Soup: Creamy Tomato	70	2	14
Rstd Red Pepper & Tomato	70	2.5	13
Wisconsin Cheddar Cheese	150	11	10
Thai Kitchen:			
Rice Noodle Soup Bowls: *Per Bowl*			
Hot & Sour	250	4	51
Lemongrass & Chili	250	3.5	52
Roasted Garlic	250	3	52
Spring Onion	260	4.5	50
Thai Ginger	260	3	52

Trader Joe's:	C	F	Cb
28 fl.oz Cans: *Per Cup*			
Chunky, Low Fat:			
Lentil with Vegetables	140	3	21
Minestrone	110	2.5	19
14.5 oz Cans: *Per 1 Cup*			
Organic: Black Bean	140	1.5	26
Lentil Vegetable	160	4	24
Split Pea	100	0	19
10.75 oz Can,			
Low Sodium, Minestrone	200	4	37
15 oz Can,			
Low Fat, Chicken Noodle, 1 cup	90	1	14
32 fl oz. Cartons: *Per 1 Cup*			
Butternut Squash	90	2	16
Carrot & Ginger	80	1	17
Creamy Corn & Rstd Pepper	110	2	23
Latin Style Black Bean	70	1	12
Sweet Potato Bisque	130	1	28
Organic: Butternut Squash	70	0	17
Tomato & Rstd Red Pepper	100	3.5	15
Low Sodium, Creamy Tomato	90	3.5	15
17.6 fl.oz Cartons: *Per Cup*			
Beef, Barley with Veggies	100	0.5	16
Chicken Noodle with Veggies	100	1	16
Whole Foods: *Per Cup*			
365 Organic:			
Chicken Noodle	100	1.5	12
Lentil	70	0	15
Minestrone	140	1.5	23
Southwestern Black Bean	120	1	23
Tomato Basil	90	2	16
Wolfgang Puck: *Per Cup*			
Organic:			
Butternut Squash	150	8	19
Chicken & Dumplings	140	7	14
Classic Minestrone	120	2.5	20
Corn Chowder	210	13	20
Free Range Chicken Noodle	90	3	11
Hearty Garden Vegetable	130	4	22
Hearty Lentil & Vegetable	150	1	28
New Engl. Clam Chowder	150	7	18
Signature Tortilla	140	3.5	21
Tomato Basil Bisque	150	6	21

Soybean Products — C F Cb

Cheeses (Soy) ~ See Page 78
Miso Soy Bean Paste:

	C	F	Cb
Cold Mountain: Light Yellow, 1 tsp	10	0	1
Mellow Red, 1 tsp	15	0	3
Red, 1 tsp	10	0	1
Miso Soup (dry mix):			
1 Tbsp., dry mix	35	1	5
1 cup, prepared	35	1	5
Natto, ½ cup, 3 oz	160	7	14
Okara (Tofu fiber residue), ½ c., 2 oz	47	1	8
Tempeh: 1 piece, 3 oz	180	8	12
Fried, 3 oz	250	14	14
Seitan *(Westsoy)*, Strips, 3 oz	120	2	4
Soybean Protein *(TVP)*, 1 oz	95	0	8
Soy Bean Paste, 1 tsp	10	0	2
Soy Beans ~ See Page 160			
Soy Drinks ~ See Page 49			

Tofu ~ Brands

Azumaya Tofu:

	C	F	Cb
Extra Firm; Firm, av., 3 oz	70	4	2
Soft (Silken), 3.2 oz	45	2	1
House Foods: *Per 3 oz*			
Premium Tofu: Extra Firm	80	4.5	2
Firm	70	4	2
Medium Firm	60	3.5	2
Soft (Silken)	60	3	2
Organic Tofu: Firm	70	4	2
Extra Firm	70	3.5	2
Ethnic: Tokusen Kinugoshi, Extra Soft	80	4	3
Sukui; Soon (Extra Soft)	45	2	2
Yaki Tofu (Broiled)	90	4	2
Mori-Nu Tofu:			
Morinaga Silken:			
Soft, 3 oz, 1" slice	45	2.5	2
Firm, 3 oz, 1" slice	50	2.5	2
Extra Firm, 3 oz, 1" slice	45	1.5	2
Organic, Silken 3 oz, 1" slice	50	2.5	2
Lite, Firm, 3 oz, 1" slice	30	1	1
Nasoya: Extra Firm, 3 oz	80	4	3
Firm, 3 oz	70	3.5	2
Silken, 3.2 oz	45	2	1
Soft, 2.8 oz	60	3	1
Tofuplus:			
Extra Firm, 3 oz	80	4	2
Firm, 3 oz	70	3	2
Sprouted, Super Firm, 3 oz	100	5	3

Supplements — C F Cb

	C	F	Cb
Aloe Vera Juice: undiluted, 2 fl.oz	5	0	1
Brewer's Yeast: Tablets, 2 tabs	4	0	0.5
Flakes, 1 heaping Tbsp, 0.3 oz	30	0.5	4
Powder, 1 heaping Tbsp, 0.5 oz	50	0.5	6
Calcium Chews: *CVS*, 1 chew	20	0	7
Trader Joe's, Chocolate, 1 chew	20	1	3
Cod Liver Oil, 1 Tbsp	125	13	0
Fiber Choice, 2 tabs	15	0	4
Fiber:			
Fibersure, 1 heaping tsp	25	0	6
Fish Oil Capsules, (1), av.	10	1	0
Flax Oil:			
Capsules (2)	10	1	0
Barlean's, softgels (3)	110	11	0
Garlic Tablets/Capsules, each	3	0	0
Glowelle:			
Beauty Drink, 8 fl.oz	100	0	24
Powder Stick (1)	50	0	12
Lecithin Granules, 1 Tbsp	55	4	0.5
Metamucil: Powder:			
Orange (Smooth Texture), 1 rounded Tbsp	45	0	12
Sugar-Free, 1 rounded tsp	20	0	5
Pink Lemonade, Sugar-Free, 1 rounded tsp	20	0	5
Fiber Wafers, (2)	120	5	17
Capsules:			
Heart & Digestive (6)	10	0	3
Strong Bones (5)	10	0	3
Protein, Powders, av., 1 oz	100	0.5	0
Seaweed: Dried, 1 oz	85	0.5	22
Soaked, drained, 1 oz	15	0.5	3
Spirulina, 1 tablet	2	0	0.5
Vitamins/Minerals: Tabs/Caps (1)	2	0	0
Vitamin E Capsules, each	5	0.5	0
Viactiv Chews, Choc. (1)	20	0.5	4

Cough & Pharmaceutical — C F Cb

	C	F	Cb
Antacids: Av., 1 tablet	4	0	1
Liquid, 1 Tbsp	6	0	1
Antacid Sodium Counts ~ See Page 280			
Cough/Cold Syrups:			
Regular: With sugar, 1 Tbsp	35	0	9
With alcohol, 1 Tbsp	46	0	9
Diabetic Tussin, Sugar Free, 1 T.	0	0	0
Cough Drops/Lozenges ~ See Page 75			
Sudafed, Syrup 1 tsp	14	0	3
Tylenol: Liquid: Child, 1 tsp	17	0	4
Extra Strength, 1 tsp	11	0	3

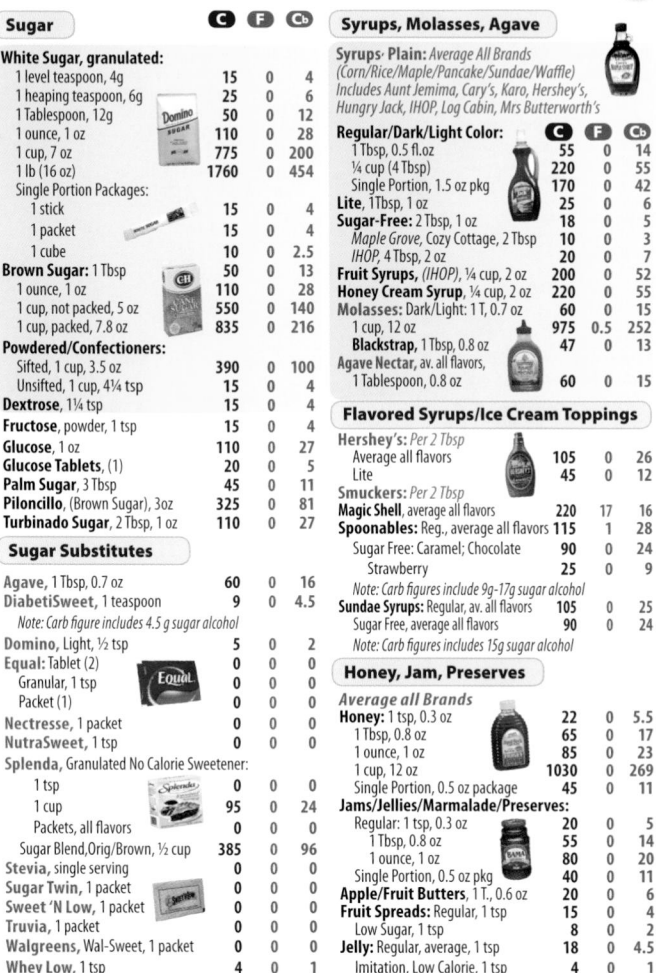

Sugar

	C	F	Cb

White Sugar, granulated:

	C	F	Cb
1 level teaspoon, 4g	15	0	4
1 heaping teaspoon, 6g	25	0	6
1 Tablespoon, 12g	50	0	12
1 ounce, 1 oz	110	0	28
1 cup, 7 oz	775	0	200
1 lb (16 oz)	1760	0	454

Single Portion Packages:

1 stick	15	0	4
1 packet	15	0	4
1 cube	10	0	2.5
Brown Sugar: 1 Tbsp	50	0	13
1 ounce, 1 oz	110	0	28
1 cup, not packed, 5 oz	550	0	140
1 cup, packed, 7.8 oz	835	0	216

Powdered/Confectioners:

Sifted, 1 cup, 3.5 oz	390	0	100
Unsifted, 1 cup, 4¼ tsp	15	0	4
Dextrose, 1¼ tsp	15	0	4
Fructose, powder, 1 tsp	15	0	4
Glucose, 1 oz	110	0	27
Glucose Tablets, (1)	20	0	5
Palm Sugar, 3 Tbsp	45	0	11
Piloncillo, (Brown Sugar), 3oz	325	0	81
Turbinado Sugar, 2 Tbsp, 1 oz	110	0	27

Sugar Substitutes

	C	F	Cb
Agave, 1 Tbsp, 0.7 oz	60	0	16
DiabetiSweet, 1 teaspoon	9	0	4.5

Note: Carb figure includes 4.5 g sugar alcohol

Domino, Light, ½ tsp	5	0	2
Equal: Tablet (2)	0	0	0
Granular, 1 tsp	0	0	0
Packet (1)	0	0	0
Nectresse, 1 packet	0	0	0
NutraSweet, 1 tsp	0	0	0

Splenda, Granulated No Calorie Sweetener:

1 tsp	0	0	0
1 cup	95	0	24
Packets, all flavors	0	0	0
Sugar Blend,Orig/Brown, ½ cup	385	0	96
Stevia, single serving	0	0	0
Sugar Twin, 1 packet	0	0	0
Sweet 'N Low, 1 packet	0	0	0
Truvia, 1 packet	0	0	0
Walgreens, Wal-Sweet, 1 packet	0	0	0
Whey Low, 1 tsp	4	0	1

Syrups, Molasses, Agave

Syrups· Plain: *Average All Brands (Corn/Rice/Maple/Pancake/Sundae/Waffle) Includes Aunt Jemima, Cary's, Karo, Hershey's, Hungry Jack, IHOP, Log Cabin, Mrs Butterworth's*

Regular/Dark/Light Color:

	C	F	Cb
1 Tbsp, 0.5 fl.oz	55	0	14
¼ cup (4 Tbsp)	220	0	55
Single Portion, 1.5 oz pkg	170	0	42
Lite, 1Tbsp, 1 oz	25	0	6
Sugar-Free: 2 Tbsp, 1 oz	18	0	5
Maple Grove, Cozy Cottage, 2 Tbsp	10	0	3
IHOP, 4 Tbsp, 2 oz	20	0	7
Fruit Syrups, (IHOP), ¼ cup, 2 oz	200	0	52
Honey Cream Syrup, ¼ cup, 2 oz	220	0	55
Molasses: Dark/Light: 1 T, 0.7 oz	60	0	15
1 cup, 12 oz	975	0.5	252
Blackstrap, 1 Tbsp, 0.8 oz	47	0	13
Agave Nectar, av. all flavors, 1 Tablespoon, 0.8 oz	60	0	15

Flavored Syrups/Ice Cream Toppings

Hershey's: *Per 2 Tbsp*

	C	F	Cb
Average all flavors	105	0	26
Lite	45	0	12

Smuckers: *Per 2 Tbsp*

Magic Shell, average all flavors	220	17	16
Spoonables: Reg., average all flavors	115	1	28
Sugar Free: Caramel; Chocolate	90	0	24
Strawberry	25	0	9

Note: Carb figures include 9g-17g sugar alcohol

Sundae Syrups: Regular, av. all flavors	105	0	25
Sugar Free, average all flavors	90	0	24

Note: Carb figures include 15g sugar alcohol

Honey, Jam, Preserves

Average all Brands

Honey: 1 tsp, 0.3 oz

	C	F	Cb
Honey: 1 tsp, 0.3 oz	22	0	5.5
1 Tbsp, 0.8 oz	65	0	17
1 ounce, 1 oz	85	0	23
1 cup, 12 oz	1030	0	269
Single Portion, 0.5 oz package	45	0	11

Jams/Jellies/Marmalade/Preserves:

Regular: 1 tsp, 0.3 oz	20	0	5
1 Tbsp, 0.8 oz	55	0	14
1 ounce, 1 oz	80	0	20
Single Portion, 0.5 oz pkg	40	0	11
Apple/Fruit Butters, 1 T., 0.6 oz	20	0	6
Fruit Spreads: Regular, 1 tsp	15	0	4
Low Sugar, 1 tsp	8	0	2
Jelly: Regular, average, 1 tsp	18	0	4.5
Imitation, Low Calorie, 1 tsp	4	0	1

Vegetables

	C	F	Cb
Alfalfa Sprouts, ½ cup, 0.5 oz	5	0	0.5
Artichokes, Globe/French:			
1 medium, 4.5 oz	60	0	13
1 large, 5.7 oz	75	0	17
Artichoke Heart, plain, 2 pieces	15	0	3
Asparagus, raw/frozen:			
Cuts & Tips, ½ cup, 4.3 oz	20	0	3
Spears, 3 medium	10	0	2
Bamboo Shoots, cooked, ½ cup, 2 oz	7	0	1
Beans, Green/Snap/String:			
10 beans (4" long), 2 oz	20	0	4
Pieces, ½ cup, 3 oz	30	0	7
Dried Beans (Kidney, Brown, Lima, Navy, Pinto/White):			
Raw: 2 Tbsp, 1 oz	95	0.5	18
1 cup, 7 oz	665	3	126
Cooked: 1 oz	35	0	7
½ cup, 3 oz	105	0	21
Bean Sprouts, average, ½ cup, 2 oz	15	0	3.5
Beets (Beetroot):			
Raw, 1 beet (2" diam.), 4 oz	35	0	8
Cooked, 1 cup, slices, 3 oz	35	0	8
Canned ~ *See Page 161*			
Beet Greens, cooked, ½ cup, 2.5 oz	20	0	4
Bell Pepper ~ *See Peppers*			
Bitter Melon/Gourd, 1 cup, 1.5 oz	15	0	1.5
Blackeye Peas, cooked, ½ cup, 3 oz	100	0.5	18
Bok Choy (Chinese Chard),			
cooked, 3 oz	10	0	1.5
Breadfruit, ¼ small fruit, 3 oz	100	0	26
Broadbeans (Fava Beans):			
Green, raw, (in pod): 4 pods			
(3.5 oz with shells, 1.2 oz beans)	30	0	6
1 cup beans, without shell, 4.5 oz	110	1	22
Mature Seeds: Raw, 1 cup, 5.3 oz	510	2.5	87
Cooked, ½ cup, 3 oz	95	0	17
Broccoflower, ⅕ head, 3.5 oz	35	0	7
Broccoli, raw, chopped,1 cup, 3 oz	30	0	6
3 Florets, 2.5 oz	25	0	5
1 Spear (5" long), 1.oz	10	0	2
1 Whole: Medium, 14 oz	135	1.5	26
Large, 21 oz	205	2	40
1 Head (no stalk), 11 oz	105	1	21
1 Stalk, small (5" long), 5.3 oz	50	0.5	10
Brocco Sprouts, ½ cup, 1 oz	15	0	2
Brussels Sprouts: Cooked, ½ cup, 2.8 oz	30	0.5	6
2 Sprouts, 1.5 oz	15	0	3
Butterbeans, cooked, ½ cup, 3 oz	90	0	16
Cabbage, average other flavors:			
Raw: 1 leaf, large, 1 oz	5	0	2
Shredded, 1 cup, 2.5 oz	15	0	4
½ large head (7" diam), 22 oz	150	1	35
Cooked, shredded, ½ cup, 2.5 oz	15	0.5	3.5

Vegetables (Cont)

	C	F	Cb
Cactus Leaf (Nopales):			
1 leaf, 4.5 oz	20	0	4
1 cup (slices), 3 oz	15	0	3
Carrots, regular thick variety:			
1 small, 4 oz	45	0	11
1 medium, 6 oz	70	0	16
1 large, 8 oz	95	0	22
Chopped, 1 cup, 4.5 oz	50	0	12
Grated, 1 cup, 4 oz	45	0	11
Slices, 1 cup, 4.5 oz	50	0	12
Sticks (4"), 4-5, 1.5 oz	20	0	4
Long thin variety, 1 medium, 2.2 oz	25	0	6
Baby: Snack size, 3 medium, 1 oz	10	0	2.5
Snack Pack, 3 oz	30	0	7
Cassava, raw, 1 cup, 2.5 oz	330	0.5	78
Cauliflower: raw: Pieces, 1 cup, 3.5 oz	25	0	5
½ medium head, 10 oz	70	0	15
Cooked, 3 florets, 2 oz	10	0	2
Celeriac, ½ cup, raw, 2.8 oz	35	0	7
Celery: 1 large stalk, 11", 2.2 oz	10	0	2
4 Strips, thin sticks, 0.5 oz	5	0	1
Chopped, 1 cup, 3.5 oz	15	0	3
Chard (Swiss), ½ cup, cooked, 3 oz	20	0	3.5
Chayote Squash: 1 medium, 7 oz	40	0	9
Pieces, 1 cup, 4.5 oz	25	0	6
Chickpeas, (Garbanzo Beans):			
Dry, 1 cup, 7 oz	730	12	121
Cooked, 1 cup, 5.8 oz	270	4	45
Chicory Greens, 1 cup, 1 oz	7	0	1.5
Chili Peppers ~ *See Peppers*			
Chinese Long Bean, slices, 1 cup, 3.2 oz	45	0	8
Chives, chopped, 1 Tbsp	1	0	0
Choy Sum, 3 oz	15	0	3
Cilantro, (Coriander), 1 cup	5	0	0.5
Collards, cooked, ½ cup, 3 oz	25	0	5
Corn, Yellow/White:			
Raw: Kernels, 1 cup, 3 oz	80	0.5	19
Ear (5"x 1¾"), 5.5 oz	155	1	37
Cooked: Kernels, ½ cup, 3 oz	77	0.5	18
Cob, small, 2.3 oz	60	0.5	14
Ear, large, 5.5 oz	120	1	28
Courgette ~ *See Zucchini*			
Cowpeas ~ *See Blackeye Peas*			
Cress, garden, raw, 1 cup, 1.8 oz	15	0	3
Cucumber, average other flavors:			
Slices, ½ cup, 2 oz	10	0	2
Green, 1 medium (9"), 11 oz	45	0	11
Persian, 1 medium (8"), 6 oz	25	0	5
Daikon Radish, ½ cup, slices, 2 oz	9	0	2
Dandelion Greens, raw, ½ cup, 1 oz	10	0	2.5
Edamame, (Immature green soybeans):			
Shelled, ½ cup, 2.6 oz	110	5	8
With shells, 10 pods, 1.3 oz	30	1	3

Vegetables (Cont)	C	F	Cb
Eggplant, raw: 4 oz	30	0	7
½ cup, 1" pieces, 1.5 oz	10	0	2
1 slice, fried, 1 oz	75	4	10
Endive, Belgian/French: Raw,			
1 medium head (6"), 2.5 oz	12	0	3
Fennel, 1 cup, sliced, 3 oz	25	0	7
Gai Choy Cabbage, cooked, 1 cup, 6 oz	20	0	3
Gai Lan, (Chinese Kale), cooked, 1 cup	35	0.5	7
Garbanzo Beans ~ See Chick Peas			
Garlic, 1 clove	4	0	1
Ginger: ¼ cup slices, 1 oz	20	0	5
Crystallized (sugared), 7 pieces, 1.5 oz	130	0	35
Horseradish, raw, 1 pod, 0.5 oz	5	0	1
Jerusalem Artichoke, raw, ½ cup	55	0	13
Jicama, raw, sliced, ½ cup, 2.3 oz	25	0	6
Kale, cooked, 2.5 oz	35	0.5	5
Kohlrabi, cooked, ½ cup, 1.8 oz	17	0	5
Leek, cooked, 1 whole, 4.5 oz	40	0	9
Lentils, green/brown: Dry, 1 oz	100	0.5	17
1 cup, 6.8 oz	675	3	115
Cooked, ½ cup, 3.5 oz	115	0.5	20
Lettuce, chopped/shredded, 2 oz	7	0	1
Butterhead, 2 leaves, 0.5 oz	2	0	0.5
Cos/Romaine, shredded, 1 cup	10	0	2
Iceberg, 1 outer leaf, 0.5 oz	2	0	0.5
1 medium head, 16 oz	75	1	16
Lima Beans, baby, cooked, ½ cup, 3 oz	105	0	20
Lotus Root, cooked, 10 slices, 3 oz	60	0	14
Mung Bean Sprouts, ½ cup, 2 oz	15	0	3
Mushrooms, average all varieties:			
Raw, diced/sliced, 1 cup, 3 oz	20	0	3
Pieces, 1 cup, 1.3 oz	8	0	1
Fried/Sauteed, 6 oz	220	16	10
Grilled, pieces, ½ cup, 2.5 oz	20	0.5	4
Shitake, dried, ½ oz package	90	0	22
Mustard Greens, raw, ½ cup, 1 oz	7	0	1
Okra: Raw, 8 pods, 4 oz	30	0	7
Cooked, ½ cup, 2.8 oz	20	0	4
Onions, Raw: 1 small, 2.5 oz	30	0	7
1 medium, 4 oz	50	0	11
1 large, 5.5 oz	65	0	15
1 jumbo, 16 oz	190	0.5	46
Chopped: ½ cup, 3 oz	35	0	8
1 Tbsp, 0.4 oz	5	0	1
Slices: 1 cup, 4 oz	50	0	12
1 medium slice (⅛"), 0.5 oz	5	0	1
1 large slice (¼"), 1.3 oz	15	0	4
Flakes, dried ¼ cup, 0.5 oz	50	0	12
Rings, breaded & fried, 2 rings	80	5	9
Scallions, ½ cup, 2 oz	15	0	3
Spring, chopped, ½ cup, 2 oz	15	0	3

Vegetables (Cont)	C	F	Cb
Parsley, chopped, ½ cup, 1 oz	10	0	2
Parsnip: 1 medium, 4 oz	85	0	20
Cooked, slices, ½ cup, 2.8 oz	55	0	13
Peas: Green, raw, ¼ cup, 1.5 oz	30	0	5
With pods, 0.5 lb	70	0	13
Snow Peas, 10 pods, 1.2 oz	15	0	3
Split: Dry, hulled, 1 oz	100	0.5	17
Cooked, 1 cup, 7 oz	230	1	42
Peppers:			
Sweet, 1 medium, 4.2 oz	30	0	7
Bell, 1 medium, 4.2 oz	30	0	7
raw, chopped, ½ cup, 2.5 oz	20	0	5
2 rings (5" diam. x ¼" thick)	3	0	1
Chili: Green/Red, 1.5 oz	20	0	5
Habanero, 1 only, 0.3 oz	10	0	2
Pigeon Peas, cooked, ½ cup, 3 oz	95	1	17
Pimientos, 3 medium, 3.5 oz	25	0	5
Poi, ½ cup, 4.2 oz	135	0	33
Potatoes:			
Raw (with skin):			
1 baby, 2 oz	45	0	10
1 small, 6 oz	135	0	30
1 medium, 8 oz	180	0	40
1 large, 12 oz	270	0	60
1 extra large, 16 oz	360	0	80
Baked, (no added fat), large, 10 oz (raw wt):			
Plain: With skin, 7 oz (cooked wt)	185	0	42
W/o skin, 5.5 oz (cooked wt)	145	0	34
With Skin/Toppings:			
With 2 tsp fat	270	8	58
With Grated Cheese, 1 oz	370	9	58
With Plain Yogurt, 2 Tbsp	260	1	60
With Sour Crm & Chives, 2 Tbsp	320	6	60
Mashed:			
With milk plus fat, ½ cup, 4 oz	120	4.5	18
KFC Style without gravy, 4 oz	90	3	15
Loaded (fat/cream/cheese/bacon):			
Side serving, 6 oz	180	9	22
Large serving, 12 oz	360	18	44
Potato Skins, baked w/ cheese topping,			
½ whole, 4 oz	240	13	22
French Fries: Small serving, 2.6 oz	250	13	30
Medium serving, 4 oz	380	20	47
Frozen, uncooked, 18 fries, 4 oz	165	5.5	28
Oven-heated, 18 fries, 4 oz	165	5.5	28
Take-Out, 1 cup, 5 oz	440	25	60
Au Gratin, ½ cup, 4.3 oz	160	9	14
Pancakes, 2 small, 2 oz	120	6.5	12
Puffs, fried, 4 puffs, 1 oz	55	2.5	8
Scalloped, 8.5 oz	220	9	26

Vegetables (Cont) | C | F | Cb

	C	F	Cb
Pumpkin:			
Raw, 1" cubes, 1 cup, 4 oz	30	0	7
Cooked:			
Baked, without fat, 4 oz	90	7	9
Mashed: 1 scoop, 2 oz	10	0	2
½ cup, 4.3 oz	25	0	6
Pumpkin Flowers, 1 cup, 1.2 oz	5	0	1
Purslane: Cooked, ½ cup, 2 oz	10	0	2
Raw, 1" cubes, 1 cup, 1.5 oz	5	0	1.5
Radicchio: 2 leaves, 0.5 oz	5	0	1
Shredded, 1 cup, 1.5 oz	20	0	4
Radishes: 1 small	0	0	0
10 medium/5 large, 1.6 oz	5	0	1
Slices, ½ cup, 2 oz	10	0	2
Rhubarb, raw, ½ cup, 2 oz	15	0	3
Rutabaga, cubes, cooked, ½ cup, 3 oz	30	0	7
Salsify, cooked, slices, ½ cup, 2.5 oz	50	0	11
Sauerkraut, ½ cup, 2.5 oz	15	0	3
Seaweed: Dried, 1 oz	5	0	2
Soaked, drained, 1 oz	15	0	1
Nori/Laver, dried, 6 sheets, 0.5 oz	35	0	5
Shallots, chopped, 1 Tbsp, 0.5 oz	5	0	1
Sorrel, raw, ½ cup, 4 oz	20	0	4
Soybeans: Dry, ½ cup, 3.3 oz	390	18	28
Mature, dry, 1 oz	120	5.5	9
Cooked, ½ cup, 3 oz	150	7.5	8
Soy Products/Tofu/Tempeh ~ See Page 156			
Spinach: Cooked, ½ cup, 3 oz	20	0	4
Creamed, average, 4.5 oz	190	15	8
Raw: 3 leaves,1 cup, 1 oz	7	0	1
1 Bunch, 12 oz	80	1.5	12
Squash:			
Summer: Raw, ½ cup, 2.5 oz	10	0	2
Cooked, slices, ½ cup, 3 oz	15	0	3
Winter, cooked:			
Acorn: Cubes, ½ cup, 3.5 oz	35	0	9
½ medium (10 oz raw weight)	115	0	30
Butternut: Cubes, ½ cup, 3.5 oz	40	0	10
¼ medium (9 oz raw weight)	115	0	30
Spaghetti, ½ cup, 1.8 oz	15	0	3
Succotash, cooked, ½ cup, 3.3 oz	110	1	23
Sweetcorn ~ See Corn			
Sweet Potatoes:			
Cooked with skin (w/o fat),			
1 medium, 4 oz	105	0	24
Without skin, mashed, ½ cup, 5.5 oz	125	0	29
Fries (Alexia, Julienne syle),			
approximately 12 pieces, 3 oz	140	5	24

Vegetables (Cont) | C | F | Cb

	C	F	Cb
Swiss Chard, cooked, chopped,1 c., 6 oz	35	0	7
Taro, cooked, ½ cup, 2.3 oz	95	0	23
Tomatoes: 1 small (2¼" diam.), 3 oz	15	0	3
1 medium (2¾" diameter), 5 oz	25	0	5
1 large (3½" diameter), 8 oz	40	0.5	9
1 extra lge (4" diam.), 12 oz	60	0.5	14
Chopped, 1 cup, 6.5 oz	35	0	8
Tomatillo: 1 medium, 1.2 oz	10	0	2
1lb quantity for recipe	135	4.5	27
Turnip: Cooked, ½ cup, 2.8 oz	15	0	4
Greens, cooked, ½ cup, 2.5 oz	15	0	3
Water Chestnuts: 5-6 nuts, 1 oz	56	0	13
Raw, slices, ½ cup, 2.3 oz	60	0	15
Canned, 1 oz	15	0	3
Watercress: 10 sprigs, 1 oz	3	0	0.5
Yams: Cooked, steamed, ½ cup, 2.5 oz	80	0	19
Baked:			
1 medium (6") 8 oz	265	0.5	63
1 large (9") 12 oz	400	0.5	94
Yardlong Bean, 1 pod, 0.5 oz	5	0	1
Yucca Root, raw, ½ cup, 3.5 oz	165	0	39
Zucchini: Raw, 1 medium, 7 oz	30	0.5	7
1 large, 12 oz	60	1	12
Cooked, slices,			
½ cup, 3 oz	15	0	4

Frozen Vegetables

	C	F	Cb
Birds Eye:			
Mixtures & Blends:			
Broccoli, Cauliflower & Carrots, 3 oz	35	0	5.5
Stir-Fry: Broccoli, 3.4 oz	35	0	6
Crisp Bean, 5.5 oz	60	0	11
Sugar Snap, 3.4 oz	40	0	7.5
Pure & Simple:			
Baby: Broccoli Florets, 1 cup, 3 oz	35	0.5	5
Gold & White Corn, ⅔ cup, 3.2 oz	105	1	22
Sweet Peas, ⅔ cup, 3 oz	80	0	14
Recipe Ready:			
Chopped Green Peppers & Onions, 2.8 oz	25	0	5
Southwest Blend, 3.3 oz	80	0	15
Sauced & Seasoned: Per 1 Cup			
Green Beans & Spaetzle,			
in Bavarian Sauce	95	4.5	10
Pasta & Veggies in Creamy Cheese Sauce	125	3	20
Steamfresh:			
Pure & Simple Blends:			
Baby Broccoli Blend, 1 cup	65	1.5	8
Baby Potato Blend, ¾ cup	50	0	10
Brocc. & Cauliflower, 1 cup, 3.4 oz	30	0.5	4.5

Frozen Vegetables (Cont)	**C**	**F**	**Cb**

Green Giant:
Create A Meal Stir Fry: *Unprepared*

	C	F	Cb
Lo Mein, 1.6 cups	130	1	27
Sweet & Sour, 1.3 cups	140	0	34
Szechuan, 1.3 cups	70	1	14
Teriyaki, 1.3 cups	60	0	14

Just for One:

	C	F	Cb
Broccoli & Cheese Sauce, 4.3 oz	40	1	7
Caulifl. & Cheese Sauce, 4.3 oz	40	1	8

Seasoned Steamers: *Per ¾ Cup, Frozen*

	C	F	Cb
Honey Dijon Carrots, 3 oz	60	2	10
Mediterranean Blend, 3 oz	80	3	11

Valley Fresh Steamers:
Prepared, with Cheese Sauce:

	C	F	Cb
Broccoli, ⅔ cup, 4 oz	60	2.5	7
Broccoli, Cauliflower & Carrots, ⅔ cup, 4.3 oz	60	2.5	8
Garden Vegetable Medley, 3.5 oz	60	0.5	12

Prepared, Without Sauce:

	C	F	Cb
Broccoli Cuts, ½ cup	15	0	3
Mixed Vegetables, ½ cup	50	0	12
Sweet Peas, ½ cup	50	0	12

Ore-Ida: *Per 3 oz Unless Indicated*
Fries:

	C	F	Cb
Classic: Golden Crinkles	120	4.5	19
Golden	130	3.5	21
Steak	110	3	19
Extra Crispy Easy, Golden Crinkles	170	6	25
Extra Crispy: Fast Food Fries	150	6	24
Golden Crinkles	160	7	22
Seasoned Crinkles	150	6	22
Tater Tots	170	9	20

Premium:

	C	F	Cb
Country Style French	130	4.5	20
Crispers	230	14	23
Golden Twirls	150	6	23
Texas Crispers	150	7	20

	C	F	Cb
Grillers: Golden Thick Cut Potatoes	130	5	19
Seasoned Thick Cut Potatoes	140	5	21
Hash Browns: Golden Patties (1)	140	8	15
Potatoes O'Brien	60	0	13
Shredded Hash Browns Pattie (1)	70	0	16
Onion: Chopped, 3 oz	20	0	5
Gourmet Rings, 2.7 oz	185	9	24
Onion Ringers, 3 oz	180	10	21
Simply: Cracked Pepper & Sea Salt, Country Style French Fries	130	4.5	22
Homestyle Wedges, all varieties	120	3.5	20
Steam n' Mash, Cut Russet, 3.5 oz	70	0	16
Tater Tots: Regular	160	8	20
Crispy Crowns	170	10	19

Canned/Bottled	**C**	**F**	**Cb**

Solids & Liquid

	C	F	Cb
Artichoke Hearts:			
Fancifoods: Plain, 1 oz (1)	8	0	1
Marinated, ¼ bottle, 1 oz	25	1.5	2
Asparagus: Drained, 3 spears	10	0	1.5
Pieces, ½ cup, 4.5 oz	25	0.5	3
Bamboo Shoots, 1 cup, 4.5 oz	25	0	4
Bean Salad, ½ cup, 4.4 oz	90	0	20
Beans: Baked, ½ cup, 4.5 oz	120	0.5	27
Butter, ½ cup, 4.5 oz	90	0	16
Green, ½ cup, 2.5 oz	15	0	3
Italian, ½ cup, 4.5 oz	30	0	6
Kidney, ½ cup 3.5 oz	105	0.5	19
Lima, ½ cup, 4.5 oz	80	0	15
Pinto, ½ cup, 4.5 oz	105	1	18
Beets: Sliced, ½ cup, 3 oz	25	0	6
Crinkle/Pickled, ½ cup	80	0	20
Carrots: Sliced, ½ cup, 2.5 oz	20	0	4
Del Monte, Honey Glazed, ½ cup	75	0	18
Corn: Kernels, ½ cup, 4.5 oz	80	0.5	18
Creamed style, ½ cup, 4.5 oz	90	0.5	23
Garbanzo/Chick Peas, ½ c, 4.2 oz	145	1.5	27
Hearts of Palm, (1), 1.2 oz	7	0	1
Mushrooms: ½ cup, 2.5 oz	20	0	4
In Butter Sauce, 2 oz	20	1	2
Onions: Cocktail (1)	0	0	0
Pickled, 1 medium, 0.5 oz	10	0	2
Peas, ½ cup, 3 oz	60	0.5	10
Peppers: Hot Chili, Jalapeno (1), 1 oz	5	0	1
Red/Green, 1 oz	5	0	1
Sweet, undrained, 2.5 oz	13	0	3
Jalapeno, with liquid, ½ cup chopped	20	0.5	3
Fried, drained, 2 Tbsp, 1 oz	60	5	3
Salsa, average all varieties, 2 Tbsp	10	0	2
Sauerkraut, drained, 1 cup, 5 oz	25	0	6
Spinach, ½ cup, 3.5 oz	25	0.5	3.5
Succotash: Cream Style, ½ cup	100	0.5	23
W/ whole kernels, undrained, ½ cup	80	0.5	18
Sweetcorn ~ *See Corn*			
Sweet Potato, ½ cup, 3.5 oz	90	0	24
Tomatoes: Sundried: Nat., 5-6 pieces	20	0	5
In Oil, drained, 6 pieces, 0.5 oz	40	2.5	4
Tomato Products ~ *See Page 144*			
Vegetables, mixed, ½ cup	45	0	8
Yams: In Light Syrup, ½ cup, 4 oz	105	0	25
Candied, ½ cup, 5 oz	170	0	46
Zucchini, in Tomato Sauce, ½ cup, 4 oz	30	0	8

Quick Guide

	C	F	Cb
Yogurt: *Average All Brands: Per 8 oz Container*			
Plain Yogurt: Whole	140	8	10
Low-Fat	145	3.5	16
Fat-Free	125	0.5	17
Fruit Flavored: Whole	225	8	32
Low-Fat	230	3	43
Fat-Free, regular	215	0.5	43
Fat-Free, no sugar added	80	0	15
Yogurt Parfait/Deli Cups:			
With Fruit Pieces: (⅔ Yogurt + ⅓ Fruit)			
Small, 8 oz cup	140	3	20
Large, 12 oz cup	210	4.5	30
With Fruit + Granola:			
Small, 8 oz cup (+ 0.75 oz Granola)	235	7	30
Large, 12 oz cup (+ 1.3 oz Granola)	400	13	58

Yogurt ~ Brands

	C	F	Cb
Activia: *Per 4 oz Container Unless Indicated*			
Fiber/Fruit flavors, average	115	2	21
Light flavors, fat free, all flav.	60	0	10
Greek, Light, Fruit Flavors	80	0	8
Alpina, Greek:			
Authentically Strained: *Per 5.3 oz*			
Fruit Flavors, average	120	0	19
Vanilla Bean	120	0	18
Artisan Granolas: *Per 6 oz*			
Plain	170	2.5	22
Fruit flavors, average	210	4.5	29
Bon Yurt: *Per 5.3 oz Container*			
Cookies & Cream	180	3.5	33
Average other flavors	150	1.5	28
Amande:			
Almond Milk Yogurt: Plain, 8 oz	170	9	19
Fruit Flavors, 6 oz	150	6	23
Vanilla, 8 oz	220	8	26
Axelrod:			
32 oz Containers:			
Low Fat, Plain, 8 oz	140	2.5	18
Nonfat, Plain, 8 oz	140	0	21
6 oz Containers:			
Low Fat, Fruit flavors, average	180	1.5	36
Nonfat, Fruit flavors, average	90	0	17
Brown Cow: *Per 6 oz Container*			
Cream Top:			
Fruit On The Bottom:			
Apricot Mango	170	6	23
Cherry-Vanilla	180	6	28
Strawberry	180	6	28

Brown Cow (Cont):	C	F	Cb
Cream Top:			
Smooth & Creamy: Plain	130	7	9
Coffee; Vanilla	160	7	19
Nonfat, Blueberry	140	0	26
Greek: *Per 5.3 oz Containers*			
Fruit On The Bottom, Fruit Flavors	130	0	19
Smooth & Creamy, Plain, nonfat	80	0	6
Cabot: *Per 8 oz Serving*			
32 oz Containers, Greek Style:			
Plain	310	22	12
Lowfat (2%): Plain	180	5	12
Strawberry; Vanilla Bean	240	4	34
Chobani: *Per 5.3 oz Containers*			
Blended: Plain	130	6	7
Coconut	150	4.5	16
Fruit Flavors, average	145	3	17
Vanilla	120	0	16
Flip: Almond Coco Loco	240	10	26
Clover Honey	190	2.5	31
Key Lime Crumble	200	6	26
Nutty for 'Nana	200	8	20
Fruit On The Bottom:			
2% Fat, Fruit Flavors, average	140	3	18
Fat Free, Fruit Flavors, average	125	0	20
Simply 100, average all flavors	100	0	15
Dannon:			
Activia ~ *See Activia*			
All Natural:			
Plain: Regular, 8 oz	150	8	11
Lowfat, 6 oz	100	2.5	12
Nonfat, 6 oz	80	0	12
Classic: Coffee, 6 oz	160	2.5	26
Vanilla, 6 oz	150	2.5	25
Creamy, Fruit Flavors, average, 4 oz	95	0.5	18
Danimals, Crunchers, all flav., 3.5 oz	100	1.5	18
Fruit On The Bottom,			
average all flavors, 6 oz	150	1.5	29
Light & Fit: All flavors, 6 oz	80	0	16
Quarts, Strawb.; Vanilla, av., 8 oz	105	0	18
Carb & Sugar Control,			
all flavors, 4 oz cup	45	1.5	3
Oikos: *Per Single, 5.3 oz Container, Unless Indicated*			
Traditional, Fruit flavors	160	4.5	19
Fat-Free: Plain	80	0	6
Fruit On Bottom, average all flav.	125	0	20
Emmi: *Per 6 oz Container*			
Swiss: Plain, lowfat	110	2.5	10
Average other flavors	110	3	28

Yogurt Brands (Cont)

	C	F	Cb
Fage:			
Total Classic: Plain, Single Serve, 7 oz	190	10	8
Fruit Flavors, average, 5.3 oz	170	6	17
Total 2%:			
Plain, Single Serve, 7 oz	150	4	8
Fruit Flavors, av., 5.3 oz	140	2.5	17
Total 0%,			
Strawberry, Single Serve, 5.3 oz	120	0	17
Horizon Organic: *Per 8 oz Cup*			
Cream On Top:			
Whole Milk: Plain	160	7	14
Vanilla	220	6	32
Fat-Free: Plain	80	0	12
Vanilla	170	0	33
Tuberz, all flavors, 1 tube	60	0.5	11
Kemps:			
Greek Style:			
Fat Free, av. all var., 5.3 oz	130	0	18
Snack Mousse, all flavors, 4.8 oz	190	2.5	31
Light, 80 Calories, av. all flavors, 6 oz	80	0	16
La Yogurt: *Per 6 oz Container*			
Low Fat: Original, average all flavors	155	1.5	29
Rich & Creamy, average all flavors	180	1.5	35
Sabor Latino, Low Fat, all flavors	185	1.5	37
LALA:			
32 oz Tubs, Plain, 8 oz	130	2.5	17
Single Serve: Fruit Flavors, av., 6 oz	150	1.5	30
Pina Colada, 6 oz	160	2	30
Liberte:			
Greek: Coconut, 5.3 oz	140	2	19
Fruit Flavors, average, 5.3 oz	135	0	22
Lucerne: *Per 6 oz Container*			
Low-Fat, av. all flavors.	170	2	32
Fat-Free: Plain	80	0	13
Light Fat-Free, fruit, 6 oz	90	0	17
Mountain High: *Per 8 oz*			
32 oz Containers:			
Original Style: Plain	170	6	19
Strawberry; Vanilla	210	6	30
Low-Fat: Plain	140	2.5	18
Strawberry; Vanilla	180	2.5	29
Fat-Free: Plain	120	0	18
Vanilla	160	0	30
Nancy's: *Per 8 oz Container*			
Natural:			
Whole Milk: Honey Yogurt, Plain	180	8	17
With Fruit on Top, av.	230	5	41
Lowfat: Lemon; Van., av.	145	3	16
Average other flavors	175	2.5	28
Organic:			
Fruit-On-Top, average	150	0	28
Low Fat, Plain	140	3	16

	C	F	Cb
Oikos ~ *see Dannon & Stonyfield*			
O Organics, Blended Low-Fat,			
average all flavors, 6 oz	160	2.5	26
Publix:			
Fat Free, Light, average all flavors, 6 oz	110	0	19
Premium Greek, av. all flavors, 5.3 oz	130	0	18
Schnucks,			
Light, average all flavors, 6 oz	110	0	20
Silk *(Dairy Free):*			
Black Cherry, 5.3 oz	160	3	26
Blueberry, 5.3 oz	140	3.5	22
Peach Mango; Strawb; Van., 5.3 oz	150	3.5	25
So Delicious:			
Cultured Coconut Milk: Plain, 4 oz	80	4.5	12
Chocolate, 6 oz	170	7	27
Pina Colada; Raspb. av., 6 oz	140	6	22
Greek: Plain, 6 oz	130	5	22
Blueberry, 6 oz	130	4.5	25
Stater Bros: *Per 6 oz Container Unless Indicated*			
Plain	105	1.5	14
Fruit on the Bottom, av. all flavors	170	1.5	34
Blended Low-Fat, av. all flavors	155	1.5	29
32 oz Tubs: Non-Fat, Plain, 8 oz	120	0	18
Low Fat, 8 oz	140	2	19
Stonyfield Organic: *Per 6 oz Container*			
Fruit On Bottom: *Per 6 oz Container*			
Fat Free: Chocolate Underground	170	0	36
Average other flavors	115	0	22
Low Fat, Fruit Varieties	130	1.5	22
Greek: *Per 5.3 oz Containers*			
Plain	80	0	6
Chocolate	140	0	23
Honey	120	0	18
Vanilla	130	0	20
Smooth & Creamy (32 oz Ctn): *Per 8 oz Serving*			
Fat Free: Plain	100	0	16
French Vanilla	170	0	33
Low Fat: Plain,	120	2	15
French Vanilla	170	2	29
Strawberry; Banilla, av.	195	2.5	36
Whole Milk: Plain	170	8	31
Stop & Shop:			
Blended, Light, Non Fat,			
average all flavors, 6 oz	90	0	16
Fruit On The Bottom,			
Low Fat, average all flavors, 6 oz	170	1.5	31
Trader Joes:			
French Village: *Per 32 oz Containers*			
Non-Fat: Plain, 8 oz	120	0	17
Vanilla, 8 oz	180	0	34
Cream Line, Plain, 8 oz	170	10	12
6 oz Container, av. all flav.	130	0	26

continued next page

Yogurt Brands (Cont) — C F Cb

Trader Joes (Cont):

	C	F	Cb
Greek Style: Plain, 8 oz	260	18	14
Apricot Mango; Honey, av., 8 oz	300	15	28
Low-Fat: With Almonds/Granola:			
Pomegranate, 4.6 oz	140	2.5	27
Vanilla, 4.6 oz	160	7	20
Organic Non-Fat:			
Plain, 5.3 oz	90	0	7
Honey; Vanilla, av., 5.3 oz	130	0	19
Squishers, Org., low fat, 1 tube, 2 oz	60	1	10
Voskos, Greek, Non-Fat, Van., 8 oz	200	0	30
Wallaby Organic, Blended,			
Low-Fat, Fruit Flavors, average, 6 oz	140	2.5	24

Wegmans: Per 6 oz Container

	C	F	Cb
Blended Lowfat, Fruit Flavors	170	1.5	33
Fruit On The Bottom, Lowfat:			
Strawberry	180	2	35
Average other Fruit Flavors	165	2	31
Greek, Non-Fat: Plain	90	0	8
Fruit flavors, average	140	0	20
Vanilla Flavored	120	0	15

Whole Foods (365):

	C	F	Cb
Non-Fat: Plain, 6 oz	90	0	13
Fruit flavors, av., 6 oz	145	0	30
Greek, non-fat, 5.3 oz	150	0	25
Whole Soy: Plain, 6 oz	150	4.5	19
Av. other flavors, 6 oz	170	3.5	33

YoCrunch: Per 6 oz Container Unless Indicated

	C	F	Cb
Cookies & Candy Crunch:			
Strawberry: With Nestle Crunch pieces	190	4	34
With Oreo Cookie pieces	170	2	29
Vanilla, with pieces, av. all flavors	180	4	32
Fruit Parfaits, with Granola, all var.	160	1	37
100 Calorie, average all flavors	100	1.5	19

Yoplait: Per 6 oz Container Unless Indicated

	C	F	Cb
Original, 99% Fat-Free, all flavors	170	1.5	33
Light: Fat-Free, Fruit flavors	90	0	16
Thick & Creamy, all flavors	100	0	21
With Granola, all flavors	190	2.5	35
Fruitful, average all flavors	170	5	24
Fruplait, average all flavors, 4 oz ctn	115	1	22
GoGurt: Av. all flavors, 1 tube, 2.3 oz	60	0.5	12
Protein, 1 tube 2.3 oz	60	0	9
Simply GoGurt, 1 tube, 2.3 oz	70	0.5	13
Twists, 1 tube, 2.3 oz	60	0.5	12

Yogurt Brands (Cont) — C F Cb

Yoplait (Cont):

	C	F	Cb
Greek, 0% Fat:			
100 Calories, Fruit Flavors, 5.3 oz	100	0	14
Blended Fruit Flavors, av., 5.3 oz	140	0	22
Thick & Creamy, all flavors	180	2.5	31
Trix, Fruit flavors, average, 4 oz cup	100	0.5	20
Whips!: Chocolate flavors,			
4 oz cup	160	4	25
Fruit flavors, 4 oz cup	140	2.5	25
Yoplait Kids, all flavors, 3 oz cup	70	1	13

Yogurt Drinks & Probiotics

	C	F	Cb
Alpina, Yogurt Smoothie,			
average all flavors, 7 oz	120	2	19
BioKult, Cultured,			
all flavors, 2.1 oz bottle	35	0	8
Cacique, Yonique,			
average other flavors, 7 fl.oz	200	1.5	35
Dannon: Activia, all flavors, 7 fl oz	160	3	27
DanActive, Strawb. Banana, 3.1 fl.oz	70	1	14
Danimals, Smoothies,			
all flavors, 3.1 fl.oz	60	0.5	11
Dan-o-nino, all flav., 3.1 fl.oz	70	0.5	15
Glen Oaks, 32 fl.oz Containers,			
average all flavors, 8 fl.oz	150	3	28

Good Belly: Per 2.7 fl.oz Bottle

	C	F	Cb
Probiotics: BigShot, all flavors	60	1	11
Plus, average all flavors	50	0	12
Straightshot, Plain, 2.7 fl oz	30	0	6
Kemps, Yo-J Drink, 16 fl.oz ctn,			
all flavors, 8 fl. oz	120	0	27

LaLa:

	C	F	Cb
Lalacult, 5 pack, 1 bottle	35	0	9
Proactive: Prune, 6.3 oz bottle	180	3	36
Average other flavors, 6.3 oz bottle	155	3.5	30
Yogurt Smoothies av. all flavors, 7 fl.oz	175	4.5	29

Lifeway:

	C	F	Cb
Kefir Smoothie:			
32 fl. oz Container: Original, 8 fl.oz	150	8	12
Lowfat: Chocolate Truffle, 8 fl.oz	160	2	25
Other flavors, 8 fl.oz	140	2	20
Ralphs,			
Smoothies, average, 7 fl.oz	200	2.5	37
Stonyfield Organic,			
Super Smoothies, av. all flav., 10 oz	230	3	40
Yakult, 2.7 fl.oz bottle	50	0	12

Cafeteria-Style Foods **C** **F** **Cb**

Average All Preparations:

	C	F	Cb
Beef Stroganoff, 5 oz	195	13	7
Beef Stroganoff, with 4 oz noodles	350	14	36
Chicken Lasagna, 1 piece	300	11	32
Chicken Chop Suey, with 4 oz rice	245	4	37
Deep Dish Burrito, 7 oz	265	13	20
Ground Beef Casserole, 2 scps, 6 oz	245	13	17
Italian Meat Sce, for Spaghetti, 5 oz	150	9	9
with 5 oz Spaghetti	350	10	49
Lasagna, 1 piece	275	11	25
Meatloaf, 3 oz	205	13	4
Ranch Beans, 2 scoops, 6 oz	350	11	45
Red Beans & Rice, 7 oz	280	9	37
Scalloped Potato/Ham, 2 scoops, 6 oz	160	6	20
Stuffed Shells in Sauce, (1)	105	3	17
Swedish Meatballs, (3)	205	12	9
Sweet & Sour Pork/Rice, 9 oz	240	3	40
Swiss Steak, w/ Mushroom Gravy, 6 oz	280	11	4
Tator Tot Casserole, 2 scoops, 6 oz	260	15	20
Tenderloin Tips/Mshrm Gravy: 5 oz	210	13	3
With 5 oz noodles	395	15	38
Tuna Noodle Casserole, 2 scoops, 6 oz	180	6	17
Turkey Tetrazzini, 2 scoops, 6 oz	195	7	17
Vegetable Lasagna, 1 piece	250	13	21

Croissants

	C	F	Cb
Unfilled, medium 1.5 oz	180	10	21
Filled: With Ham (2 oz), garnish	280	14	24
With Ham (2 oz), Cheese (2 oz)	470	30	20
With Chick (2 oz) Cheese (2 oz)	470	30	20
With Turkey/Ham/Cheese (2 oz ea.)	580	36	20
Au Bon Pain: Ham & Cheese	390	21	35
Spinach & Cheese	290	17	28

7-Eleven ~ See Page 236

Bagels

	C	F	Cb
Plain: Large, 4 oz (without filling)	320	2	65
With 2 oz Cream Cheese	500	27	54
With 2 oz Lox (Smoked Salmon)	400	4	65

Also see Bagels Section ~ Page 54
Fast-Foods Restaurants ~ Page 175
Au Bon Pain ~ Page 179
Bruegger's ~ Page 185
Einstein Bros Bagels ~ Page 199

Sandwiches **C** **F** **Cb**

No Spreads Unless Indicated:
Includes 2 Slices Bread ~ 3 oz

	C	F	Cb
BLT, (5 strips Bacon, 2 Tbsp Mayo)	600	40	46
Breaded Chicken & Garnish	540	28	46
Chicken Salad, with Mayo., 5 oz	580	30	44
Chopped Liver, Egg Mayonnaise	630	25	44
Corned Beef with Mustard, 5 oz	560	28	44
Egg Salad, with Mayonnaise	570	29	49
Egg Salad Club, with Bacon & Mayo,	780	53	49
Grilled Cheese, (3 oz)	540	30	44
Ham, (4 oz), Cheese (4 oz), & Mayo.	910	56	44
Lobster Salad, (4 oz), w/ Mayo.	530	25	45
Overstuffed Tuna Salad, (7 oz)	870	39	75
Philly Cheese Steak Sandwich	550	23	42
Reuben, (6 oz Beef/Pastrami,			
2 oz Cheese, 2 Tbsp Dressing)	920	60	28
Roast Beef, (4 oz), with Mustard	460	12	45
Roast Pork, (4 oz), with Apple Sauce	500	16	55
Shrimp Salad Club, w/ Bacon & Mayo	800	57	48
Sloppy Joe with Sauce, (7 oz)	600	30	45
Steak Sandwich, (5 oz cooked)	680	32	41
Triple Cheese Melt, (4 oz)	720	45	46
Tuna Salad, (5 oz), with Mayonnaise	610	30	49
Turkey Breast, (5 oz), w/ Mayo.	460	18	44
Turkey Breast, (5 oz), with Mustard	360	7	44
Turkey Club, with Bacon & Mayo.	830	38	31
Vegetarian, with Avocado & Cheese	820	49	72

7-Eleven ~ Page 236
Schlotzsky's ~ Page 237
Subway ~ Page 245

Wraps & Roll-Ups

Average All Types
Meat/Chicken/Fish/Veggie:

	C	F	Cb
Small, approximately 9 oz	500	25	48
Regular, approximately 15 oz	830	40	80
Large, approximately 22 oz	1400	70	134

Fast-Foods Restaurants ~ Page 175
Au Bon Pain ~ Page 179
Sonic Drive-In ~ Page 241
Subway ~ Page 245
WAWA ~ Page 254

Fair & Carnival Foods | C | L | Cb

Barbeque Chicken/Meats:

Item	C	L	Cb
Chicken, ½ chicken, 15 oz	740	24	34
Grilled Chicken Pita, with dressing	680	19	82
Teriyaki Chicken, on stick, w/ dress.	250	6	4
Pork Ribs, 18 oz	1360	68	21
Turkey Leg: Regular, 19 oz	1135	54	0
Caveman (2lb Turkey Leg, with 1lb Bacon)	2360	177	3
Bacon: Fried, on-a-stick, with syrup	230	16	5
Choc-covered Bacon, 4.5 oz dish	640	43	30
Beef Stew over Rice, 2 cups	440	14	61
Butter Balls, deep fried, 4 Balls	460	38	24
Cheese Curds, Breaded & fried, Culver's, 6.7 oz	670	38	54
Corn Dogs: Regular, 4 oz	250	14	23
Jumbo, 6 oz	375	21	36
Pretzel-Wrapped Dog	300	16	30
Papa Pup, on-a-stick	400	24	32
Pronto Pup, on-a-stick	170	9	16
Corn On The Cob, 8"(1), 16 oz	200	1	42

Finger Foods:

Item	C	L	Cb
Artichoke, fried, 9 pieces	250	14	24
Chicken Nuggets, (6)	340	17	26
Chicken Strips, (4), 4.5 oz	445	21	33
Onion Rings, 3 rings	310	13	40
Onion Flower	1320	72	140
Shrimp, Fried, 10-12 pieces, 5 oz	555	30	36
Spam, deep-fried in batter, 2 pieces	330	24	18

Gator:

Item	C	L	Cb
Big Gator, Nuggets/Hushpuppies	550	31	54
Stick Gator, 1 sausage	250	20	4

Greek:

Item	C	L	Cb
Baklava, 2" square	245	13	32
Falafel, 11.6 oz	660	27	85
Greek Salad, 14 oz	520	48	17
Gyro, 7.5", 12 oz	680	40	55
Spanakopita, 8 oz	200	7.5	23

Hamburgers:

Item	C	L	Cb
⅓ Pound Burger, 7.5 oz	670	41	26
Cheeseburger, 6 oz	550	36	25

Hot Dogs: With Bun

Item	C	L	Cb
Regular: No extras	215	14	28
With Chili, 6 oz	450	32	32
With Chili & Cheese, 7.3 oz	500	36	31
⅓ Pound Hot Dog	550	41	31
Foot Long Hot Dog	470	26	41
Jumbo, Bratwurst/Kielbasa, average	800	60	28

Fair & Carnival Foods (Cont) | C | F | Cb

Mexican:

Item	C	F	Cb
Burrito, with Bean/Beef, 17 oz	1100	41	104
Carne Asada, 14.5 oz	820	44	58
Cheese Quesadilla, 1.8 oz	480	27	40
Chicken Taco, 3.3 oz	210	12	16
Fish Taco, 5 oz	270	13	31
Jalapeno Pepper, choc-covered (3)	270	15	31
Nachos with Cheese, 9" plate	860	59	70
Tamale, 3.5 oz	180	8	21
Taquito, 5 oz	370	17	43

Pizza:

Item	C	F	Cb
Pizza Bread, Pepperoni, ½ loaf, 12 oz	1115	32	151
Pizza on-a-stick, 1 piece	535	28	55
Personal Pizza: Per 7"			
Cheese	670	24	80
Pepperoni	795	35	80
Ham & Pineapple	800	31	87

Potatoes & Fries:

Item	C	F	Cb
Australian Battered Potatoes	1290	66	155
Baked Potato, 14 oz	435	0.5	100
Fries: French, 7 oz	560	24	79
Cheese Fries, 10 oz	645	38	62
Chili Fries, 10 oz	700	36	83
Curly Fries, 7 oz	620	30	78
Jamaican Jerk Fries, 7 oz	640	34	77
Sweet Potato, baked, 14 oz	405	0.5	97
Tornado, on-a-stick	210	15	18

Salads/Sides:

Item	C	F	Cb
Chili, 1 cup	280	11	24
Cole Slaw, 5 oz	350	21	37
Pickle, whole (6")	30	0	8
Potato Salad, 5 oz	290	15	35

Sandwiches: 7½" Roll

Item	C	F	Cb
Ham, 11 oz	645	39	47
Hot Pastrami, 9 oz	760	17	62
Roast Beef, 11 oz	620	36	46
Philadelphia Cheese Steak, 13 oz	680	36	49
Turkey, 11 oz	665	24	65

Drinks:

Item	C	F	Cb
Icee, 16 fl.oz	235	0	59
Shakes, average, 16 fl.oz	690	33	85
Slushies: Horchata, 16 fl.oz	280	8	50
Lemonade, 18 fl.oz	210	0	52
Orange Julius, 20 fl.oz	490	10	96
Strawberry Julius, 20 fl.oz	430	0	98
Soft Frozen Lemonade, 12 fl.oz	300	0	78
Smoothies, Berry Flavors, 16 fl.oz	350	1	80

Fair & Carnival Foods (Cont)

Cakes, Pastries:	C	F	Cb
Funnel Cake, Plain (1)	760	44	80
Toppings:			
Apple Cinnamon, 2 oz	85	3	16
Cinnamon & Sugar, 2 tsp	40	0	10
Strawberry & Cream, 2 oz	70	0	16
Cheesecake on-a-stick, 6 oz	655	47	56
Churro, (1), 9", 1.6 oz	170	8	22
Cream Puff, 4.3 oz	500	43	22
Fried Twinkie, (1)	420	34	45
Puff-on-a-Stick, (4), 8.6 oz	995	86	44
Strawberry Crepe, 4.3 oz	280	14	36
Twinkie Dog, (Sundae)	500	14	89
Candied Apple, 7 oz	330	0	80
Cookies:			
Sweet Martha, (1), 0.8 oz	90	4	14
Deep Fried: Oreos, tray (5)	890	48	108
Cookie Dough on stick, 3 pieces	670	32	89
Cotton Candy:			
Small, 1 oz	110	0	27
Large, 2.3 oz	250	0	62
Family Size, 5.5 oz	610	0	151
Dirt Dessert, 1 cup, 9.3 oz	405	12	69
Donuts, Jumbo Twist, (1), 7.5 oz	905	49	109
Fried Dough/FryBread:			
Plain: 7", 3.7 oz	390	19	47
9", 4¾ oz	510	25	61
Toppings: Cinnamon Sugar, 2 tsp	40	0	10
Butterscotch; Caramel, 2 Tbsp	115	0	29
Hot Fudge, average, 2 Tbsp	110	4	22
Cheese Powder, 2 tsp	70	3	2
Honey, 1 Tbsp, 0.8 oz	65	0	17
Fudge, 1.5 oz	200	11	25
Ice Cream & Frozen Treats:			
Deep-fried Klondike Bar, w/ syrup	430	16	18
Dippin' Dots Ice Cream, 6 oz cup	380	20	44
Frozen Banana, choc. coated, 5 oz	240	4	53
Frozen Yogurt, in sugar cone, 14 oz	475	2	94
Ice Cream: Small, sugar cone, 10 oz	775	42	83
Large, sugar cone, 14 oz	935	54	99
Sherbet, 8 oz	270	4	59
Snow Cone, with 3 oz syrup	270	0	68
Strawberry, Choc. Dipped, 1 piece	125	7	15
Popcorn:			
Plain: Small, 3 oz	450	24	48
Large, 6 oz	900	48	96
Kettle Corn: Small, 5 oz	600	15	110
Large, 10 oz	1200	30	220
Pretzels, Soft, 4.5 oz	340	2	70
S'more, on stick	275	14	27

Stadium Foods

	C	F	Cb
Burgers:			
Bacon Burger, 8.3 oz	470	25	34
Cheeseburger, 8.3 oz	450	23	33
Hamburger, 7.8 oz	400	19	33
French Fries, 6.4 oz	470	34	39
Fruit Cup, 6 oz	80	0	20
Hot Dogs:			
Chili Dog, 7.7 oz	520	29	45
Hot Dog, 6.4 oz	465	21	50
Jumbo Dog, 6 oz	440	25	38
Kraut Dog with Sauerkraut, 7.8 oz	490	27	41
Individual Pan Pizza (6"): Per Pizza			
BBQ Chicken	630	24	71
Cheese	630	27	71
Pepperoni	660	30	70
Nachos, 40 chips, with 4 oz cheese	1100	59	132
Sandwiches:			
Chicken: With Bacon, 8.3 oz	530	31	41
With Cheese, 8.3 oz	510	29	40
Without Cheese, 7.7 oz	460	25	40
Polish Sausage Sandwich, 7 oz	565	33	45
Snacks:			
Brownie, 2.5" x 4.5"	360	18	44
Cheese Sauce, 1.3 oz	100	8	4
Cheetos, 2.8 oz package	440	28	42
Chocolate Chip Cookie, 2.3 oz	280	12	40
Churro, (1), 10", 2 oz	210	10	26
Doritos, Nacho, 2.8 oz package	390	20	48
King Size Candy:			
Butterfinger, 3.8 oz	480	18	75
Nestle Crunch, 2.8 oz	390	21	85
Lay's, Chips, 2.8 oz package	440	28	42
Peanuts, in shell, 8 oz	930	80	24
Popcorn: Small (9 cup size)	575	35	56
Large (15 cup size)	950	58	93
Pretzel, Soft, Reg., 5.5 oz	490	3.5	101
Red Vines, 5 oz box	500	0	117
Snow Cone: With 3 oz syrup	270	0	68
With 6 oz syrup	540	0	136
Beverages:			
Orange Juice, 12 fl.oz	180	0	21
Beer:			
Heineken, 16 fl.oz	200	0	16
Miller: Draft, 16 fl.oz	195	0	17
Lite, 16 fl.oz	125	16	4
Jack Daniels, Punch, 12 fl.oz	235	0	34
Wine, White, 9 fl.oz	190	0	6
Soda, (with ½ ice), average:			
20 fl.oz	160	0	40
32 fl.oz	260	0	65
Starbuck's, Coffee, Frappuccino, 9.5 fl.oz	200	3	37

Asian & Chinese Dishes

	C	F	Cb
Appetizers:			
Crab Cake, 2.3 oz	125	10	1
Dumplings: *Per Dumpling*			
Pork: Steamed	80	4.5	5
Fried	90	6	5
Vegetable, steamed	35	1	5
Egg Rolls, Mini, 3 rolls	100	3	11
Spring Roll:			
Small, 1.5 oz	85	4	9
Medium, 3 oz	170	8	17
Large, 5 oz	290	15	29
Wonton, 1 only	75	4	5
Soup: Egg Flower, bowl 12 oz	90	2	16
Hot & Sour Soup, bowl 12 oz	110	3.5	14
Rice: Plain, 1 cup, 6.5 oz	320	2	66
2 Cups, 13 oz	640	4	132
Fried: 1 cup, 5 oz	365	11	55
Large dish, 16 oz	950	28	67
Noodles, Chinese Egg, cooked, 1 cup	200	4	37
Entrees & Mains: *Per Serving*			
Almond Chicken, 6 oz	270	10	21
BBQ Pork, 5.5 oz	440	23	15
Beef in Black Bean Sauce, 8.5 oz	390	17	17
Broccoli Beef, 6 oz	370	21	13
Chicken & Broccoli, 5.5 oz	160	8	10
Chicken Skewers, 3 oz	210	9	18
Chop Suey:			
Chicken, 5 oz	140	9	2
Pork, 5 oz	170	12	3
Chow Mein, Beef/Chicken, 8 oz	390	12	59
Crab Puff/Rangoon, 1 dumpling	190	11	13
Crispy Fried Chicken, 8 oz	485	33	12
Egg Drop Soup: With Noodles, 1 cup	110	3	16
Without Noodles, 1 cup	60	3	4
Egg Foo Yung with Sauce, 1 cup	270	15	16
Kung Pao Chicken, 5.5 oz	240	15	12
Lemon Chicken, 5 oz	525	21	57
Lo Mein, stir-fried, 8 oz	705	42	49
Omelet, Chicken/Shrimp, 16 oz	990	82	10
Orange Chicken, 5.5 oz	500	27	42
Steamed Whole Fish,			
½ Sockeye Salmon	646	36	23
Sweet & Sour:			
Fish, 20 oz	1160	58	106
Pork, 5.5 oz	400	23	35
Vegetable Combo, with oil, 6 oz	367	5	66
Vegetables, Steamed, without oil, 6 oz	135	1	29
Sauces: Mandarin Sauce 1.5 oz	70	0	17
Potsticker Sauce, 1.5 oz	35	0	8
Bubble Tea, average, 12 fl oz	280	0.5	68
Fortune Cookie, each	32	0.5	7

Cajun & Creole

	C	F	Cb
Alligator, cooked, 4 oz	160	2	0
Baked Herb Chicken, 1 serving	850	53	2
Bouillabaisse	400	15	10
Cajun Fried Turkey, 1 serving	630	25	0
Cocktail Sauce, 2 Tbsp	30	0	6
Couche-Couche, ½ cup	80	0	17
Crawfish Bisque, 1 serving	500	10	10
Crawfish, cooked, 2 oz	45	0.5	0
Creole Jambalaya,			
1 serving	550	30	15
Frog Legs, steamed (2)	45	0	0
Guinea Fowl, flesh, 4 oz, cooked	160	4	0
Hogshead Cheese, ¼ cup	80	5.5	0
Jambalaya, Shrimp & Crabmeat	520	14	12
Red Beans & Rice, 1 serving	400	17	52
Roasted Quail, with Bacon, on Toast	550	25	15
Remoulade Sauce, 2 Tbsp, 1 oz	110	11	2
Shrimp Creole, 1 serving	450	20	10
Stuffed Smothered Steak,			
with 1 cup Rice	890	50	50
Turtle, cooked, 3 oz	120	3	0

Canadian

	C	F	Cb
Bagels, Montreal-Style:			
Plain, 100g/3.5 oz	300	2	60
Poppyseed, 100g/3.5 oz	310	4	58
Sesame, 100g/3.5 oz	320	6	56
Bannock: Plain 33g/1.2 oz	120	3	20
With currants/raisins, 85g/3 oz	215	9	32
Meals:			
Baked Beans in Maple Syrup,			
1 cup, 250g/8.8 oz	320	1	62
Donnairs (*Pizza Delight*):			
Famous, regular, 250g/8.8 oz	510	21	60
Super, regular, 310g/11 oz	685	34	62
Poutine:			
A&W, 330g/12 oz	610	33	58
Boston Pizza, regular, 400g/14 oz	610	30	67
Burger King, Classic, 330g/11.6 oz	680	36	72
Harvey's, 240g/8.5 oz	730	41	63
McDonald's, 1 serving	510	29	44
Swiss Chalet,			
Chalet -Style, 340g/12 oz	150	12	195
Shish Taouk:			
Chicken, 1 skewer, 200g/7 oz	270	25	9
Wrap, 455g/16 oz	1150	12	195
Tassot:			
Beef, 283g/10 oz	430	28	12
Goat, 100g/3.5 oz	360	36	9
Toutiere, 170g/6oz	600	42	35

Canadian (Cont)

	C	F	Cb
Pastries:			
Beaver Tails:			
Cheese & Garlic, 80g/2.8 oz	390	30	28
Cinnamon & Sugar, 80g/2.8 oz	315	13	30
Butter Tart, mini, 1 tart	120	3	16
May West,			
Original, 54g/1.9 oz	240	11	34
Nanaimo Bar, 56g/2 oz	270	16	30
Snacks: Maple Syrup Taffy, 40g/1.4 oz	130	0	33
Potato Chips: Dill Pickle Flav., 40g	160	10	15
Ketchup Flavor, 50g/1.8 oz	260	16	26

French Foods

	C	F	Cb
Blanquette d' Agneau, (Lamb Stew)	800	30	17
Brioche, 1 cake	280	14	34
Bouillabaisse	400	15	10
Coq au Vin, leg/thigh	700	28	31
Coquilles St. Jacques	320	13	36
Crème Brulée, 1 serving	460	40	21
Baguette, 3 slices, 2.2 oz	150	1	35
Creme Caramel, (Caramel Custard)	260	10	38
Crepe Suzette, 1x6" crepe with sauce	220	10	13
Duck a l'Orange, ¼ duck, 22 oz	970	44	19
Escargot, (Snails), in garlic butter (6)	200	10	4
Frog Legs, fried, 4 medium pairs	400	20	10
Lamb Noisettes, fried, 2 chops	500	40	1
Potage Creme Crecy, (Carrot Soup)	360	18	14
Salade Nicoise, (Tuna/Olives/Vegs)	450	13	14
Veal Cordon Bleu, (Veal/Ham)	650	25	18
Vichyssoise, (Potato /Leek Soup), 1 c.	200	9	15
Baguette & French Stick ~ Page 54			

German

	C	F	Cb
Beef: Goulash with Veggies	520	20	46
Weiner Schnitzel, 1 medium	750	35	38
Chicken: Fried, Viennese-style	530	20	28
Livers with Apple/Onion, 6 oz	460	28	10
Herring, pickled: Rollmops, 4 oz	260	16	3
With Sour Cream, 4 oz	310	20	3
Pork, Sauerbraten (Pot Roast)	650	35	15
Sausage: Bratwurst, grilled, 6 oz	450	37	2
Hot Sausage Curry	300	7	6
Cakes:			
Black Forest, 1 slice	380	16	30
Bavarian Bread Dumpling, 3 small	330	10	28
Kugelhupf Cake, 1 large slice, 4 oz	400	23	40
Torte: Linzer (Almond/Raspb. Jam)	430	18	58
Sacher (Chocolate/Apricot Jam)	260	12	23

Greek

	C	F	Cb
Baklava Pastry: Small	240	13	32
Large, 3.8 oz	400	21	45
Calamari, deep fried, 1 cup	300	13	17
Chicken Kebob Plate	345	13	8
Dolmades, 2 rolls, 6 oz	200	5	13
Galactobureko, 1 only			
(Filo, Custard, Pastry in Syrup)	360	15	48
Greek Chicken Salad	400	18	9
Gyros: 6" Pita, 8 oz	475	32	35
7½" Pita, 12 oz	680	40	55
Hummus & Pita, 4 oz	260	12	30
Kataifi, (Filo, Nut, Pastry in Syrup)	350	11	56
Moussaka, Small serving, 8 oz	350	22	22
Large serving, 16 oz	700	44	44
Soup, Avgolemono (Egg & Lemon			
with Chicken & Rice), 1 cup	85	6	5
Souvlaki, (Lamb), each, 2 oz	120	6	1
Stuffed Tomatoes, (2)	250	12	17
Taramasalata, 1 T., 0.5 oz	40	3	2
Tyropita, (Filo/Cheese Pastry)	350	26	31

Hawaiian

	C	F	Cb
Ahi Tuna, grilled w/o fat, 6 oz fillet	220	2	0
Chicken Long Rice, 1 cup, 7 oz	240	14	14
Gyoza, 1 only	55	2	6
Haupia, (Coconut Pudd.), 1 pce, (4"x 2½")	120	6	17
Hawaiian Sweet Bread, ½" slice, 2 oz	180	4.5	29
Kalua: Chicken, 4 oz	280	16	0
Pork, 4 oz	350	24	0
Kim Chee, (pickled cabbage), ½ cup, 4 oz	20	0	5
Kulolo (Taro Pudding), 1 slice	125	5	19
Lau Lau:			
Chicken (1), 7 oz	280	21	3
Pork (1), 7 oz	320	26	5
Loco Moco (rice/burger/egg/gravy)	650	27	63
Lomi Salmon, ¼ cup, 4 oz	20	1	2
Malasadas, (Donut), 2 oz	240	13	26
Manapua, (Char Siu Pork Bun), 2.3 oz	180	8	25
Poi ,(mashed cooked taro), 1 cup., 8.5 oz	270	0.5	65
Poke, average all types, 4 oz	90	1	0
Portuguese Sausage, 2 oz	180	15	2
Potato Salad, ½ cup, 5 oz	170	10	17
Shave Ice, (Matsumoto), all flavors:			
With Ice Cream, 1 large	300	4	64
With Beans, 1 large	290	0	72
Spam Musubi:			
With Regular Spam	265	11	34
(4 oz rice+1.3 oz Spam/7-Eleven Hawaii)			
Homemade, w/ Lite Spam (50% less fat)	220	5	34
Taro Pancake Mix, ⅓ cup (makes 2)	140	2	26

Hawaiian (Cont)

Plate Lunches:	C	F	Cb
Chicken Katsu: (9 oz:) With Rice	1110	48	108
+ Macaroni Salad, ¾ cup	1360	68	123
or Tossed Salad + 2Tbsp Fr. Dress.	1240	61	111
Hamburger, (5 oz): With Rice	710	24	81
Gravy + Macaroni Salad	1135	49	112
Mahi Mahi, (7 oz): With Rice	650	12	90
+ Macaroni Salad + Tartar Sce	1150	58	109
or Macaroni Salad, w/o Tartar ce	935	34	108
or Tossed Salad + 3 Tbsp Fr. Dress.	815	27	96
or Tossed Salad, without dressing	670	12	93
Teri Beef, (5 oz): With 2 scoops Rice	790	23	94
+ Macaroni Salad, ¾ cup	1095	47	113
or Tossed Salad, without dressing	800	23	95

Indian & Pakistani

Per Serving, Meat dishes allow 4 oz meat/serving

	C	F	Cb
Aloo Samosa, each	155	12	12
Alu Gosht Kari, (Meat/Potato Curry)	600	40	23
Chicken Korma	500	35	6
Chicken Pilaf	700	53	50
Chicken Tikka	260	16	2
Chicken Vindaloo	400	20	8
Chapati/Roti, 7" diameter, 1 piece	60	0.5	11
Dahl, (Lentil Puree):			
1 cup, without oil	230	1	37
1 Tbsp Tadka (oil topping)	120	13	0
Dhakla, (Lentil Dish), 1" square, 1 oz	105	5	13
Dhansak, ½ cup	105	3.5	11
Gosht Kari	460	25	17
Lamb Pilaf	520	35	40
Lassi, (Sweet or Mango), 1 cup, 8 oz	160	4	24
Masala Gosht, (Beef/Tomato/Gravy)	400	25	18
Mulligatawney Soup	300	15	8
Murgh Tikka, 1 cup	300	4	7
Naan Flatbread, 2 oz	160	3.5	29
Pappadum, 1 large/2 small	50	3	5
Pesrattu, (Lentil Crepe), 9", 2.6 oz	130	5	15
Pork Vindaloo Curry, without Rice	620	47	3
Rajmah, 1 cup	225	5	35
Rogan Josh,			
without Rice/Potatoes	500	30	3
Shahi Korma, (Braised Lamb)	430	28	3
Tandoori Chicken:			
Breast	260	13	5
Leg/Thigh portion	300	17	6

Italian Dishes

Entrees:	C	F	Cb
Baked Ziti: Small	370	27	32
Regular	575	42	49
Breadstick, 2 oz piece	120	2.5	25
Broccoli Fettucine Alfredo, regular	815	23	125
Bruschetta, 2 slices	380	17	53
Calzones, av. all varieties	840	34	101
Cannelloni, 1 tube, 6 oz	280	15	18
Cheese Breadstick, 2.4 oz piece	180	8	20
Cheese Ravioli, with sauce	495	17	65
Chicken Alfredo	775	29	82
Chicken Parmigiana, 11 oz	520	22	16
Chicken Scallopine, dinner	1110	71	68
Eggplant Parmigiana	900	39	78
Fettucine Alfredo: Lunch, 9 oz	885	65	63
Dinner, 15 oz	1475	108	104
Linquine & Seafood, dinner	1130	71	79
Manicotti Formaggio	800	38	57
Meat Lasagne:			
Small, 10 oz	440	23	39
Large, 16 oz	700	36	60
Meat Ravioli	725	22	102
Minestrone Soup, 1 bowl	110	2	18
Penne Rustica: Lunch	1300	71	76
Dinner	1540	80	101
Ravioli, over-stuffed, average	990	67	57
Panini Sandwich:			
Chicken, 16 oz	900	38	81
Meats, average, 18 oz	940	39	81
Vegetarian, 15 oz	750	31	83
Pizza, Ready-To-Eat ~ *See Page 135*			
Spaghetti & Meatballs:			
With Tomato Sauce: Kids	500	20	58
Medium/Lunch	1080	63	89
Large/Dinner	1430	81	119
With Meat Sauce: Kids	550	25	56
Medium/Lunch	1300	79	84
Large/Dinner	1700	103	110
Veal Marsala, dinner	1320	66	132
Veal Parmigiana, dinner	1270	65	116
Vegetable Primavera	610	8	116
Salad,			
Caprese , 11 oz	445	34	10
Desserts:			
Gelato: Vanilla (Milk Base), ½ cup	200	15	18
Choc. Hazelnut (Milk), ½ cup	370	29	26
Water Base, ½ cup	100	0	25
Lemon Ice,	180	0	45
Tiramisu, 1 piece, 5 oz	400	29	30
Further listings ~ *See Fast-Foods Section*			

Japanese

	C	F	Cb
Sashimi: (Sliced Raw Seafood/Beef)			
Ika (Squid), 4 oz	105	2	0
Hamachi (Yellowtail), 4 oz	165	6	0
Maguro (Yellowfin Tuna), 4 oz	120	1	0
Niku (Beef), 5 oz	200	10	0
Saba (Mackerel), 4 oz	160	7	0
Suzuki (Sea Bass), 4 oz	110	0.5	0
Tako (Octopus), 4 oz	95	1	0
Sushi Rice: Cooked, 1 Tbsp	25	0	5
1 cup, 5.3 oz	380	3	82
Sushi (Maki) Rolls: *Per Piece*			
Average all types (California Rolls; Cream Cheese with Crab; Eel; Salmon; Shrimp; Tuna; Yellowtail; Vegetable)			
Small (1.2" diam. x 1.2" high), 0.8 oz	25	0.5	3.5
Medium (1¾" diam. x 1¾" high), 1.6 oz	50	1	7
Large (2¼" diam. x ⅞" high), 2 oz	60	1.5	9
Sushi Packs: *Per Pack*			
Average all types: 6 large pieces	370	5	55
9 medium pieces	360	6	60
12 small pieces	265	3	45
Futomaki (thick roll), 6 pieces	380	5	72
Hand Roll (Cone), 4 oz	120	2	18
Inari (rice filled soybean pocket), 4 pces	420	9	73
Sushi-Nigiri, (fish on rice), average all varieties, 1 piece	70	0.5	12
Sushi Plate: Assorted: 6 pieces	420	3	36
Combination (Sushi & Sushi Rolls) 2 Sushi + 6 small & 3 medium rolls	400	7	72
Dipping Sauces: Average, 2 Tbsp	30	0	7
Ginger Vinegar Dressing, 2 Tbsp	20	0	5
Edamame: (young green soybeans):			
Boiled beans (no pods), 4 oz	160	7	12
Steamed (in pods), 4 oz	60	3	5
Katsu-don, Pork with Rice	1100	39	141
Miso Soup, with Tofu pieces, 1 cup	85	3	11
Sake Wine, (16% alcohol), 3 fl.oz	115	0	7
Seaweed Salad, 1.5 oz	20	2	0
Sukiyaki, (Beef/Tofu/Veggies), 8 oz	400	24	32
Tempura:			
3 large shrimp & veggies	320	18	25
1 shrimp only	60	4	3
Teppan Yaki, (Steak, Seafood & Veggies), 10 oz serving	470	30	15
Teriyaki: Beef, 4 oz	350	25	4
Chicken, 4 oz	260	9	7
Salmon, medium, 6 oz	270	8	3
Yakatori, 1 skewer, 2.5 oz	140	5	1

Kosher/Deli Foods

	C	F	Cb
Bagel/Bialy, 1 small, 2 oz	160	2	32
Beiglach, (Cheese Knish)	350	17	35
Blintzes: Average, 1 only	120	1	25
With Sour Cream & Preserves	370	10	30
Borscht, (Without Sour Cream): 1 cup	85	3	14
Diet/Reduced Calorie, 1 cup	30	1	7
Cabbage Roll, (meat/rice), 5 oz	170	6	21
Chicken Broth: 1 cup	80	8	0
With vegetables	100	8	5
With noodles	150	9	16
Lowfat, plain, 1 cup	25	1	0
Cholent, 1 medium serving, 1 cup	350	16	48
Chopped Liver: 1 serving, 3 oz	110	6	1
With Egg Salad, ¼ cup	100	7	3
Farfel, dry, ½ cup	90	0.5	21
Gefilte Fish Balls:			
Regular, 2 oz	55	2	4
With Jelled Broth	80	2	6
Cocktail size, 1 oz	30	1	2
Sweet: Medium, 2 oz	65	2	4
With Jelled Broth	95	2	9
Hallah, (Yeast Bread), 1 slice, 1 oz	85	2	14
Herring: Smoked, 2 oz	120	8	0
In Sour Cream, 2 oz	150	10	0
Kasha, cooked, ½ cup	100	0.5	20
Kipfel, (Vanilla/Almdond Cookie), 1 pce	60	2	7
Knaidlach ~ *See Matzo Balls*			
Knish: Kasha/Potato, 1 only	130	4	22
Cheese, 1 only	350	17	35
Kreplach, beef, 1 piece	40	1	4
Kugel, potato/noodle, 1 serving	300	20	25
Latkes, (Potato Pancake): 2 oz	200	11	22
3 Latkes w/ Sour Cran Apple Sauce	750	25	95
Lochshen: Plain, 1 cup	130	2	26
Pudding, 1 cup	380	13	48
Lox, (Smoked Salmon), 2 oz	65	2	0
Mandelbrot, (Almond Bread), 1 slice, ¼" thick	45	2	5
Matzo, 1 oz board	110	0.5	21
Matzo Balls: 2 small, or 1 large, 2"	90	3	12
Extra large ball, 3"	180	6	24
Matzo Ball Soup:			
Cup w/ 2 small or 1 large ball	150	5	27
Bowl w/ Chkn & Noodles	325	13	34
Jerry's Deli, large bowl	560	17	56
NY Cheesecake, 4 oz	350	24	26
Pierogi, potato/cheese, 1 piece	90	4	11
Reuben S'wich, w/ ½ lb Corned Beef	920	60	28
Schmaltz, (Rend'd Chicken Fat), 1 T.	90	10	0

Restaurant & International Foods

Korean Food

	C	F	Cb
Bibimbab, (Veg. & Beef on Rice), 1 cup	565	15	89
Bulgogi, (Barbeque Beef), 3.5 oz	325	12	15
Galbi (Short Ribs), 16 oz	975	61	16
Gujeolpan, (Pancake with Meat & Vegetables), 1 cup with 1 pancake	340	11	39
Japchae, (Noodle w/ Veggies & Meat), 1¼ cups	365	19	34
Sides:			
Kimchee, (Cabbage Relish), ½ cup	30	0	6
Namool, (Assorted Vegetables), 1 cup	125	6.5	4
Soups: Per Serving			
Muguk, (Radish & Chive Soup), 6 oz	105	7	6
Samgyetang, (Ginseng Chkn Soup):			
Without Chicken Skin, 1 cup	520	11	60
With Chicken Skin, 1 cup	725	35	60
Yuk Gae Jang, (Spicy Beef Soup), 1¼ cups	180	13	5

Lebanese/Middle East

	C	F	Cb
Baba Ghannouj, 2 Tbsp, 1 oz	70	6	2
Baklava, (Pastry, Nuts, Syrup), 1 pastry, 13/4 oz	245	18	18
Cabbage Rolls, (Cabb. Leaf, Meat, Rice), 1 roll, 3 oz	100	3	12
Cous Cous, (Semolina, Milk, Fruit, Nuts), 1 cup	400	21	43
Falafel, (Chick Pea Fritter), Fried, 1 medium, 1 oz	60	4	4
Hummus, ¼ cup, 2.2 oz	105	3	5
Fried Kibbi, (Wheat, Meat Pinenuts), 1 piece, 3 oz	180	8	15
Kafta, (Ground Lamb, Ssge on Skewer), 1 skewer, 1.5 ozoz	85	5	2
Kibbeh Naye, (raw Lamb, Bulgur & Spice) 1 cup, 9 oz	450	18	28
Lebanese Omelet, 1 serving, 4 oz (Egg, Spinach, Pinenuts, Onion)	200	12	13
Pilaf, (Rice, Onion, Raisins, Apr., Spice) 1 cup	400	4	60
Shawourma, (Spit-Roast Beef), 4 oz serving	280	15	2
Shish Kabob, 1 stick, 2.5 oz	130	7	2
Spinach Pie, 1 piece, 3.5 oz	290	21	20
Sweet Almond Sanbusak, (Pastry, Almonds, Spices), 1 piece	200	15	11
Tabouli, 1 serving, 4 oz	125	7	13
Tahini Sauce, average, 1 Tbsp	90	8	2

Mexican

	C	F	Cb
Burritos *(Taco Bell):* Bean	370	10	56
Supreme Beef	420	16	53
Chili, plain, ¼ cup	90	6	8
Chili con Carne: With Beans, 1 cup	310	17	15
Without Beans, 1 cup	370	28	10
Chimichangas, Beef, 5 oz	400	19	43
Chorizo Sausage, 2 oz	265	23	0
Churro, (1), 1.5 oz	150	8	18
Corn Chips, ½ cup, 1 oz	160	10	17
Enchilada, average	330	10	49
Fajitas, Chicken	200	7	20
Guacamole, average, 2 Tbsp, 1 oz	45	4	2
Horchata: *(Don Jose)*, 1 cup, 8 fl.oz	140	4	25
Cacique, 1 pint bottle, 16 fl.oz	320	7	62
Margarita, with 1.5 oz Tequila	160	0	6
Masa, (Pre-mixed for Tamales), 1 oz	80	5	9
Menudo:			
With Hominy, 1 cup	240	9	19
Without Hominy, 1 cup	170	9	2
Nachos: With cheese, peppers, 1 portion, 6-8 nachos, 7 oz	600	33	60
With cheese, beans, peppers, 1 portion, 6-8 nachos, 9 oz	570	31	56
Del Taco: Regular, 4 oz	300	19	30
Macho Nachos, 17 oz	1000	56	94
Taco Bell, BellGrande®, 10.8 oz	780	40	84
Nopal Cactus Salad, 1 cup	130	9	11
Papas Fritas, (1), 6 oz	325	18	40
Piloncillo, (Brown Sugar):			
1 Tbsp, 0.5 oz	50	0	13
Cone, small, 3", 3 oz	325	0	81
Quesadilla, Cheese	490	28	39
Queso Fresco, ¼ cup	80	4.5	2
Refried Beans, ¾ cup, 6 oz	160	5	26
Rice Pudding, (Arroz Con Leche), 4 oz	140	3	24
Soup, Black Bean, 1 bowl	200	3	34
Tacos *(Taco Bell):*			
Crunchy: Regular	170	10	12
Supreme	200	12	15
Soft: Crispy Potato	270	13	31
Grilled Steak	250	14	19
Taco Salad with Salsa	840	52	85
Taco Sauce, average, ¼ cup	15	0	3
Taco Shell, regular	50	2	8
Tamales, Beef/Chicken, av. 4.5 oz	250	11	27
Taquitos, Beef & Cheese, 4.5 oz	330	15	36
Tostada *(Taco Bell)*	250	10	29
Tortilla, Corn, 6" diameter	70	1	14
Tortilla Chips, 1 oz	150	8	18
Soup, Black Bean, 1 bowl	200	3	34

Extra Food Listings ~ See Fast Food Section
(Examples: Del Taco, Taco Bell, Taco Cabana, Taco Time)

Mexican (Cont) **C F Cb**

Breads:

	C	F	Cb
Bolillos, 1 roll, 3.5 oz	240	4	42
Mexican Cornbread, 4" square	210	11	19
Pan de Leche, 1 roll, 1.3 oz	110	2.5	20
Telera, 2 oz	150	1.5	19

Cakes, Cookies, Pastries Pan Dulce:

	C	F	Cb
Banderilla, 1 piece	140	10	8
Bigotes, 7"	570	22	44
Capirotada, (Bread Pudding), 10 oz	810	38	107
Cinnamon Cookies, 2	125	8	13
Concha, av. all varieties:			
Small (3" diameter), 2.5 oz	250	8	38
Medium (4" diameter), 3.5 oz	350	11	53
Large (5" diameter), 5.5 oz	550	18	84
Cream Puff, with Custard, 4.3 oz	255	14	25
Cuernos, (Horns), 3 oz	340	17	41
Donut, large, 4", 3.5 oz	440	21	58
Elotes, 3.5 oz	450	24	51
Empanadas, average all varieties:			
Medium, 3 oz	300	14	42
Large, 4 oz	400	19	56
Fiesta Cookie, (1), 2.3 oz	280	8	47
Galletas Mixtas:			
Small, 1 oz	100	2.5	16
Medium, 2 oz	200	5	32
Large, 3 oz	300	7.5	48
Guayaba, 3.3 oz	360	14	53
Jelly Roll, (1), 3.3 oz	240	4	46
Mantecadites, 4.5 oz	670	42	64
Mini Cupcake, (1),1.8 oz	180	8	25
Muffins/Nino Enbuelto, large, 6 oz	465	11	48
Nuez, 3.3 oz	380	17	52
Ojo de Buey, 4 oz	360	15	45
Orejas, 1 medium, 3 oz	310	15	38
Pan Dulce, 1 bun	330	10	45
Panquecitos, 2.5 oz	260	11	36
Piedras, 4 oz	470	15	76
Polvorones: Small, 1.5 oz	180	9	24
1 large, 3 oz	370	18	48
Pound Cakes, mini, 3.5 oz	380	16	52
Puerquitos, 3.5 oz	350	12	55
Rebanadas, 3.5 oz	390	18	51
Roles De Canela, (Cinn. Roll), 4.5 oz	490	15	81
Roscas, 1 piece, 2.8 oz	360	18	44
Semitas (Bimbo), 1 piece, 2.2 oz	210	6	33
Sopapillas, (flaky pastry puffs): 1 piece	100	7	10
With Honey & Cream	200	14	18
Strawberry Crema Roll, 2.5 oz slice	240	5	45

Extra Food Listings ~ See CalorieKing.com

Polish **C F Cb**

	C	F	Cb
Cabbage Rolls, w/ Sour Cream, 2 small	220	10	30
Chicken Casserole, w/ Mshrms, 1 cup	520	27	5
Kielbasa, (Sausages, Onions, fried), 2 large	350	28	2
Meatballs, in sour cream, 3 x 1½" balls	300	16	11
Pierogi, Fruit/Vegetables, 3"ball	80	2	15
Pork Goulash, (Pork/Vegetable Stew)	550	21	38
Pot Roast, with Vegetables	630	21	28

Soul Foods

	C	F	Cb
Breakfast Sausage, fried, 2 patties	250	17	0
Brunswick Stew, 1 cup, 8.5 oz	320	14	19
Cornbread, homemade, 3 oz	200	7.5	28
Fatback, 0.5 oz	110	11	0
Ham Hock, pickled, 3 oz	200	12	0
Hog Maw, 1 oz	70	4.5	4
Hominy, cooked, ¾ cup	110	0.5	25
Hush Puppies, 5 pieces	260	12	35
Kale, cooked, ½ cup	20	0.5	4
Opossum, roasted, without bone, 3 oz	190	9	0
Oxtail, cooked, without bone, 2 oz	85	4.5	0
Pig's Ear, ¼ ear	50	3	0
Pig's Foot, ½ foot	70	4.5	0
Pig's Tail, ⅓ tail	115	10	0
Poke Salad, cooked, ½ cup	16	0.5	3
Pork Brains, braised, 3 oz	115	8	0
Pork Chitterlings, simmered, 3 oz	260	25	0
Pork Cracklings, 0.5 oz	80	6	0
Pork Neck Bones, cooked, no bone, 2 oz	100	4.5	0
Pork Skin, 1 cup	70	4.5	0
Pork Tongue, ⅓ tongue	75	5.5	0
Sousemeat, 1 oz	60	4.5	0
Succotash, ½ cup	80	1	17
Sweet Potato Pie, ⅛ of 9" pie	250	12	34
Tripe, 2 oz	55	2	0
Vienna Sausage:			
2 small, 1 oz	90	8	1
1 small, 0.5 oz	45	4	0.5

OLD McDONALDS FARM
128 FOR PEOPLE WHO WANT BETTER

Brooklyn

Spanish

	C	F	Cb
Arroz Abanda, (Fish with Rice)	340	8	31
Arroz Con Pollo, (Rice/Chkn Salad)	500	23	50
Clams Marinara, 8 clams	330	16	22
Cochifrito, (Lamb with Lemon/Garlic)	650	25	5
Cochinillo Asado, (Rst Suckling Pig), 2 slices	300	15	3
Cocido Madrileno, (Madrid-Style Boiled Dinner)	450	27	18
Flan de Leche, (Caramel Custard)	325	9	52
Fritadera de Ternera, (Sauteed Veal)	450	27	2
Gazpacho, 1 bowl	60	0	15
Mole Poblano, ½ cup	205	14	16
Paella a la Valenciana, (Chicken & Shellfish Rice)	900	42	70
Pollo a la Espanola, (Chicken)	475	30	4
Ternera al Jerez, (Veal with Sherry)	660	29	6
Zarzuela, (Fish & Shellfish Medley)	530	27	40

Thai Foods

	C	F	Cb
Appetizers: Satay Pork, 1 oz	100	4	2
Spring Roll, 1.3 oz	110	6	13
Soups: Tom Yam (Hot & Sour): Spicy Shrimp/Seafood:			
1 cup	100	4	6
1 bowl	160	7	10
Vegetarian, 1 cup	50	0	11
Curries: Chicken with Ginger, 1 cup	390	34	4
Thick Red Curry with Beef, 1 cup	600	50	7
Thai Chicken Curry, 1 cup	340	23	4
Massaman Curry, 1 cup	680	57	8
Green Curry with Pork, 1 cup	480	44	5
Pad Thai, large serving, 18 oz	990	38	125
Fish: Steamed with Spicy Thai Sce	450	8	46
Crispy Fried, 5 oz	290	15	9
Spicy Chicken, stir-fry	450	22	14
Spicy Garlic Tofu, stir-fry	340	18	18
Sticky Thai Rice: Plain 1 cup, 6 oz	170	0.5	36
With Coconut & Sesame Seeds, 1 cup	880	28	120
Stir-fried Rice Noodles, 1 cup 5.5 oz	270	9	40
Stir-fried Vegetables, 1 cup	100	3	18
Salads: Green Papaya Salad	160	4	40
Spicy Prawn, 9 shrimp	170	3	15
Thai Beef Salad, 1 serving	260	9	15
Thai Chicken, 1 serving	330	9	17
Thai Noodle, 1 serving	410	13	45
Satay Chicken & Peanut Sauce, 1 satay stick	390	24	20
Sauce, Peanut Satay, ½ cup, 4 oz	160	10	13

Vietnamese

	C	F	Cb
Banh Cuon, (Steam Rice w/ Pork), 1 roll	105	7	8
Bo Nuong, (Beef Satay), 2 sticks	265	9	4
Bo Xao Dau Phong, (Ginger Beef with Onion, Fish Sce)	750	30	10
Ca Chien Gung, (Whole Snapper/Ginger)	600	16	6
Canh Chay, (Vegetable/Tofu Soup)	80	3	13
Cari Chicken, 1 cup	475	29	16
Cari Chicken, with Rice Noodle, 1 cup curry & 1 cup noodles	660	29	60
Cari Chicken, with Steamed Rice, 1 cup curry & 1 cup rice	650	29	55
Cuu Xao Lan, (Curried Lamb and Veggies in Coconut)	900	40	80
Ga Chien, (Crisp Chick + Plum Sauce)	900	40	105
Ga Nuong, (Chicken Satay + Sauce)	240	10	4
Ga Xao Rau, (Marinated Chicken Braised with Vegetables)	800	26	100
Gio Lua, (Lean Pork Pie), ⅛ of pie	245	12	0
Goi Cuon, (Cold Spring Rolls), 1 roll	60	1	7
Rau Cai Xao Chay, (Stir Fried Veggies)	400	15	65
Thit Bo Vien, (Beef Balls), 6 balls	225	14	2
Thit Heo Goi Baup Cai, (Spicy Cabb. Rolls with Pork), 1 roll	200	7	11
Soup: Per Bowl, ½ Cup			
Bun Bo Hue, (Hot & Spicy Soup):			
Without Pork Feet	340	9	35
With Pork Feet	830	45	35
Chicken & Rice Noodle Soup	400	3	55
Pho Bo, (Beef Noodle Soup)	410	7	59
Pho Ga, (Chicken Noodle Soup)	460	6	58
Pho Tai, (Rare Beef & Noodle Soup)	440	7	73
Salad, Goi Du Du, (Green Papaya), ½ cup	155	3	29
Sauce, Nuoc Cham (Hot Sauce)	5	0	1

Gourmet & Miscellaneous

	C	F	Cb
Ants Eggs/Larvae, 1 Tbsp	20	0	0
Ants, chocolate coated, 3 Tbsp	140	7	2
Bee Maggots, canned, 3 Tbsp	65	2	0
Caviar, black/red, 1 Tbsp	40	3	0
Caterpillars, canned, 2 oz	60	4	0
Frog Legs, fried, 1 pair (large)	125	7	0
Haggis, boiled, 4 oz	350	24	22
Locusts, roasted, 1 oz	35	1	0
Silkworms, raw, 1 oz	60	2	0
Snails in garlic butter, 6 large	200	10	4
Snake, roasted, 4 oz	160	6	0

Fast - Foods & Restaurants

©2013 Allan Borushek

Nutritional data is based on U.S. outlets

For More Restaurants & Full Nutritional Data ~ See CalorieKing.com

	Page		Page		Page
A&W; Applebee's	176	Hungry Howie's Pizza	206	Round Table Pizza	233
Arby's	177	In-N-Out Burger	206	Rubio's Fresh Mexican Grill	233
Atlanta Bread Co.	178	IHOP	206	Ruby Tuesday	234
Au Bon Pain	178	Jack in the Box; Jack's	207	Runza	235
Auntie Anne's	179	Jamba Juice; Jersey Mike's	208	Ryan's Grill; 7-Eleven	236
Back Yard Burgers; Baja Fresh	180	Jimmy John's; Johnny Rockets	209	Salad Works; Sarku Japan	236
Baskin-Robbins	181	KFC	210	Sandella's Flatbread Cafe	236
Big Apple Bagels	182	Krispy Kreme; Krystal	211	Schlotzsky's	237
Biggby; Blimpie	182	La Rosa's Pizzeria; La Salsa	212	Shakey's; Shari's	238
Bob Evans	183	Little Caesars; Lone Star	213	Sheetz	239
Bojangles; Boston Market	184	Long John Silver's	213	Sizzler; Skyline Chili	240
Boston Pizza Canada	184	Macaroni Grill	214	Smoothie King	241
Braum's; Bruegger's	185	Manhattan Bagel	214	Snappy Tomato; Sonic Drive-In	241
Buca di Beppo	185	Marie Callender's; Max & Erma's	215	Souplantation	242
Burgerville	186	McAlister's Deli	216	Southern Tsunami	242
Burger King	186	McDonald's	216	Starbucks	243
California Kitchen; Captain D's	187	Mimi's Cafe	218	Steak Escape	244
Caribou Coffee; Carl's Jr	187	Mr. Goodcents; Mr. Hero	218	Steak 'n Shake; Subway	245
Carvel; Cheesecake Factory	188	Mrs Fields Cookies	219	Sweet Tomatoes	242
Charley's Grilled Subs	188	My Favorite Muffin	219	Swiss Chalet	246
Chevy's Fresh Mex	188	Nathan's Famous; Ninety Nine	219	Taco Bell	247
Chick-Fil-A; Chili's	189	Noodles & Co; O'Charley's	220	Taco Cabana	248
Chipotle; Chuck E. Cheese	190	Nothing But Noodles	220	Taco Del Mar	248
Church's Chkn; Cici's; Cinnabon	190	Olive Garden	221	Taco John's; Taco Mayo	249
Claim Jumper	191	Old Spaghetti Factory	221	Taco Time	250
Coldstone Creamery	191	On The Border; Orange Julius	221	TCBY	250
Cosi; Cousins Subs	191	Outback Steakhouse	222	TGI FRiday's	251
Culver's; D'Angelo's	192	Panda Express	222	ThunderCloud; TJ Cinnamons	251
Dairy Queen	193	Panera Bread; Papa Gino's	223	Tim Hortonss	252
Daphne's Greek Caffe; Davanni's	193	Papa John's; Papa Murphy's	224	Togo's Eatery	252
Del Taco; Denny's	194	Pei Wei Asian; Pepe's Mexican	224	Tropical Smoothie Cafe	253
Dippin' Dots; Donato's Pizza	195	Perkins	225	Tubby's	253
Domino's Pizza	196	Peter Piper Pizza; P.F. Chang's	226	Uno Chicago Grill	253
Don Pablos; Dunkin' Donuts	197	Pita Pit; Pizza Hut	227	Villa Italian Italian; Vocelli Pizza	254
Eat'N Park	198	Pizza Ranch	228	Wahoo's Fish Taco	254
Edo Japan; Einstein Bros	199	Popeye's; Port of Subs	228	WAWA	254
El Pollo Loco; Fatburger	200	Pret A Manger	229	Wendy's	255
Fazoli's	201	Pretzelmaker	229	Whataburger; White Castle	256
Firehouse Subs; Five Guys	201	Qdoba; Quiznos Subs	230	Wienerschnitzel	257
Flame Broiler; Freshens	201	Rally's/Checker; Ranch 1	231	Winchell's; Wing Street	257
Godfather's Pizza	202	Red Hot & Blue; Red Lobster	231	Woody's Bar-B-Q	257
Gold Star Chili; Golden Corral	202	Red Robin	232	Yoshinoya; Z Pizza	258
Great American Bagel Co	203	Roly Poly	232	Zaxby's	258
Green Burrito	203				
Great Steak & Potato Co	203				
Haagen-Dazs; Hardee's	204				
Hissho Sushi	205				
Hot Dog On A Stick	205				

Fast - Foods & Restaurants

A&W® (Jan '15)

Burgers:

	C	F	Cb
Hamburger	380	19	33
Cheeseburger	420	21	37
Double Cheeseburger	680	38	44
Original: Bacon Cheeseburger	530	30	39
Bacon Double Cheeseburger	760	45	45
Papa Burger	690	39	44

Sandwiches:

	C	F	Cb
Crispy Chicken	550	25	52
Grilled Chicken	400	15	31
Chicken Strips, 3 pcs	500	29	32

Hot Dogs: Plain

	C	F	Cb
Plain	310	19	23
Coney Chili Dog	340	20	26
Coney Chili Cheese Dog	380	23	28

Fries/Sides:

	C	F	Cb
French Fries: Small/Kids, 2.5 oz	200	8	28
Regular, 4 oz	310	12	45
Large, 5.5 oz	430	17	61
Cheese Fries: 6 oz	390	18	50
Chili Cheese Fries, 7 oz	410	17	52
Cheese Curds, Regular, 5 oz	570	40	27
Corn Dog Nuggets: 5 pieces	180	8	20
8 pieces	280	13	32
Onion Rings, Breaded: Reg., 4 oz	350	16	45
Large, 5.5 oz	480	27	62
Dipping Sauces: BBQ, 1 oz	40	0	10
Honey Mustard, 1 oz	100	6	12
Ranch, 1 oz	160	17	2

Sweets & Treats:

	C	F	Cb
Polar Swirl: M&M; Oreo, av.	700	25	107
Reese's	740	31	97
Sundaes: Chocolate	320	8	53
Caramel; Hot Fudge, av.	345	10	56
Soft Serve Cone, Vanilla, 5.5 oz	260	7	41

Floats:

	C	F	Cb
A&W Root Beer: Medium, 20 oz	350	5	77
Large, 32 oz	640	10	136
Diet, Medium, 20 oz	170	5	30
Freeze, A&W Root Beer, 16 oz	370	8	68
Milkshakes: Strawb., Small, 16 oz	670	29	90
Chocolate; Vanilla, average:			
Small, 16 fl.oz	710	30	98
Medium, 20 oz	890	38	123
Smoothies: Pineapple Banana, 16 oz	400	6	85
Strawberry, 16 oz	360	6	70
Strawberry Banana, 16 oz	390	6	78

Sodas:

	C	F	Cb
A&W Root Beer: Reg., 20 oz	270	0	72
Diet, 20 oz	0	0	0
Pepsi: Small, 16 oz	200	0	56
Regular, 20 oz	250	0	70

Applebee's® (Jan '15)

Appetizers: As Served

	C	F	Cb
Cheese Quesadillas	1160	74	85
Chicken Quesadillas	1330	76	91
Chili Cheese Nachos	1420	87	118
Crunchy Onion Rings	1290	56	181
Grilled Chicken Wonton Tacos	480	14	48
Mozzarella Sticks (9)	780	39	73
Queso Blanco	150	62	99
Queso Blanco with Chili	1150	68	103

Chicken: Includes Standard Sides

	C	F	Cb
Chicken Fried Chicken	1150	56	104
Chicken Tenders: Basket	1100	63	98
Platter	1430	80	123
Crispy Orange Chicken	1520	49	208

FreshBurgers: Without Fries

	C	F	Cb
Cheeseburger	940	60	51
Classic Burger	790	48	49
Cowboy Burger	1290	74	101
Mushroom Swiss	1100	79	47
Quesadilla Burger	1400	105	43

Pasta: As Served

	C	F	Cb
Chicken Broccoli Alfredo	1120	55	96
Shrimp Scampi Linguine	1010	53	98
Three-Cheese Chicken Penne	1000	46	91

Sandwiches: Without Sides

	C	F	Cb
Applebee's Reuben	980	54	74
Oriental Chicken Rollup	1160	61	119
Roast Beef, Bacon & Mshrm Melt	860	45	57

Seafood: As Served

	C	F	Cb
Blackened Tilapia	470	18	45
Double Crunch Shrimp	1200	56	142
Hand-Battered Fish & Chips	1700	125	96
New England Fish & Chips	1690	126	92

Sizzling Entrees: Includes Sides

	C	F	Cb
Bourbon Street Chicken & Shrimp	610	27	39
Bourbon Street Steak	730	43	38

Skillet Fajitas:

	C	F	Cb
Chicken	1290	46	144
Shrimp	1170	45	145
Steak	1330	48	146

Continued Next Page...

Applebees® cont... (Jan '15)

Steaks & Toppers: Without Sides

	C	F	Cb
House Sirloin, 9 oz	330	17	1
New York Strip, 12 oz	480	25	1
Ribeye, 12 oz	670	47	4
Shrimp 'N Parmesan Sirloin	560	33	5
Steak Combos: With Fried Shrimp	670	37	38
With Grilled Shrimp	470	28	3
With Honey BBQ Chicken	620	18	38
Toppers: Grilled Onions	45	2.5	5
Sauteed Garlic Mushrooms	130	13	3
Shrimp 'N Parmesan	230	17	4

Weight Watchers & Have it All: Includes Sides

Napa Chicken & Portobellos	490	16	37
Signature Sirloin w/ Garlic Shrimp	500	23	31
WW Chicken Frescadi	460	13	45
WW Lemon Parmesan Shrimp	480	14	65
WW Roma Pepper Steak	530	29	27

Salads: Regular, Without Dressing

Fiesta Chicken, Chopped	700	32	66
Fried Chicken	680	41	30
Oriental Grilled Chicken	590	20	53
Pecan Crusted Chicken	890	46	78

Sides: As Served

Chili Bowl	400	24	17
Garlic Mashed Potatoes	250	14	29
House Salad, without Dressing	230	15	12
Loaded Baked Potato	400	23	41
Loaded Mashed Potatoes	460	31	31

Soups: Per Bowl

Chicken Noodle	170	4.5	18
Chicken Tortilla	220	9	24
Clam Chowder	380	26	24
French Onion	370	23	25
Tomato Basil	290	17	29

Desserts: As Served

Butter Pecan Blondie	1150	62	135
Shooters: Chocolate Mousse	480	25	44
Hot Fudge Sundae	430	21	54
Strawberry Cheesecake	390	24	38
Triple Choc. Meltdown	960	52	122

Arby's® (Jan '15)

Sandwiches:

	C	F	Cb
Beef 'n Cheddar: Classic	450	20	45
Mid	560	27	45
Roast Beef: Classic	360	14	35
Mid	460	21	35
Max	560	27	35
Ultimate Angus:			
Philly	590	27	48
Three Cheese & Bacon	630	30	45
Chicken:			
Chicken Bacon & Swiss, Crispy	600	29	49
Crispy Chicken	540	27	48
Turkey:			
Roast Turkey & Swiss	700	28	77
Roast Turkey, Ranch & Bacon	800	35	76
Wraps:			
Roast Turkey & Swiss	520	27	38
Roast Turkey, Ranch & Bacon	620	34	38

Chicken:

Chicken Cordon Bleu Sandwich, Crispy	620	31	47
Chicken Tenders, 3 tenders	350	17	25
Chicken Tenders, 5 tenders	590	28	42

Optional/Regional Menu:

Homestyle Fries: Small	360	17	49
Medium	480	22	66
Large	610	28	82
Melts: Arby's	340	13	37
Ham & Swiss	300	9	35

Kids Meals:

Curly Fries, 2.75 oz	240	13	28
Jr Roast Beef Sandwich	210	8	22
Jr Turkey & Cheese Sandwich	220	6	23
Prime Cut Chkn Tenders, (2), 3 oz	230	11	17

Fries:

Curly Fries: Small, 4.5 oz	400	22	47
Medium, 6 oz	540	29	62
Large, 7 oz	630	35	74

Snack 'N Save:

Jalapeno Bites: 5 bites	280	16	31
8 bites	460	25	49
Mozzarella Sticks: 4 sticks	420	21	35
6 sticks	620	32	52
Potato Cakes: 3 cakes	340	20	37
4 cakes	460	27	50
Steakhouse Onion Rings, 5 rings	410	20	51
Turnovers: Apple with Icing	430	18	64
Cherry Turnover with Icing	390	13	64

Continued Next Page...

Arby's® cont... (Jan '15)

Market Fresh Salads: Without Dressing

	C	F	Cb
Chopped Farmhouse:			
Crispy Chicken	420	23	24
Roast Turkey	230	13	8
Dressings: *Per 1.5 oz packet*			
Balsamic Vinaigrette	130	12	5
Buttermilk Ranch	210	22	2
Dijon Honey Mustard	180	16	8
Breakfast: Per Serving			
Biscuits: Bacon, Egg & Cheese	470	27	35
Ham, Egg & Cheese	420	21	34
Sausage, Egg & Cheese	620	43	36
Croissants: Bacon, Egg & Cheese	400	26	25
Ham, Egg & Cheese	350	20	24
Sausage, Egg & Cheese	550	42	26
Sourdoughs:			
Bacon, Egg & Cheese	480	22	45
Ham, Egg & Cheese	430	16	44
Sausage, Egg & Cheese	630	38	46
Wraps: Bacon, Egg & Cheese	500	27	42
Ham, Egg & Cheese	410	20	41
Sausage, Egg & Cheese	630	41	43
Sauces: Arby's, 0.5 oz	15	0	3
Bronco Berry, 1 oz	60	0	15
Cheddar Cheese, 1.5 oz	50	3.5	4
Horsey, 0.5 oz	50	5	3
Marinara, 1 oz	25	0.5	3
Spicy Three Pepper, 0.5 oz	25	1	3
Tangy BBQ, 1 oz	45	0	11
Dipping Sauces: Buffalo, 1 oz	10	1	1
Honey Mustard, 1 oz	140	13	5
Ranch, 1 oz	100	11	1
Shakes: Per Regular Size			
Chocolate, 22 oz	570	15	99
Vanilla, 22 oz	470	15	75
Sodas: Without Ice			
Average all flavors:			
Small, 16 fl.oz	200	0	50
Medium, 22 fl.oz	280	0	70
Large, 32 fl.oz	400	0	100
Iced Tea, no added sugar, 18 fl.oz	5	0	1

Atlanta Bread Co® (Jan '15)

Signature Sandwiches:
As Per Menu Board Components

	C	F	Cb
ABC Special on French Baguette	780	37	62
Chicken Salad	630	34	45
Curry Chicken Salad	650	42	44
Fresh Caprese	570	29	51
Roast Beef	510	16	56
Salmon Banh-Mi on Ciabatta	560	12	77
Tuna	620	39	40
Paninis:			
Cuban	740	31	77
Grilled Caprese	570	29	51
NY Hot Pastrami	830	58	39
Steakhouse	800	39	68
Pizza:			
BBQ Chicken	870	24	99
Buffalo Chicken	970	42	87
Four Cheese	940	41	85
Margherita	740	25	84
Pepperoni	690	23	85
White	740	25	84
Salads: With Dressing			
Balsamic Bleu	390	18	52
Buffalo Chicken	720	60	13
Caesar	540	47	20
House Salad	430	36	18
Montamore Berry	360	25	24

For Complete Menu & Data ~ see CalorieKing.com

Au Bon Pain® (Jan '15)

Bagels: Per Bagel

	C	F	Cb
Asiago Cheese	370	8	56
Cinnamon Crisp	410	7	77
Everything	300	2	58
Honey 9 Grain	310	2	63
Jalapeno Double Cheddar	320	8	52
Cream Cheese Spreads:			
Garden Vegetable, 1.5 oz	100	6	2
Honey Pecan, 2 oz	200	16	10
Lite Cream Cheese, 1.5 oz	90	8	3

Continued Next Page... ...

Au Bon Pain® cont... (Jan '15)

Breakfast Sandwiches:	C	F	Cb
2 Egg on a Bagel	430	12	58
With Bacon	510	17	58
With Cheese	480	16	58
Egg Whites & Cheddar	230	9	22
Smoked Salmon & Wasabi, on Onion Dill	410	10	62

Cafe Sandwiches: *Per Whole Sandwich*			
Black Angus Roast Beef & Cheddar	510	18	52
Black Forest Ham & Cheddar	640	17	92
Classic Chicken Salad	450	12	60
Grilled Chicken	480	15	55
Tuna Salad	470	14	60
Turkey & Swiss	740	30	79

Signature Sandwiches: *Per Whole Sandwich*			
Black Angus Roast Beef & Herb Cheese	520	14	71
Caprese	550	27	52
Chipotle Turkey & Avocado	670	32	60
Turkey Club	600	24	52

Wraps: Chicken Caesar	600	31	50
Thai Peanut Chicken	540	17	72
Veggie & Hummus	670	38	66
Waldorf Turkey	650	32	63

Harvest Rice Bowls:			
Roasted: Angus Steak Teriyaki	610	14	91
Mayan Chicken	580	17	80

Soups: *Per Medium 12 oz Bowl*			
Baked Stuffed Potato	380	24	33
Chicken Gumbo	190	9	22
Corn & Green Chili Bisque	270	16	26
Cream of Chicken & Wild Rice	270	15	20
Italian Wedding	180	10	15
Vegetarian Chili	270	2.5	47
Wild Mushroom Bisque	190	9	23

Specialty Soups: *Per 12 fl.oz Bowl*			
Beef & Vegetable Stew	340	19	26
Macaroni & Cheese	530	29	46
Turkey Chili	340	9	44

Au Bon Pain® cont... (Jan '15)

Salads: *Without Dressing*	C	F	Cb
Chicken Caesar Asiago	250	10	19
Chicken Cobb, with Avocado	410	24	13
Southwest Chicken	350	12	40
Thai Peanut Chicken, 10.5 oz	190	5	19
Tuna Garden, 12 oz	270	12	20
Turkey, Apple, Brie & Spinach	430	25	30

Dressings: Balsamic Vinaig., 2 oz	110	9	7
Bleu Cheese, 2 oz	310	33	2
Caesar, 2 oz	270	28	4
Sesame Ginger, 2 oz	230	20	12
Thai Peanut, 2 oz	160	8	20

Bakery: *Per Item*			
Brownie Bites, 1.4 oz	160	7	22
Cakes: Red Velvet Cupcake, 3 oz	400	22	46
Pound Cakes: Iced Lemon, 4.5 oz	470	21	66
Marble, 4 oz	450	24	54
Cookies: English Toffee, 2.3 oz	320	16	42
Choc. Dipped Shortbread, 2.6 oz	390	23	43
Croissants: Almond, 4.1 oz	500	31	48
Apple & Cinnamon, 3.4 oz	240	8	38
Chocolate, 4 oz	470	25	57
Raspberry Cheese, 4 oz	360	16	48
Sweet Cheese, 3.9 oz	430	23	48
Muffins: Blueberry, 4.7 oz	490	19	78
Berry, Low-Fat, 4.5 oz	290	3	61
Carrot Walnut, 5 oz	540	25	73
Raisin Bran, 5.5oz	420	11	78
Beverages: Caffe Latte, 16 fl.oz	140	7	12
Caramel Macchiato, 16 fl.oz	280	7	45
Peach Iced Tea, 24 fl.oz	270	0	67
Strawberry Smoothie, 16 fl.oz	290	0	68

For Complete Nutritional Data – see CalorieKing.com

Auntie Anne's® (Jan '15)

Pretzels: *With Butter*	C	F	Cb
Cinnamon Sugar	470	12	84
Jalapeno	330	5	63
Original	340	5	65
Original Stix, 6 sticks	340	5	65
Pepperoni	480	16	65
Sour Cream & Onion	360	5	68
Sweet Almond	390	6	74

Continued Next Page ...

Auntie Anne's® cont... (Jan '15)

Dipping Sauces:

	C	F	Cb
Caramel Dip, 1.5 oz	130	3	23
Cheese Dip; Hot Salsa Cheese, av., 1 oz	95	8	3
Light Cream Cheese, 1.3 oz	80	6	1
Marinara, 2 oz	45	1	7
Sweet Glaze, 1.4 oz	130	0	32
Sweet Mustard, 1.3 oz	60	2	10

Beverages: Per Serving

Frozen Lemonade Mixer: *Per 16 fl.oz*
| Blue Raspberry; Strawberry, av. | 235 | 0 | 60 |

Back Yard Burgers® (Jan '15)

Burgers:

	C	F	Cb
American Cheeseburger, ⅓ lb	780	48	46
Bacon Cheddar	870	55	47
Black Jack	890	62	44
Bleu Cheeseburger: ⅓ lb	730	43	46
Double ⅔ lb	1170	77	46
Cheddar Cheeseburger: ⅓ lb	790	48	47
Double ⅔ lb	1295	87	48
Classic Burger, ⅓ lb	680	39	46
Jr Burger	530	27	47
Mushroom Swiss	790	48	45
Pepper Jack, ⅓ lb	770	48	46
Swiss Cheeseburger: ⅓ lb	790	48	46
Double ⅔ lb	1290	87	46

Chicken:

	C	F	Cb
Sandwiches: Blackened Chicken	530	23	51
Chicken Club	700	41	48
Chicken Tender	660	33	64
Grilled Chicken	345	4.5	46
Wraps: Blackened Chicken	295	14	27
Grilled Chicken	205	4	24

Specialities:

Back Yard Dog	320	18	29
Chicken Tender Basket	465	25	33
Chili Cheese Dog	635	45	32
Loaded Smoked Sausage	575	39	30
Original Smoked Sausage	450	28	32
Veggie Burger (just "Veggie")	400	13	67

Turkey Burgers: Classic | 595 | 36 | 46 |
Turkey Club	750	53	45
Wild Turkey Burger	705	48	45
Wild Turkey Wrap	385	26	23

Fries:

Seasoned: Regular, 6 oz	700	49	64
Large, 9 oz	1050	73	96
Sweet Potato, Regular, 5 oz	555	43	43

Back Yard Burgers® cont... (Jan '15)

Salads:
Without Dressing Unless Indicated

	C	F	Cb
Chicken: Blackened	555	37	17
Grilled	450	26	16
Caesar, Blackened Chkn w/ drsg	770	64	17
Chopped, Blackened Chkn w/ drsg	1010	68	58

Dressings: Per Serving

Bleu Cheese	220	24	1
Gorgonzola Vinaigrette	170	15	6
Honey Mustard	240	23	7
Ranch	150	15	2

Desserts: Per Serving

Cobblers: Apple	360	14	59
Blackberry	285	7.5	51
Cherry	345	12	59
Pecan	740	26	119

Shakes: Per 12 fl.oz

Chocolate	760	36	100
Strawberry/Vanilla	730	32	100

Baja Fresh® (Jan '15)

	C	F	Cb

Burritos: With Standard Menu Board Components

	C	F	Cb
Baja: With Carnitas	830	45	67
With Chicken	790	38	65
With Steak	850	46	67
Bean & Cheese: With Carnitas	1010	42	98
With Chicken	970	35	96
With Steak	1030	43	97
Vegetarian, without Meat	840	33	96
Mexicano: With Carnitas	830	20	119
With Chicken	790	13	117
With Steak	860	21	118
Ultimo: With Chicken	880	38	84
With Steak	950	44	85
Vegetarian, Grilled Veggie	800	33	94

Fajitas: As Served, Without Tortilla Chips

Chicken, with Corn Tortillas	860	24	105
Chicken, with Flour Tortillas	1140	33	147

Nachos: As Served

Regular: With Cheese	945	54	82
With Chicken	1010	55	82
With Steak	1060	59	82

Continued Next Page...

Baja Fresh® cont... (Jan '15)

Quesadillas: With Grilled Flour Tortilla and Standard Menu Board Components

	C	F	Cb
With Cheese	1200	78	84
With Chicken	1330	80	84
With Steak	1430	87	84
Vegetarian	1260	78	96

Tacos: With Standard Menu Board Components

	C	F	Cb
Americano, Soft Taco: Carnitas	250	12	21
Chicken	230	10	20
Crispy Wahoo	250	13	27
Grilled Wahoo, with black beans	180	1	30
Original Baja, average all varieties	215	6.5	28

Salads: With Standard Menu Board Components Without Dressing

Baja Ensalada:

	C	F	Cb
With Carnitas	370	18	20
With Chicken	310	7	18
With Shrimp	230	6	18
With Steak	450	18	18

Tostada:

	C	F	Cb
With Carnitas	1180	62	100
With Shrimp	1120	55	99
With Steak	1230	63	98

For Complete Nutritional Data ~ see CalorieKing.com

Baskin Robbins® (Jan '15)

Cones:

	C	F	Cb
Cake	25	0	5
Fresh-Baked Waffle	130	3.5	24
Sugar	45	0.5	9

Ice Creams: Per 4 oz Scoop

Classic Flavors: Cherries Jubilee

	C	F	Cb
Cherries Jubilee	220	11	26
Chocolate	240	14	26
Jamoca Almond Fudge	260	15	28
Mint Chocolate Chip	250	16	23
Nutty Coconut	300	19	28
Old Fashioned Butter Pecan	280	18	25
Oreo Cookies 'n Cream	260	15	28
Peanut Butter 'n Chocolate	320	20	30
Pistachio Almond	270	19	21
Pralines 'n Cream	270	14	32
Rainbow Sherbet	130	2	27
Reese's P'nut Butter Cup	300	17	32
Vanilla	260	16	27
Very Berry Strawberry	200	11	23
World Class Chocolate	260	16	25

Baskin Robbins® cont... (Jan '15)

Ice Creams (Cont): Per 4 oz Scoop

	C	F	Cb
Seasonal Flavors: Baseball Nut	260	14	29
Creole Cream Cheese	230	13	24
Fudge Brownie	290	19	28
German Chocolate	300	17	34
Rum Raisin	240	11	30
Strawberry Cheesecake	260	13	31

Grab-N-Go:

	C	F	Cb
Brownie a la Mode, 2.77 oz slice	260	13	36

Soft Serve:

	C	F	Cb
Cups: Vanilla: Kid's, 3 oz	130	4.5	18
Regular, 6 oz	250	9	37
Large, 9 oz	380	14	55

Parfaits: *Per Regular 15 oz Size*

	C	F	Cb
M&M's	820	31	124
Oreo	740	27	114
Reese's	990	63	86
Snickers	780	25	127
Strawberry 'n Almonds	600	27	76

31 Below' Mix-In: Per 16 oz Medium Cup

	C	F	Cb
Butterfinger	840	32	127
Choc. Chip Cookie Dough	860	30	132
Heath	860	43	106
Oreo	750	28	110
Reese's P'nut Butter Cup	830	40	100

Sundaes:

	C	F	Cb
Banana Royale	620	28	87
Brownie	920	47	119
Choc. Chip Cookie Dough	990	43	138
Classic Banana	1010	34	173
Made with Snickers	1000	46	138
Two Scoop	530	29	61
Warm Brownie	820	43	101

Beverages:

Fruit Blast: *Per Medium, 24 fl.oz*

	C	F	Cb
Mango	500	1.5	123
Strawberry Citrus	350	0	87

Milk Shakes: *Per Medium, 24 fl.oz*

	C	F	Cb
Choc. with Choc. Ice Cream	930	40	129
Chocolate Chip	890	44	109
Strawb. w/ Strawb. Ice Cream	780	31	109

Smoothie: *Per Medium, 24 fl.oz*

	C	F	Cb
Mango Banana	630	2	150
Strawberry Banana	520	1	126
Tropical Banana	550	1.5	132

Big Apple Bagels® (Jan '15)

Bagels:

	C	F	Cb
Regular flavors, average all, 5 oz	340	2	70

Choice Bagels: Per Bagel

	C	F	Cb
Blueberry Cobbler	390	8	70
Cheddar Nacho	350	6	60
Cinnamon Bun	400	8	70
Cinnamon Danish	395	8	72
Quiche Lorraine	355	8	54
Strawberry White Chocolate	365	4	72
Swiss Melt	370	8	58
White Chocolate Swirl	395	8	70

Cream Cheese: Per 2 Tbsp, 1 oz

Plain	90	9	2
Plain, Lite	60	4.5	3
Other varieties, average	90	8	2
Whipped: Classic Plain	70	7	1
Brown Sugar Cinnamon	70	5	5
Reduced-Fat Spring Veggie	60	5	2

Overstuffed Sandwich,

Manhattan Club	1120	40	120

Specialty Sandwiches:

All-American Duo	750	28	78
Big Apple Club	795	37	75
Chicken Caesar	610	19	78
Turkey Club	780	34	75

Toasted Sandwiches:

Cafe Chicken Melt	815	32	80
Roast Beef Parmesan Grinder	585	15	76
Tuna Melt	640	23	75

Breakfast,

Morning Classic	485	11	73

For Complete Nutritional Data ~ see CalorieKing.com

Biggby Coffee® (Jan '15)

Hot Drinks:

	C	F	Cb

Per Tall, 16 fl.oz, w/o Whipped Cream & Sugar Unless Indicated

Caffe au Lait:

With 2% Milk	100	4	9
With Non-Fat Milk	65	0	9
With Soy	90	3	11
Caffe Latte: With 2% Milk	175	7	16
With Non-Fat Milk	115	0	16
With Soy	160	5	19
Cappuccino: With 2% Milk	105	4.5	10
With Non-Fat Milk	70	0	10
With Soy	95	3	11
Chai Latte: With 2% Milk	315	7.5	51
With Non-Fat Milk	255	0	51
Dark Hot Chocolate: With 2% Milk	400	15	54
With Non-Fat Milk	340	8	54

Biggby Coffee® cont... (Jan '15)

Cold Drinks: Per Tall, 16 fl.oz

	C	F	Cb

Creme Freeze: With Whipped Cream

Banana Berry	535	15	95
Chocolate Chip, 2% Milk	820	33	131
Mango	670	15	125

Freeze Specials,

Almond Blizzard Creme Freeze,			
2% milk & Whipped Cream	570	17	97

For Complete Menu & Data ~ see CalorieKing.com

Blimpie® (Jan '15)

Cold Deli Subs:

	C	F	Cb

Per Regular, 6" White Sub, with Standard Menu Board Toppings

Blimpie Best	450	18	47
BLT	430	22	43
Club	410	13	49
Ham & Swiss	410	14	47
Roast Beef & Provolone	430	15	44
Tuna without Cheese	460	21	41
Turkey & Provolone	410	14	47

Wraps: Includes Dressing

Chicken Caesar	590	26	56
Southwestern	490	18	57

Hot Deli Subs: Per 6" White Sub with Standard Menu Board Toppings

Meatball Parmigiana	560	29	47
Pastrami	430	16	42
VegiMax	520	21	55

Salads: Regular, Without Dressing

Buffalo Chicken	200	8	11
Garden	30	0	6
Tuna	270	19	6
Ultimate Club	270	14	11

Dressings & Sauces: Per 1.5oz

Creamy Caesar	210	21	2
Creamy Italian	180	18	4

Soups: Per 8.6 oz Serving

Chicken Noodle	130	4	18
Cream of Broccoli with Cheese	250	19	13
Harvest Vegetable	100	1	19
New England Clam Chowder	170	3	28
Vegetable Beef	80	2	13

Desserts:

Brownie	230	10	28
Cookies: Oatmeal Raisin	160	8	23
Sugar	320	15	42

For Complete Nutritional Data ~ see CalorieKing.com

Bob Evans® (Jan '15)

	C	F	Cb
Starters:			
Breaded Garlic Mushrooms, 11 oz	460	18	63
Country Fair Cheese Bites	950	66	49
Fruit Plate w/ Low Fat Strawb Yog.	355	2	84
Sandwiches & Burgers:			
Big Farm Burgers: Regular	725	42	50
Bacon Cheeseburger	900	58	51
Favorite Burger	835	51	48
Smokehouse Burger	1170	78	65
Sandwiches: *Per Full Sandwich*			
Farm Favorites: Chicken, Fried	660	26	61
Chicken, Grilled	520	17	48
Farm-Grill: Chicken Club, Fried	670	27	61
Chicken Club, Grilled	535	18	48
Pot Roast	650	36	49
Slow Rstd Knife & Fork Turkey	755	39	62
Turkey Bacon Melt	555	25	48
Dinners: Without Sides Unless Indicated			
Beef:			
Country Fried Steak w/ Gravy	605	41	42
Meatloaf, 1 slice	345	23	15
Chicken:			
Chicken-N-Noodles, Deep-Dish	665	30	72
Chicken Pot Pie, slow roasted	860	56	63
Wildfire Gr. Chkn Breast, 5.2 oz	220	4	15
Fish: *A la Carte*			
Gr. Garlic Butter Salmon, 8 oz	255	9	1
Grilled Wildfire Salmon, 8.5 oz	310	9	15
Potato-Crusted Flounder, 5 oz	245	12	13
Turkey, Slow-Roasted, 3 oz	95	3	2
Side Dishes:			
Baked Potato, Plain, 10 oz	195	0	50
Bread & Celery Dressing, 6 oz	295	16	29
Coleslaw, 3.5 oz	210	14	19
French Fries, 7 oz	495	21	71
Hash Browns, Shredded, 4.5 oz	315	9	53
Home Fries, 5 oz	180	6	28
Loaded Baked Potato, 12 oz	395	16	53
Loaded Home Fries, 5 oz	270	16	22
Macaroni & Cheese, 7 oz	280	15	24
Mashed Potatoes, 5 oz	190	9	24
Gravy: Beef, 2.3 oz	20	1	2
Chicken, 2 oz	50	4	3
Country, 3 oz	55	2	8

Bob Evans® cont... (Jan '15)

	C	F	Cb
Sauces:			
Hollandaise, 1 oz	25	1	3
Wildfire BBQ, 1 oz	60	0	15
Soups: Per Bowl			
Beef Vegetable	165	3	25
Cheddar Baked Potato	330	19	26
Tomato Basil, with Saltines	460	37	36
Salads: Large, Without Dressing			
Cobb, 14.5 oz	515	31	10
Cranberry Pecan Chicken, 14 oz	620	36	34
Heritage Chef, 12.5 oz	400	25	11
Wildfire Grilled Chicken, 13.5 oz	390	13	37
Dressings: Per 3 oz			
Blue Cheese	410	44	5
Buttermilk Ranch	290	29	3
Sweet Italian	255	23	12
Breakfast:			
Hotcakes: *With Set Menu Items*			
Cinnamon Supreme Hotcakes	1170	34	203
Double Chocolate	1110	35	191
Fruit & Nut Multigrain	990	21	186
Omelets: Border Scramble	630	45	15
With Egg Lites	415	23	14
Farmer's Market	535	38	13
Western	495	35	7
Pot Roast Hash, 14.5 oz	760	53	29
Shredded Loaded Hash Browns, 6.7 oz	520	25	57
Sunshine Skillet, 11.5 oz	435	24	38
Fit From The Farm:			
Breakfast:			
Be Fit Breakfast	350	3	68
Veggie Omelet w/ Fruit/Toast/Jelly	310	6	43
Salad: Apple Cranberry Spinach, with Reduced Fat Raspb. Drssng	365	14	47
Kid's Menu: French Fries, 4.5 oz	320	13	46
Fried Chicken Strips (1), 1.5 oz	135	8	10
Mac & Cheese, 7 oz	300	9	45
Mini Chsebgr (1)	275	15	21
Plenty-O-Pancakes, Plain, w/o Topping, 11.5 oz	710	18	130
Smiley Face Potatoes, 3 oz	270	16	29
Sundae, Fudge Blast, 4 oz	185	7	29
Dessert: Coconut Cream Pie, 7 oz sl.	515	29	59
French Silk Pie, 5.5 oz slice	660	44	60
Peanut Butter Brownie Bites (8)	930	45	122

183

Bojangles® (Jan'15)

Biscuit:

	C	F	Cb
Plain	280	14	33
Bacon, Egg & Cheese	550	37	35
Cajun Filet	515	28	45
Country Ham	355	18	33
Egg & Cheese	515	34	35
Gravy Biscuits	390	20	43
Sausage	420	27	33
Steak	555	35	44

Dinner:

	C	F	Cb
2 Breast	1380	80	77
1 Leg, 2 Thighs	1470	95	86
3 Wing	1090	67	83

Sandwiches:

	C	F	Cb
Cajun Filet: Regular	495	27	43
Club	640	39	44
Grilled Chicken: Regular	375	15	33
Club	520	27	34

Fixins': Per Individual Serve Unless Indicated

	C	F	Cb
Bo-Tato Rounds	230	14	24
Cole Slaw	255	20	18
Dirty Rice	165	6	24
Macaroni & Cheese	240	7	33
Mashed Potatoes 'N Gravy	150	6	21
Seasoned Fries: Individual	215	14	20
Medium size	300	20	27
Picnic size	530	35	49

Salads: Chicken Supreme

	C	F	Cb
	460	18	33
Garden	190	9	9
Grilled Chicken	305	11	11

Sweets:

	C	F	Cb
Bo-Berry Biscuit (1)	375	15	55
Cinnamon Twist (1)	270	12	36
Sweet Potato Pie	410	23	48

For Complete Nutritional Data ~ see CalorieKing.com

Boston Market® (Jan'15)

Sandwiches:

Per Whole With Set Menu Board Toppings

	C	F	Cb
All-White Chicken Salad	890	56	62
Meatloaf Carver	950	39	93
Roasted Turkey Carver	850	46	62
Rotisserie Chicken Carver	750	34	62

Individual Meals: Without Sides Or Bread

	C	F	Cb
St Louis Style BBQ Ribs, half	1180	74	67
Meatloaf, regular, 7.6 oz	510	29	26
Rotisserie Chicken, half, 12 oz	640	23	2

Boston Market® cont... (Jan'15)

Salads:

Per Whole, With Dressing, Without Cornbread

	C	F	Cb
Chicken Caesar, 10.8 oz	440	29	16
Mediterranean, 13.4	550	39	14
Southwest Santa Fe, 13.7 oz	530	30	30

Sides:

	C	F	Cb
Creamed Spinach, 6.3 oz	250	20	11
Fresh Steamed Vegetables, 4.8 oz	70	4	7
Fresh Vegetable Stuffing, 5.5 oz	220	10	30
Garlic Dill New Potatoes, 4.5 oz	100	2	20
Garlicky Lemon Spinach, 6 oz	110	9	7
Green Beans, 4.3 oz	90	6	9
Macaroni & Chse, 7.4 oz	280	11	33
Mashed Potatoes: Regular, 7.oz	240	10	32
Loaded, 7 oz	310	16	31
Sweet Potato Casserole, 7.4 oz	430	12	79

Soups:

	C	F	Cb
Chicken Noodle, 14 oz	230	8	22
Chicken Tortilla	410	22	33

Desserts:

	C	F	Cb
Apple Pie, 5.8 oz slice	430	21	59
Chocolate Brownie (1), 4.7 oz	530	26	74
Chocolate Cake, 1 Slice, 5.4 oz	580	32	67

For Complete Nutritional Data ~ see CalorieKing.com

Boston Pizza® Canada (Jan'15)

Starters:

	C	F	Cb
Oven Roasted Wings, 8.4 oz	580	37	7
Poutine, 14 oz	610	30	67
Spinach & Artichoke Dip, 13.7 oz	660	35	65

Gourmet Pastas: Full Order, Without Garlic Toast

	C	F	Cb
Boston's Lasagna	790	23	107
Montréal Smoked Meat Pasta	890	16	142
Spicy Sausage Arrabiata Penne	1230	54	142

Gourmet Pizza: Per Individual Pizza

Classic Crust:

	C	F	Cb
Boston Royal	710	30	69
Deluxe	730	33	65
Hawaiian	660	24	72
Pepperoni	630	30	60

Original Crust:

	C	F	Cb
Bacon Double Cheeseburger	830	44	64
The Meateor	750	38	58

Continued Next Page...

Updated Nutrition Data ~ www.CalorieKing.com
Persons with Diabetes ~ See Disclaimer (Page 22)

Boston Pizza® Canada cont... (Jan '15)

Sandwiches: Without Sides	C	F	Cb
BBQ Pulled Pork	1070	57	92
Boston Brute	800	24	108
Buffalo Chicken	920	35	119
Chipotle Chicken Club	710	35	57
NY Striploin Steak Sandwich	1060	51	95
Smoked Meat	910	59	40
Salads: Full Order With Dressing			
Crispy Chkn Pecan	1170	88	46
Santa Fe	710	51	64
Desssert:			
NY Cheesecake	600	32	76
The Panookie, with ice cream	880	38	133

For Complete Nutritional Data ~ see CalorieKing.com

Braum's® ~ see CalorieKing.com

Bruegger's® (Jan '15)

Bagels:	C	F	Cb
Chocolate Chip, 4 oz	330	3.5	65
Jalapeno Cheddar, 5.5 oz	440	9	75
Plain, 4.1 oz	300	2	60
Sesame; Whole Wheat, av., 4 oz	310	3.5	61
Breakfast Bagel S'wiches: Plain Bagel, with			
Standard Toppings			
Smoked Salmon	460	10	66
Spinach & Cheddar Omelet	490	16	63
Western	670	34	67
Deli Sandwiches: With Standard Toppings			
BLT on Hearty White Bread	720	42	62
Chicken Breast on Plain Bagel	550	6	81
Garden Veggie on Plain Bagel	360	2	72
Ham On Honey Wheat Bread	500	13	62
Hot Paninis: On Ciabatta With Standard Toppings			
Four Cheese & Tomato	570	26	59
Harvest Turkey	690	24	84
Primo Pesto Chicken	560	19	58
Roast Beef Cheddar Melt	630	26	72
Turkey, Artichoke, Mozzarella	520	14	61
Signature & Classic Sandwiches: With Standard			
Toppings			
Herby Turkey on Sesame Bagel	570	15	75
Leon. da Veggie on Asiago Parm. Bagel	490	14	70
Thai Peanut Chicken on Plain Bagel	580	11	91
Turkey Chipotle Club on Wheat Bread	400	17	36

Bruegger's® cont... (Jan '15)

Cafe Salads: Without Dressing	C	F	Cb
Blue Apple, 7 oz	300	14	20
Chicken Almond, 11 oz	260	14	8
Chicken Caesar, 6 oz	190	7	11
Dressings: Balsamic Vinaig., 1 oz	60	6	3
Caesar, 1 oz	80	7	2
Ranch	90	10	1
Dessert Bars:			
Chocolate Chunk Brownie, 2.7 oz	340	17	42
Marshmallow Chew, 2.7 oz	290	7	54
Toffee Almond, 2.7 oz	350	17	44

For Complete Menu & Data ~ see CalorieKing.com

Buca di Beppo® (Oct '13)

Antipasti:	C	F	Cb
Bruschetta, 5.4 oz	230	10	4
Fried Calamari, 5.7 oz	330	21	19
Fried Mozzarella, 14.7 oz	940	42	77
Baked Pasta Specialties: Per Small Size			
Baked Rigatoni, 16.9 oz	830	40	79
Baked Ziti, 11.3 oz	650	25	74
Lasagna, 12 oz	480	24	31
Entrees: Per Small Size			
Chicken Glorioso, 11.8 oz	480	22	24
Chicken Limone, 6.4 oz	360	25	2
Chicken Saltimbocca, 8.2 oz	450	32	10
Prosciutto Stuffed Chicken, 11 oz	670	36	33
Veal Parmigiana, 10 oz	400	19	25
Specialty Pasta: Per Small Size			
Chicken & Sausage Ziti, 12.5 oz	800	45	67
Chicken Carbonara, 14 oz	860	46	72
Linguine Fruttie Di Mare, 14 oz	550	11	75
Shrimp Florentine, 11 oz	660	29	68

Burgerville® (Jan '15)

Burgers:	C	F	Cb
Original Hamburger, with Spread	330	17	30
Cheeseburger, with Spread	380	21	30
Dble Beef Chseburger, w/ Spread	480	28	30
Half Pound Colossal Cheeseburger,			
with Spread	800	46	41
Pepper Bacon Chsebgr, w/ Mayo	670	41	37
Tillamook Chseburger, with Mayo	600	35	40
Sandwiches:			
Crispy Chicken, with Spread	590	29	60
Deluxe Crispy Chicken, with Spread	750	42	61
Turkey Club, with Mayo & Cheese	610	38	38
French Fries: Small, 2.8 oz	220	11	28
Regular, 5 oz	400	19	50
Large, 6.5 oz	510	25	65

Burger King® (Jan '15)

Grilled Whoppers:
Without Cheese, With Mayo

	C	F	Cb
Whopper	650	37	50
Double Whopper	900	56	50
Triple Whopper	1160	75	50
Whopper JR.	300	16	27

Flame Broiled Burgers: With Standard Toppings

	C	F	Cb
Bacon Cheeseburger	290	13	27
Cheeseburger	270	12	27
Double Cheeseburger	360	19	27
Hamburger	230	9	26

Chicken & Fish Sandwiches: With Standard Toppings

	C	F	Cb
Original Chicken, with Mayo	640	36	53
Spicy Crispy Chicken, with Mayo	640	38	57
Chicken Nuggets: 4 pieces	190	11	13
6 pieces	280	17	20
10 pieces	470	29	34
20 pieces	950	57	67
Big Fish, with Tartar Sce	530	27	54

Chicken Strips:

	C	F	Cb
Honey BBQ: 3 pieces	410	17	42
5 pieces	690	28	72

Dipping Sauces: Per 1 oz

	C	F	Cb
BBQ; Sweet & Sour, average	45	0	11
Buffalo	80	8	2
Honey Mustard	90	6	8
Ranch; Zesty Onion Ring, average	145	15	2

Sides:

	C	F	Cb
French Fries: salted:			
Small, 4.3 oz	340	15	49
Medium, 5.8 oz	410	18	58
Large, 7 oz	500	22	72
Fresh Apple Slices, 2 oz	30	0	7
Onion Rings: Small (15)	320	16	41
Medium (20)	410	21	53
Satisfries, small	270	11	41

Garden Fresh Salads: With Dressing

	C	F	Cb
Chicken BLT:			
With TenderCrisp Chicken	640	45	30
With TenderGrill Chicken	440	29	11
Chicken Caesar:			
With TenderCrisp Chicken	650	43	39
With TenderGrill Chicken	450	27	20

Dressings: Per 1.8 oz Packet

	C	F	Cb
Ken's: Apple Cider Vinaigrette	210	18	10
Avocado Ranch	170	17	4
Honey Mustard	220	18	13

Burger King® cont... (Jan '15)

Breakfast:

	C	F	Cb
Biscuits: Bacon, Egg & Cheese	450	27	33
Ham, Egg & Cheese	430	23	35
Sausage, Egg & Cheese	550	36	34
Burritos:			
Sausage	310	19	22
Southwestern	600	38	43
Croissan'wich:			
Bacon Egg & Chse	370	21	31
Egg & Cheese	330	18	31
Ham Egg & Cheese	390	20	33
Double Croissan'wich:			
Bacon, Egg & Cheese	440	27	32
Ham, Bacon, Egg & Cheese	470	27	34
Ham, Egg & Cheese	480	26	36
Ham, Sausage, Egg & Cheese	600	39	35
Sausage, Bacon, Egg & Cheese	580	39	33
Sausage, Egg & Cheese	790	57	35
French Toast Sticks:			
3 pieces	230	11	29
5 pieces	380	18	49
Hash Browns: Small, 3 oz	250	16	24
Medium, 6 oz	500	33	48
Large, 8 oz	670	44	65
Muffin Sandwiches:			
Bacon, Egg & Cheese	300	14	27
Ham, Egg & Cheese	310	13	29
Sausage, Egg & Chse	430	26	28
Platters:			
Pancake, with Sausage & Syrup	660	31	83
Ultimate Breakfast, 18 oz	1420	79	139
Kid's, Oatmeal	170	3	32

Desserts:

	C	F	Cb
Cookies: Chocolate Chip (2)	330	15	47
Oatmeal Raisin (2)	310	13	46
Pies: Dutch Apple Pie	340	14	51
Hershey's Sundae Pie	310	19	32

Shakes:

	C	F	Cb
Chocolate: Small, 12 fl.oz	580	17	97
Medium, 16 fl.oz	760	21	131
Large, 20 fl.oz oz	980	24	174
Vanilla: Small, 12 fl.oz	550	16	91
Medium, 16 fl.oz	730	20	124
Large, 20 fl.oz	930	23	163

Beverages:

	C	F	Cb
Coca Cola Classic: Small, 20 fl.oz	190	0	51
Medium, 30 fl.oz	290	0	77

For Complete Nutritional Data ~ see CalorieKing.com

Updated Nutrition Data ~ www.CalorieKing.com
Persons with Diabetes ~ See Disclaimer (Page 22)

Captain D's Seafood® (Jan '15)

Fish: Without Sides

	C	F	Cb
Breaded Flounder, 1 piece	235	14	12

From The Grill: Without Sides

	C	F	Cb
Grilled Steak Tips, 1 kabob			
Popcorn Shrimp	485	27	48
Seasoned Tilapia, 1 pce	225	9	0.5
Shrimp Scampi, 1 serving	655	35	64
Stuffed Crab	140	10	10

Other Favorites:

	C	F	Cb
Cheese Sticks, 1order	500	32	34
Jalapeno Poppers, 1 order	1160	75	102

Seafood:

	C	F	Cb
Butterfly Shrimp (6)	330	24	22
Popcorn Shrimp	485	27	48
Stuffed Crab, 1 piece	140	10	10

Side Dishes:

	C	F	Cb
Baked Potato (1)	210	0	47
Cole Slaw, 1 order	180	12	15
French Fries, 1 serving	365	26	29
Hushpuppy (1)	80	4	9
Dessert, Chocolate Cake, 1 order	300	10	48

Caribou Coffee® (Jan '15)

Without Whipped Cream Unless Indicated

Classic Hot Coffees: Per Medium

	C	F	Cb
Coffee Of The Day, with 2% Milk	90	3.5	9
Espresso, 4 oz	0	0	0
Cappuccino, with 2% Milk	110	4.5	10
Latte, with 2% Milk	180	7	17
Macchiato, with 2% Milk	20	1	1

Hot Chocolate: Per Medium, With Whipped Cream

	C	F	Cb
Milk Chocolate, 2% Milk	550	33	51

Specialty, Mint Condition,

	C	F	Cb
Milk Chocolate, 2% Milk	570	31	67

Cold Beverages: Per Medium

	C	F	Cb
Iced Americano	5	0	0
Iced Latte, with 2% Milk	90	3.5	9
Iced Mocha, Milk Choc., 2% Milk	320	10	47

Coolers: Per Medium, With Whipped Cream

	C	F	Cb
Caramel	500	16	88
Chocolate	620	24	97
Vanilla	480	16	85

Smoothies: Per Medium

	C	F	Cb
Mango Orange Key Lime	450	0	113
Strawberry Banana	380	0	88
White Peach Berry	330	0	80

Snowdrift: Per Medium, With Milk Chocolate

	C	F	Cb
Cookies & Cream, with 2% Milk	610	17	98
Mint, with 2% Milk	480	12	80

Carl's Jr.® (Jan '15)

California menu only. Please check instore for further nutritional information.

Charbroiled Burgers:

	C	F	Cb
Big Hamburger	480	18	56
Famous Star with Cheese	670	37	57
Kid's Hamburger	270	10	33
Super Star with Cheese	930	56	59
The Big Carl	920	58	56
Western Bacon Cheeseburger	1090	69	74

½ lb Thickburgers: Original

	C	F	Cb
Original	1050	72	62
Guacamole Bacon	1210	89	57
Low-Carb	670	56	9
Western Bacon	990	55	73

Chicken Sandwiches:

	C	F	Cb
Charbroiled: BBQ Chicken	390	7	50
Chicken Club	580	28	46
Santa Fe Chicken	560	27	46
Spicy Chicken Sandwich	460	24	47

Chicken Tenders, hand breaded,

	C	F	Cb
5 pieces, without Sauce	440	21	21
Chicken Stars, 6 pieces, w/o Sce	260	16	18
Fish, Ch'broiled Atl. Cod S'wich	390	11	52

Turkey Burgers: Regular

	C	F	Cb
Regular	490	22	43
Jalapeno	500	22	43
Teriyaki	480	14	56

Breakfast: Bacon & Egg Burrito

	C	F	Cb
Bacon & Egg Burrito	570	34	38
Breakfast Burger	800	43	68
Hash Brown Nuggets: Small, 3.8 oz	350	23	32
Medium, 4.2 oz	390	26	36
Large, 6 oz	560	37	52
Loaded Breakfast Burrito	790	50	53
Sourdough Breakfast Sandwich	450	23	40
Steak & Egg Burrito	650	36	44

Fries:

	C	F	Cb
Chili Cheese, 11.2 oz	810	46	80
CrissCut Fries, 5 oz	450	29	42
Natural Cut: Medium, 6 oz	430	21	55
Large, 6.5oz	460	22	59
Onion Rings, 4.5 oz	530	28	61

Salads: Without Dressing or Croutons

	C	F	Cb
Chicken: Crispy	350	16	29
Original Grilled	280	12	26
Garden, Side	110	4.5	14

Dressings: Per 2 oz Package

	C	F	Cb
Blue Cheese	320	34	1
House	220	22	3
Low-Fat Balsamic	35	1.5	5

Malts, with Ice Cream:

	C	F	Cb
Oreo Cookie	790	41	94
Other flavors, average	770	37	99

Shakes, with Ice Cream:

	C	F	Cb
Oreo Cookie	720	40	79
Vanilla; Choc.; Strawb. av	700	36	85

Fast - Foods & Restaurants

Carvel® (Jan '15)

Carvelanche: Per Small, 16 oz

	C	F	Cb
Butterfinger	850	45	104
M&M's; Reese's, average	880	48	99

Classic Sundaes: Per Small, 12 oz

	C	F	Cb
Caramel	700	36	84
Hot Fudge	540	30	60
Strawberry	610	34	67

Sundae Dashers: Per Small, 12 oz

	C	F	Cb
Banana's Foster	660	23	105
Fudge Brownie	850	45	102
Mint Chocolate Chip	770	42	95
Peanut Butter Cup	1060	60	95
Strawberry Shortcake	580	29	74

Take Home Treats: Brown Bonnet

	C	F	Cb
	390	23	43
Flying Saucers: Chocolate	230	10	33
Deluxe, with Sprinkles	350	16	49

Thick Shakes: Per 16 oz

	C	F	Cb
Chocolate	650	27	93
Strawberry	600	31	70
Vanilla	660	31	86

Thick Shake Floats: Per 16 oz

	C	F	Cb
Chocolate	790	34	109
Strawberry	750	39	85
Vanilla	810	39	102

Checkers®

Same Menu & Data as Rally's ~ See Page 231

Cheesecake Factory® (July '14)

10" Cheesecake: Per Slice

	C	F	Cb
Chocolate Raspberry Truffle	1210	n/a	106
Original: W/ Strawberries	940	n/a	71
Low Carb	640	n/a	41
Reese's P.B. Chocolate Cake	1690	n/a	173

Small Plates & Snacks: Per Dish, As Served

	C	F	Cb
Crispy Crab Bites	350	n/a	10
Ssg. & Ricotta Flatbread	440	n/a	34
Vietnamese Tacos	860	n/a	150

Glamburgers & Sandwiches: Without Sides

	C	F	Cb
Chicken Almond Salad	1480	n/a	83
Factory Burger	730	n/a	52
Turkey Burger	1130	n/a	57

Specialties: Per Dish, As Served

	C	F	Cb
Crispy Chicken Costoletta	2540	n/a	103
Famous Factory Meatloaf	1560	n/a	115
White Chicken Chili	580	n/a	41

Salads: As Served, Includes Dressing

	C	F	Cb
Herb-Crusted Salmon	760	n/a	22
Santa Fe Salad	1690	n/a	98
Skinnylicious Spicy Chicken	430	n/a	40

Charley's Grilled Subs® (Jan '15)

Subs: Regular 7½" Includes Standard Toppings, Without Sauce or Dressings Unless Indicated

	C	F	Cb
Bacon 3 Cheese Steak	635	32	55
Buffalo Chicken, with Sauce	525	16	59
Chicken Bacon Club	570	25	54
Chicken Cordon Blue	570	18	55
Chicken Teriyaki, with Sauce	520	16	59
Italian Deli Deluxe	585	28	53
Mushroom Swiss Steak	520	19	57
Philly Cheesesteak	520	19	56
Philly Chicken	515	16	58
Philly Steak Deluxe	525	19	58
Sicilian Steak	640	31	53
Turkey Cheddar Melt	470	12	53
Ultimate Club	560	23	54

Salads: Cheese or Dressings not included

	C	F	Cb
Grilled Chicken; Gr. Teriyaki/Buffalo, av.	210	7	13

Fries: Large

	C	F	Cb
	635	55	55
Cheddar	525	30	55
Cheddar Bacon	555	30	55

Breakfast:

Omelets:

	C	F	Cb
Bacon; Ham, av.	410	28	9
Veggie	355	23	13

Sandwiches:

	C	F	Cb
Bacon/Ham, Egg & Cheese, av.	540	23	55
Sausage, Egg & Cheese	605	29	54
Steak, Egg & Cheese	620	25	55

For Complete Menu & Data ~ see CalorieKing.com

Chevys Fresh Mex® (July '14)

Burritos: As Served

	C	F	Cb
Fajita Carnitas	1260	51	144
Fajita Chicken	1240	46	142
Fajita Steak	1300	54	142

Fresh Mex Combos: As Served

	C	F	Cb
Chevys Super Cinco	1920	100	171
Mar Y Tierra Combo	1230	54	108
Taste of Chevys	1480	68	155

Fresh Mex Innovations: As Served

	C	F	Cb
Enchiladas: Chipotle Chicken	1070	65	93
Farmers' Market	1130	72	101
Shrimp & Crab	1250	80	94

Tacos: As Served

	C	F	Cb
Mesquite Grilled: Chicken	980	28	123
Steak	1050	38	123
Fish	920	27	123

Grande Salads: Without Dressing Unless Indicated

	C	F	Cb
Sizzling Fajita Chicken w/ dressing	1220	90	51
Santa Fe Chopped	660	39	26
Tostada Steak	1560	100	91
Soup, Tortilla, 1 bowl	420	18	38
Tortilla, El Machino, 6"	140	4	22
Tortilla Chips	430	20	56

Chick-fil-A® (Jan '15)

Breakfast:

	C	F	Cb
Bagel, Chicken, Egg & Cheese	480	20	48
Biscuits: Chicken	440	20	48
Bacon, Egg & Cheese	450	23	44
Sausage, Egg & Cheese	670	44	44
Burritos: Chicken	440	19	43
Sausage	500	28	40
Chick-n-Minis, 1 box, 3 pieces	280	11	30
Cinnamon Cluster	430	17	63
Hash Browns, 2.7 oz	240	15	25
Oatmeal: Multigrain w/ toppings	290	11	50
Without toppings	140	3	28

Chick-fil-A Sandwiches: Without Sauce

Grilled Chicken	320	5	40
Grilled Chicken Club	440	14	41
Regular Chicken	440	18	41

Cool Wrap, Grilled Chicken,

without dressing	340	13	30

Chicken:

Chick-n-Strips, breaded, 4 count	470	24	21
Nuggets: Breaded, 8 count	270	13	10
12 count	400	19	15

Salads: Without Dressing or Toppings

Asian	330	13	24
Cobb	430	22	22
Grilled Market	200	5	17

Condiments:

Charred Tom. Crispy Bell Peppers	80	6	6
Garlic & Butter Croutons, 0.5 oz	70	3	9
Harvest Nut Granola, salad portion	60	3	8

Dressings:

Buttermilk Ranch, 1.5 oz	280	30	2
Honey Mustard, fat-free	100	0	23
Light Italian, 1.5 oz	25	1.5	3

Sauces: BBQ

	45	0	11
Buffalo, 0.8 oz	10	0	1
Buttermilk Ranch, 0.8 oz	110	12	1
Chick-fil-A, 1 oz	140	13	6
Honey Roasted BBQ, 0.5 oz	60	5	2

Sides:

Chicken Salad Cup, 6 oz	360	24	7
Cole Slaw, medium	360	31	19
Waffle Potato Fries: Small	310	16	37
Medium	400	21	48
Large	520	27	63
Dessert, Chocolate Chunk Cookie	330	14	45
Milkshakes: Chocolate, large	730	27	110
Vanilla, large	650	27	89
Sundaes: Cookie	400	13	66
Mini Sundae	170	3.5	33

Chili's® (Jan '15)

Appetizers: As Served

	C	F	Cb
Bottomless Tostada Chips w/ Salsa	910	46	113
Classic Nachos: Chicken, regular	970	61	43
Fajita Beef, regular	1090	71	41
Sthwst Eggrolls w/ Avocado Ranch	800	41	82

Triple Dipper:

Big Mouth Bites w/ Ranch	770	52	47
Orig. Chicken Crispers	630	42	30
Hot Spin. & Artichoke Dip w/ Chips	600	40	48

Burgers: As Served, with Fries

Classic Bacon	1350	80	104
Oldtimer, with Cheddar Cheese	1180	65	102
Southern Smokehouse Bacon	1550	89	130

Chicken: As Served, with Set Sides

Chicken Crispers, without Sauce	1300	63	131
Monterey Chicken	900	46	56

Fresh Mex:

Bowls:

Chipotle Chicken	940	43	83
Chipotle Steak	1020	59	83
Margarita Shrimp	820	27	114

Enchiladas: With Rice & Black Beans

Beef	1190	55	117
Chicken: W/ Green Chile Sauce	1070	41	113
With Sour Cream Sauce	1170	53	112
Top Shelf: Beef Short Rib	1190	62	107
Jalapeno BBQ Chicken	1210	51	126

Tacos: With Rice & Black Beans

Crispy Chicken	1480	66	154
Spicy Shrimp	1010	45	122

Ribs: Full Rack, As Served

Original	1580	84	130
Memphis Dry Rub	1690	92	134

Quesadillas: As Served

Bacon Ranch Chicken	1690	125	69
Bacon Ranch Beef	1800	135	68

Sides: Homestyle Fries

	390	17	55
Loaded Mashed Potatoes	380	23	32
Mashed Pot. w/ Black Pepper Gravy	310	17	35
Southwest Mac 'n' Cheese	490	30	38
Sweet Potato Fries	430	18	64

Salads: Includes Dressing

Boneless Buffalo Chicken	1020	67	55
Caribbean with Sseared Shrimp	680	27	79
Quesadilla Explosion	1430	95	84

Sweet Stuff: Per Slice

Cheesecake	750	47	69
Molten Chocolate Cake	1160	63	145

For Complete Menu & Data ~ see CalorieKing.com

Chipotle® (Jan '15)

Tortillas:

	C	F	Cb
Burrito Size Flour Tortillas (1)	300	10	46
Taco Size: Crispy Corn Tortilla (3)	210	7.5	30
Soft Corn Tortillas (Taco), (3)	210	0	45
Soft Flour Tortillas (Taco), (3)	255	3	39

Meal Components:

	C	F	Cb
Barbacoa, 4 oz	165	7	2
Black/Pinto Beans, average, 4 oz	120	1	22
Brown Rice, 4 oz	200	7	32
Carnitas, 4 oz	220	13	0.5
Cheese, 1 oz	100	7.5	1
Chicken, 4 oz	180	7	0.5
Fajita Vegetables, 2.5 oz	20	0.5	4
Guacamole, 3.5 oz	200	19	7
Lettuce, 1 oz	5	0	0
Steak, 4 oz	190	6.5	2

Condiments:

	C	F	Cb
Salsa: Chili Corn, 3.5 oz	80	1.5	16
Green Tomatillo, 2 oz	20	0	3
Red Tomatillo, 2 oz	25	1	4
Tomato, 3.5 oz	20	0	4
Sour Cream, 2 oz	115	10	1
Extras, Chips, serving, 4 oz	570	27	73

Chuck E. Cheese® (Jan '15)

Appetizers:

	C	F	Cb
Buffalo Wings, Traditional (1)	80	5	0
Cheesy Breadstick, with Marinara, and Light Ranch Dressing	110	6	9

Oven Baked Sandwiches:

	C	F	Cb
Ham & Cheese	620	24	70
Italian Sub	730	36	70

Pizzas: Per Medium Slice

	C	F	Cb
BBQ Chicken	145	4	21
Canadian Bacon & Pineapple	160	4	22
Cheese	150	4	21
Pepperoni	180	7	21
Super Combo	180	7	22
Veggie Combo	160	5	22

Platters: Sandwich, ½ Platter

	C	F	Cb
	185	8	20
Veggie, ⅛ Platter	130	11	7

French Fries,

	C	F	Cb
W/ Ketchup & Light Ranch, 8 oz	645	33	83

Desserts: Apple Dessert Pizza, 1 sl.

	C	F	Cb
	105	1	21
Chocolate Cake (8"), 1 slice	290	13	41
Cinnamon Stick, w/ Toppings (1)	70	2	11

Church's Chicken® (Jan '15)

Chicken: Per Serving

	C	F	Cb
Original: Breast, 1 piece	200	11	3
Leg, 1 piece	110	6	3
Thigh, 1 piece	330	23	8
Wing, 1 piece	300	18	7
Spicy: Breast, 1 piece	320	20	12
Leg, 1 piece	180	11	8
Thigh, 1 piece	480	35	20
Wing, 1 piece	430	27	17
Tender Strips, average, 1 piece	120	6	6

Sides: Per Small Serving

	C	F	Cb
Baked Macaroni & Cheese, 6.3 oz	260	8	24
Cajun Rice, 6 oz	290	17	27
Cole Slaw, 4.15 oz	150	10	15
French Fries, 1.6 oz	140	6	19
Honey Butter Biscuits (1), 2 oz	240	12	28
Mashed Potatoes & Gravy, 6 oz	110	2	17
Okra, 1.95 oz	170	11	17
Sweet Corn Nuggets (6), 3.5 oz	240	7	40

Sauces: Per Packet

	C	F	Cb
BBQ; Sweet & Sour, av.	40	0	10
Creamy Jalapeno	125	13	2
Honey Mustard	140	13	4
Ranch	140	15	2

Cici's Pizza® (Jan '15)

Buffet: Per ⅒ of 12" Pizza

	C	F	Cb
Alfredo	125	2.5	19
BBQ	155	3	25
Beef	165	4	21
Cheese; Ham & Pineapple, av.	150	4	21
Pepperoni & Jalapeno	155	4	20
Sausage	150	3.5	20
Spin. Alfredo; Zesty Ham & Chedd.	125	3.5	19

To-Go: Per ⅒ of 15" Pizza

	C	F	Cb
Alfredo	170	4	23
BBQ	250	6.5	36
Beef	210	6.5	25
Sausage	235	10	25
Spinach Alfredo	165	5.5	23
Zesty Pepperoni	190	8	23

Cinnabon® (Jan '15)

Baked Goods: Cinnabon Bites (6)

	C	F	Cb
	620	24	88
Cinnabon Stix (5)	390	21	46
Caramel Pecanbon (1)	1080	50	147
Bites (6)19	800	39	100
Classic Cinnabon (1)	880	36	127
Frosting Cup, 1.4 oz	180	11	20

Claim Jumper® (Jan '15)

Appetizers: As Served

	C	F	Cb
Southwest Eggrolls	1190	53	114
Three Cheese Potatocakes (3)	1075	71	80

Burgers & Sandwiches: Without Sides

	C	F	Cb
Grilled Cobb Sandwich	1210	78	78
Widow Maker Burger	1370	87	84

Calzones: Specialty

	C	F	Cb
Specialty	1430	80	137
Traditional	1350	66	140

Meals:

Favorites: *With Menu Set Sides & Toppings*

	C	F	Cb
Country Fried Steak	2030	107	189
Giant Stuffed Chicken Baker	990	34	118
Meatloaf & Mashed Potatoes	1300	75	117

Pasta: Black Tie Pasta

	C	F	Cb
Black Tie Pasta	1535	84	126
Parmesan Crusted Chicken	975	47	83

Pizza: Calif. Works, Classic Crust

	C	F	Cb
Calif. Works, Classic Crust	1295	64	127
Steakhouse, Flatbread	820	47	65

Specialties: *With Roasted Vegetables*

	C	F	Cb
BBQ Baby Back Pork Ribs, Full Rack	1745	111	111
Roasted Tri-Tip	800	47	19

Seafood: *With Menu Set Sides & Sauces*

	C	F	Cb
Fish & Chips	1195	74	82
Tilapia Bianca	1165	80	56

Entree Salads: Without Dressing Or Bread

	C	F	Cb
Calif. Citrus Chkn, Charbroiled	865	53	58
Seared Ahi Spinach	515	24	31

Soups: Per Bowl

	C	F	Cb
New England Clam Chowder	525	45	23
Potato Cheddar	710	61	31

Sweets: Choc. Motherlode Cake

	C	F	Cb
Choc. Motherlode Cake	2770	144	340
Italian Lemon Cake	1240	62	158

Coldstone Creamery® (Jan '15)

Ice Creams:

	C	F	Cb
Amaretto: Like it	330	20	33
Love it	530	31	53
Gotta have it	790	47	80
Chocolate: Like it	320	20	33
Love it	520	31	53
Gotta have it	780	48	79

Hot Stone:

	C	F	Cb
Brownie A La Cold Stone, 11 oz	810	55	99
Chocolate Lava Meltdown, 9 oz	730	36	97
Churro Caramel Crave, 8.6 oz	700	33	98

Sorbet:

	C	F	Cb
Strawberry Mango: Like it	220	0	55
Love it	350	0	87
Gotta have it	520	0.5	131

For Complete Nutritional Data ~ See CalorieKing.com

Cosi® (Jan '15)

Flatbread Pizza: Individual

Original Crust:

	C	F	Cb
Chicken & Spinach	940	37	102
Margherita	805	30	94
Pepperoni	855	33	92
Sausage	810	27	93
Traditional Cheese	715	21	92

Melts: With Original Flatbread, without Toppings

	C	F	Cb
Chicken TBM	680	28	52
Pesto Chicken	660	25	51
Steakhouse Gorgonzola	690	43	45

Bowls: With Original Flatbread

	C	F	Cb
Adobo Chicken with Avocado	725	20	106
Korean BBQ Pork	755	23	99
Stuffed Portobello	670	20	102

Soup: Per Regular, Without Flatbread

	C	F	Cb
Chicken Noodle	105	3	12
Tomato Basil	395	36	16

Salads: Includes Dressing

	C	F	Cb
Cobb, with Sherry Shallot Dressing	705	53	20
Greek, with Italian Dressing	535	47	20
Signature, w/ Sherry Shallot Drsng	660	45	51
Steakhouse, with Blue Chse Drsng	655	53	15

Breakfast:

Sandwiches: Coswi Club Squagel

	C	F	Cb
Coswi Club Squagel	560	21	64
Sausage & Pepper Frittata	780	42	65
Western Croissant	560	32	43

Wraps: Santa Fe

	C	F	Cb
Santa Fe	470	28	30
Steak & Egg	510	33	27

Cousins Subs® (Jan '15)

Subs: Per 7½" Italian Bread

	C	F	Cb
BLT, with Mayo	600	36	49
Cheese Steak	675	33	50
Chicken Cheddar Deluxe, w/ Mayo	680	37	52
Club, with Mayo	715	39	53
Double Cheese Steak	1085	58	50
Ham & Provolone, wth Mayo	675	39	51
Italian Special, with Dressing	895	56	51
Philly Cheese Steak	695	38	51
Roast Beef & Cheddar, with Mayo	705	35	51
Tuna with Mayo Blend	690	40	51
Turkey Breast w/ Mayo	530	31	53

French Fries: Small, 2.8 oz

	C	F	Cb
Small, 2.8 oz	250	13	30
Medium, 4 oz	365	19	43
Large, 5.3 oz	485	25	57

Salad, Almond Berry Chicken,

	C	F	Cb
without dressing	180	13	8

For Complete Nutritional Data ~ see CalorieKing.com

Culver's® (Jan '15)

ButterBurgers:

		C	F	Cb
Original: Single		360	16	39
Double		490	24	39
Triple		620	32	40
Cheddar with Bacon, Single		480	26	39
Cheese: Single		430	22	40
Double		630	36	41
Culver's Bacon Deluxe: Single		580	36	42
Double		780	50	43
Culver's Deluxe: Single		540	33	42
Double		740	47	43
Mushroom & Swiss, Single		460	24	40
Sourdough Melt, Single		420	21	36
Corn Dog, Kids		210	13	17
Chicken Tenders, Breaded, 4 pcs		540	24	42

Sandwiches: Beef Pot Roast

	C	F	Cb
Beef Pot Roast	410	16	41
Crispy Chicken	440	14	57
Grilled Reuben Melt	670	35	49
North Atlantic Cod Filet	640	36	51
Pork Tenderloin	600	30	74
Shaved Prime Rib	660	40	44

Sides:

	C	F	Cb
Chili Cheddar Fries	670	31	77
Mashed Potatoes, w/ Gravy, reg.	140	2	25
Wisconsin Cheese Curds, 5.3 oz	510	25	51

Dinners: With Fries, Cole Slaw & Bread Roll

	C	F	Cb
Butterfly Jumbo Shrimp, 6 pieces	1120	55	130
Fried Chicken, 2 pieces	1590	87	119
North Atlantic Cod, Fried, 2 pieces	1480	100	107

Soup:

	C	F	Cb
Broccoli Cheese, 10.5 oz	220	12	17
Chicken Noodle, 10.5 oz	110	2	14
Potato with Bacon, 10.5 oz	240	10	28

Salads: Without Dressing

	C	F	Cb
Chicken Cashew w/ Gr. Chicken	460	24	19
Cranberry Bacon Bleu, with Grilled Chicken	360	13	17
Garden Fresco w/ Gr. Chicken	360	13	20
Side Salad	55	2	6

Dressings:

	C	F	Cb
Chunky Bleu Cheese, 1.8 oz	310	33	2
French Dressing, 1.8 oz	190	13	19
Ranch, 1.75 oz	230	24	3
Sesame Ginger, 2 oz	70	0	16

Culver's® cont... (Jan '15)

Concrete Mixers: Per Medium

	C	F	Cb
Chocolate	950	46	121
Cookie Dough	1010	56	113

Sundaes: Per 2 Scoops

	C	F	Cb
Banana Split w/ Whipped Cream	1060	60	121
Caramel Cashew	1000	51	122
Fudge Pecan	1040	64	107

Beverages: Chocolate Malt, med.

	C	F	Cb
Chocolate Malt, med.	885	42	114
Chocolate Shake, medium	840	42	104

D'Angelo's® (Jan '15)

Toasted & Hot Sandwiches: Per Medium Size, Menu Board Toppings Only, w/out Bread

	C	F	Cb
BLT	1120	34	5
Classic Veggie	350	23	16
Italian Toasted	840	69	16
Meatball & Cheese	770	59	25

Add Sandwich Bread: Per Medium Size

	C	F	Cb
Classic Italian Sub	310	3.5	58
Multigrain Sub	310	3.5	60
Pokket	160	0	34

Wraps: Menu Board Toppings, Without Wraps

	C	F	Cb
Buffalo Chicken, Whole	520	36	17
Chicken Caesar, Whole	620	42	25

Add Wraps: Wheat, 4 oz

	C	F	Cb
Wheat, 4 oz	310	8	55
Flour Tortilla Wrap, 4 oz	310	9	49

Dressings: Caesar, 1.5 oz

	C	F	Cb
Caesar, 1.5 oz	200	21	3
Greek, 1.5 oz	210	24	1
Ranch, 1.5 oz	150	15	2

Salads: Entree Size, without Bread

	C	F	Cb
Caesar, with Dressing	630	53	28
Chicken Caesar, with Dressing	770	55	30
Chicken Cobb, w/o Dressing	310	17	11
Greek, w/o Dressing	240	13	17

Soup: Per Bowl

	C	F	Cb
Extreme Broccoli & Cheddar	370	28	18
Hearty Beef Stew	330	12	34
Main Lobster Bisque	540	43	24
New England Clam Chowder	480	27	46

For Complete Menu & Data ~ see CalorieKing.com

Updated Nutrition Data ~ www.CalorieKing.com
Persons with Diabetes ~ See Disclaimer (Page 22)

Dairy Queen® (Jan '15)

Burgers & Sandwiches:

		C	**F**	**Cb**
Burgers:				
Cheeseburger: Original		380	19	34
Double		580	34	35
GrillBurgers:				
¼ lb Bacon Cheese		620	36	41
½ lb Burger, with Cheese		770	46	43
½ lb Flame Thrower		1010	71	39
¼ lb Mushroom Swiss		560	33	39
Sandwiches: Crispy Chicken		610	30	50
Grilled Chicken		360	16	32
Baskets:				
Chicken Quesadilla, Iron Grilled		1160	60	110
Chicken Strips: 4 pce w/ Country Gravy		1030	53	105
6 piece, with Country Gravy		1260	66	121
Hot Dogs: Beef		290	17	22
Beef, Chili & Cheese		380	24	23

Salads: Without Dressing

		C	**F**	**Cb**
Chicken BLT: Crispy Chicken		520	31	26
Grilled Chicken		380	19	11
Sides:				
DQ French Fries, regular, 4 oz		310	13	43
DQ Onion Rings, 4 oz		360	16	47
Desserts: *Per Medium*				
Blizzard Treats: Banana Cream Pie		770	28	117
Butterfinger		740	26	114
Cookie Dough		1020	40	148
Heath		920	41	126
Oreo Cookies		790	30	117
Reese's Peanut Butter Cups		740	31	101
Strawberry CheeseQuake		690	28	92
DQ Blizzard Cakes (10"):				
Oreo, 1⁄10 cake		760	33	104
Reese's P'nut Butter Cup, 1⁄10 cake		720	33	94
DQ Dipped Cone, Chocolate, med.		470	22	61
DQ Sundaes: *Per Medium, 8.3 oz*				
Caramel		430	11	74
Hot Fudge		440	15	67
Strawberry		350	10	56
Malts: *Per Medium*				
Caramel		830	25	134
Chocolate		790	26	130
Strawberry		700	22	107
Moo Latte: *Per Medium, With Whipped Topping*				
Cappuccino		570	19	90
French Vanilla		630	19	107
Mocha		660	25	102

For Complete Nutritional Data ~ see CalorieKing.com

Daphne's Greek Cafe® (Jan '15)

Starters:

	C	**F**	**Cb**
Fire Feta & Warm Pita	400	19	43
Hummus & Warm Pita	330	13	44

Pita Sandwiches: With Sides, Without Tzatziki Sauce

	C	**F**	**Cb**
Chicken	480	16	43
Crispy Shrimp	450	19	51
Falafel	560	25	72
Gyros	730	47	52

Plates: Without Sides, Pita Bread or Tzatziki

Mix & Match:	**C**	**F**	**Cb**
Crispy Shrimp	150	8	9
Falafel	260	15	29
Fresh-Carved Gyros	420	37	9
Grilled Chicken Kabob	120	4	3
Grilled Steak Kabob	120	4	4

Classic Greek Salads: With Dressing, W/O Pita & Sce

	C	**F**	**Cb**
Crispy Shrimp	440	31	25
Falafel	540	37	45
Grilled Chicken	460	28	18
Dressings: Greek	120	12	4
Gorgonzola	170	16	4
Sides: Fire Roasted Vegetables	60	3	6
French Fries	320	16	40
Moroccan Carrot-Walnut	180	13	16
Multigrain Pita Chips	170	5	27
Pita Bread	240	5	39
Seasoned Rice	250	6	47
Tabouli Salad	220	15	20

Davanni's® (Jan '15)

Half Hoagies: Includes 6" White Bun and Standard Toppings

	C	**F**	**Cb**
Assorted	490	30	39
Cheese	500	31	39
Chicken & Bacon w/ Honey Mstrd	505	22	46
Chicken Parmigiana	445	16	40
Club	495	27	40
Pastrami	470	27	40
Roast Beef	470	25	39
Southwestern Chicken	535	26	43
Tuna Melt	645	44	42
Turkey Bacon Chipotle	565	33	39
Veggie	445	24	43

Pasta: As Served, With Garlic Toast

	C	**F**	**Cb**
Chicken Florentine, half portion	570	23	56
Lasagna, half portion	625	43	37

continued next page...

Fast - Foods & *Restaurants*

Davanni's® cont... (Jan '15)

Pizzas: Per Slice

	C	F	Cb
Five Meat: Thin Crust	255	13	19
Traditional Crust	305	13	30
Solo, Thin Crust	655	36	44
Veggie: Thin Crust	220	10	19
Traditional Crust	275	10	30
Works: Thin Crust	265	14	19
Traditional Crust	315	15	30

Del Taco® (Jan '15)

Breakfast:

	C	F	Cb
Burritos: Breakfast	290	13	28
½ lb Sausage & Egg	500	26	38
½ lb Steak & Egg	460	20	40
Egg & Cheese	400	17	38
Hash Brown Sticks: 5 pieces	230	17	18
8 pieces	360	27	28
Quesadilla, Bacon & Egg	410	22	32

American Grill:

	C	F	Cb
Burgers: Cheeseburger	430	22	40
Double Del Cheeseburger	720	48	40
Crinkle Cut Fries: Kids, 3 oz	160	10	17
Regular, 4 oz	210	13	22
Medium, 6 oz	320	19	34
Macho, 8.8 oz	470	28	49
Chili Cheddar Fries, 10.5 oz	570	34	41

Burritos:

	C	F	Cb
Classic Grilled Chicken	530	33	40
Macho Beef	960	43	71
Macho Chicken	870	30	100
Macho Combo	940	34	100
Nachos: 4 oz	300	19	30
Macho, Steak or Chicken, 19 oz	1040	53	101

Quesadillas:

	C	F	Cb
Cheddar: Spicy Jack, average	460	27	32
Chicken Cheddar/Spicy Jack, av	550	31	35

Tacos:

	C	F	Cb
Al Carbon, Chicken or Steak, av.	150	4.5	19
Bacon Ranch Grilled Chicken, 4 oz	240	13	17
Beer Battered Fish	280	17	27
Macho	300	17	16
Regular	130	7	9
Salads: Deluxe Beef Taco	820	47	66
Deluxe Chicken	770	43	64
Desserts: Cinnamon Churro, 1.8 oz	220	15	23
Caramel Cheesecake Bites, 2 Bites, 4.3 oz	460	28	43

Premium Shakes: Per 16 oz

	C	F	Cb
Chocolate	560	11	105
Strawberry; Vanilla, average	520	11	95

Denny's® (Jan '15)

Breakfast:

Favorites: Without Side Choices

	C	F	Cb
Banana Pecan P'cakes w/- Syrup	750	14	131
Blueberry P'cakes & Egg Whites	590	18	85
Cinnamon P'cakes, Hash Browns, & Fried Eggs	970	49	114
Moons Over My Hammy, & Hash Browns	910	58	56
Peanut Butter Cup Pancakes, Hash Bowns & Fried Egg	1500	92	144

Omelettes: With Hash Browns, without Bread

	C	F	Cb
Meat Lovers	1020	73	37
Loaded Veggie	520	36	25
Ultimate	870	63	37

Skillets: As Served

	C	F	Cb
Hearty Breakfast	990	46	36
Santa Fe, 14 oz	710	52	30
Ultimate, 15 oz	740	56	34

Slams:

	C	F	Cb
All American, w/- Hash Browns	950	78	20
Fit Slam	390	10	54
French Toast, 15 oz	780	45	66
Lumberjack, w/o side choices, 17oz	1000	60	73
The Grand Slamwich, with Hash Browns, 20 oz	1340	89	83
Sides: Buttermilk Biscuit (1)	190	9	24
English Muffin, w/o Margarine (1)	140	1	25
Hash Browns, 5 oz	210	12	26

Pancakes: Without Margarine, Syrup or Toppings

	C	F	Cb
Buttermilk, 2 cakes	340	4	67
Hearty Wheat, 2 cakes	310	1.5	64

Lunch:

Burgers: Without Sides, Unless Indicated

	C	F	Cb
Bacon, Avocado Cheeseburger	970	64	50
Bacon Slamburger	880	49	55
Double Cheeseburger	1120	67	49
Mushroom Swiss	720	38	51

Sandwiches: Without Sides

	C	F	Cb
Bacon Lovers BLT	680	46	40
Chicken Salad	610	34	50
Club	810	39	75
The Super Bird	580	30	43

continued Next Page...

Denny's® cont... (Jan '15)

Dinners: W/out Sides Unless Indicated **C** **F** **Cb**

	C	F	Cb
Bourbon Chicken Skillet, 22 oz	890	30	78
Brooklyn Spag. & Meatballs, 23 oz	1220	61	108
Chicken Strips, with Bread, 10 oz	760	29	84
Fish & Chips, w/ French Fries, 23 oz	1330	73	132
Slow-Cooked Pot Roast, 16 oz	690	33	91
T-Bone Steak, with bread:			
12 oz	820	35	24
With Breaded Shrimp, 15 oz	1050	59	56

Dinner Sides:

	C	F	Cb
Broccoli, 3 oz	25	0	4
French Fries, salted, 6 oz	510	28	59
Golden-Fried Shrimp, 6 pieces	190	8	20
Hash Browns, 1 serving	210	12	26
Mac 'n Cheese, 3 oz	140	9	9
Mashed Potatoes, 1 serve	100	3	20
Red-Skinned Potatoes, 4 oz	205	9	28

Soups: Per Bowl, Without Bread

	C	F	Cb
Broccoli & Cheddar	370	16	48
Chicken Noodle	140	4	17
Vegetable Beef	170	4	23

Salads: With Dressing, w/out Bread, Unless Indicated

	C	F	Cb
Caesar, 8 oz	450	29	38
Cranb. Apple Chicken, 14 oz	450	14	46
Fried Chicken Strip Cobb Salad, with Bread, 19 oz	1060	56	91

Dressings: Per 1 oz

	C	F	Cb
Bleu Cheese	110	11	1
Caesar	100	10	0
French	75	5	8
Honey Mustard	120	10	8
Ranch	120	13	0

Desserts: As Served

	C	F	Cb
Apple Pie, 7 oz	480	22	67
Banana Split, 15 oz	810	31	125
Caramel Apple Crisp, 13 oz	740	21	134
Hot Fudge Brownie à la Mode, 9 oz	830	37	122
NY Style Cheesecake, 5 oz	510	34	43

Toppings: Caramel, 1.5 oz

	C	F	Cb
Caramel, 1.5 oz	190	1	44
Hot Fudge, 1.5 oz	150	6	23
Strawberry, 1.5 oz	60	0	14

Beverages:

	C	F	Cb
Lemonade Iced Tea, 15 oz	70	0	19
Strawberry Lemonade, 15 oz	200	0	50

For Complete Nutritional Data ~ see CalorieKing.com

Dippin' Dots® (Jan '15)

Flavored Ices: Per ½ Cup, 3 oz **C** **F** **Cb**

	C	F	Cb
Rockin' Cherry with Popping Candy	130	0.5	30
Sour Blue Razz	60	0	14
Other varieties	100	0	26

Frozen Yogurt: Per ½ Cup

	C	F	Cb
Strawberry Cheesecake, ½ cup	100	0	21
YoDots: Cookies 'N Cream	100	1.5	16
Chocolate & Vanilla	70	0	12
Cookie Dough	110	2	19

Ice Cream: Per ½ Cup

	C	F	Cb
Banana Split	160	8	20
Choc. Chip Cookie Dough	230	11	32
Mint Chocolate	170	8	21
Strawberry	160	8	18

Donatos Pizza® (Jan '15)

Pizzas: **C** **F** **Cb**

Signature: Thin Crust, ¼ Large Pizza

	C	F	Cb
Classic Trio	630	32	51
Founder's Favorite	660	34	51
Hawaiian	540	24	52

Signatures: Thicker Crust, ¼ Large Pizza

	C	F	Cb
Founder's Favorite	730	33	70
Mariachi Beef	600	23	70
Mariachi Chicken	610	21	70
Pepperoni	670	30	69
Serious Cheese	650	23	69
The Works	690	32	70
Vegy	560	21	69

Signature Subs: On White

	C	F	Cb
Big Don: Italian	670	33	63
Marinara	610	25	65
Sausage Italian	950	56	64
Sausage Marinara	890	48	64
Buffalo Chicken	680	27	66
Chicken Bacon Cheddar	810	39	65
Meatball	930	52	74

Signature Subs: On Wheat

	C	F	Cb
Buffalo Chicken	680	27	67
Steak Hoagie: Marinara Sauce	670	30	66
Mushroom Gravy	650	30	63
Turkey Club	700	30	64

Stromboli: Deluxe

	C	F	Cb
Deluxe	790	35	82
Pepperoni	930	46	83
Three Meat	920	44	83

Desserts: Apple Timpano, 1 slice

	C	F	Cb
Apple Timpano, 1 slice	200	3.5	37
Cinnamon Timpano, 1 slice	260	10	37
Cinnamon Twists (2 sticks)	230	4	45

For Complete Nutritional Data ~ see CalorieKing.com

Fast - Foods & *Restaurants*

Domino's® (Jan '15)

	C	F	Cb
12" Hand Tossed: *Per Slice, ⅛ Pizza, Includes Base Sauce and Cheese*			
Bacon, Beef & Sausage	275	14	27
Beef, Green Pepp., On. & Mshrm	200	8	25
Black Olives, Green Peppers, Onions, Mushrooms, Tomatoes	190	7	25
Ham & Pineapple	200	6.5	25
Pepperoni	215	9	25
Pepperoni & Sausage	240	11	26
Sausage	230	10	26
Sliced Ital. Ssg, Beef & Pepperoni	265	14	25
14" Thin Crust: *Per Slice, ⅛ Pizza, Includes Base Sauce and Cheese*			
Bacon, Beef & Sausage	325	19	21
Beef, Green Pepp., On. & Mshrm	220	12	19
Black Olives, Green Peppers, Onions, Mushrooms & Tomatoes	210	11	19
Ham & Pineapple	220	10	21
Pepperoni	240	13	19
Pepperoni & Sausage	275	16	20
Sausage	260	15	21
14" Brooklyn: *Per Slice, ⅙ Pizza, Includes Base Sauce and Cheese*			
Beef, Green Pepp., On. & Mushroom	270	13	26
Black Olives, Green Peppers, Onions, Mushrooms, Tomatoes	250	12	26
Ham & Pineapple	265	12	29
Pepperoni	290	15	26
Pepperoni & Sausage	340	19	27
Sausage	320	18	28
12" Feast Hand-Tossed: *Per Slice, ⅛ Pizza*			
America's Favorite	250	12	27
Bacon Cheeseburger	270	13	26
Deluxe	230	10	27
ExtravaganZZa	290	14	28
MeatZZa	280	14	27
Ultimate Pepperoni	260	13	25
14" Feast Hand Tossed: *Per Slice, ⅙ Pizza*			
America's Favorite	350	17	36
Bacon Cheeseburger	380	19	36
Deluxe	320	14	36
ExtravaganZZa	390	19	37
MeatZZa Feast	380	19	36
Ultimate Pepperoni	360	18	34
12" Legends Thin Crust: *Per ¼ Party Pizza*			
Buffalo Chicken	380	22	26
Cali Chicken Bacon Ranch	490	33	28
Fiery Hawaiian	390	22	32
Memphis BBQ Chicken	370	19	33
Philly Cheese Steak	360	21	26

Domino's® cont... (Jan '15)

	C	F	Cb
Chicken Wings: *W/out Dipping Sauce*			
Barbeque, 4 wings	250	13	14
Hot, 4 wings	200	13	5
Chicken Dipping Cups: *Per 1.5 oz Container*			
Blue Cheese	240	25	2
Kicker Hot	50	4.5	3
Mango Habanero	80	0	20
Ranch	200	21	2
BreadBowl Pasta: *Per ½ Bowl*			
Chicken Alfredo, 10.85 oz	700	26	93
Chicken Carbonara, 11.6 oz	740	28	94
Italian Sausage Marinara, 11.85 oz	730	27	97
Pasta Primavera, 11 oz	670	24	94
Oven Baked Sandwiches: *Per Sandwich*			
Buffalo Chicken with Blue Cheese	830	41	74
Chicken Bacon Ranch	870	45	72
Chicken Parmesan	750	30	73
Italian	820	41	70
Italian Sausage & Peppers	860	45	74
Mediterranean Veggie	680	29	72
Philly Cheese Steak	690	28	70
Sweet & Spicy Chicken Habanero	800	32	83
Salads: *Per Serving Without Dressing*			
Garden Fresh	70	3.5	5
Grilled Chicken Caesar	90	3.5	5
Salad Dressings & Condiments: *Per 1.5 oz Package*			
Blue Cheese	240	25	2
Buttermilk Ranch	230	24	2
Creamy Caesar	210	21	2
Golden Italian	210	22	2
Light Italian	20	1	3
Bread Side Items:			
Breadsticks: 1 stick, without sauce	110	6	11
8 sticks, without sauce	880	48	88
Cheesy Bread:			
1 stick, without sauce	120	6	11
8 sticks, without sauce	960	48	88
Bread Dipping Sauces: *Per Container*			
Garlic, 1 oz	250	28	0
Marinara, 2 oz	25	0	5
Cinna Stix:			
1 stick, without icing	120	6	14
8 sticks, without icing	960	48	112
Sweet Icing, Dipping Cup	250	2.5	57
Dessert, Chocolate Lava Crunch Cake	350	17	47

196

Updated Nutrition Data ~ www.CalorieKing.com
Persons with Diabetes ~ See Disclaimer (Page 22)

Don Pablos® (Jan '15)

Start The Fiesta: Per Entire Plate **C** **F** **Cb**

Don's Boneless Wings: *Without Bleu Cheese Dressing*

	C	F	Cb
Buffalo	750	48	49
Chipotle Honey BBQ	1010	59	94
Flautas, without Guacamole	505	29	40
Taquitos, without Guacamole	560	39	28
Optional Guacamole, #30 scoop	70	6	1

Nachos:

	C	F	Cb
Cantina: With Chicken	1060	46	108
With Beef	1185	55	109

Quesadillas: *Without Guacamole*

	C	F	Cb
Cheese, small	950	66	50
Mesquite Grilled, Steak, small	860	53	54

Dips: *Without Chips or Tortillas*

	C	F	Cb
Bowls: Queso Blanco	1080	88	14
Prairie Fire Bean	715	43	53

Entrees: Per Meal, Without Sides

	C	F	Cb
Burritos: Chicken	1025	53	79
Fajita Steak	1025	50	79
Carnitas: Pork	815	31	88
Cold Set, Side	185	11	24
Chimichangas: Chicken	785	37	64
Spicy Beef De Oro	1360	79	89

Don's Combos: *Without Sides*

	C	F	Cb
Cinco Combo	1175	66	64
El Matador	960	54	59
Mexicano	715	43	31
Numero uno Favorito	870	45	65
Presidente	1010	54	70

Enchiladas: Cadillac Chicken

	C	F	Cb
Cadillac Chicken	875	43	60
Cadillac Steak	1015	53	65

Sizzlin' Fajitas: *With Proteins, Onions & Peppers*

	C	F	Cb
Combo - Steak & Chicken	580	28	34
Mesquite-Grilled: Chicken	570	27	58
Steak	680	36	36

Fajita Fixin's: 7" Flour Tortilla (3)

	C	F	Cb
7" Flour Tortilla (3)	375	11	60
Corn Tortillas (4)	60	1	12
Guacamole, #30 scoop	70	6	4
Sour Cream, #30 scoop	80	8	2
Tortilla Chips (13), 1 serving	190	2	39

Fresh Salads: Without Dressing

	C	F	Cb
Caesar: With Chicken	815	27	96
With Steak	945	38	99

Southwest: *Without Extra Dressing*

	C	F	Cb
With Buffalo Sauce	950	57	73
With Chipotle-Honey BBQ Sauce	1215	67	118

Sides:

	C	F	Cb
Mexican Rice, 3 oz	120	2	23
Refritos, 5 oz	215	7	27
Seasoned French Fries, 7 oz	345	16	46
Seasoned Vegetables, 6 oz	110	5	16

Dunkin' Donuts® (Jan '15)

Bagels:

	C	F	Cb
Plain; Onion; Wheat, average	310	1	64
Blueberry; Cinnamon Raisin, av.	320	1	67
Everything	340	3	67
Sesame Seed	350	4.5	65
Sour Cream & Onion	330	1.5	66

Danish: Apple Cheese

	C	F	Cb
Apple Cheese	330	16	41
Cheese	330	17	39
Strawberry Cheese	320	16	40

Donuts: Apple 'n Spice

	C	F	Cb
Apple 'n Spice	270	14	32
Bavarian Kreme	270	15	31
Boston Kreme	310	16	39
Bow Tie Donut	310	15	39
Chocolate Frosted Cake	370	23	45
Chocolate Kreme Filled	370	21	42
French Cruller	220	15	18
Jelly	270	14	32
Old Fashioned Cake	320	22	33
Powdered Cake	340	22	38
Strawberry Frosted	280	15	32
Sugar Raised	230	14	22
Vanilla Kreme Filled	380	23	42

Muffins:

	C	F	Cb
Blueberry: Regular	460	15	76
Reduced Fat	410	10	75
Chocolate Chip	550	21	83
Coffee Cake	590	24	86
Corn; Honey Bran Raisin, av.	450	15	73

Munchkins: Jelly Filled (4)

	C	F	Cb
Jelly Filled (4)	320	16	36
Plain Cake; Cinnamon Cake (4)	240	14	24

Sandwiches: On French Roll Unless Indicated

	C	F	Cb
Bacon Ranch Chicken	660	27	69
BBQ Chicken	590	19	74
Chicken Salad Croissant	580	38	42
Ham & Cheese	440	14	54
Roast Beef	460	16	54
Texas Toasted Grilled Cheese	510	30	41
Tuna Salad: Melt on Croissant	680	47	42
On a Plain Bagel	570	24	69
On English Muffin	400	24	34
Turkey Cheddar Bacon	460	14	55

Continued Next Page... …

Fast - Foods & *Restaurants*

Dunkin' Donuts® cont... (Jan '15)

	C	F	Cb
Breakfast:			
Hash Browns, 9 pieces	200	11	22
Oatmeal:			
Original, w/ Dried Fruit Topping	270	4	54
Brown Sugar Flavored Oatmeal, with Dried Fruit Topping	300	4	61
Bagels:			
Bacon, Egg & Cheese	460	11	67
Egg & Cheese	410	7	67
Ham, Egg & Cheese	440	8	67
Sausage, Egg & Cheese	620	26	67
Big N' Toasted, Regular	530	28	43
Biscuits: Bacon, Egg & Cheese	470	27	38
Chicken	540	28	51
Sausage, Egg & Cheese	630	43	38
Croissants: Bacon, Egg & Cheese	480	27	40
Egg & Cheese	440	24	40
Ham, Egg & Cheese	460	25	40
Sausage, Egg & Cheese	650	43	41
Egg White Flatbreads:			
Turkey Sausage	280	8	32
Veggie	280	10	32
English Muffins:			
Bacon, Egg & Cheese	290	10	32
Ham, Egg & Cheese	280	8	34
Sausage, Egg & Cheese	450	26	32
Wake-Up Wraps:			
Egg & Cheese	150	8	13
Egg White Turkey Sausage	150	6	14
Egg White Veggie	150	7	14
Ham, Egg & Cheese	170	8	14
Sausage, Egg & Cheese	260	17	14
Hot Beverages: Per Medium Size			
Chocolate: Original	320	11	58
Mint	310	10	52
Dunkaccino	350	16	51
Cold Beverages: Per Medium Size			
Coolatta: Orange, 24 fl.oz	310	0	80
Strawberry Fruit, 24 fl.oz	350	0	86
Vanilla Bean, 24 fl.oz	630	9	138
Iced Coffee: Per Medium Size, Without Cream			
Regular, without sugar	15	0	2
Caramel Mocha	180	0	41
Peppermint Mocha	190	0.5	46
Lattes: Per Medium, With Whole Milk			
Caramel Mocha	260	0.5	53
Caramel Swirl	350	9	55

Eat 'N Park® (Jan '15)

	C	F	Cb
Breakfast:			
Bananas Foster French Toast, 2 slices	495	15	82
Omelettes: Ham & Cheese	535	35	5
Meat Lover's	725	55	3
Pancakes:			
Buttermilk: Plain (1)	75	1	15
Blueberry (1)	85	1	17
Scramblers:			
All-American w/ sausage	705	39	55
Skinny	355	14	32
Waffles: Belgian (1)	280	12	35
Strawberry (1)	375	17	48
Appetizers:			
Fried Cheese Sticks	535	36	26
Fried Ravioli	455	31	30
Grilled Chicken Quesadilla	905	56	52
Onion Rings Basket	365	24	34
Burgers:			
Black Angus:			
American Grill	615	37	30
Mushroom & Onion	575	31	31
Superburger	1085	73	28
Classic: Black Angus	455	22	28
Black Angus Bacon Cheeseburger	570	31	28
Black Angus Cheeseburger	505	26	28
Garden Burger	290	5	43
Original, Superburger	565	38	27
Sandwiches: With Menu Board Standard Add-Ins			
BLT	490	15	65
Buffalo Chicken Wrap	835	48	61
Chargrilled Chicken	345	7	31
Gourmet Grilled Cheese	795	58	27
Hot Turkey	500	8	71
Santa Fe Turkey	740	50	31
Shredded Pot Roast	530	31	28
Turkey Club	835	49	51
Whale of a Cod Fish	880	42	76
Dinners: Without Sides			
Baked Chicken Parmigiana:			
W/ Marinara Sauce	960	38	99
W/ Meat Sauce	985	41	95
Baked Lemon Sole, 2 fillets	390	19	11
Chicken Fillets, 5 pieces	530	26	28
Cod Floridian, 2 fillets	240	3	8
Mile-High Meatloaf	900	57	59
Smothered Ground Sirloin Steak	445	27	8
Spaghetti Marinara	695	8	129
Spaghetti with Meat Sauce	835	16	146
Whitefish w/ Mac & Cheese 2 fillets	750	34	58

Continued Next Page....

Eat 'N Park® cont... (Jan '15)

Salads: Without Dressing

	C	F	Cb
Buffalo Chicken	610	33	42
Garden	95	3	16
Grilled Chicken	445	20	30
Steak	740	46	33

Dressings: Per 2 oz

Bleu Cheese	245	25	3
Citrus Lime Vinaigrette	70	6	13
French, Fat Free	75	0	18
House Ranch	215	21	4
Poppy & Sesame Seed	390	32	26

Desserts:

Ice Cream, 2 scoops	230	12	27
Pies: Apple Pie, 1 slice	525	27	67
Blackberry Pie, 1 slice	565	28	75
Coconut Cream Pie, 1 slice	490	27	55
Dutch Apple Pie, 1 slice	375	14	61
Sundaes: Caramel Fudge	400	19	56
Oreo	505	21	74

Edo Japan® (Jan '15)

Bento Box: Without Teriyaki Sauce

	C	F	Cb
Beef Yakisoba, 20.3 oz	840	29	102
Chicken Yakisoba, 20.5 oz	790	24	102
Sizzling Shrimp, 22 oz	790	15	122
Sukiyaki Beef, 20.3 oz	880	27	120

Teriyaki Dishes: Without Teriyaki Sauce

Chicken, 15 oz	570	11	80
Chicken & Shrimp	640	14	82
Sukiyaki Beef, 14.8 oz	580	15	80

Soup: Per 33 oz Bowl

Beef Udon	750	16	117
Chicken Udon	700	12	117

Maki Sushi: Per 6 Pieces

California Roll, 7.6 oz	430	17	61
Spicy Tuna Roll, 6.5 oz	300	2.5	54

Nigiri Sushi: Per 1 Piece

Ebi (Steamed Prawn), 1.7 oz	70	0.5	12
Salmon Sashimi, 0.7 oz	30	1.5	1

Einstein Bros® (Jan '15)

Breakfast:

	C	F	Cb
Egg Paninis: Spinach & Bacon	820	50	59
Green Chili & Turkey Sausage	690	32	62
Egg Sandwiches: Ham & Swiss	480	15	58
Turkey Sausage & Cheddar	530	19	59
Wraps: Santa Fe	660	33	60
Spicy Elmo	670	37	56

Bagels:

Thintastic:			
Everything	180	2	34
Other varieties, average	160	1	32
Classics, Plain; Everything, average	265	1.5	56
Gourmet Bagels: Apple Cinnamon	350	6	69
Green Chile	350	8	63
Power Protein	290	5	53
Six-Cheese	330	6	56
Spinach Florentine	320	6	56
Signature Bagels: Asiago Cheese	290	4	54
Blueberry	300	1	65
Chocolate Chip	280	2.5	56
Cinnamon Sugar	300	5	59
Cranberry; Onion, average	270	1	60
Garlic	270	2.5	56
Poppy Seed; Sesame	280	3	56
Potato	270	4	52

Bagel Dogs:

Original	610	31	62
Asiago	620	32	62

Open Facce Deli Melts:

Ham & Swiss	490	15	60
Chicken & Mozzarella	530	15	61
Turkey & Cheddar	490	15	60

Lunch Paninis:

Italian Chicken	720	36	59
Turkey Club	770	40	60

Wraps:

Buffalo Chicken	610	30	60
California Chicken	680	34	64
Chipotle Turkey	640	29	69

Cream Cheese: Per 1.3 oz Schmear

Reduced Fat:			
Garlic Herb/Garden Veggie	130	11	6
Honey Almond; Strawberry, av.	150	11	12
Plain	150	15	2
Onion and Chive	150	13	6

Fast - Foods & Restaurants

El Pollo Loco® (Jan '15)

	C	F	Cb
Bowl:			
Pollo	610	10	87
Ultimate Double Chkn	970	34	94
Chicken Burritos:			
Chicken Avocado, 17.9 oz	950	53	74
Poblano Avocado, 18.6 oz	910	39	93
Ranchero, 17.3 oz	860	38	86
Spicy Chipotle, 17 oz	860	35	86
Flame-Grilled Chicken: Skin On			
Breast	220	9	0
Leg	90	4	0
Thigh	220	15	0
Wing	90	5	0
Salads:			
Premium: Without Dressing			
Avocado Bacon	900	46	81
Chicken Tostada & Shell	860	42	77
Grilled Chicken	240	8	19
Signature Chicken: Without Dressing			
Mexican Cobb, 14.3 oz	520	25	38
Ultimate Double, 12.9 oz	340	9	19
Dressings: Per Container			
Creamy Cilantro: 1.3 oz	190	20	1
Light, 1.5 oz	70	5	6
Ranch, 1.5 oz	230	24	2
Soup:			
Chicken Tortilla with Tortilla Strips:			
Small, 10.8 oz	210	9	19
Large, 23.6 oz	450	19	40
Sides:			
Black Beans, 6 oz	200	0	35
Cole Slaw, 4 oz	130	10	9
Corn Cobbette, 2 pieces, 6.2 oz	160	5	25
French Fries, 3.8 oz	330	17	40
Gravy, 1 oz	10	0	2
Macaroni & Cheese, 5.5 oz	250	15	22
Mashed Potatoes, 5 oz	110	1.5	23
Pinto Beans, 6 oz	200	4	29
Tortilla Chips & Guacamole, 7.5 oz	740	46	77
Condiments:			
Pico de Gallo, 1.5 oz	15	1	2
Salsa: Avocado, 1.5 oz	30	2.5	2
House; Roja, av.,1.5 oz	15	0	3
Sour Cream, 1.3 oz	80	7	1
Dessert, Cheesecake Chimichanga	380	21	39

For Complete Nutritional Data ~ see CalorieKing.com

Fatburger® (Jan '15)

	C	F	Cb
Burgers: Without Extras			
Burgers: Small	400	21	37
Medium	590	31	46
Large	850	41	69
Turkeyburger	480	21	50
Veggieburger	510	20	60
Hot Dogs: Without Extas			
Chili Cheese	480	27	35
Regular Hot Dog	320	15	32
Sandwiches: Without Extras			
Chicken: Crispy	560	27	53
Grilled	430	14	42
Fish	560	31	55
Fries: Fat Fries; Skinny Fries, av.	385	17	53
With Chili, average	485	23	57
With Chili & Cheese, average	595	32	58
Add-Ons: American Cheese, 1 slice	70	5	1
Cheddar Cheese, 1 slice	110	9	1
Mayonnaise, 1 serving	90	10	1
Relish, 1 serving	20	0	5
Sides: Chili Cup	200	11	10
With Cheese & Onions	320	20	12
Onion Rings	540	29	64
Shakes: Chocolate	910	45	115
Cookies & Ice Cream	1180	59	163
Maui Banana	940	44	126
Peanut Butter	950	53	114
Strawberry; Vanilla, average	885	44	112

For Complete Nutritional Data ~ see CalorieKing.com

Fazoli's® (Jan '15)

	C	F	Cb
Oven-Baked Pasta: Per Serving			
Baked Ziti	660	27	70
Chicken Broccoli Penne	870	41	74
Chicken Parmigano	870	35	91
Penne Romano	850	42	74
Penne with Creamy Basil Chicken	870	42	72
Spaghetti	570	20	69
Twice-Baked	700	31	69
Top It Options:			
Asiago Mushrooms, 2.5 oz	120	11	3
Broccoli, 2.5 oz	60	4.5	3
Italian Meatballs, 3 oz	250	18	6
Italian Sausage, 2 oz	200	16	3
Roasted Chicken, 3.6 oz	110	2.5	1

Continued Next Page....

Fazoli's® cont... (Jan '15)

Lighter Options Baked Pasta:

	C	F	Cb
Baked Spaghetti	330	10	43
Chicken Mushroom Alfredo	400	23	45
Three Cheese Baked Ravioli	430	28	25

Samplers: Per Serving

Classic Sampler	870	25	121
Spicy Sampler	1010	34	125
Ultimate Sampler Platter	1120	29	165

Submarinos:

Fazoli's Original	790	37	42
Smoked Turkey Basil	740	33	40
Turkey Club Italiano	730	28	41

For Complete Nutritional Data ~ see CalorieKing.com

Firehouse Subs® (Jan '15)

	C	F	Cb

Hot Subs: Per Medium White Sub, With Standard Toppings and Dressings

Ham	740	37	71
Roast Beef	710	36	54
Turkey	670	35	58
Veggie	720	45	60
Specialty: Club on a Sub	780	43	64
Engineer	685	35	61
Hero	770	37	64
Hook & Ladder	700	37	64
Italian	915	57	64
Meatball	815	50	60
Chili, Bowl	335	18	25

Under 500 Calorie Salads: With Dressing

Chopped: With Chicken Salad	425	26	23
With Grilled Chicken	335	16	19
With Honey Ham	405	19	33
With Turkey	345	17	21
Hook & Ladder	375	18	27
House, without meat	240	16	17
Italian, with Grilled Chicken	485	32	18

Five Guys® (Jan '15)

Burgers:

	C	F	Cb
Bacon Burger	780	50	39
Bacon Cheeseburger	920	62	40
Cheeseburger	840	55	40
Hamburger	700	43	39

Little Burgers:

Little: Bacon Burger	560	33	39
Bacon Cheeseburger	630	39	40
Cheeseburger	550	32	40
Hamburger	480	26	39

Five Guys® cont... (Jan '15)

Dogs:

	C	F	Cb
Bacon Dog; Cheese Dog	620	42	40
Bacon Cheese Dog	695	48	41
Hot Dog	545	35	40

Fries:

Little Fry, 8 oz	525	23	72
Regular, 15 oz	955	41	131

Flame Broiler® (Jan '15)

Bowls: With White Rice

	C	F	Cb
Beef	620	11	74
Chicken	600	14	68
Chicken & Veggie	510	14	49
Half & Half	610	13	71
The Works	520	13	52

Plates: With White Rice

Beef	840	18	94
Rib	1100	44	95
The Works	700	19	63

Freshens® (Jan '15)

Smoothies: 100% Juice (20 fl.oz)

	C	F	Cb

Blended Fruit Classics:

Bangin' Berry	370	0	90
Caribbean Craze; Maui Mango	330	0	81
Feelin' Peachy; Mango Me Crazy	310	0	78
Jmcn Jammer; Ornge S'prise, av.	320	2	70
Peach On The Beach	280	3	61
Pom-Tastic; Purple Rein, av.	320	0	80
Tropical Therapy	480	6	109
Wild Strawberry	340	0	87
Protein: Peanut Butter	500	12	76
Power-Up	560	14	73

Crepes:

Breakfast, Denver, with Bacon	510	27	28

Savory Golden Crepes:

Chipotle Ranch Turkey	430	24	27
Pesto Chicken	350	12	30

Flatbreads: BBQ Chicken, 10.4 oz

BBQ Chicken, 10.4 oz	570	15	75
California Club, 11 oz	640	38	38
Roasted Vegie, 10 oz	440	22	41

Rice Bowls: Bangkok Thai, 15.7 oz

Bangkok Thai, 15.7 oz	570	12	87
KC BBQ, 16.8 oz	620	22	79
Mediterranean, 16 oz	650	37	71

Dessert Crepes:

Cheesecake Supreme	450	23	51
Nutella Supreme	520	21	75

Godfather's Pizza® (Jan '15)

Golden Crust Pizza: Per Slice

	C	F	Cb
Cheese: Medium, ⅛ pizza	220	8	25
Large, ⅒ pizza	250	9	28
Combo: Medium, ⅛	290	13	27
Large, ⅒ pizza	330	15	30
Super Combo: Medium, ⅛ pizza	320	15	28
Large, ⅒ pizza	370	18	31

Original Crust Pizza:

Cheese: Mini, ¼ pizza	150	4	20
Medium, ⅛ pizza	260	7	34
Jumbo, ¹⁄₁₂ pizza	350	10	44
Combo: Mini, ¼ pizza	200	8	21
Medium, ⅛ pizza	350	14	36
Jumbo, ¹⁄₁₂ pizza	480	20	47
Super Combo: Mini, ¼ pizza	220	9	22
Medium, ⅛ pizza	350	14	36
Jumbo, ¹⁄₁₂ pizza	520	23	48

Thin Crust Pizza:

Cheese: Medium, ⅛ pizza	170	8	15
Large, ⅒ pizza	210	10	17
Combo: Medium, ⅛ pizza	240	13	17
Large, ⅒ pizza	280	16	20
Super Combo: Medium, ⅛ pizza	290	16	19
Large, ⅒ pizza	330	19	20

Calzones: Per Medium Calzone

Cheese	1660	51	200
Combo	1450	40	200
Pepperoni	1410	39	195

Sides:

Breadstick (1)	110	2	20
Cheesestick, medium, ⅛	200	7	24
Garlic Toast: 1 piece	150	9	15
With Cheese, 1 piece	210	12	16
Hot Chicken Wings (4), breaded	180	12	4
Potato Wedges, 4 oz	175	8	24

Gold Star Chili® (Jan '15)

Burritos & Burrito Bowls:

	C	F	Cb
Gold Star Chili	970	33	126
Grilled Chicken Bowl	905	29	111

Coneys:

Cheese	310	19	21
Coney	225	12	21
Sriracha Coney	315	19	21

Ways, Regular:

2-Way	395	10	54
3-Way	680	34	55
4-Way, Bean	825	34	81
5-Way	895	34	82
Ways, Super 5-Way	1180	48	122

Gold Star Chili® cont... (Jan '15)

Double Deckers:

	C	F	Cb
Beef & Bacon	625	31	49
Double Bacon	585	35	40
Ham & Beef	645	27	48
Turkey & Bacon	590	30	44
Sandwich, Crispy Chicken	355	20	24

Salads: Without Dressing

Cafe	305	13	34
With Crispy Chkn	495	25	43
With Grilled Chkn	410	16	35

Fries: Regular

Cheese	575	30	59
Chili Cheese	680	36	63
Firehouse	425	16	64

Golden Corral® (Jan '15)

Breakfast:

	C	F	Cb
Bacon & Cheese Quiche, 1 slice	290	21	15
Corned Beef Hash, Grilled, 1 cup	440	28	26
Creamed Chipped Beef, 1 cup	320	18	20
French Toast, Plain, 1 slice	200	6	29
Hash Brown Casserole, 1 cup	260	10	28
Sausage Links (1)	120	11	1
Sausage Patties (1)	170	15	1

Meals: Without Sides

Hot Buffet:

Awesome Pot Roast, 1 cup	320	14	16
Baked Fish w/ Shrimp & Sce, 3 oz	160	10	2
Baked Florentine Fish, 1 piece	180	12	2
BBQ: Chicken Leg Quarter, 1 pce	490	22	21
Pork, 3 oz	170	8	5
Bone-In Catfish, 3 oz	210	14	7
Bourbon Street Chicken, 3 oz	170	9	4
Lasagne, 1 piece	430	26	21
Pork Meatloaf, 1 sl.	200	11	10
Roast Beef, 3 oz	110	3	0
Salisbury Steak (1)	130	4.5	9
Sirloin Steak, 3 oz	150	6	0

Salad Buffet: Per ½ Cup Unless Indicated

Caesar, without dressing, 1 cup	110	8	8
Cajun Potato	230	17	15
Chicken	240	20	3
Coleslaw	110	9	6
Seafood	140	10	9
Spinach Bacon, 1 cup	120	9	4
Tuna	190	13	5

Dressings: Balsamic Vinaig., 2 T.

Balsamic Vinaig., 2 T.	20	0	5
Caesar, 2 Tbsp	150	15	2
Ranch, 2 Tbsp	110	12	2

Updated Nutrition Data ~ www.CalorieKing.com
Persons with Diabetes ~ See Disclaimer (Page 22)

(The) Great American Bagel Co® (Jan '15)

Bagels:	C	F	Cb
Asiago Cheese	520	16	72
Cheddar Herb	390	8	66
Cinnamon Raisin	380	3.5	76
Jalapeno Cheddar	370	7	63
Plain	360	4	71
Spinach Tomazzo	640	20	86
Tomazzo	520	13	77
Paninis: On Regular Baguette			
Chicken Pesto	770	35	70
Ham & Swiss	600	26	58
Philly Beef	920	40	92
Turkey Club	680	29	67
Sandwiches: Asiago Omelet	720	29	80
BLT	550	17	72
Chicken Parmigiana	740	22	81
Ham	460	9	71
Roast Beef	465	9	71
Turkey	435	5	72
Cream Cheese Filling: Per 1 oz			
Plain	100	10	1
Strawberry; Vegetable, average	90	8	4
Pastries:			
Cookies: Chocolate Chunk, 4 oz	110	3.5	19
Oatmeal Raisin, 4 oz	120	5	18
Muffins: Blueberry, 4.25 oz	430	16	64
Banana Nut, 4.25 oz	430	18	61

Green Burrito® (Jan '15)

Burritos:	C	F	Cb
Bean & Cheese	440	15	56
Beef, Bean & Cheese	470	18	52
California: Chicken	470	21	45
Steak	480	21	44
Chicken Especial	550	22	59
Mexicano: Chicken	520	20	57
Steak	540	19	56
Specialties:			
Super Nachos:			
Chicken	920	47	95
Ground Beef	970	51	95
Taco Salad: Chicken	800	43	70
Ground Beef	850	47	70
Steak	810	43	69
Tacos: Crispy Taco	220	13	21
Ground Beef, hard shell	210	12	16
Southwest Chicken, soft	310	21	19
Street Tacos: Chicken	150	7	15
Steak	160	7	14
Sides: Beans, 6.25 oz	250	6	35
Chips, 2 oz	300	17	35
Guacamole, 1.4 oz	60	5	3

(The) Great Steak & Potato Company® (Jan '15)

Breakfast Sandwiches:	C	F	Cb
Bacon, Egg & Cheese	600	36	39
Sausage, Egg & Cheese	700	47	39
Steak, Egg & Chse	590	31	41
Burgers:			
Bacon Cheeseburger	680	45	33
BBQ Cheeseburger	570	28	50
Cheeseburger	600	39	33
Chili Burger	550	27	47
Hamburger	550	34	32
Philly Cheeseburger	570	32	37
Sandwiches: 7"			
Bacon Cheddar Cheesesteak	620	23	60
Buffalo Chicken Philly	800	42	66
Chicagoland Cheesesteak	640	25	61
Chicken Bacon Ranch	860	47	65
Chicken Cordon Bleu	580	15	77
Great Steak Cheesesteak	720	34	60
Gyro	600	32	53
Orig. Philly Cheesesteak	540	17	60
Reuben	690	33	61
Turkey Philly	570	19	63
Super Steak Cheesesteak	720	34	62
Ultimate Chicken Philly	620	23	65
Veggie Delight	530	21	67
Wisconsin Inside-Out	550	26	55
Baked Potatoes:			
The Great Potato: Chicken	430	19	42
Ham	420	19	45
Steak	440	20	39
The King	480	29	30
Turkey	390	16	41
Fries:			
Great Fry: Kids	270	13	36
Regular	440	20	60
Large	540	25	72
Coney Island Fry, Regular	590	29	72
King Fry, regular	570	31	64
Nacho Fry, regular	490	23	64
Salads: Without Dressing			
Great Salad: Grilled Chicken	380	22	16
Grilled Ham	370	22	20
Grilled Steak	370	23	13
Grilled Turkey	340	19	15
Salad Dressings: Ranch, 1 oz	170	18	1
Thousand Island, 1 oz	130	12	4

Fast - Foods & Restaurants

Haagen-Dazs® (Jan '15)

Classic Flavors: Per ½ Cup	C	F	Cb
Butter Pecan	300	22	20
Caramel Cone	320	20	30
Chocolate Chocolate Chip	300	19	26
Chocolate Chip Cookie Dough	300	18	30
Chocolate Peanut Butter	340	23	26
Coffee; Green Tea	250	17	20
Dulce de Leche	270	16	27
Mint Chip	280	18	25
Pineapple Coconut	230	13	25
Rocky Road	290	17	29
Rum Raisin	240	16	21
Strawberry	240	15	22
Vanilla Swiss Almond	290	19	24
Vanilla Bean	270	17	24
White Chocolate Raspb. Truffle	280	16	31

Frozen Yogurt: Per ½ Cup	C	F	Cb
Coffee	180	2.5	31
Vanilla	170	2.5	29
Vanilla Raspberry Swirl	150	1	31

Gelato: Per ½ Cup	C	F	Cb
Black Cherry Amaretto; Limoncello	240	9	35
Cappuccino	230	10	32
Sea Salt Caramel	270	11	38
Stracciatella	270	13	34

Sorbet: Per ½ Cup	C	F	Cb
Mango	150	0	38
Orchard Peach	130	0	33
Raspberry; Zesty Lemon, av.	115	0	29

Ice Cream Bars/Cones ~ See Page 109

Hardee's® (Jan '15)

Burgers:	C	F	Cb
Big Hot Ham 'N' Cheese	410	18	31
Cheeseburgers: Small	330	15	32
Double, 7 oz	420	22	33
Hamburger, Small	280	12	32
Original Turkey Burger	390	17	31
Thickburgers:			
Original, 1/3 lb	850	54	56
Bacon Cheese, ⅓ lb	890	59	54

Hardee's® cont... (Jan '15)

Burgers (Cont):	C	F	Cb
Thickburgers (Cont):			
Double, ⅔ lb	1200	81	58
Frisco, ⅓ lb	880	59	46
Little Thickburger	580	39	33
Little Thick Cheeseburger, 6 oz	430	23	33
Low-Carb, ⅓ lb	470	36	9
Monster, ⅔ lb	1330	95	51
Mushroom 'N' Swiss, ⅓ lb	710	41	52
Six Dollar	980	66	63

Sandwiches:	C	F	Cb
Chicken: Charbroiled BBQ Chicken	330	6	50
Charbroiled Chicken Club	540	31	38
Hand Breaded Chicken Fillet	530	32	38
Fish, Charbroiled Cod	380	18	39

Breaded Chicken Tenders: Without Sauce	C	F	Cb
3 pieces, 4.5 oz	260	13	13
5 pieces, 7.5 oz	440	21	21

Fried Chicken Pieces:	C	F	Cb
Breast, 5.2 oz	370	15	29
Leg, 2.4 oz	170	7	15
Thigh, 4.3 oz	330	15	30
Wing, 2.3 oz	200	8	23

Sides:	C	F	Cb
Coleslaw, 4 oz	170	9	21
Green Beans4.7 oz	60	3.5	6
Mashed Potatoes & Gravy, 5 oz	80	1	15

Fries & Onion Rings:	C	F	Cb
Beer Battered Onion Rings, 4.5 oz	410	24	45
Natural Cut Fries: Small, 4 oz	360	18	47
Medium, 5.85 oz	490	24	63
Large, 6.8 oz	530	26	69

Kids Meals: Includes Kid's Fries & Small Drink	C	F	Cb
Cheeseburger	550	26	61
Chicken Tenders	400	19	37
Hamburger	500	22	61

Breakfast:	C	F	Cb
Biscuits: Bacon, Egg & Cheese	460	26	38
Biscuit 'N' Gravy	460	26	49
Chicken Fillet	550	32	47
Cinnamon 'N Raisin	300	15	40
Country Fried Steak	510	31	44
Loaded Omelet	490	28	40
Monster	730	49	40
Sausage and Egg	560	37	39

Continued Next Page...

Updated Nutrition Data ~ www.CalorieKing.com
Persons with Diabetes ~ See Disclaimer (Page 22)

Hardee's® cont... (Jan '15)

Breakfast (Cont):

	C	F	Cb
Big Country Platter, Bacon, without syrup, jam & butter	880	43	93
Bowl, Low Carb	660	52	10
Burritos:			
Country Fried Steak & Eggs	580	29	45
Loaded	580	34	46
Frisco Breakfast Sandwich	450	19	45
Sandwiches, Frisco	450	19	45
Sunrise Croissants:			
With Bacon	440	30	27
With Ham	450	28	30
With Sausage	590	44	28
Texas Toast Sandwiches:			
Bacon, Egg & Cheese	240	15	13
Ham, Egg & Cheese	260	13	14
Sausage, Egg & Cheese	380	29	14
Breakfast Sides:			
Grits	100	3	16
Hash Rounds: Small, 2.9 oz	260	15	23
Medium, 4.2 oz	370	22	33
Large, 5.8 oz	510	30	45
Desserts:			
Apple Turnover w/o Cinn. Sugar	270	13	35
Chocolate Chip Cookie (2), 2 oz	240	10	36
Single Scoop Ice Cream:			
Bowl, 4 oz	240	13	27
Cone, 4.4 oz	290	13	37
Drinks:			
Hot Chocolate	150	3	18
Ice Cream Malts: *Per 14.6 oz Cup*			
Chocolate	780	35	99
Strawberry	770	35	97
Vanilla	780	35	98
Ice Cream Shakes: *Per 14 oz Cup*			
Chocolate; Strawberry, average	705	34	86
Vanilla	700	33	86

For Complete Nutritional Data ~ see CalorieKing.com

Hissho Sushi® (Jan '15)

Starters: Per Serving

	C	F	Cb
Baby Octopus Salad, 3.5 oz	150	2	18
Spring Rolls: Regular (2), 4.9 oz	135	2	18
Garden (2), 4.9 oz	130	3	23
Grilled Chicken (2), 4.9 oz	140	4	19
Ocean Salmon (2), 4.9 oz	150	5	16
Ocean Tuna (2), 4.9 oz	155	4	16

Hissho Sushi® cont... (Jan '15)

Maki Sushi:

	C	F	Cb
Rolls: *Per 6 Pieces Unless Indicated*			
Blazing California	265	2	53
Boston	265	2	53
California	275	3	56
Crab Salad	270	3	53
Crunchy	285	3	53
Dynamite: Salmon	295	5	51
Shrimp	285	3	52
Tuna	290	4	49
Yellowtail	295	4	51
Inari	285	4	54
Nippon Favorite: Salmon, 16 pcs	330	2	65
Tuna, 16 pieces	330	2	64
Philadelphia	345	10	56
Snow Crab	280	3	56
Sushicado: Salmon, 12 pieces	510	7	92
Shrimp, 6 pieces	300	3	56
Specialty Items: Per 4 Pieces			
Rolls:			
Caterpillar	330	5	60
Grande Finale	280	5	48
Living Color	250	3	43
Mango Tango	250	5	37
Salmon Lover	305	8	42
Sriracha Party	450	8	77
Tempura Shrimp	255	3	52
TNT: Salmon	290	4	52
Shrimp	280	2	52
Tuna	290	3	50
Wasabi Crunch	335	7	53

Hot Dog on a Stick® (Jan '15)

Menu Items:

	C	F	Cb
American Cheese on a Stick	260	16	21
Beef Hot Dog on a Bun	380	20	33
Turkey Hot Dog on a Stick	240	13	23
Veggie Dog on a Stick	220	8	24
Pepperjack Cheese on a Stick	240	14	19
Sides, French Fries, 4.5 oz	400	21	49
Dessert, Funnel Cake Sticks, (10)	210	8	31
Beverages: Per Regular Size, 16 fl.oz			
Lemonade: Original	150	0	38
Sugar Free	15	0	3
Lime	230	0	57

Hungry Howie's Pizza® (Jan '15)

Counts may vary in Florida.

	C	F	Cb
Pizzas: Per Slice			
BBQ Chicken: Small, ⅙ pizza	210	6	27
Medium, ⅛ pizza	240	8	30
Large, ⅒ pizza	260	8	32
X-Large, ⅒₂ pizza	300	9	39
Calzones: Per ½ Sub			
Deluxe Italian	660	23	81
Ham & Cheese	590	15	68
Steak & Cheese	610	18	81
Turkey Club	660	18	80
Veggie	610	19	83
Wings: Asian, 5 wings	440	28	11
Original Howie, 5 wings	400	29	0
Salads: Per Regular			
Antipasto	170	10	10
Chef	140	8	9
Garden	140	8	9
Greek	140	7	15
Dressings: Per 1 oz			
Creamy Italian	120	12	2
Greek	110	11	2
Ranch	180	19	1
Thousand Island	140	14	4

In-N-Out Burger® (Jan '15)

	C	F	Cb
Burgers:			
Hamburger: With Onion	390	19	39
With Mustard/Ketchup, w/o Spread	310	10	41
Protein Style w/ Lettuce Wrap, w/o Bun	240	17	11
Cheeseburger: With Onion	480	27	39
With Mustard/Ketchup, w/o Spread	400	18	41
Protein Style w/ Lettuce Wrap, w/o Bun	330	25	11
Double Double: With Onion	670	41	39
With Mustard/Ketchup, w/o Spread	590	32	41
Protein Style w/ Lettuce Wrap, w/o Bun	520	39	11
French Fries, 4.5 oz	395	18	54
Drinks: Milk, 10 fl.oz	180	6	18
Coca-Cola, 16 fl.oz	195	0	54
Dr Pepper; 7-Up, av., 16 fl.oz	200	0	53
Lemonade, 16 fl.oz	180	0	40
Root Beer, 16 fl.oz	220	0	60
Shakes:			
Chocolate, 15 fl.oz	590	29	72
Strawberry, 15 fl.oz	590	27	81
Vanilla, 15 fl.oz	580	31	67

IHOP® (Jan '15)

	C	F	Cb
Pancakes:			
Buttermilk: With Menu Toppings			
Full Stack (5)	750	22	115
Short Stack (3)	470	15	69
Chocolate Chocolate Chip (4)	710	23	110
Double Blueberry (4)	690	17	118
Strawberry Banana (4)	760	17	137
Condiments:			
Syrup: Blueberry; Maple, 1 fl.oz	110	0	27
Boysenberry; Strawberry, 1 fl.oz	100	0	26
Sugar-Free Syrup, 1 fl.oz	15	0	6
French Toast & Waffles: W/ Toppings Unless Indicated			
French Toast: Original	720	30	92
Berry Berry Brioche	770	29	114
Strawberry Banana	880	28	138
Waffle, Belgian	500	24	60
Crepes:			
Cheese Blintzes:			
With Blueberry Topping	1160	65	114
With Strawberry Topping	1150	65	113
Chicken, Bacon & White Cheddar	1080	67	53
Chicken Florentine	870	48	57
German Crepes	840	45	90
Hearty Omelettes: Without Pancakes or Sides			
Big Steak	1260	90	47
Garden	910	76	15
Hearty Ham & Cheese	1040	79	17
Spinach & Mushroom	980	82	21
Breakfast Combinations: As Served, w/o Syrup			
Biscuits & Gravy Combo with Country Gravy	1380	88	106
Breakfast Sampler	1180	74	77
Chicken Fried Chicken & Eggs, with Country Gravy	1160	65	94
Chorizo & Egg	1480	93	105
T-Bone Steak & Eggs, 12 oz	1240	65	73
Sandwiches: Without Sides			
Baja Fish, with Tartar Sauce	750	33	87
Chicken Clubhouse Super Stacker	1150	76	62
Melts: Full Sandwich, without Sides			
Ham & Egg	1280	77	81
Spinach, Rstd Red Pepp. & Cheese	1380	91	84
Dinner Classics: With Set Sides, excluding Baked Potato, Salad or Soup			
Chkn Fried Chkn, w/ Country Gravy	760	37	84
Pot Roast	950	46	83
T-Bone Steak, 12 oz	950	48	66

Jack in the Box® (Jan '15)

Sandwiches & Burgers:	C	F	Cb
Bacon Ultimate Cheeseburger	905	56	44
Cheeseburger	320	14	32
Hamburger	280	11	32
Jumbo Jack:			
With Cheese	570	30	45
Without Cheese	490	23	44
Junior Bacon Cheeseburger	385	21	32
Sirloin Cheeseburger	930	65	48
Sourdough Jack	660	41	40
Ultimate Cheeseburger	820	49	44
Chicken & Fish:			
Chicken Sandwich	415	21	42
With Bacon	470	25	42
Chicken Strips: Crispy, 4 pieces	565	24	53
Grilled, 4 pieces	250	7	5
Fish Sandwich	380	14	45
Jack's Spicy Chkn S'wich	530	20	61
With Cheese	600	25	62
Sourdough Gr. Chicken Club	535	26	38
Breakfast:			
Biscuit: Bacon, Egg & Cheese	410	25	26
Sausage, Egg & Cheese	535	38	27
Breakfast Jack: Regular	285	11	30
With Bacon	310	14	30
Croissants: Sausage	560	39	32
Supreme	450	27	32
Hash Brown Plank	185	13	17
Meaty Burrito, with salsa	600	36	40
Sandwiches: Extreme Sausage	645	45	32
Sourdough	410	21	35
Ultimate	520	25	42
Snacks & Sides:			
Bacon Cheddar Pot. Wedges	680	41	58
Chiquita Apple Bites, w/ Caramel Dip	70	0	17
Egg Rolls (3), w/o sauce	440	22	46
Mozzarella Cheese Sticks:			
3 Pieces	280	16	22
6 Pieces	560	33	43
Stuffed Jalapenos:			
3 Pieces	220	12	21
7 Pieces	510	29	49
Onion Rings (8), 4.3 oz	450	28	45
Seasoned Curly Fries, med., 4.5 oz	430	25	46
Better For You:			
Chicken Fajita Pita, without Salsa	365	13	42
Chicken Teriyaki Bowl	690	6	134
Grilled Chicken Strips, w/ Teriyaki Dipping Sce	310	8	15

Jack in the Box® cont... (Jan '15)

Salads: No Dressing or Condiments	C	F	Cb
Chicken Club with Grilled Chicken	370	20	11
Grilled Chicken	250	10	13
Southwest Chicken, with Grilled Chicken Strips	355	15	27
Croutons	70	3	9
Dressings: Creamy Southwest	190	19	3
Ranch	250	25	5
Low Fat Balsamic Vinaigrette	30	1.5	4
Sauces:			
Dipping Sauce: Barbecue, 1 oz	40	0	10
Buttermilk, 1 oz	130	13	3
Frank's Red Hot Buffalo, 1 oz	10	0	1
Sweet & Sour, 1 oz	45	0	11
Tartar, 1 oz	150	16	2
Sandwich Sauce:			
Mayo-Onion, 0.5 oz	90	10	0
Peppercorn Mayo, 1.5 oz	280	31	1
Sundried Tomato Sauce, 0.6 oz	80	8	1
Desserts:			
Chocolate Overload Cake	300	7	57
Churros, Mini (5)	345	18	42
New York Style Cheesecake	310	17	32
Shakes: 16 oz, with Whipped Topping			
Chocolate	780	38	103
Oreo Cookie	795	43	92
Strawberry	760	38	97
Vanilla	685	38	78

For Complete Nutritional Data ~ see CalorieKing.com

Jack's® (Jan '15)

Sandwiches:	C	F	Cb
Big Bacon Cheeseburger	610	41	31
Big Jack Burger	530	33	35
Cheeseburger	380	21	31
Chicken Fillet Sandwich	490	24	40
Double Big Jack Cheese Burger	850	59	35
Double Cheeseburger	540	33	31
Grilled Chicken Sandwich	380	16	32
Hamburger	340	18	31
Chicken, Chicken Fingers, 3 pieces	300	14	14
Fries, regular	310	13	42
Breakfast: Egg & Cheese Biscuit	360	21	31
Sausage, Egg & Cheese Biscuit	520	35	32
Steak Biscuit	480	28	43

For Complete Menu & Data ~ see CalorieKing.com

Jamba Juice® (Jan '15)

	C	**F**	**Cb**
Coconut Water Fruit Refreshers:			
Island Strawberry, medium	320	1.5	76
Pina Colada, medium	380	8	74
Tropical Mango, medium	300	1.5	69
Freshly Squeezed Juice: Per 16 fl.oz			
Carrot Cayenne	180	0.5	42
Purely Carrot	130	0.5	30
Purely Orange	220	1	52
Tropical Kick-Start	210	1	50
Smoothies: Per 16 fl.oz			
Classic: Banana Berry	280	1	67
Mango-A-Go-Go	300	1.5	69
Peach Pleasure	280	1	65
Strawberry Surf Rider	320	1	78
Make It Light:			
Aloha Pineapple	190	0	40
Caribbean Passion	150	0	34
Razzmatazz	180	0	41
Tasty Bites:			
Artisan Flat Bread: *Per Flatbread*			
Four Cheese	420	16	46
Sweet 'n Spicy	390	10	53
Baked Goods: *Per Item*			
Apple Cinnamon Pretzel	380	4	76
Cheddar Tomato Twist	240	4.5	41
Cheesy Pretzel	310	10	42
Jalapeno Pretzel	280	6	43
Pesto Twist	290	10	40
Sourdough Parmesan Pretzel	410	10	67
Sweet Belgian Waffle	310	15	41
Breakfast Wraps:			
Spinach 'n Cheese	240	8	30
Turkey Sausage 'n Cheese	320	16	29
Steel-Cut Oatmeal: *With Soymilk*			
Plain	220	3.5	44
Add: Banana	270	3.5	57
Blueberries	230	3	46
Pineapple	240	0	49
Strawberries	225	0	45
Toasted Bistro Sandwiches:			
Cheddar, Provolone & Havarti	330	14	32
Ham, Jarlsberg & Dijon	290	8	33
Roast Chkn, Cheddar & Hon. Dijon	290	7	34
Acai Bowls: *Per 12 fl.oz*			
Berry	370	6	80
Primo	440	11	80
Tropical	320	8	80

Jersey Mike's Subs® (Jan '15)

	C	**F**	**Cb**
Cold Subs: Per Regular, on White, without Vinegar, Oil or Mayo Unless Indicated			
#1 BLT	550	23	63
#2 Jersey Shore Favorite	565	15	70
#3 American Classic	560	15	69
#5 Super Sub	580	16	71
#6 Roast Beef & Provolone	720	22	67
#7 Turkey Breast & Provolone	535	12	67
#8 Club Sub with Mayonnaise	895	49	70
#9 Club Supreme w/ Mayonnaise	940	49	70
#10 Albacore Tuna	915	56	70
#13 Original Italian	680	24	72
#14 Veggie	670	29	69
Hot Subs: Per Regular on White Roll			
#15 Meatball & Cheese	830	42	75
#17: Chicken Philly	685	22	71
Steak Philly	620	21	71
#18 Grilled Chicken Parmesan	545	14	64
#19 BBQ Beef	750	18	87
#20 Pastrami & Swiss	665	21	70
#43: Chipotle Chicken	965	52	74
Chipotle Steak	945	51	84
#56: Big Kahuna Steak	675	25	72
Big Kahuna Chicken	735	26	72
Cold Wraps: With Flour Tortilla, w/o Vin./Oil or Mayo			
#1 BLT	580	29	59
#2 Jersey Shore Favorite	580	22	64
#3 American Classic	580	22	63
#5 Super Sub	600	22	65
Salads: Without Dressing			
Chef, 16 oz	255	10	16
Grilled Chicken Caesar, 12.5 oz	510	35	11
Tossed, 12 oz	50	0.5	11
Tuna, 18 oz	690	60	15
Dressings: Per 2 Tbsp, 1 oz			
Caesar	150	15	2
Chipotle Mayo	180	20	0
Golden Italian	110	11	3
Ranch	120	12	2
Russian	160	16	4
Desserts: Cookie, Choc Chip, 1.5 oz	190	9	22
Chocolate Brownie, 4 oz	470	21	79
Drinks: Mountain Dew, 22 oz	310	0	84
Mug Root Beer, 22 oz	290	0	79
Tropicana Twister Orange, 22 oz	360	0	96

Updated Nutrition Data ~ www.CalorieKing.com
Persons with Diabetes ~ See Disclaimer (Page 22)

Jimmy John's® (Jan '15)

Subs: (8")

Figures Based on French Bread w/ Standard Toppings & Mayo, Unless Indicated

	C	**F**	**Cb**
#1 Pepe	600	31	58
#2 Big John	510	23	55
#3 Totally Tuna, without mayo	690	35	61
#4 Turkey Tom	480	21	56
#5 Vito with Italian Vinaigrette	610	32	60
#6 Vegetarian	660	39	60
JJBLT	570	32	55

Giant Club Sandwiches: Figures Based on French Bread w/ Standard Toppings & Mayo, Unless Indicated

#7 Gourmet Smoked Ham	760	35	70
#8 Billy Club	790	37	68
#9 Italian Night w/ Mayo & Vinaig.	935	54	72
#10 Hunter's Club	800	38	66
#11 Country Club	750	34	69
#12 Beach Club	810	43	71
#13 Gourmet Veggie Club	970	60	72
#14 Bootlegger	660	27	66
#15 Club Tuna w/o dressing	1000	56	73
#16 Club Lulu	720	35	66
#17 Ultimate Porker, with 9-grain wheat bread	730	36	67

Plain Slims: Figures Based on French Bread without Toppings, Dressing or Mayo

Slim 1 Ham & Cheese	540	13	76
Slim 2 Roast Beef	450	5.5	73
Slim 3 Tuna Salad	785	36	78
Slim 4 Turkey Breast	420	3	74
Slim 5 Salami Capicola & Cheese	625	23	75
Slim 6 Double Provolone	580	21	75

Sides:

Jimmy Chips: BBQ, 1 oz	150	8	17
Jalapeno, 1 oz	150	8	17
Regular, 1 oz	150	9	16
Sea Salt & Vinegar, 1 oz	150	8	17
Thinny, 1 oz	130	5	19
Jumbo Kosher Dill Pickle	20	0	4

Johnny Rockets® (Jan '15)

Original Hamburgers: No Substitutes

	C	**F**	**Cb**
Hamburger #12	950	60	57
Original Burger	850	54	53
Rocket: Single	930	59	53
Double	1400	96	53
Route 66	980	67	49
Smoke House: Single	1080	65	67
Double	1640	109	67
Streamliner	400	10	56
Chicken Tenders, without Sauce	880	56	42

Hot Dogs: With Condiments & Bun

Regular	550	24	63
Chili Cheese Dog	770	51	42

Rocket Melts: Without Sides

Patty Melt, on Rye Bread	880	54	53
Tuna, w/ Cheddar & White Bread	810	52	45

Sandwiches:

BLT, on White Bread	480	26	49
Chicken Club, on White Bread	920	36	77
Grilled Chicken, on Hambgr Bun	520	25	49
Tuna Salad, on White Bread	750	48	47

Breakfast: With Menu Set Components

French Toast with Bacon	560	20	77
Omelette, 3 egg	1150	72	92
Pancakes with Bacon	570	19	85
Patty & 2 Eggs	1370	89	90
The Works	1000	70	55

Starters:

Chili Bowl, 9 oz	610	48	17
Fries: American Fries, 7 oz	480	19	69
Bacon Cheese Fries, 13 oz	830	44	82
Cheese Fries, 12 oz	740	37	82
Chili Cheese Fries, 14 oz	1000	56	93
½ Rings & ½ American Fries, 8 oz	660	29	80
Onion Rings, 8 oz	880	40	90
Rocket Wings, Traditional, without Dressing, 7 wings	660	49	19

Desserts: Apple Pie | 620 | 34 | 74

Super Sundae w/ Hot Fudge, 11 oz	660	41	65

Beverages:

Coke, 20 oz	240	0	67
Fanta Orange, 20 oz	270	0	74
Minute Made Lemonade, 20 oz	240	0	65

Deluxe Shakes:

Chocolate Vanilla Twist, 12 oz	910	50	102
Oreo Cookies & Cream, 12 oz	1030	61	110
Strawberry Banana, 11.5 oz	900	50	99

Fast - Foods & Restaurants

KFC® (Jan '15)

Chicken Pieces: Per Piece	C	F	Cb
Original Recipe: Breast, 5.8 oz	320	14	13
Drumstick, 1.8 oz	120	7	3
Thigh, 3.4 oz	290	21	8
Whole Wing, 2 oz	140	8	5
Original Recipe Bites: 6 Bites	200	9	7
10 Bites	330	15	12
Extra Crispy: Breast, 6.4 oz	490	29	20
Drumstick, 2 oz	160	10	5
Tenders: 5 pieces	630	33	28
10 pieces	1260	66	56
Thigh, 3.8 oz	370	26	15
Whole Wing, 2 oz	210	15	8
Kentucky Grilled:			
Breast, 4.3 oz	220	7	0
Drumstick, 1.5 oz	90	4	0
Thigh, 2.5 oz	170	10	0
Whole Wing, 1.3 oz	80	4.5	1
Spicy Crispy:			
Breast, 6.2 oz	520	34	23
Drumstick, 2 oz	150	10	5
Thigh, 3.5 oz	350	27	11
Whole Wing, 1.7 oz	160	12	6

Strips & Filet:	C	F	Cb
Extra Crispy Tenders:			
2 Strips, 4 oz	250	13	11
3 Strips, 6 oz	380	20	17

Wings: Without Dipping Sauce	C	F	Cb
Fiery Buffalo, Hot	70	4	5
Honey BBQ, Hot	80	4	4
Hot	70	4	3

Dipping Sauces: Per 0.9 oz Container	C	F	Cb
Bacon/Creamy Ranch	140	15	1
Creamy Buffalo	70	7	2
Honey BBQ	40	0	9
Honey Mustard	120	10	6
Orange Ginger	50	0	11
Sweet & Sour	45	0	12

KFC Famous Bowls & Pot Pie:	C	F	Cb
Famous Bowl: Snack Size, 7 oz	280	13	27
19 oz	650	26	73
Chicken Pot Pie, 14 oz	790	45	66

KFC® cont... (Jan '15)

Sandwiches: With Sauce	C	F	Cb
Chicken Littles	310	18	23
Colonal's Original	450	20	41
Crispy Twister	610	32	52
Doublicious	530	27	42
Honey BBQ	320	3.5	47

Value Boxes:	C	F	Cb
Drumsticks: Original	400	22	37
Extra Crispy	450	25	39
Grilled	380	19	34
Thighs: Original	540	32	42
Extra Crispy	660	41	49
Grilled	460	25	34
Wings: Fiery Buffalo	510	28	50
BBQ	540	28	57
Hot	490	27	45

Salads: Without Dressing or Croutons	C	F	Cb
Caesar, Side	40	2	2
Crispy Chicken BLT	350	18	18
Crispy Chicken Caesar	330	17	16
House Side Salad	15	0	3

Dressings & Add-Ins:	C	F	Cb
Creamy Parmesan Caesar, 2 oz	260	26	4
Light Italian, 1 oz	15	0.5	2
Original Ranch Fat Free, 1.5 oz	35	0	8
Croutons, Parm. Garlic, 1 pouch	70	3	8

Sides: Per Single Portion	C	F	Cb
BBQ Baked Beans, 4.5 oz	210	1.5	41
Biscuit, 2 oz	180	8	23
Cole Slaw, 4.2 oz	170	10	19
Corn on the Cob (3"), 2.5 oz	70	0.5	16
Cornbread Muffin, 2 oz	210	9	28
Macaroni & Cheese, 4.8 oz	170	6	22
Mashed Potatoes, with Gravy, 5 oz	120	4	19
Potato Wedges, 3.8 oz	290	15	35

Desserts:	C	F	Cb
Apple Turnover, 2.9 oz	230	10	32
Reese's Peanut Butter Pie, 2.6 oz	310	19	31
Sweet Life Sugar Cookie, 1.1 oz	160	7	21

Kilwins® ~ see CalorieKing.com

Kolache® ~ see CalorieKing.com

Updated Nutrition Data ~ www.CalorieKing.com
Persons with Diabetes ~ See Disclaimer (Page 22)

Krispy Kreme® (Jan '15)

Doughnuts:	C	F	Cb
Apple Fritter, 3.5 oz	390	20	50
Chocolate Iced Cake, 2.5 oz	280	16	32
Chocolate Iced Custard Filled, 3 oz	350	22	35
Choc. Iced, Kreme Filled, 3.2 oz	340	17	42
Cinnamon Apple Filled	330	21	31
Cinnamon Bun	220	12	27
Cinnamon Twist	230	12	30
Dulce de Leche	310	17	37
Glazed: Chocolate Cake	330	22	32
Chocolate Iced, 2.2 oz	240	12	32
With Sprinkles	250	12	34
Choc. Iced Glazed Cruller, 2.5 oz	300	18	34
Cinnamon	190	10	23
Cruller	250	17	23
Kreme Filled	370	23	38
Lemon Filled	340	21	35
Maple Iced	230	11	31
Original	190	11	21
Sour Cream	360	22	42
Powdered: Cake	260	16	26
Strawberry Filled	330	22	30
Sugar	180	11	19
Traditional Cake	230	15	20
Doughnut Holes: Orig. Glazed (5)	200	9	27
Glazed Cake, Chocolate (4)	190	10	24

Kool Kreme:

Doughnut Shakes: Per 17 oz			
Chocolate	750	24	117
Vanilla	730	23	113
Doughnut Sundae,			
Original Glazed, 7 oz	450	17	69

Chiller Beverages: Without Whipped Cream Topping

Orange You Glad; Very Berry, average:			
12 fl.oz	175	0	43
20 fl.oz	295	0	71

Kremey Chillers: Includes Whipped Cream Topping

Berries & Kreme: 12 fl.oz	620	28	92
20 fl.oz	960	40	150
Oranges & Kreme: 12 fl.oz	630	28	92
20 fl.oz	970	40	150

For Complete Menu & Daa ~ See CalorieKing.com

Krystal® (Jan '15)

Burgers:	C	F	Cb
Big Angus: Original	550	35	46
Dble, w/ Bacon & Cheese	850	59	48
Krystal:			
Original	130	6	20
Double	290	13	33
Bacon Cheese	200	11	20
Chik Club	320	16	29
Double Cheese	350	17	34
Pups: Chili Cheese	230	14	16
Corn	240	14	22
Plain	150	8	15
Fries:			
Chili Cheese, 8.25 oz	570	29	62
Regular, Medium, 4.25 oz	310	13	46
Chik'n Bites, Small, 3 oz	200	7	20
Salad, Crispy Chicken, 11 oz	370	21	20
Breakfast Items:			
Biscuits:			
Bacon, Egg & Cheese	440	24	34
Chik	400	18	43
Gravy	350	18	41
Plain	260	13	32
Sausage	420	28	32
Sandwich, Krystal Sunriser	200	11	16
Scramblers:			
Original: With Bacon	330	16	27
With Sausage	420	26	27
4-Carb Scrambler,			
With Sausage	620	52	3
Desserts:			
Apple Turnover, fried	220	8	34
Lemon Icebox Pie	320	9	56
Drinks: Per 16 fl.oz, with ¼ ice			
Coca-Cola, Classic	120	0	32
Diet Coke	0	0	0

For Complete Menu & Data ~ see CalorieKing.com

For Menu Updates,
Check Author's Website
www.CalorieKing.com

Fast - Foods & *Restaurants*

LaRosa's Pizzeria® (Jan '15)

Pizzas:

	C	F	Cb
Focaccia Style: *Per Slice, 1/10 of Medium Pizza*			
Florentine	240	13	24
Roma	300	18	23
Hand Tossed: *Per Slice, 1/8 of Medium Pizza*			
Cheese	230	8	29
Double Pepperoni	300	14	29
Big 4: Meat	325	15	29
Pick 4	280	11	30
Veggie	240	7	30
Multigain Wheat: *Per 1/2 of 12" Pizza*			
Pepperoni-Sausage	190	11	14
Average other varieties	125	5	15
Pan Crust: *Per Slice, 1/8 of Medium Pizza*			
Cheese	300	16	30
Double Pepperoni	370	22	30
Big 4: Meat	325	15	29
Pick 4	280	11	30
Veggie	240	7	30
Traditional Crust: *Per Slice, 1/8 of Medium Pizza*			
Cheese	200	10	19
Double Pepperoni	280	16	20
Big 4: Meat	285	16	20
Pick 4	240	12	20
Veggie	200	8	21
Calzones: *Per Calzone, No Dipping Sauce*			
Cheese & Pepperoni	960	45	101
Cheese	840	34	101
Philly Cheesesteak	870	39	90
Sausage Pelucci	1040	52	92
Classic Hoagys: *Baked Meatball*	700	29	75
Original Steak	740	33	69
Pasta Dinner: *Without Bread, Soup or Salad*			
Cheese Ravioli	660	26	80
Lasagna, with Meat Sauce	735	38	61
Spaghetti: With Alfredo Sauce	975	50	104
With Meatballs	870	28	119
With Meat Sauce	700	18	104
With Traditional Sauce	640	12	113
Ziti Chicken Alfredo	980	42	102
Ziti Sausage Pelucci	765	20	115
Appetizers: *Garlic Fries, 11 oz*	630	34	74
Four Taste Sampler, 6.6 oz	475	26	48
Fried Cheesesticks, 6.2 oz	450	22	45
Garlic Bread, 2 pcs, 2.6 oz	300	14	38
Kitchen Chips, 10 oz	570	27	71
Onion Twists, 10 oz	910	57	91
Rondo: Pepperoni, 4.6 oz	545	36	35
Spinach/Cheese, av., 4.5 oz	405	22	35

For Complete Nutritional Data ~ see CalorieKing.com

La Salsa Fresh Mexican® (Jan '15)

Appetizers:

	C	F	Cb
Salsa & Chips: Regular, 14.5 oz	700	32	87
W/ Guacamole, 14.5 oz	970	55	103
Chips (15), 1.4 oz	200	10	25
Nachos:			
Black Beans: With Carnitas	1570	83	141
With Chicken	1600	83	148
With Steak	1580	84	142
Pinto Beans: With Carnitas	1560	83	139
With Chicken	1590	83	146
With Steak	1565	84	139
Burritos: *Without Chips*			
Black Beans & Cheese	1100	48	132
With Carnitas	1205	51	132
With Chicken	1240	52	139
Pinto Beans & Cheese	1070	48	115
With Chicken	1200	52	122
With Steak	1175	54	115
Baja Fish Burrito	875	53	58
California Steak w/ Black Beans	815	35	89
Overstuffed Grilled Burrito:			
With Carnitas	1200	59	108
With Chicken	1260	59	110
With Steak	1290	66	109
Grande, Black Beans:			
With Carnitas or Chicken, average	810	34	92
With Steak	820	35	91
Tacos: *Without Chips*			
Baja Fish	395	22	29
Baja Shrimp	320	19	30
Guadalajara Carnitas	320	15	30
Mexico City, Chicken or Steak, av.	190	4	27
Quesadillas: *Without Chips*			
Classic: Carnitas	960	58	57
Chicken	955	57	58
Steak	965	59	57
Grande, Pinto Beans,			
with choice of meat, average	1130	61	90
Grande, Black Beans,			
with choice of meat, average	1140	61	91
Favorites: *Without Chips*			
Stuffed Fajita Quesadilla			
With Carnitas or Chicken, av.	860	51	54
With Shrimp	800	49	54
With Steak	885	55	53
Fire Roasted Bowls:			
Black Beans: W/ Chicken	730	32	74
With Steak	735	34	73
Without Meat	630	29	71
Pinto Beans: W/ Chicken	730	32	73
With Steak	720	34	70
Without Meat	620	29	69

Updated Nutrition Data ~ www.CalorieKing.com
Persons with Diabetes ~ See Disclaimer (Page 22)

Little Caesars® (Jan '15)

14" Pizza: Per Slice, ⅛ Pizza

	C	F	Cb
Optional: 3 Meat Treat	340	17	32
Hula Hawaiian: W/ Ham	280	9	35
W/ Canadian Bacon	280	9	35
Ultimate Supreme	320	13	33
Veggie	270	10	33
Hot-N-Ready:			
Deep Deep Dish: Cheese	360	15	41
Pepperoni	390	18	41
Round Pizza:			
Cheese	250	9	32
Pepperoni	280	11	32

Caesar Wings: Per Wing

BBQ: Regular	80	5	3
Spicy	70	5	1
Buffalo, Mild or Hot	70	5	0
Garlic Parmesan	90	7	1
Lemon Pepper	90	8	1
Oven Roasted	70	5	0

Caesar Dips: Per 1 oz Container Unless Indicated

BBQ; Buffalo Ranch	160	17	2
Buffalo	100	10	2
Buttery Garlic, 0.5 oz	130	14	0
Cheezy Jalapeno	140	15	2
Ranch	170	18	2

Bread: Per Piece

Crazy Bread, 1 stick	100	3	15
Crazy Sauce, 4 oz	45	0	10
Italian Cheese Bread	130	6	13
Pepperoni Cheese Bread	150	8	13

Lone Star Steakhouse® (Oct '12)

Appetizers: Per Serving

	C	F	Cb
Chicken Tenders: Original, 3.5 oz	320	19	27
Buffalo Style, 3.5 oz	300	19	23
Lone Star Wings, mild, 3.5 oz	305	20	5
Spin. & Artichoke Dip, 3.5 oz	160	13	4.5
Texas Rose, 3.5 oz	285	19	25

Meals: Without Sides, Toppings & Sauce

Mesquite Grilled Steaks:

Chopped Steak, 9.6 oz	710	52	0
Five Star Filet, 6 oz	335	18	2
NY Strip, 9.6 oz	525	28	0
Texas Ribeye, 12.5 oz	710	40	5.5

Lone Star® cont... (Oct '12)

Meals: (Cont): Without Sides, Toppings & Sauce

Ribs Combo:

	C	F	Cb
Baby Back Ribs:			
With Chicken, 10.5 oz	740	30	46
With Sirloin, 10.2 oz	655	33	7.5
Grilled Pork Chops: 3.5 oz	190	10	0
5.9 oz	315	16	0
Seafood:			
Fried Shrimp Entree, 11.7 oz	865	40	97
Grilled Shrimp: 3.5 oz	60	2	5.5
11 oz	190	7	17
Lobster Tail, 3.5 oz	150	1	14
Lobster & Lobster, 4 oz	165	1	15
Sweet Bourbon Salmon: 6oz	240	11	0
9 oz	360	16	0

Burgers:

Bubba, 15.7 oz	1085	57	67
Bacon Bleu,13.5 oz	820	37	51
Cheeseburger, 14 oz	895	45	50
Lonestar, 12.2 oz	640	27	48
Swiss & Mushroom, 15.2 oz	845	38	53
Chili, 10 oz bowl	345	18	14

Salads: Per Serving, Includes Dressing

Dinner, Caesar, 6.3 oz	145	11	8
Grilled Chicken Caesar	480	24	19
Lettuce Wedge	395	34	10
Steakhouse	710	53	2

Sides: Per Serving

Garlic Mashed Potatoes, ½ cup	130	5	19
Macaroni & Cheese: 3.5 oz	80	4	8
8 oz	185	9	18
Steak Fries, 8 oz	610	26	86
Texas Rice, 8 oz	100	3.5	14

Long John Silver's® (Jan '15)

	C	F	Cb
Chicken Tenders, 1 piece 2 oz	170	8	11
Sandwiches & Tacos:			
Ciabatta Jack: Chicken Sandwich	660	33	57
Fish Sandwich	550	30	48
Baja: Fish Taco (1), 7oz	580	39	41
Chicken Taco (1), 6.2 oz	530	33	40

Continued Next Page....

Fast - Foods & *Restaurants*

Long John's® cont... (Jan '15)

Seafood:

	C	F	Cb
Baked Cod, 1 piece, 6 oz	160	1	1
Battered: Alaskan Pollock, 1 piece, 3.2 oz	230	14	14
Cod, 1 piece, 3 oz	280	19	6
Shrimp, 3 pieces, 1.5 oz	130	7	5
Crab Cake, 1 cake, 2.2 oz	280	15	26
Snack Box: Breaded Clam Strips	280	16	20
Popcorn Shrimp, 3 oz	330	12	26

Sauces & Condiments:

	C	F	Cb
Dipping Sauces: BBQ, 1 oz	40	0	10
Cocktail, 1 oz	25	0	6
Honey Mustard, 1 oz	100	6	12
Louisiana Hot Sauce, 1 tsp	0	0	0
Ketchup, 1 pouch, 1 oz	30	0	0
Malt Vinegar, 0.5 oz	0	0	0
Tartar, 0.5 oz packet	40	4	2

Sides:

	C	F	Cb
Breaded Mozzarella Sticks (3)	170	10	12
Broccoli Cheese Soup, 1 bowl, 7.5 oz	220	18	8
Clam Chowder, 1 bowl	230	16	16
Cole Slaw, 4 oz	200	15	15
Corn Cobbette w/ Butter Oil, 3.5 oz	150	10	14
Crumblies, 1 oz	150	13	8
Fries, 3.7oz	350	17	44
Hushpuppy, 2 pups, 1.5 oz	160	13	18
Jalapeno Cheddar Bites (5), 1 oz	240	16	18
Rice, 5 oz	180	1	37

For Complete Menu & Data ~ see CalorieKing.com

Macaroni Grill® (Jan '15)

(n/a = not available)

Tapas & Antipasti: Per Whole Appetizer as Served

	C	F	Cb
Calamari Fritti	760	51	33
Goat Cheese Peppadew Peppers	350	13	55
Mac & Chse Bites w/ Dip	920	71	44
Spicy Ricotta Meatballs	440	35	14
Stuffed Mushrooms	390	n/a	19

Meals: Per Whole Entree, as Served

	C	F	Cb
Carne: Calabrese Steak	1650	n/a	41
Chianti Pork Chop	960	n/a	38
Chicken: Caprese	720	34	40
Marsala	790	35	61
Milanese	1410	99	80
Scallopine	1110	77	51
Under a Brick	1590	n/a	20

Macaroni Grill® cont... (Jan '15)

Meals (Cont): Per Whole Entree

	C	F	Cb
Classics: Eggplant Parmesan	1340	n/a	103
Fettuccine Alfredo	1040	n/a	86
Lasagna Bolognese	1110	78	69
Mom's Meatballs: W/ Bologn.	1130	81	83
With Pomodoro	970	67	79
Pasta: Cannelloni Bolognese	930	n/a	39
Carmela's Chicken	1030	62	82
Lobster Ravioli	600	35	36
Mama's Trio	2040	135	123
Mushroom Ravioli	930	60	53
Penne Rustica	930	43	78
Pesce: Grilled Salmon	1030	n/a	53
Parmesan-Crusted Sole	1330	82	94

Flatbreads: Per Whole Meal, as Served

	C	F	Cb
Farmhouse	1370	n/a	147
Margherita	1280	n/a	148
Pesto Primavera	1210	n/a	149
Smashed Meatball	1420	n/a	149

Kids: Chkn Tenders w/ Broccolini

	C	F	Cb
Kids: Chkn Tenders w/ Broccolini	360	n/a	47
Macaroni & Cheese	540	32	44
Pepperoni Pizza	630	24	72
Spaghetti & Meatballs, w/ Sauce	460	25	45

Salads: Includes Dressing

	C	F	Cb
Bibb & Blue	480	44	17
Parmesan Crusted Chicken	870	n/a	73
Side Caesar	240	21	8
Warm Spinach & Shrimp	370	25	14

Soups: Minestrone, 8 oz bowl

	C	F	Cb
Soups: Minestrone, 8 oz bowl	160	n/a	28
Pomodorina, 8 oz bowl	170	n/a	12

Dessert: Gelato, Vanilla

	C	F	Cb
Dessert: Gelato, Vanilla	310	13	42
Homemade Choc. Cake	940	58	101
Lemon Passion	740	46	77
New York Style Cheesecake	690	40	70
Tiramisu	600	42	54

Manhattan Bagel® (Jan '15)

Bagels: Per Bagel

	C	F	Cb
Blueberry, 3.8 oz	300	1	65
Chocolate Chip, 3.8 oz	290	3	58
Cinnamon Raisin, 4 oz	330	1	70
Egg; Jalapeno Cheddar, av., 4 oz	320	2	67
Everything; Poppy, av 4.3 oz	335	3	68
Pumpernickel, 3.5 oz	240	2	53
Salt, 4.3 oz	320	1	68

Cream Cheese: Plain, 1.3 oz

	C	F	Cb
Cream Cheese: Plain, 1.3 oz	120	12	2
Plain, Red.-Fat, Whipped, 1.3 oz	110	9	4

Updated Nutrition Data ~ www.CalorieKing.com
Persons with Diabetes ~ See Disclaimer (Page 22)

Manhattan Bagel® cont... (Jan '15)

Breakfast: On Plain Bagel

Egg & Cheese	195	13	76
Egg Bacon & Cheese	225	25	70
Egg, Pork Roll & Cheese	280	31	71
Omelet Wrap, Egg, Chse,Ham	355	29	54

Deli Sandwich:

Big City BLT on Multigrain bread	205	25	48
Wall St Roast Beef on Cheddar Roll	300	8	76

Grilled Sandwich: Bronx Bomber

Chicken Cuban	200	14	49
	315	24	48
Pastrami Reuben on Marble Rye	310	40	56
Tuna Melt Panini	255	31	46

Salad: Without Dressing

Garden Market, 10 oz	335	26	25
NY Deli Chef, 14 oz	450	49	25

Marie Callender's® (Jan '15)

Appetizers: Per Serving

	C	F	Cb
Crispy Chicken Tenders, 12.9 oz	870	47	72
Crispy Green Beans, 10.5 oz	810	52	75
Mozzarella Sticks, 8.6 oz	690	42	46

Burgers and Sandwiches: With Fries

Original Burger	1290	87	84
Albacore Tuna Melt	1430	92	99
Grilled Ham Stack	1260	81	96
Roasted Turkey Croissant Club	1450	97	95

Main Meals: Per Complete Meal as Served

Comfort Classics:

Artichoke & Mushroom Chicken	1070	74	38
Callender's Fish & Chips	1280	92	85

From The Grill: Gr. Rosemary Chkn

	900	49	43
Gr. Atlantic Salmon, Cajun style	630	37	25
St. Louis BBQ Ribs	1090	72	58

Pasta Perfecto: Includes Garlic Bread

Chicken & Broccoli Fettuccini	1540	87	119
Double Shrimp Pasta	1500	96	97
Pies, Chicken Pot Pie, w/out sides	1140	79	70

Fresh Crisp Salads: Includes Dressing

Chinese Salad	910	33	107
Gorgonzola, Pecan & Field Greens	990	53	79
Traditional Caesar, with Chicken	700	43	28

Sides: Cornbread,

with Honey Butter, 3 oz	340	21	33
French Fries, 4 oz	380	20	45
Loaded Mashed Potatoes, 6.2 oz	340	23	23
Macaroni & Cheese, 6.4 oz	230	9	26

Soups: Per Bowl

Chicken Noodle	130	0.5	22
Clam Chowder	270	13	22
Hearty Vegetable	90	3	13
Split Pea & Ham	220	13	17

Marie Callender's® cont... (Jan '15)

Breakfast: As Served

	C	F	Cb
Griddle Greats:			
Belgian Waffles	600	19	99
Buttermilk Pancake Stack	720	30	99
Old Fashioned French Toast	830	31	123
Hashers: Country	1320	82	90
Tex-Mex	1180	71	99
Homestyle Choices:			
Country Fried Steak & Eggs	1580	70	179
Grilled Ham & Eggs	1170	47	146
Marie's Magnificent Six:			
With Bacon	750	36	80
With Sausage	910	52	81
Omelettes: BTA	1610	84	160
Denver	1380	65	149
Spanish	1550	78	165
Quiche: Bacon, 1 slice	990	79	45
Ham, 1 slice	1030	83	39

Desserts: Per Slice Unless Indicated

Pies: Apple	630	39	66
Banana Cream, with Meringue	510	24	66
Chocolate Cream, with Meringue	570	26	77
Coconut Cream with Meringue	590	29	75
Razzleberry	630	39	71

For Complete Nutritiona Data ~ see CalorieKing.com

Max & Erma's® (Jan '15)

Munchies:

	C	F	Cb
Black Bean Roll-Ups, w/- dressing	730	36	90
Wings: Buffalo (6), w/o dressing	530	47	4
Sweet Chili (6), w/o dressing	490	31	33

Burgers: With Fries

Aunt Patty, Emma	1550	100	106
Aunt Patty, Max	1760	114	106
Daily Double	1270	69	98
Garbage, Emma	1660	102	110

Salads: Entrée Size, w/ Dressing, w/out Breadstick

Apple Pecan, with Chicken	1060	59	87
Caesar: Without Chicken	670	57	28
With Chicken	880	67	28
Sides: Onion rings	280	17	28
Herb Rice	250	1.5	51

Sweet And Treats:

Banana Cream Pie	990	61	107
Triple Choc. Cake, with Ice Cream	1270	65	157

215

McAlister's Deli® (Jan '15)

Sandwiches: Per Whole Sandwich

	C	F	Cb
Classic: Grilled Chicken	680	37	46
Harvest Chicken Salad	760	53	51
The Italian	760	36	51
Tuna Salad	540	27	45
Veggie Pita	590	40	45
Club: Black Angus	810	40	68
Grilled Chicken	750	33	73
McAlister	770	36	73
Grilled Sandwiches:			
Four Cheese Griller	800	43	64
Smoky Pepper Jack Turkey	800	39	72
Spicy Southwest Chicken	930	52	74
Sweet Chipotle Chicken	650	20	75
Hot Sandwiches:			
California Turkey Reuben	850	50	66
French Dip	540	20	43
Ham Melt	590	25	44
Reuben	780	41	62
Roast Beef Melt	580	25	41
The Big Nasty	780	24	67
The New Yorker	740	30	51

McDonald's® (Jan '15)

Beef Burgers/Sandwiches:

	C	F	Cb
Bacon Clubhouse Burger	720	40	52
BBQ Ranch Burger	340	15	37
Big Mac Burger	530	27	47
Cheeseburger	290	11	33
Double: Cheeseburger	430	21	35
Daily Double	430	33	34
Jalapeno Double	430	23	35
Hamburger	240	8	32
McDouble: Regular	380	17	34
Bacon	440	22	35
McRib	500	26	44
Quarter Pounder: With Cheese	520	26	42
Bacon Habanero Ranch	610	31	47
Deluxe	540	27	45
Double, with Cheese	740	42	43
Chicken & Fish Sandwiches:			
Filet-O-Fish	390	19	39
McChicken	360	16	40
Premium: Crispy Chicken Classic	510	22	55
Crispy Chicken Club	670	33	58
Grilled Chicken Classic	350	9	42
Grilled Chicken Club	510	20	44

McDonald's® cont... (Jan '15)

Premium McWraps:

	C	F	Cb
Crispy: Chicken & Bacon	630	32	56
Chicken & Ranch	610	31	56
Chicken Sweet Chili	540	23	61
Grilled: Chicken & Bacon	480	19	42
Chicken & Ranch	450	18	42
Chicken Sweet Chili	380	10	47
Snack Wraps:			
Crispy Chicken: Chipotle BBQ	340	15	37
Honey Mustard	340	16	34
Ranch	360	20	32
Grilled Chicken: Chipotle BBQ	260	8	30
Honey Mustard	260	9	27
Ranch	280	13	25
Chicken McNuggets:			
4 pieces	190	12	12
6 pieces	280	18	18
French Fries: Kids, 1.3 oz	110	5	15
Small, 2.6 oz	230	11	30
Medium, 3.9 oz	340	16	44
Large, 5.9 oz	510	24	67
Ketchup, packet	10	0	2
Sauces: Chipotle BBQ, 1 oz	50	0	11
Creamy Ranch, 0.8 oz	110	12	1
Spicy Buffalo, 0.8 oz	35	3	1
Sweet 'N Sour; Tangy BBQ, 1 oz	50	0	12
Breakfast:			
Bagel, Steak, Egg & Cheese	670	35	56
Big Breakfast: With Regular Biscuit	740	48	51
With Hotcakes	1090	56	111
Biscuits:			
Bacon Egg & Cheese: Reg. Bisc.	460	26	38
Large Biscuit	520	30	43
Sausage with Egg: Regular Bisc.	510	33	36
With Large Biscuit	570	37	42
Southern Style Chicken:			
Regular Biscuit	410	20	41
Large Biscuit	470	24	46
Steak & Egg, regular biscuit	540	32	38
Burrito, Sausage	300	16	26
Cinnamon Melts, 4 oz	460	19	66
Fruit & Yogurt Parfait	150	2	30
Fruit & Maple Oatmeal:			
With Brown Sugar	290	4	58
Without Brown Sugar	260	4	49

continued Next Page...

McDonald's® cont... (Jan '15)

Breakfast (Cont):

	C	F	Cb
Hash Brown, (1), 2 oz	150	9	15
Hotcakes: Plain (3)	350	9	60
With 2 pats Margarine & Syrup	610	18	105
With Sausage, Margarine & Syrup	780	33	106
McGriddles: Bacon, Egg & Cheese	460	21	48
Sausage	420	22	44
Sausage, Egg & Cheese	550	31	48
McMuffins: Egg	300	13	31
Sausage	370	23	29
Sausage with Egg	450	28	30
Steak & Egg	430	23	31

Happy Meals:

4 Chicken McNuggets:

	C	F	Cb
+ Fries + Apple Slices	320	17	31
+ Fries + 1% Low Fat Milk	410	20	39
+Apple Slices +1% Low Fat Milk	310	14	28

Hamburger:

	C	F	Cb
+Fries + Apple Juice	440	13	67
+Fries + Fat Free Choc Milk	480	13	50
+ Apple Slices + GoGurt Strawb Yog.	380	8	61

Cheeseburger:

	C	F	Cb
+Fries + Apple Juice	480	16	69
+Fries + Fat Free Choc Milk	530	16	71
+Apple Slices & Fat-Free Choc Milk	435	11	60

Mighty Kids Meals:

With 6 Chicken McNuggets:

	C	F	Cb
+Fries+ Apple Juice	470	23	54
+ Apple Slices+ Fat-Free Choc Milk	425	18	45

With McDouble:

	C	F	Cb
+Fries + Apple Juice	570	23	70
+ Apple Slices + 1% Low-Fat Milk	495	20	50

Premium Salads: Without Dressing

	C	F	Cb
Bacon Ranch: Without Chicken	140	7	10
With Crispy Chicken	390	22	14
With Grilled Chicken	230	8	10
Southwest: With Crispy Chicken	450	22	42
With Grilled Chicken	290	8	28

Salad Dressings: Per Package

	C	F	Cb
Newman's Own: Ranch, 2 fl.oz	170	15	9
Low-Fat: Balsamic Vinaig., 1.5 fl.oz	35	2.5	3
Family Recipe Italian, 1.5 fl.oz	50	2.5	7
Snacks: Apple Slices	15	0	4
Yoplait Go-Gurt	50	0	9

McDonald's® cont... (Jan '15)

Desserts & Shakes:

	C	F	Cb
Baked Apple Pie, 2.7 oz	250	13	32
Cookies: Choc. Chip Cookie (1)	160	8	21
Oatmeal Raisin (1), 1 oz	150	6	22
McFlurry: M&M Candies, 12 fl.oz	650	23	96
Oreo Cookies, 12 fl.oz cup	510	17	80
Soft Serve: Kiddie Cone	45	1.5	7
Vanilla Reduced Fat, Cone	170	4.5	27

Sundaes:

	C	F	Cb
Hot Caramel, 6.4 oz	340	8	60
Hot Fudge, 6.3 oz	330	9	53
Strawberry, 6.3 oz	280	6	49

Shakes: Chocolate; Strawberry, average:

	C	F	Cb
12 fl.oz cup	555	16	91
16 fl.oz cup	695	20	114
22 fl.oz cup	850	24	140
Vanilla: 12 fl.oz	530	15	86
16 fl.oz	660	19	109
22 fl.oz	820	23	135

Smoothies, all flavors:

	C	F	Cb
Small, 12 fl oz	210	0.5	50
Medium, 16 fl oz	260	1	60
Large, 22 fl oz	340	1	77
Milk: 1% Low-Fat, 8 fl.oz	100	2.5	12
Fat-Free Chocolate Milk	130	0	23
Juice: Apple, 6.8 fl.oz box	100	0	23
Orange: Small, 12 fl.oz	150	0	34
Medium, 16 fl oz	190	0	44
Large, 22 fl.oz	280	0	65

Soda: With Ice, approx. 30%

Coca-Cola or Sprite:

	C	F	Cb
Child, 12 fl.oz cup	100	0	29
Small, 16 fl.oz cup	140	0	38
Medium, 21 fl.oz cup	205	0	55
Large, 30 fl.oz cup	280	0	76
Diet Coke	0	0	0

Hi-C Orange Lavaburst:

	C	F	Cb
Child, 12 fl.oz	110	0	31
Small, 16 fl.oz	160	0	43
Medium, 21 fl.oz	230	0	61
Large, 30 fl.oz	310	0	84

Powerade, Mountain Berry Blast:

	C	F	Cb
Childs, 12 fl.oz	60	0	15
Small, 16 fl.oz	80	0	21
Medium, 21 fl.oz	150	0	39
Large, 30 fl.oz	220	0	58
Iced Tea, regular	0	0	0
Sweet Tea, small, 16 fl oz	150	0	36

McCafe Coffees ~ Next Page

Fast - Foods & Restaurants

McDonald's® cont... (Jan '15)
McCafe:

Hot Chocolate:

	C	F	Cb
Whole Milk: Small, 12 fl oz	360	13	50
Medium, 16 fl oz	440	16	61
Large, 20 fl oz	540	20	73
Nonfat Milk: Small, 12 fl oz	280	3.5	50
Medium, 16 fl oz	340	3.5	61

Hot Mocha:

	C	F	Cb
Whole Milk: Small, 12 fl oz	340	11	49
Medium, 16 fl oz	410	14	60
Large, 20 fl.oz	500	19	72
Nonfat Milk: Small, 12 fl oz	270	3.5	49
Medium, 16 fl oz	330	3.5	60
Large, 20 fl.oz	390	4	73

Iced Coffee:

	C	F	Cb
Regular: Small, 16 fl.oz	140	4.5	23
Large, 22 fl.oz	190	7	31
Mocha: Small, 12 fl.oz	290	11	41
Large, 22 fl.oz	480	16	70

Mimi's Cafe® (Jan '15)

Breakfast:

Benedicts: *With Potatoes*

	C	F	Cb
Original	1030	68	55
Slow-Smoked Ham Croissant	1020	70	53

Omelettes: *With Potatoes Unless Indicated*

	C	F	Cb
Andouille Sausage & Red Pepper	800	52	36
Bacon Avocado	900	66	35
Egg White & Veggie, with Fruit	300	12	21
Hickory-Smoked Ham & Cheese	730	49	31

Griddle: *Includes Fresh Fruit*

	C	F	Cb
Brioche French Toast	800	22	132
Cinnamon Roll French Toast	1120	37	179
Orange Crème French Toast	620	22	97

Lunch & Dinner: Without Side Choices

Burgers:

	C	F	Cb
Bacon Avocado Sourdough	1160	73	76
Brioche Cheeseburger	650	36	54
Brioche, Bacon & Egg Chseburger	980	63	56

Craft Sandwiches:

	C	F	Cb
Chicken Cordon Bleu	990	49	58
West Coast Reuben	1270	72	80

Entrees:

	C	F	Cb
Bouillabasse	610	25	57
French Pot Roast	830	47	56
Grilled Atlantic Salmon	750	52	42
Slow-Roasted Turkey	680	25	58
Sides: Broccoli/Green Beans, av.	80	6	6
Mashed Potatoes	300	14	37

Mr. Goodcents® (Jan '15)
Cold Subs:
Per 8" Wheat Bread Sub With Standard Toppings

	C	F	Cb
Centsable	440	17	55
Italian Sub	630	37	52
Mr. Goodcents Original	510	24	54
Oven Roasted Chicken Breast	340	6	52
Penny Club	350	5	53
Pepperoni	685	42	52
Roast Beef	340	6	52
Tuna Salad	475	20	59
Veggie Sub	295	4	57

Toasted Sub: *Per 8" Wheat Bread Sub With Standard Toppings*

	C	F	Cb
Chicken Bacon Ranch, w/ Cheddar	665	30	57
Chkn Chipotle Chsesteak, w/ P.Jack	660	29	63
Meatball with Mozzarella	760	37	70

Pasta:

	C	F	Cb
Alfredo Sauce	1235	42	183
Chicken Alfredo	1380	45	187
Chicken Parmesan	1090	12	190
Marinara Sauce, with Meatballs	1205	27	197
Bread Stick, 1 piece, 2 oz	170	8	23

Mr. Hero® (Jan '15)
7" Hot Subs & Burgers:

Burgers:

	C	F	Cb
Cheeseburger	775	55	47
Classic Gourmet HERO burger	990	72	45
Romanburger	860	62	48

Subs:

Chicken,

	C	F	Cb
Grilled Chicken Philly	540	22	48

Deli Subs: *Per 7" Sub with Menu Board Toppings*

	C	F	Cb
Original Italian	640	39	47
Tuna & Cheese	725	54	44
Turkey	470	20	46
Ultimate Italian	675	40	46

Steak Subs:

	C	F	Cb
Hot Buttered Cheesesteak	670	42	45
Zesty Bacon & Swiss	615	32	42

Taste Buddies: *Per 4½" Sandwich with Menu Board Toppings*

	C	F	Cb
Bacon Cheeseburger	430	30	33
Grilled Italiano	440	32	32
Tuna 'n Cheese	485	38	31
Zesty Chicken	495	25	48

Sides:

	C	F	Cb
Mozzarella Sticks, w/ Marinara Sce	565	43	12
Onion Petals, w/ Tangy Sce, 5.8 oz	595	37	58
Fries: Potato Waffer, w/o Sce, 5.8 oz	430	30	38
With Cheese Sauce, 1.5 oz	485	34	42
Zesty Fries, 5.6 oz	595	37	58
Desserts: Oreo Cookie Cheesecake	260	17	24
Snickers Cheesecake	270	18	23
Strawb. Swirl Cheesecake	280	19	22

Updated Nutrition Data ~ www.CalorieKing.com
Persons with Diabetes ~ See Disclaimer (Page 22)

Mrs Fields Cookies® (Jan '15)

Brownies: Per 2.15 oz Brownie	C	F	Cb
Butterscotch Blondie	260	10	38
Double Fudge; Pecan Fudge, av.	265	14	33
Special Walnut Fudge & Blondie	260	13	35
Toffee Fudge; Walnut Fudge, av.	265	14	33
Brownie Bites:			
Double Fudge (3)	200	10	27
Toffee Fudge (3)	200	11	26
Coffee Cake,			
Choc. Chip, small, 2.35 oz	240	11	30
Cookies:			
Bite Size Nibblers: Cinn. Sugar (3)	180	8	25
Peanut Butter (3)	170	9	19
Semi-Sweet Chocolate (3)	170	8	23
Triple Chocolate (3)	160	8	22
White Chunk Macadamia (3)	180	9	22
Butter (1)	200	8	29
Cut Out (1)	280	11	44
Debra's Special (1)	200	9	27
Oatmeal, Raisins and Walnuts (1)	200	9	27
Peanut Butter (1)	200	12	24
Semi-Sweet: Chocolate (1)	210	10	29
With Walnuts (1)	220	11	28
Triple Chocolate (1)	210	10	28
White Chunk Macadamia (1)	230	12	28
Muffins: Per 2 oz			
Blueberry	190	9	24
Chocolate Chip	200	10	26

For Complete Nutritional Data ~ see CalorieKing.com

My Favorite Muffin® (Jan '15)

Jumbo Muffins: Per 5.8 oz	C	F	Cb
Regular: Blueberry	505	24	66
Choc. Chip; Cinn Swirl Cheesecake	635	33	82
Deep Dish Apple Pie	530	24	75
Pumpkin Spice	545	24	78
Fat Free: Blueberry	325	0	78
Chocolate Marble	375	0	87
Cinnamon Bun	505	0	126

Nathan's Famous® (Jan '15)

Burgers:	C	F	Cb
Bacon Cheeseburger, 5 oz	900	61	43
Double Beefburger, 10 oz	1030	73	41
Hamburger, 5 oz	620	38	41
Super Cheeseburger, 5 oz	960	67	48
Nathan's Famous Hot Dogs: With Natural Casings			
Original, 3.5 oz	290	17	24
Cheese Dog, 5.5 oz	390	25	30
Chili Dog, 5.5 oz	420	28	30
Chili Cheese, 6.5 oz	460	31	33
Corn Dog, on a stick, 3.2 oz	380	21	39

Nathan's Famous® cont... (Jan '15)

Chicken:	C	F	Cb
Chicken Tenders, Krispy,			
3 pieces, 6.3 oz	520	31	32
Grilled: Chicken Sandwich, 8.2 oz	470	21	43
Chicken Caesar Wrap, 9.2 oz	570	22	57
Krispy: Chicken Sandwich, 8.8 oz	620	32	59
Homestyle Sandwich, 8.5 oz	660	37	58
Fries:			
French: Regular, 7.5 oz	510	34	42
Large, 11.5 oz	780	52	64
Family, 15.5 oz	1050	70	86
Cheese: Regular, 9 oz	570	38	46
Large, 13.5 oz	860	58	70
Philly Cheesesteak, 14.4 oz	680	33	52

New York Fries® ~ See CalorieKing.com

Ninety Nine (Jan '15)

Standout Starters: As Served	C	F	Cb
Boneless Wings & Skins Sampler	1630	110	73
Fried Mozzarella	770	36	74
Outrageous Potato Skins	1130	84	45
Burgers: Without Sides			
All Star Steakburger	1300	97	52
Bacon & Cheese Steakburger	1010	68	43
BBQ BLT Burger	1330	80	101
West Coast Turkey Burger	740	40	47
Sandwiches: Without Sides			
Honey BBQ Chicken Wrap	930	40	94
Triple-Decker Turkey Club	940	38	110
Meals: Served With Menu Set Sides Unless Indicated			
Chicken Caesar Crowd Pleaser	2700	210	67
Fish & Chips	1840	123	122
Macadamia Crusted Chicken	1130	69	80
New England Shoreline Combo	2190	144	161
Prime Rib: 12 oz, without sides	740	36	2
18 oz, without sides	1210	66	3
Smothered Sirloin Tips, w/o sides	1010	56	12
Salads: As Served			
Chicken Caesar	830	54	50
Fire Grilled SW Cobb	890	58	30
Tropical Chicken	740	40	58
Sides:			
Double Bleu Iceberg Wedge	460	42	9
Honey Butter Bisc., w/ Honey Butter	210	8	29
Loaded Baked Potato,			
with Butter & Sour Cream	580	34	52
Dessert,			
Little Midnight Fudge Hero	490	25	60

Fast - Foods & *Restaurants*

Noodles & Company® (Jan '15)

Noodles & Pasta: Regular Size	C	F	Cb
Buttered Noodles	930	39	115
Bangkok Curry	480	14	78
Indonesian Peanut Saute	810	17	150
Japanese Pan Noodles	620	15	111
Mushroom Stroganoff	930	44	105
Pad Thai	800	19	145
Penne Rosa, with Parmesan	700	25	97
Spaghetti & Meatballs	1020	54	98
Steak Stroganoff	1170	59	107
Wisconsin Mac & Cheese	1040	42	125
Sandwiches: BBQ Pork	540	16	69
Mmmeatball	790	49	57
Spicy Chkn Caesar,			
without Dressing	370	14	40
The Veggie Med	320	12	43
Salads: Per Regular Size			
Chinese Chicken Chop Salad	510	26	42
Grilled Chicken Caesar	550	34	25
Pork Med Salad	340	13	44
Spinach & Fresh Fruit Salad	600	38	46
Soups: Per Regular Size			
Chicken Noodle	350	10	43
Thai Curry	450	15	65
Tomato Basil Bisque	450	31	36
Extras: Cheesy Garlic Bread (3)	300	16	28
Cucumber Tomato Salad	90	0	21
Margherita Flatbread	330	14	37
Potsticker (6), without sauce	340	10	45

Nothing But Noodles® (Jan '15)

Noodle Bowls:	C	F	Cb
American: Beef Stroganoff	510	31	33
Buttery Noodles	650	44	46
Santa Fe Pasta	705	54	40
Southwest Chipotle	715	58	41
Spicy Cajun Pasta	660	50	44
Asian: Pad Thai Noodles	600	10	118
Sesame Lo Mein	410	11	64
Spicy Japanese Noodles	420	8	74
Thai Peanut	570	20	89
Italian: Basil Pesto	575	42	36
Cappelini Primavera	500	28	56
Fettuccini Alfredo	725	56	36
Margherita Pasta	475	31	36
Marinara Pasta	485	11	77
Three-Cheese Macaroni	445	21	45

For Complete Menu & Data ~ see CalorieKing.com

O'Charley's® (Jan '15)

Appetizers: As Served	C	F	Cb
Chicken Tenders, Chipotle	1160	40	107
Over-Loaded Potato Skins	1400	109	44
Spicy Jack Cheese Wedges (7)	720	48	44
Top Shelf Combo Platter	1880	132	74
Chicken & Pasta: Without Sides Unless Indicated			
Bruschetta Chicken	340	10	14
Cajun Chicken Pasta	1150	59	97
Chckn Tenders, Buffalo w/o sides	1070	64	31
Prime Rib Pasta	1400	94	80
Classic Combos: Without Sides			
Panko-Crusted Shrimp,			
with Battered Cod	1060	58	69
Steak & Chicken Tenders	1030	67	26
Steak & Grilled Atlantic Salmon	750	47	3
Steak & Panko-Crusted Shrimp	780	42	41
Steak & Shrimp Scampi	700	51	9
Hand-Crushed Burgers: Without Sides			
Better Cheddar Bacon	1000	58	3
Wild West Burger	1290	94	4
Steaks & Ribs: Without Sides			
O'Charley's:			
Baby Back Ribs:			
Full Rack	1460	85	96
Half Rack	730	43	48
Slow Roasted Prime Rib:			
8oz	830	70	3
16 oz	1460	120	3
Coastal Favorites: Without Sides			
Grilled Atlantic Salmon, 9 oz	500	31	1
Hand Battered Fish & Chips: Reg.	1460	91	6
Large	1810	127	7
Panko Crusted Shrimp Dinner	560	24	3
Sides: Bacon Smashed Potatoes	350	16	44
Broccoli	110	8	3
French Fries, side	400	24	40
Loaded Baked Potato	490	27	53
Sweet Potato Fries	280	19	27
Salads: Per Full Salad, With Dressing Unless Indicated			
California Chicken, w/out Dressing	980	63	68
Southern Fried Chicken Salad	1620	114	50
Southern Pecan Chicken Tender	1600	114	89
Signature Soup: Per Cup			
Chicken Harvest	120	7	11
Chicken Tortilla	100	4	11
Overloaded Potato	260	15	24
Desserts:			
Double Crust Peach Pie, 1 slice	570	35	64
Ooey Gooey Caramel Pie, 1 slice	640	39	76

For Complete Menu & Data ~ see CalorieKing.com

Olive Garden® (Jan '15)

Appetizers:		C	F	Cb
Bruschetta		680	22	104
Classic Calamari		680	44	47
Spicy Shrimp Scampi Fritta		560	37	34
Stuffed Mushrooms		380	30	13

Entrees:

Lunch:

	C	F	Cb
Chicken Alfredo	1030	70	59
Eggplant Parmigiana	520	26	68
Fettuccine Alfredo	700	45	56
Five Cheese Ziti al Forno	740	42	62
Lasagna Classico	610	37	34
Spaghetti with Meatballs	740	35	67
Seafood Alfredo	760	46	58

Dinner:

	C	F	Cb
Eggplant Parmig.	790	39	86
Fettucini Alfredo	1090	68	92
Five Cheese Ziti al Forno	1150	66	98
Lasagna Classico	960	58	54
Ravioli di Portobello	810	47	73
Stuffed Chicken Marsala	950	59	34
Tour of Italy	1500	93	91
Desserts: Black Tie Mousse Cake	770	52	77
Tiramisu	470	27	52
Zeppoli	810	28	119

Old Spaghetti Factory® (Jan '15)

Appetizers: As Served	C	F	Cb
Shrimp, Spinach & Artichoke Dip	590	40	39
Sicilian Garlic Cheese Bread	1320	77	111

Entrees, Lunch/Dinner:

Classics:

	C	F	Cb
Spaghetti: With Clam Sauce, 15 oz	810	31	107
With Marina Sauce, 15 oz	560	5	108
With Meat Sauce, 15 oz	650	11	108
With Sicilian Meatballs, 21 oz	1040	36	115

Factory Favorites:

	C	F	Cb
Chicken Parmigiana, 18 oz	750	29	70
Spinach & Cheese Ravioli, 11 oz	470	16	63
Spinach Tortellini w/ Alfredo Sce	940	56	86

Managers Favorites:

	C	F	Cb
Marinara: Clam, 15 oz	690	18	107
Meat, 15 oz	600	8	108
Mushroom, 16.5 oz	610	10	109

Signature Selection:

	C	F	Cb
Chicken Penne, 18.8 oz	870	38	102
Baked Chicken, 16.5 oz	950	55	61
Crab Ravioli, 11 oz	810	45	73

On the Border® (Jan '15)

Appetizers: As Served	C	F	Cb
Border Sampler	2090	143	101
Fajita Quesadillas: Chicken	1190	83	55
Steak	1220	89	54

Burritos: Includes Rice, Without Beans & Sauce

	C	F	Cb
Classic Chicken	910	36	96
Classic Shredded Beef	1070	41	95

Chimichangas: Includes Rice, Without Beans & Sauce

	C	F	Cb
Chicken Tinga	1430	90	104
Ground Beef	1580	105	106

Enchiladas: With rice, Without Beans

	C	F	Cb
Barbacoa	1090	48	99
La Bandera	920	39	95
Suiza	960	44	99

Fajita Grill: Without Rice, Beans, Tortillas or Condiments

	C	F	Cb
Monterey Ranch Chicken	660	44	11
The Ultimate	1040	85	20

Fresh Grill: Served As Listed

	C	F	Cb
Carne Asada	980	59	64
Queso Chicken	820	40	63
Jalapeno- BBQ Salmon	570	15	54

Salads: Without Dressing

	C	F	Cb
House, side size	160	6	22
Grande Taco Salad: Chkn Tinga	1190	70	85
With Ground Beef	1330	84	86

Sides: Per Serving

	C	F	Cb
Black Beans	170	1.5	29
Mexican Rice	280	4.5	54
Pico de Gallo	10	0	1
Sour Cream	60	5	2

Dressings: Per Serving

	C	F	Cb
Ranch Dressing	230	24	2
Smoked Jalapeno Vinaigrette	250	24	8

For Complete Nutritional Data ~ see CalorieKing.com

Orange Julius® (Jan '15)

Julius Originals: Per Small Size	C	F	Cb
Berry Pomegranate	330	0	83
Mango Pineapple	350	0	87
OrangeBerry	250	0	63
Strawberry Banana	400	6	87

Premium Fruit Smoothies: Per Medium Size

	C	F	Cb
Berry Pomegranate	380	0	91
Pina Colada	340	0	80
Strawberry	300	0.5	71

Light Smoothies: Per Medium Size

	C	F	Cb
Orange	170	0	41
Strawberry	200	0	50
Tripleberry	210	0	55
Boost, Banana, Small drink	30	0	7

Fast - Foods & Restaurants

Outback Steakhouse® (Jan '15)

Aussie-Tizers: Per Whole Dish, With Selected Dressing/Sauce

	C	F	Cb
Alice Springs Chicken Quesadilla:			
Small, serves 2	930	63	51
Regular, serves 4	1540	94	91
Aussie Cheese Fries:			
Small, serves 3	1215	91	70
Regular, serves 6	1910	134	126
Bloomin' Onion, serves 6	1950	160	117
Coconut Shrimp, serves 2	615	35	54
Crab Stuffed Mushrooms, serves 4	395	17	15
Seared Ahi Tuna, small, serves 2	330	16	15

Burgers & Sandwiches: Without Sides

	C	F	Cb
Aged Cheddar Bacon Burger	960	70	33
Classic Cheeseburger:			
With American Cheese	745	47	37
With Cheddar Cheese	805	52	36
With Swiss Cheese	810	53	37
Cripsy Chicken Sandwich	765	41	68
Prime Rib Dip	935	62	44
The Bloomin Burger	985	68	48

Combinations: Without Sides

	C	F	Cb
Filet & Lobster Tail	730	52	3
Ribs & Chicken On The Barbie	585	28	19
Sirloin & Coconut Shrimp	595	30	36
Sirloin & Grilled Shrimp	495	28	7

Outback Favorites: Without Sides

	C	F	Cb
Alice Springs Chicken, 8 oz	750	44	15
Baby Back Ribs, full order	1045	69	23
Grilled Chicken on the Barbie	310	4	11
Maple Mustard Glazed Pork Chops	365	14	13
New Zealand Rack of Lamb	595	39	1
No Rules Parmesan Pasta: Plain	880	51	73
With Grilled Chicken , 5 oz	1120	60	76
With Grilled Chicken & Shrimp	1310	70	80
With Grilled Shrimp	1070	61	77
Teriyaki Steak Tenderloin	445	10	43

Straight From The Sea: Without Sides

	C	F	Cb
Lobster Tails, with Butter, 4 oz	485	28	2
Royal Port Tilapia	750	49	7

Outback Steakhouse® cont... (Jan '15)

Signature Steaks: Without Sides

	C	F	Cb
New York Strip, 14 oz	765	49	0
Outback Special: 6 oz Sirloin	255	13	0
9 oz Sirloin	380	19	0
12 oz Sirloin	510	25	0
Porterhouse, 22 oz	1110	78	5
Ribeye, 14 oz	760	49	0
Victoria's Filet: 6 oz	220	9	0
8 oz	300	12	0

Dinner Salads: Without Dressing Unless Indicated

	C	F	Cb
Asian Sesame, with Seared Ahi & Dressing	490	32	32
Aussie Chicken Cobb:			
Crispy	800	50	44
Grilled	475	23	17
Caesar: Chicken, with Dressing	695	39	20
Shrimp, with Dressing	585	40	22

Soups: Clam Chowder, 1 bowl

	C	F	Cb
Clam Chowder, 1 bowl	695	45	45
French Onion, 1 bowl	465	31	28

Add Ons: Blue Cheese Crumb Crust

	C	F	Cb
Blue Cheese Crumb Crust	305	29	6
Grilled Shrimp	240	16	6
Horseradish Crumb Crust	280	26	10
Lobster Tail	315	23	2
Sauteed Mushrooms	145	7	11

Sides: Aussie Fries

	C	F	Cb
Aussie Fries	380	20	45
Blue Cheese Pecan Side Salad, with Dressing	545	43	30
Blue Cheese Wedge, w/ Dressing	435	38	16
Dressed Baked Potato	350	13	50
Fresh Seasonal Mixed Veggies	95	3	11
Garlic Mashed Potatoes	300	16	32
Sweet Potato, w/ Honey Butter & Br. Sugar	470	18	73

Desserts: Per Single Serving

	C	F	Cb
Carrot Cake, ½ dish	320	15	45
Chocolate Thunder, ¼ of dish	395	27	35
Classic Cheesecake, w/o sce, ½ slice	165	12	11

For Complete Menu & Data ~ see CalorieKing.com

Panda Express® (Jan '15)

Appetizers:

	C	F	Cb
Chicken Egg Roll (1), 3 oz	200	10	20
Chicken Potsticker (3), 3.3 oz	220	6	20
Cream Cheese Rangoon (3), 2.4 oz	190	8	24
Veggie Spring Rolls (2), 3.4 oz	160	8	27

Continued Next Page...

Updated Nutrition Data ~ www.CalorieKing.com
Persons with Diabetes ~ See Disclaimer (Page 22)

Panda Express® cont... (Jan '15)

Entrees:

	C	F	Cb
Beef: Beijing Beef, 5.6 oz	690	35	59
Broccoli Beef, 5.4 oz	120	9	12
Shanghai Angus Beef, 5.4 oz	220	19	16
Chicken Breast: Honey Sesame	420	22	40
String Bean, 5.6 oz	160	13	13
Sweet & Sour, 5.8 oz	380	14	46
SweetFire, 5.8 oz	440	15	47
Shrimp: Crispy Shrimp (6), 3.5 oz	260	13	26
Honey Walnut Shrimp, 3.7 oz	370	23	35

Rice & Noodles: Per Serving

	C	F	Cb
Chow Mein, 9.4 oz	490	22	65
Fried Rice, 9.3 oz	530	16	82
Steamed White Rice, 8 oz	380	0	87

Panera Bread® (Jan '15)

Bagels:

	C	F	Cb
Asiago Cheese	330	6	55
Cinnamon Crunch	420	6	81

Breakfast Sandwiches, Grilled:

	C	F	Cb
Asiago Cheese Bagel, with Bacon, Egg & Cheee	610	28	55
Bacon, Egg & Cheese on Ciabatta	520	25	43
Sausage, Egg & Cheese on Ciabatta	550	29	44

Cafe Sandwiches: Per Full Sandwich

	C	F	Cb
Sierra Turkey, on Asiago Cheese Foccacia	770	33	79
Smoked Turkey Breast on Country	430	4	67
Tuna Salad on Honey Wheat	510	16	64

Signature Sandwiches: Per Full Sandwich:

	C	F	Cb
Asiago Steak on Asiago Chse Demi	780	34	67
Bacon Turkey Bravo on Tomato Basil	790	27	85
Napa Almond Chicken Salad, on Sesame Semolina	690	24	92

Hot Paninis: Per Full Panini

	C	F	Cb
Chipotle Chicken on Artisan French	840	38	72
Frontega Chicken on Focaccia	780	30	84
Tomato & Mozzarella on Ciabatta	750	27	95

Salads: Full Size, With Dressing, without Bread

	C	F	Cb
Asian Sesame Chicken	420	22	25
Caesar, with Chicken	440	26	19
Greek	360	32	13
Thai Chicken	490	19	42

Panera Bread® cont... (Jan '15)

Soups: Per Bowl, w/o Bread

	C	F	Cb
All Natural Low Fat Chicken Noodle	130	2	23
Baked Potato	340	24	27
Broccoli Cheddar	330	21	23
Cream of Chicken & Wild Rice	310	20	24
New England Clam Chowder	720	62	31
Vegetarian Creamy Tomato	450	32	33

Pastries & Sweets:

	C	F	Cb
Bear Claw, 4.5 oz	550	28	66
Cheese Pastry, 3.8 oz	400	22	44
Chocolate Pastry, 3.5 oz	410	23	47
Cobblestone, 7 oz	570	15	100
Oatmeal Raisin Cookie, 3.3 oz	400	14	62

Muffins: Apple Crunch, 5 oz

	C	F	Cb
Apple Crunch, 5 oz	450	12	80
Pumpkin, 6 oz	590	22	91
Wild Blueberry, 4.5 oz	440	17	66

Papa Gino's® (Jan '15)

Appetizers: Per Small Serving

	C	F	Cb
BBQ Chicken Tender (2), 5.2 oz	360	18	33
Buffalo Chicken Tender (2), 5.4 oz	390	25	22
Chicken Tender (2), 4.4 oz	350	3	24
Toasted Ravioli (2), 7.9 oz	570	32	62

Burgers: Cheeseburger, 6.7 oz

	C	F	Cb
Cheeseburger, 6.7 oz	570	32	37
Classic Double, 12.8 oz	1040	67	43
Hamburger, 6.3 oz	520	28	36

French Fries, small, 5 oz

	C	F	Cb
French Fries, small, 5 oz	230	14	33

Pastas: Per ⅙ of Order

	C	F	Cb
Mac & Cheese, 8.8 oz	520	30	44
Ravioli, 10 oz	450	17	56
Spaghetti & Meatballs, 10.5 oz	540	29	52

Pizzas:

Thin Crust: Per slice, ⅛ of Large Pizza

	C	F	Cb
Boss BBQ Chicken	340	12	41
Cheese	230	7	32
Meat Combo	330	16	32
PapaRoni	340	16	32
Pepperoni	280	11	32
Super Veggie	250	8	35
Works	330	14	34

Subs: Per Small Sub

	C	F	Cb
BLT	690	35	67
Italian	590	24	64
Meatball Parmesan	790	38	79
Steak & Cheese	710	33	63
Super Steak	750	33	72
Tuna	730	39	64
Turkey Club	600	22	67

Papa John's® (Jan '15)

Pizzas:

	C	F	Cb
Original Crust (14"): Per ⅛ of Large 14" Pizza			
Double Bacon 6 Cheese	350	14	38
Spicy Italian, 5.25 oz	380	18	38
Spinach Alfredo, 4 oz	280	10	36
The Meats, 3.8 oz	370	17	38
The Works, 5.5 oz	330	14	39
Thin Crust (14"): Per ⅛ of Large 14" Pizza			
Double Bacon 6 Cheese	290	16	22
Spicy Italian, 4 oz	320	20	22
Spinach Alfredo, 2.8 oz	220	12	21
The Meats, 3.8 oz	310	19	22
The Works, 4.3 oz	270	15	23

Wings: Without Dipping Sauce

	C	F	Cb
BBQ, 2 wings, 2.5 oz	190	12	6
Spicy Buffalo, 2 wings, 2.5 oz	170	13	3

Dipping Sauces: Per 1 oz Container

	C	F	Cb
Barbeque	45	0	11
Blue Cheese	160	16	1
Buffalo	15	0.5	2
Ranch	100	10	1

Sides: Without Dipping Sauce

	C	F	Cb
Breadsticks (2)	290	4.5	53
Cheesesticks (4)	370	16	41
Parmesan Breadsticks (2)	340	10	54

Papa Murphy's® (Jan '15)

Pizzas:

	C	F	Cb
Original Crust: Per 1/12 of Family Size Pizza			
BBQ Chicken	330	12	36
Cheese	270	10	29
Chicken Garlic	320	13	30
Classic Italian	350	18	31
Cowboy	335	16	30
Gourmet Vegetarian	300	13	31
Hawaiian	295	11	33
Murphy's Combo	350	17	31
Papa's Favorite	350	17	31
Pepperoni	320	15	31
Rancher	325	15	31
Specialty of the House	310	14	30
Vegetarian	280	12	32
Stuffed Pizzas: Per 1/16 of Family Size Pizza			
5 Meat	370	16	38
Big Murphy	370	15	39
Chicago Style	365	15	39
Chicken and Bacon	370	12	38

Papa Murphy's® cont... (Jan '15)

Pizzas (Cont):

	C	F	Cb
Thin Crust: Per ⅛ of Large Pizza			
Cheese	180	9	16
Hawaiian	195	9	19
Pepperoni	215	12	16

Salads: Per Whole Salad, Without Dressing or Croutons

	C	F	Cb
Club, 13 oz	280	16	12
Garden, 14.5 oz	190	11	15
Italian, 13 oz	265	19	13

Pei Wei Asian Diner (Jan '15)

Perfect Additions: W/out Sauce

	C	F	Cb
Crab Wontons (4)	340	20	26
Crispy Potstickers (4)	300	16	25
Traditional Edamame, small	160	7	10
Vegetable Spring Rolls (4)	460	20	52
Sauces: Potsticker	50	3	3
Sweet Chile	130	0	32
Thai Peanut Dipping Sauce	160	10	15

Lettuce Wraps: With Sauce

	C	F	Cb
Korean Steak	510	32	33
Thai Chicken	530	30	29
Traditional Chicken	670	33	69

Wok Fresh Classic Entrees: Per Small Serving, with Rice

	C	F	Cb
Honey Seared: With Chicken	1070	31	164
With Shrimp	1010	30	161
With Steak	1080	33	164
Original:			
With Chicken	1580	50	228
With shrimp	1470	48	222
With Steak	1610	53	228
Fried Rice:			
With Chicken	870	24	122
With Shrimp	790	22	121
With Steak	900	29	125
Pei Wei Spicy:			
With Chicken	960	23	158
With Steak	1120	32	185

Soup: Hot & Sour, 1 Cup — 70 / 2.5 / 6
Thai Wanton, 1 Cup — 80 / 2 / 11

Salads: Per Per Small, Without Dressing

	C	F	Cb
Asian Chopped Chicken	260	10	22
Pei Wei Spicy Chicken	650	27	78
Wok Roasted Vegetable	410	26	40

Pepe's Mexican. ~ *see CalorieKing.com*

Updated Nutrition Data ~ www.CalorieKing.com
Persons with Diabetes ~ See Disclaimer (Page 22)

Perkins® (Jan '15)

Breakfast: C F Cb

Classic: Eggs Benedict,

	C	F	Cb
w/- Engl. Muffin & Hash Brn	**1220**	54	148
Eggs & Canadian Bacon,			
w/- Fruit Cup & Wh. Bread Tst	**630**	32	48

Griddle Greats: Belgian Waffles,

With Wh. Butter & Pwdr Sgr	**470**	23	57
W/ Glazed Blueb., Pwdr. Sugar,			
and Non Dairy Topping	**640**	18	112
W/ Glazed Strawb. Pwdr. Sugar,			
and Non Dairy Topping	**580**	18	97
Berry Blueberry Pancakes,			
w/ Non-Dairy Topping & Sgr.	**860**	24	145
Brioche French Toast Platter	**890**	47	74

Omelettes: With Fruit Cup & White Bread Toast

Everything	**840**	46	65
Farmers	**950**	60	61
Granny's Country	**1260**	53	149

Hearty Extras:

Breakfast Potatoes, 5 oz	**250**	12	32
English Muffin, w/ butter, 2.7 oz	**230**	11	28
Fruit Cup, 4 oz	**50**	0	12
Hash Browns, 4 oz	**490**	13	87
Oatmeal,			
w/ 2% Milk & Br. Sugar	**330**	6	60
Sausage Links (4)	**460**	44	2

Burgers: With Standard Toppings, Without Any Side Choices

BBQ Bacon Supreme	**900**	52	56
Cheeseburger	**780**	46	46
Hamburger	**620**	33	44
Tangler	**1040**	69	56

Melts: Without any Side Choices

Chicken Strips	**1380**	90	89
Country Club	**1050**	64	66
Reuben Melt, on Rye	**1100**	63	75

Sandwiches: With Standard Toppings, Without Any

Kickin' Chicken	**990**	57	80
Triple Decker Club	**910**	56	57
Sides, French Fries, 7 oz	**570**	36	56

Wrap, Ham & Turkey BLT

with French Fries	**1080**	69	89

Perkins® cont... (Jan '15)

Lunch & Dinners: C F Cb

Fork Worthy Entrees: With Bread Roll, Without Sides

	C	F	Cb
Chicken Pot Pie	**1480**	101	90
Chicken Strips,			
with Honey Mustard Sauce	**1040**	58	80
Country Fried Steak	**760**	44	62
Grilled Pork Chops	**740**	43	25
Homestyle Pot Roast	**450**	25	23
Mushroom 'n Swiss Chicken on Rice	**750**	34	57
Tilapia Grille, with Tartar Sauce	**550**	30	26
Turkey & Dressing,			
with Cranberry Sauce & Gravy	**670**	29	59
Tuscan Gr. Chicken on Herb Rice	**560**	21	51

Sides:

Baked Potato, with Sour Cream,			
& Whipped Butter, 8.6 oz	**390**	22	42
Broccoli Florets, 4 oz	**35**	0	5
Dinner Roll & Butter	**180**	12	17
French Fries, 7 oz	**570**	36	56
Macaroni & Five Cheese, 5.2 oz	**300**	16	26
Mashed Potatoes & Gravy, 8.6 oz	**290**	16	32
Sauteed Spinach, 4.1 oz	**70**	3.5	4
Side Salad with Croutons,			
and Ranch Dressing, 6.5 oz	**300**	25	15
Vegetable Medley, side, 4 oz	**110**	8	6

Soups: Per Bowl, With Crackers & Croutons

Homestyle Chicken Noodle	**310**	7	43
Tomato Basil	**480**	26	49

Salads: Without Bread or Dressing Unless Indicated

Chef Deluxe	**470**	28	17
Chicken & Spinach	**790**	54	23
Honey Mustard Chicken Crunch			
with Honey Mustard Dressing	**1040**	67	67

Dessert: Per Slice

Muffins: Apple Cinnamon, 6.4 oz	**570**	31	66
Banana Nut, 6.4 oz	**700**	40	78
Chocolate Chocolate Chip, 6.4 oz	**660**	34	78

Pies:

Caramel Apple, 7.2 oz	**500**	22	68
Chocolate French Silk,			
with Whipped Cream, 6 oz	**760**	54	66
Southern Pecan, 5.5 oz	**670**	33	86
Wildberry, no sugar added, 7 oz	**470**	27	50

Fast - Foods & Restaurants

Peter Piper Pizza® (Jan '15)

Appetizers:

	C	F	Cb
Boneless Wings: *Per 10 oz Serving*			
Mild Buffalo	1010	67	56
Sweet BBQ	1130	58	110
Cheddar Bacon Roll (1)	350	18	34
Garlic Cheese Bread, 3.25 oz	390	17	45
Handmade Breadsticks, with Marinara Sauce (6)	1000	9	198
Dipping Sauces:			
BBQ	240	0	60
Buffalo	120	9	6
Ranch	320	36	2
Sweet Chili	200	0	46
Xtra Hot Buffalo	90	6	5

Signature Pizzas: Per Slice

Original Crust: *Per ⅛ of Large 14" Pizza*	C	F	Cb
5 Meat Supreme	390	18	39
Buffalo Ranch	400	20	37
California Veggie	290	9	41
Cheddar & Bacon	540	28	45
Cheese	310	11	39
Chicago Classic	330	12	40
Double Pepperoni Parmesan	310	15	27
Extreme Pepperoni	260	13	26
New York 3 Cheese w/ Pepperoni	480	25	40
Pizza Mexicana	390	18	39
The Werx	340	14	40
Original Crust: *Per ½ of Extra Large 16" Pizza*			
5 Meat Supreme	340	16	34
Buffalo Ranch	340	17	32
California Veggie	250	7	36
Cheddar & Bacon	480	25	39
Cheese	270	9	33
Chicago Classic	290	11	35
Double Pepperoni Parmesan	400	19	35
Extreme Pepperoni	340	16	34
New York 3 Cheese w/ Pepperoni	410	21	34
Pizza Mexicana	340	15	34
The Werx	290	11	35

Salads: Without Dressing

	C	F	Cb
Apple Harvest	270	16	27
Caesar, small	140	8	5
Chopped House, small	210	6	35
Mandarin Cranberry, small	150	6	26

Peter Piper® ...cont (Jan '15)

Dessert:

	C	F	Cb
Cinnamon Crunch, 3 pieces	380	9	69
Vanilla Soft Serve: Cone	200	6	35
Cup	180	6	31

P.F. Chang's® (Jan '15)

Starters: Per Whole Dish

	C	F	Cb
Crispy Green Beans, without sauce	760	55	63
Crispy Bean Sauce, 2 oz	310	33	3
Egg Rolls (4), without sauce	560	20	75
Lettuce Wraps: Chicken (4)	530	24	47
Vegetarian (4)	610	36	39
Pork Dumplings:			
Pan-Fried, with sauce, (6)	420	20	39
Steamed, with sauce, (6)	390	17	39
Salt & Pepper Calamari	710	37	69
Shrimp Dumplings:			
Pan-Fried, with sauce, (6)	300	11	34
Steamed, with sauce, (6)	290	6	37
Spring Rolls, without Sauce, (4)	330	11	50

Specialties:

Beef: *Per Whole Meal, Without Rice*	C	F	Cb
A La Sichuan	680	32	54
Mongolian	720	39	31
Shaking	800	49	42
Chicken: *Per Whole Dish, Without Rice*			
Almomnd & Cashew	640	25	46
Cantonese-Style Lemon	750	37	47
Chang's Spicy	820	34	73
Moo Goo Gai Pan	420	15	21
Seafood: *Per Whole Meal, Without Rice*			
Asian Grilled Salmon	610	35	17
Hunan-Style Hot Fish	650	32	42
Oolong Chilean Sea Bass	560	38	10
Salt & Pepp. Prwns	590	30	34
Sauce, 2 oz	70	1.5	13
Walnut Shrimp with Melon	1380	104	74
Vegetarian Plates: *Without Rice*			
Coconut Curry Vegetables	1050	77	47
Ma Po Tofu	1030	70	44

Continued Next Page...

Updated Nutrition Data ~ www.CalorieKing.com
Persons with Diabetes ~ See Disclaimer (Page 22)

P.F. Chang's® cont... (Jan '15)
Specialties (Cont):
Wok Classics: *Without Rice*

	C	F	Cb
Crispy Honey Chicken	1140	49	114
Crispy Honey Shrimp	760	28	108
Kung Pao Combo	830	49	46
Kung Pao Scallops	830	48	44
Sweet & Sour Pork	710	25	94

Noodles Meins & Rice:

Fried Rice, with Beef	1240	28	203
Lo Mein Pork	760	24	104
Singapore Street Noodles	920	21	127

Sides: *Per Small Dish*

Shanghai Cucumbers	70	3	7
Sichuan-Style Asparagus	90	4	11
Spinach with Garlic	120	8	8

Soups:

Hot & Sour: 1 cup	80	2.5	11
1 bowl	380	11	48
Egg Drop: 1 cup	50	2	8
1 bowl	260	9	39

Desserts: *Per Whole Dish*

Banana Spring Rolls	950	38	143
New York Style Cheesecake	900	57	83
Tiramisu	250	11	25

Pita Pit® ~ *See CalorieKing.com*

Pizza Hut® (Jan '15)   C F Cb
Hand-Tossed Style: *Per ⅛ of 12" Pizza*

	C	F	Cb
Cheese Only	210	8	26
Chicken Supreme	210	7	26
Meat Lover's	300	16	26
Pepperoni	230	10	25
Pepperoni Lover's	270	13	26
Supreme	260	12	27
Super Supreme	270	13	27
Ultimate Cheese Lover's	230	9	26
Veggie Lover's	200	7	27

Pan: *Per ⅛ of 12" Pizza*

Cheese Only	240	10	26
Chicken Supreme	230	9	27
Meat Lover's	320	18	26
Pepperoni	260	13	26
Pepperoni Lover's	300	16	26
Supreme	280	14	27
Super Supreme	300	15	27
Ultimate Cheese Lover's	260	12	26
Veggie Lover's	220	9	27

Pizza Hut® cont... (Jan '15)
Personal Pan: *Per 6" Pizza*

	C	F	Cb
Chicken Supreme	590	25	68
Meat Lover's	850	48	68
Pepperoni	620	28	68
Pepperoni Lover's	730	37	68
Supreme	730	38	69
Super Supreme	760	40	70
Ultimate Cheese Lover's	630	29	67
Veggie Lover's	540	20	69

Thin 'n Crispy: *Per ⅛ of 12" Pizza*

Cheese Only	190	8	22
Chicken Supreme	190	6	23
Meat Lover's	280	16	22
Pepperoni	210	10	21
Pepperoni Lover's	260	14	22
Supreme	230	12	23
Super Supreme	250	13	23
Ultimate Cheese Lover's	210	10	21
Veggie Lover's	180	6	23

P'Zone: *Per ½ P'Zone*

Classic	470	17	61
Meaty	550	24	61
Pepperoni	460	16	60

Stuffed Crust: *Per ⅛ of 14" Pizza*

Cheese Only	310	13	35
Meat Lover's	440	25	35
Supreme	380	19	36
Ultimate Cheese Lover's	340	15	35
Veggie Lover's	300	11	37

Wings: *Per 2 Pieces, Without Dipping Sauce*

Bone Out: Buffalo, all flav., 2.5 oz	190	9	18
Honey BBQ, 3 oz	220	8	27
Crispy Bone In:			
Buffalo, all flavors, 2.5 oz	230	15	16
Honey BBQ, 3 oz	260	14	24
Traditional: Buffalo, all flav, 2 oz	110	6	8
Garlic Parmesan, 2 oz	180	16	1
Dipping Sauces: Blue Chse, 1.5 oz	230	24	2
Ranch, 1.5 oz	220	23	2

Pastas, Tuscani: *Per ½ Pan*

Chicken Alfredo	520	27	46
Meaty Marinara	450	21	44

Desserts: Cinnamon Sticks, 2 pcs

Cinnamon Sticks, 2 pcs	160	4.5	2
Hershey's: Choc. Dunkers, 2 pcs	190	8	27
Chocolate Sauce, 1.5 oz	120	2.5	24
White Icing Dipping Cup, 2 oz	170	0	44

Fast - Foods & *Restaurants*

Pizza Ranch® (Jan '15)

Pizza:

Breakfast, average all varieties

	C	F	Cb
⅛ of medium pizza	200	12	13

Original Crust: *Per 1/10 Slice of Medium Pizza*

	C	F	Cb
Bacon Cheeseburger	240	9	29
BLT	280	14	29
Bronco	250	10	29
Buffalo Chicken	240	9	28
California Chicken	260	11	28
Chicken Bacon Ranch	270	12	28
Chicken Broccoli Alfredo	230	8	28
Garlic Cheese	240	11	27
Italian Sausage	230	8	29
Pepperoni	240	9	29
Prairie (Veggie)	220	7	30
Roundup	240	9	30
Stampede	250	9	30
Sweet Swine	220	6	30
Texan Taco	270	9	37

Thin Crust: *Per 1/8 Slice of Medium Pizza*

	C	F	Cb
BBQ Chicken	180	7	16
Beef & Blue	220	13	13
BLT	250	16	14
Cheese	190	10	12

For Complete Menu & Data ~ see CalorieKing.com

Pollo Tropical® ~ See CalorieKing.com

Popeye's® (Jan '15)

Chicken Pieces: Mild & Spicy With Skin

	C	F	Cb
Breast, average	430	27	14
Leg, average	165	10	5
Thigh, average	270	20	8
Wing	210	14	8

Nuggets: 4 pieces, 1.8 oz

	C	F	Cb
4 pieces, 1.8 oz	150	9	10
6 Pieces 2.7 oz	230	14	14

Tenders: Mild, 3 pieces, 4.5 oz

	C	F	Cb
Mild, 3 pieces, 4.5 oz	340	14	26
Spicy, 3 pieces, 4.5 oz	310	15	16

Sandwiches & Wraps: Each

	C	F	Cb
Blackened BBQ Chicken Po'Boy	340	7	49
Chicken & Sausage Jambalaya	220	11	20
Chicken Po'Boy	660	34	61
Loaded Chicken Wrap	310	13	33
Shrimp Po' Boy	690	42	66

Seafood: Catfish Fillets, 5 oz

	C	F	Cb
Catfish Fillets, 5 oz	460	29	27
Butterfly Shrimp (8)	290	17	21
Popcorn Shrimp, 3 oz	330	9	28

Popeye's® ... cont (Jan '15)

Sides:

	C	F	Cb
Biscuit, 2 oz	260	15	26
Cajun Fries, regular, 3 oz	260	14	30
Cajun Rice, regular, 4.3 oz	170	5	25
Cole Slaw, regular, 4.9 oz	220	15	19
Corn on the Cob (1), 7.8 oz	190	2	37
Mashed Potatoes, regular, 5 oz	110	4	18
Onion Rings (12)	560	38	50
Red Beans & Rice, regular, 5.2 oz	230	14	23

Breakfast:

Biscuits: Bacon

	C	F	Cb
Bacon	400	25	37
Chicken	490	26	47
Egg	510	29	41
Egg & Sausage	690	45	43
Sausage	540	36	41
Sausage & Gravy	510	33	42
Grits	370	5	80
Hashbrowns	360	20	41

Desserts:

	C	F	Cb
Hot Sweet Potato Pie 3.4 oz	350	19	41
Mardi Gras Cheesecake, 3 oz	310	19	32
Mississippi Mud Pie, 3 oz	280	7	51
Sliced Pecan Pie, 3.4 oz	410	21	52

Port of Subs® (Jan '15)

Figures Based on West Coast Outlets

Cold Submarine S'wiches: Per 5" Sub with Cheese, Lettuce, Tomato Vinegar, Oil, Salt & Oregano

	C	F	Cb
#1 Ham, Salami, Capicolla Pepperoni, Provolone	435	18	42
#2 Ham & Turkey, Provolone	355	9	43
#3 Salami & Turkey, Provolone	390	13	43
#4 Ham, Salami, Provolone	385	14	42
#5 Smoked Ham, Turkey, Cheddar	370	10	43
#6 Vegetarian, 3 Chse	450	21	45
#7 Roast Beef, Prov.	365	10	42
#8 Turkey, Provolone	360	8	44
#10 Rstd Chicken Breast, Provolone	350	8	42
#11 Ham, American Cheese	405	14	44
#12 Salami, Provolone	395	16	42
#13 Peppered Pastrami Turkey, Swiss	375	12	43
#15 Salami, Pepperoni, Provolone	405	18	42
#16 BLT	470	26	39
#17 Tuna, Provolone	475	25	43
#18 Roast Beef, Turkey, Provolone	360	9	43

Continued Next Page...

Updated Nutrition Data ~ www.CalorieKing.com
Persons with Diabetes ~ See Disclaimer (Page 22)

Port of Subs® ... cont (Jan '15)

Figures Based on West Coast Outlets **C** **F** **Cb**

Light Submarine S'wiches: Per 5" Sub, w/out Cheese, Oil or Mayo

	C	F	Cb
#2 Ham Turkey	305	5	42
#5 Smoked Ham & Turkey	315	6	43
#6 Vegetarian	250	5	42
#7 Roast Beef	315	6	42
#8 Turkey	310	5	44
#9 Peppered Pastrami	265	4	41
#10 Roasted Chicken Breast	300	4	42
#18 Roast Beef & Turkey	310	5	43

Wraps: With 12" Flour Tortilla, Cheese, Lettuce, Tomato, Onion, Vinegar, Oil, Salt & Oregano

	C	F	Cb
#4 Ham, Salami, with Provolone	600	28	56
# 8 Turkey, with Provolone	565	21	59
#11 Ham, with American Cheese	615	27	58

Fresh Salads: With Lettuce, Tomato & Onion, w/o Dressing

	C	F	Cb
Caesar: With Parmesan, 6 oz	35	0	11
Add Grilled Chicken, 10 oz	190	3	10
Garden, 10 oz	70	2	11
Grilled Chicken, 10 oz	190	3	10

Salad Dressings:

	C	F	Cb
Blue Cheese, 1.5 oz	220	23	2
Ranch, 1.5 oz	260	28	2
Fat Free Ranch, 1.5 oz	50	0	13

Sides: Per Regular, 8 oz

	C	F	Cb
Caesar Bow Tie Pasta Salad, 8 oz	355	18	37
Potato Salad	325	13	52

Desserts:

	C	F	Cb
Brownie, 4.5 oz	535	12	96
Chocolate Chunk Cookie, 4.5 oz	560	29	72

Pret A Manger® (Jan '15)

Baguettes: Per Pack **C** **F** **Cb**

	C	F	Cb
Albacore Tuna & Cucumber	490	28	35
Brie, Tomato & Basil	540	17	72
Chicken Mozzarella	620	19	73
Roast Beef & Parmesan	350	15	70

Hot Food: Per Pack

	C	F	Cb
Crispy Bacon Mac & Cheese	470	26	38
Melts: Chicago's Angus Beef	610	23	55
Toasties: Ham & Cheese	540	24	49
Mozzarella & Pesto	450	16	52
Wraps: BBQ Pulled Pork	650	20	96
Holiday Turkey	540	12	79
New York Meatball	600	22	60
Pret's Buffalo Chicken	560	24	55

Pret A Manger® ... cont (Jan '15)

Sandwiches: Per Pack **C** **F** **Cb**

	C	F	Cb
Albacore Tuna Salad	510	29	39
California Club	490	25	44
Crayfish & Arugula	360	16	36
Lebanese Chicken Flatbread	380	16	40
Pret's: Egg Salad & Arugula	420	25	37
Holiday Lunch	490	9	74

Soups: Per Medium

	C	F	Cb
Butternut Squash & Apple	225	12	30
Chicken Noodle	150	4	14
Creamy Chicken & Veggie	225	11	26
Moroccan Lentil	450	18	53
Thai Chicken Curry	140	5	18
Tomato Feta	195	11	18

Salads: Per Pack, Without Dressing

	C	F	Cb
Baja Crayfish Pot	170	7	15
California Tuna	490	30	32
Kale Chicken Caesar	360	15	22
Pret's Cobb	430	22	35

Dressings:

	C	F	Cb
Balsamic Vinaigrette	140	15	2
Caesar	170	17	3
Lemon Shallot Vinaigrette	100	10	2
Skinny	50	0	10

Bakery: Per Pack

	C	F	Cb
Croissants: Almond	410	23	41
Pain au Chocolate	300	15	34
Muffins: Blueberry	420	20	54
Cranberry Orange	370	12	62
Yogurt Pots: Banana & Honey	310	9	41
Blueberry & Granola	320	12	33
Pomegranate & Honey	150	3	21

Pretzelmaker® (Jan '15)

Pretzels: Per Serving **C** **F** **Cb**

	C	F	Cb
Bites: Plain, salted, large, 3.5 oz	250	1	52
Cinnamon Sugar, 3.8 oz	330	4	65
Whole: Caramel Crunch, 4.2 oz	300	4	58
Cinnamon Sugar, 3.9 oz	330	4	65
Garlic; Salted, average, 4.2 oz	310	4	60
Iced Cinnamon Swirl, 3.9 oz	330	4	65
Ranch, 4.2 oz	320	4.5	60
Pretzel Dogs: Mini (6)	300	19	23
Jalapeno	410	19	32
Rolls, Pepperoni (1)	560	22	73

Continued Next Page...

Pretzelmaker® cont... (Jan '15)

Sauces: Per Single Portion

	C	F	Cb
Caramel	140	0	35
Cheddar Cheese	80	5	4
Cream Cheese	200	20	2
Honey Mustard	80	0	20
Icing	180	0	45
Ketchup	20	0	4
Mustard	10	0	1
Nacho Cheese	80	5	4
Pizza	20	0.5	6

Beverages: Per 20 fl.oz Unless Indicated

Blended Drinks:

	C	F	Cb
Cool Cappuccino	640	21	107
Lemon Twist	540	16	99
Mango Madness	520	16	89
Mocha Mania	620	20	106
Power Pomegranate	490	16	86
Strawberry Bananza	650	20	115
Lemonade: Original, 44 oz	380	0	91
Strawberry; Raspberry, 20 oz	290	0	74

Qdoba® (Jan '15)

Burritos: Each with Flour Tortilla, Cilantro-Lime Rice, Black Beans, Salsa Verde, Sour Cream and Shredded Cheese

	C	F	Cb
Grilled Chicken	1070	39	121
Pulled Pork	1040	33	130
Seasoned Ground Beef	1120	45	122

Signature Flavors: With Flour Tortilla, 3-Cheese Queso, Pinto Beans, Lettuce, Guacamole & Sour Cream

Grilled Chicken	925	40	91
Grilled Steak	935	41	91
Pulled Pork	895	34	100
Seasoned Ground Beef	975	46	92

Grilled Quesadillas: With Flour Tortilla, Shredded Cheese, Pice de Gallo and Fajita Vegetables

Grilled Chicken	980	54	61
Shredded Beef	980	51	66

3-Cheese Nachos: Per Serving, with Tortilla Chips, 3-Cheese Queso, Salsa Roja, Guacamole & Sour Cream

Grilled Chicken	1120	64	95
Pulled Pork	1090	58	104

Qdoba® cont... (Jan '15)

Tacos: Each, With Lettuce, Cheese, Guacamole, Pico de Gallo & Sour Cream

Crispy Shell: Grilled Chicken	C	F	Cb
Crispy Shell: Grilled Chicken	250	16	12
Pulled Pork	235	14	15
Seasoned Ground Beef	265	19	13
Shredded Beef	245	16	14

Taco Salads: With Crunchy Flour Tortilla Bowl, Lettuce, Black Bean & Corn Salsa, Shredded Cheese, Sour Cream, Guacamole & Cilantro Lime Dressing

Grilled Chicken	1035	64	70
Pulled Pork	985	58	78
Seasoned Ground Beef	1085	70	71

Chips & Dip: Includes Tortilla Chips

3- Cheese Queso	750	42	81
3-Cheese Queso, Guac. & Salsa Roja	955	56	98

Breakfast Burritos: With Flour Tortilla

Chorizo, Egg & Potato:			
With 3-Cheese Queso Sauce	925	42	87
With Shred. Chse & Salsa Roja	1070	52	89

Quiznos Subs® (Jan '15)

Subs: Per Regular, with Standard Menu Toppings on White Italian Roll

All Natural Chicken:	C	F	Cb
Baja Chicken	860	38	74
Chicken Carbonara	950	48	71
Honey Bourbon Chicken	610	11	84
Mesquite Chicken	910	43	72
Steak:			
Black Angus Steak	860	32	83
Double Swiss Prime Rib	830	38	78
French Dip	910	48	80
Peppercorn Prime Rib	880	48	75
Deli Classics:			
Classic Italian	870	47	74
Honey Bacon Club	860	39	85
Italian Meatball	1110	59	86
Spicy Monterey Turkey	630	20	78
The Traditional	760	37	73
Tuna	790	37	74
Veggie Guacamole	760	43	71

Grilled Flatbreads: Per Small

Basil Pesto Chicken	360	15	37
Chicken Bacon Ranch	480	25	37
Honey Bourbon Chkn	290	6	45
Sonoma Turkey	450	26	36

Continued Next Page...

Quiznos Subs® cont... (Jan '15)

Wraps: Includes Dressing

	C	F	Cb
BBQ Ranch Chicken	510	15	64
Honey Mustard Chicken	580	21	63

Salads: Per Large, without Dressing

Honey Mustard Chicken	290	14	13
Peppercorn Caesar Chicken	180	6	13

Savory Soups: Per Regular Bowl, with 2 Crackers

Broccoli Cheese	180	9	17
Chicken Noodle	140	4.5	19

Desserts:

Choc. Chunk Cookie	390	19	54
Chocolate Brownie	310	16	40
Cinnamon Sugar Cookie	400	17	58
Oatmeal Raisin Cookie	360	12	58

Rally's/Checkers® (Jan '15)

Burgers/Sandwiches:

	C	F	Cb
Big Buford	570	36	31
Bacon Double Cheese	650	42	32
Cheese Double Cheese	510	31	31
Chili Cheeseburger	320	15	30
Rallyburger	390	22	32

Classic Wings: Buffalo, 5 pieces

Buffalo, 5 pieces	335	18	2
Honey BBQ, 5 pieces	390	17	18
Parmesan Garlic, 5 pieces	480	35	1

Fries:

Fries, medium, 4.2 oz	420	27	40
Chili Cheese, 7.8 oz	550	34	48
Fully Loaded, 7.4 oz	640	44	51

Ranch One® (Jan '15)

Sandwiches:

	C	F	Cb
Chicken & Cheese	390	12	40
Chkn Philly, 9.3 oz	410	13	40
Grilled Classic Chicken, 9.4 oz	680	47	37
Original Crispy Chicken, 11.5 oz	640	31	60

Other Favorites:

Chicken Fajita, 10 oz	540	24	53
Chicken Platter, with Rice, 11.9 oz	270	6	28
Popcorn Chicken: Small, 5.5 oz	310	10	30
Large, 7.5 oz	420	14	40
Kids, 2 oz	120	4	11

Salads: Completed

Grilled Chicken Caesar, 13.3 oz	430	30	14
Southwest Chicken, 17.5 oz	680	43	44

Fries: Medium, 5.8 oz

Medium, 5.8 oz	380	19	43
Kids, 4.3 oz	280	14	31
Cheese: Medium, 7.3 oz	490	27	46
Large, 11 oz	760	44	66

Red Hot & Blue® (Jan '15)

Entrees: Per Serving

	C	F	Cb
Delta Double:			
With Memphis Chicken	900	54	12
With Pulled Pork	795	60	9
Five Meat Treat	935	63	15
Ribs, Half Slab: Dry	935	72	14
Sweet	950	71	22

Sandwiches: Regular, Without Sides

Beef Brisket	390	15	37
Carolina Chopped Pork	360	14	34
Pulled Pork	370	15	37

Salads: Without Dressing

Grilled Chicken Caesar Salad	770	46	47
Pulled Chicken Salad	295	8	14
Smokehouse Salad	670	36	36
Southern Fried Chicken Salad	710	31	60

Soup, Memphis Corn Chowder,

1 bowl	270	12	23

Sides:

BBQ Beans	255	2	48
Mashed Potatoes with Gravy	310	14	44
Memphis Fries, 6 oz	345	19	38
Potato Salad	405	28	33

Red Lobster® (Jan '15)

Lunch Menu: Without Condiments, Dipping Sauces or Optional Side Dishes.

Seaside Starters:

	C	F	Cb
Chilled Jumbo Shrimp Cocktail	120	0.5	0.5
Crispy Calamari & Vegetables	1650	109	133
Lobster Pizza	680	31	66
Shrimp Nachos	1200	72	98

Lunch Classics:

Cajun Chicken Linguini Alfredo, lunch serve	720	35	54
Crab Linguine, lunch serve	810	46	64
Crunchy Popcorn Shrimp	380	18	38
Garlic Shrimp Scampi	100	4.5	1
Sailor's Platter	320	10	6
Walleye:			
Beer-Battered	590	37	26
Blackened	220	4.5	2
Fried	290	15	6

Lighthouse/Fresh Fish Menu: *Without Sides*

Maine Lobster, steamed	230	1.5	0
Parmesan Crusted Tilapia	370	16	17
Snow Crab Legs	180	2	0
Wood-Grilled Peppercorn Sirloin	300	11	3

Continued Next Page...

Fast - Foods & *Restaurants*

Red Lobster® cont... (Jan '15)

Dinner Menu: Without Condiments, Dipping Sauces Or Optional Side Dishes Unless Indicated

	C	F	Cb
Seaside Starters:			
Lobster, Artich. & Seafood Dip	1040	61	93
Lobster, Crab & Seafood,			
Stuffed Mushrooms	430	26	20
Mozzarella Cheesesticks	780	43	64
Sweet Chili Shrimp	1140	79	79
Soup: *Per Cup*			
Creamy Potato & Bacon	250	18	19
Lobster Bisque	290	23	15
New England Clam Chowder	200	15	11
Lobster & Signature Combinations:			
Live Main Lobster, steamed,			
with Corn & Potatoes	420	4.5	35
Rock Lobster Tail	170	1	1
Ultimate Feast w/- Rice Pilaf	600	18	52
Shrimp & Classic Combinations:			
Parrot Isle Jumbo C'nut Shrimp	860	57	64
Shrimp Linguini Alfredo, full sve	1250	66	107
Walt's Favorite Shrimp	580	28	57
Side Dishes:			
Baked Potato: Plain	200	0.5	43
Blue Cheese Crumbles	80	6	1
Cheddar Bay Biscuit	160	10	16
Coleslaw	260	20	17
Creamy Lobster Mashed Potatoes	380	24	30
Fresh Broccoli	50	0.5	7
French Fries	360	17	47
Garden Salad	70	1.5	13
Wild Rice Pilaf	170	3	32
Salads: Includes Dressing			
Caesar Salad: With Chicken	660	53	15
With Shrimp	640	53	16
Sauces: Per Dinner Menu			
Cocktail Sauce	45	0	11
Honey Mustard Dipping Sauce	190	17	8
Tartar Sauce	210	21	4
100% Pure Melted Butter	300	33	0
Desserts:			
Carrot Cake	600	36	63
Chocolate Wave	1490	81	172
Key Lime Pie	580	22	88
New York-Style Cheesecake			
with Strawberries	590	41	48
Warm Apple Crostada	620	30	79
Warm Chocolate Chip Lava Cookie	1070	51	142

For Complete Nutritional Data ~ see CalorieKing.com

Red Robin® (Jan '15)

Nutritional Information varies between restaurants. Please refer to Red Robin's website for further information

	C	F	Cb
Appetizers:			
Chili Con Queso	725	37	61
Creamy Artichoke & Spinach Dip	770	44	63
Guacamole,			
Salsa & Chips	845	36	99
Towering Onion Rings,			
w/ Ranch Dressing & Mayo	2725	164	274
Warm Pretzel Bites, w/ Beer Chse	635	19	96
Yukon Chips & French Onion Dip	825	62	50
Jump Starters:			
Jalepeno Coins, fried, w/out Dress.	490	31	47
Swt Potato Fries, w/out Dressing	285	15	35
Zucchini, Breaded & Fried,			
without Dressing	215	15	17
Entrees: With Standard Menu Components			
Arctic Cod Fish & Chips	1055	65	75
Clucks & Fries	1285	76	95
Clucks & Shrimp Combo	905	54	62
Ensenada Chicken Platter, 1 piece	230	9	14
Prime Rib Dip	735	27	75
Red's Nantucket Seafood Scatter	1205	72	92
Gourmet Burgers:			
A.1. Peppercorn	1380	83	96
All Am. Patty Melt	1180	80	71
Bleu Ribbon	1375	85	100
Burnin' Love	890	52	61
Fiery Ghost Style Big Tavern	790	44	59
Guacamole Bacon	990	61	50
Prime Chophouse	1460	87	116
Red Robin with Swiss	865	51	56
Sauteed Mushroom	840	49	52
Whiskey River BBQ	1390	89	94
Sandwiches & Wraps:			
Baja Turkey Club Sandwich	890	47	48
BLTA Croissant	785	49	45
Caesars Chicken Wrap	765	42	54
Whiskey River BBQ Chicken Wrap	820	39	69

Continued Next Page... ...

Updated Nutrition Data ~ www.CalorieKing.com
Persons with Diabetes ~ See Disclaimer (Page 22)

Red Robin® cont... (Jan '15)

Soups:

	C	F	Cb
Chicken Tortilla: *Includes Tortilla Strips*			
1 Cup	205	11	17
1 Bowl	400	19	35
Clam Chowder: *Includes Garlic Bread*			
1 Cup	325	19	23
1 Bowl	605	39	37
French Onion: *Includes Garlic Bread*			
1 Cup	245	14	20
1 Bowl	415	19	44
Salads: *Without Bread or Dressing*			
Avo-Cobb-O	545	30	19
Crispy Chicken Tender	820	47	45
Simply Grilled Chicken	480	15	43
S'west Grilled Chicken,			
with Baja Veges, side	670	36	41
Whiskey River BBQ Chicken	825	40	72
Desserts:			
Gooey Chocolate Brownie Cake	795	28	132
Mountain High Mudd Pie	1390	59	194
Milkshakes:			
Classic: Banana	715	30	101
Chocolate	725	30	101
Smoothie: Chillin' Mango	225	0	58
Groovy	365	4	84
Hawaiian Heart Throb	375	2	91

Roly Poly® (Jan '15)

Wraps:

Per 6" White Tortilla Unless Indicated

	C	F	Cb
Chicken: Basil Cashew Chicken	300	10	30
Catalina Chicken	315	11	28
Chicken Caesar	310	11	30
Chicken Fajita	315	9	28
Cobb Salad	255	12	27
Oriental Chicken	230	4	29
Santa Fe Chicken	305	11	28
Ham & Smoked Pork:			
Italian Classic	335	12	32
Key West Cuban Mix	330	9	44
Peachtree Melt	310	11	27
Pork Melt	310	11	26
Porky's Nightmare	320	12	28
Tuna: Classic Tuna Melt	340	17	26
Popeyes Tuna on Wheat	305	10	31
Texas Tuna	310	12	30
Thai Hot Tuna	290	11	30
Turkey: California	330	12	30
Tuscan	220	2	31

Round Table Pizza® (Jan '15)

Appetizers:

	C	F	Cb
Boneless Wings:			
With BBQ Sauce,			
8 pieces	565	14	73
With Buffalo Sauce, av., 6 pcs	440	14	42
Garlic Bread: 1 piece	70	3.5	9
With Cheese, 1 piece	100	6	9
Garlic Parmesan Twists, 1 twist	170	5	26
Pizzas: *Per ½ of Large 14" Pizza*			
Original Crust: Cheese	230	9	25
Chicken & Garlic Gourmet	250	11	25
Gourmet Veggie	240	10	27
Guinevere's Garden Delight	220	8	26
Hawaiian	220	8	26
Italian Garlic Supreme	270	14	25
King Arthur Supreme	270	13	26
Maui Zaui, with Polynesian Sce	260	10	29
Montague's All Meat Marvel	290	15	25
Smokehouse Combo, Chicken	290	14	26
Triple Play Pepperoni	250	12	24
Pan Crust: Cheese	300	11	38
Chicken & Garlic Gourmet	340	13	39
Gourmet Veggie	320	12	41
Guinevere's Garden Delight	300	10	39
Hawaiian	300	10	40
Italian Garlic Supreme	360	16	39
King Arthur Supreme	340	14	39
Maui Zaui w/ Polynesian Sauce	340	12	43
Montague's All Meat Marvel	350	15	37
Smokehouse Combo, Chicken	370	16	40
Triple Play Pepperoni	330	14	36
Skinny Crust: Cheese	190	9	17
Chicken & Garlic Gourmet	220	11	18
Gourmet Veggie	200	10	20
Guinevere's Garden Delight	180	8	19
Hawaiian	190	8	20
Italian Garlic Supreme	240	14	18
King Arthur Supreme	240	13	19
Maui Zaui w/ Polynesian Sauce	220	10	22
Montague's All Meat Marvel	260	15	18
Smokehouse Combo, Chicken	250	14	20
Triple Play Pepperoni	220	12	17
Sandwiches:			
Chicken Club	800	43	59
Ham Club	740	40	60
RT Veggie	630	32	65
Turkey Club	720	38	59
Turkey Sante-Fe	730	40	57

For Complete Nutritional Data ~ see CalorieKing.com

Rubio's Mexican Grill® (Jan '15)

Burritos: Each With Flour Tortilla, without Chips

	C	F	Cb
Beef:			
Baja Grilled, with Steak	640	28	52
Especial, w/ Steak	890	34	107
Chicken:			
Baja Grilled, w/ Chkn	600	25	52
Especial, with Chicken	850	31	106
Seafood: Beer Battered Fish	850	53	68
Blackened Atlantic Salmon	710	33	74
Classic Grilled Shrimp	690	33	70
Grilled Pacific Mahi Mahi	690	31	74
Veggies & More: Bean & Cheese	710	31	74
Grilled Veggie	750	40	82

Enchiladas: With Black Beans & Citrus Rice

	C	F	Cb
Two Cheese, with Fire-Rstd Sauce	800	38	83
Two Chicken, with Fire-Rstd Sauce	770	30	84
Two Shrimp, with Verde Sauce	800	34	87

Tacos: Each, with Corn Tortilla

	C	F	Cb
Grilled Gourmet: Chicken	320	19	19
Steak	330	20	19
Seafood, Blackened:			
Atlantic Salmon	230	11	22
Pacific Mahi Mahi	220	10	22
Seafood, Grilled:			
Atlantic Salmon	230	10	21
Pacific Mahi Mahi	220	10	22
Regal Springs Tilapia	220	11	17

Sides:

	C	F	Cb
Black Beans: Regular, 4 oz	130	2	22
Large, 12 oz	380	4	64
Chips: Regular, 1.8 oz	210	2	43
Large, 4 oz	460	5	96
Citrus Rice: Regular, 3 oz	150	2	29
Large, 8 oz	400	6	78
Mexican Rice: Regular, 3 oz	140	2	27
Large, 8 oz	360	5	71
No Fried Pinto Beans: Reg., 4 oz	130	1	21
Large, 12 oz	370	3	62

Salad & Bowls: Entree Size, Includes Dressing

	C	F	Cb
Chipotle Ranch: With Grilled Chkn	480	34	20
With Grilled Mahi Mahi	490	35	20
With Grilled Tilapia	510	38	19

Salsas: Per 1 oz

	C	F	Cb
Mango, Picante, Tomatillo, average	20	0.5	3
Other Varieties	10	0	1

Ruby Tuesday® (Jan '15)

Shareables: Per Serve, w/out Sauce

	C	F	Cb
BBQ Chicken Flatbread	130	6	12
Cheese Fries	265	16	22
Fire Wings	180	11	4
Fried Mozzarella	135	8	11
Shrimp Fondu, with chips	300	18	25
Spinach Artichoke Dip, with chips	300	18	28
Thai Spring Rolls	130	6	14

Burgers: With Fries

	C	F	Cb
Avocado Turkey	1380	77	112
Buffalo Chicken	1235	63	123
Chicken BLT	1245	61	123
Ruby's Classic	1305	76	104
Smokehouse	1600	92	129
Turkey	1215	65	110
Triple Prime: Original	1355	80	109
Bacon Cheddar	1575	97	109
Cheddar	1515	92	109

Fit & Trim Choices: Without Sides

	C	F	Cb
Chicken Bella	425	20	17
Grilled Salmon	425	23	9
Hickory Bourbon:			
Chicken	355	10	25
Salmon	485	23	25
Top Sirloin	445	27	15
Sides: Green Beans	70	4	5
Grilled Zucchini	40	2	4
Roasted Spaghetti Squash	55	3	6
Steamed Broccoli	50	2	7

Fresh All Natural Chicken: Without Sides

	C	F	Cb
Chicken Bella	330	15	7
Chicken Fresco	350	20	8
Hickory Bourbon Chicken	250	5	16
Smoky Mountain Chicken	550	28	16

Ribs & Chops: Without Sides

	C	F	Cb
BBQ Baby-Back Ribs, Half-Rack	470	24	21
Hickory Bourbon-Glazd Pork Chops	885	42	57

Seafood: Without Sides

	C	F	Cb
Grilled Salmon	330	18	0
Herb-Crusted Tilapia	400	24	11
Jumbo Skewered Shrimp	275	15	0
New Orleans Seafood	315	14	6

Smart Eating: Without Sides

	C	F	Cb
Blackened Tilapia	200	7	2
Grilled Chicken Wrap	495	17	47
Plain Grilled Chicken	190	5	0
Turkey Burger Wrap	585	28	45

Continued Next Page...

Updated Nutrition Data ~ www.CalorieKing.com
Persons with Diabetes ~ See Disclaimer (Page 22)

Ruby Tuesday® cont... (Jan '15)

Pasta & More: Without Sides

	C	F	Cb
Cajan Jambalaya	960	44	88
Chicken & Broccoli	1435	87	100
Chicken & Mushroom Alfredo	1170	58	95
Parmesan Chicken	1285	67	113
Parmesan Shrimp	1015	47	97

Steakhouse Steaks: Without Sides

Black Fire New York Strip	505	28	6
Rib Eye	840	67	6
Top Sirloin	350	22	6

Salads: Without Dressing

Carolina Chicken	1100	47	54
Grilled: Chicken	750	28	47
Salmon	730	40	37

Dressing: Per 1 oz

Balsamic Vinaigrette	40	2	5
Blue Cheese	180	19	1
Honey Mustard; Thsnd Island, av.	85	8	5
Italian; Signature Parmesan, av.	140	15	1
Ranch	90	9	1

Fresh Sides:

Baked Potato: Plain	250	3	51
Loaded	555	29	52
French Fries	480	24	54
Garlic Cheese Biscuit	110	5	12
Mashed Potatoes	265	15	29
Onion Rings	340	19	37
Rice Pilaf	160	3	30
Sweet Potato Fries	330	12	54

Kid's Menu: Includes Fries

Chicken Breast	335	14	27
Chicken Tenders	585	24	36
Grilled Cheese Sandwich	660	29	80

Desserts:

Blondie for One	545	24	77
Cake, Double Chocolate	815	31	124
Cookies: Chocolate Chip	180	9	24
White Choc. Macadamia Nut	200	12	23
Cupcakes: Carrot Cake (1)	325	16	45
Red Velvet (1)	285	11	45
New York Cheesecake	760	60	89
Tiramisu	555	30	69

For Complete Menu ~ see CalorieKing.com

Runza® (Jan '15)

Burgers:

	C	F	Cb
¼ lb BBQ Bacon & Swiss	530	32	26
¼ lb Bacon Cheeseburger Deluxe	510	31	26
	540	34	26
¼ lb French Onion	490	29	26
¼ lb Jalap.; Legend Supreme, av.	525	34	26
¼ lb Spicy Jack Hamburger	570	38	23
¼ lb Swiss Mushroom	480	29	24
Runza Way: ¼ lb Cheeseburger	420	22	28
¼ lb Hamburger	370	18	26
½ lb Double Cheeseburger	670	39	30
½ lb Double Hamburger	570	31	26

Sandwiches:

Grilled: BBQ Chicken	400	11	40
Buffalo Chicken	360	11	37
Deluxe Chicken	360	10	37

Sides:

French Fries: Small	220	11	29
Medium	320	15	41
Large	460	23	60
Frings: Medium	330	18	39
Large	470	25	55
Onion Rings: Medium	320	19	35
Large	550	31	58

Salads:

Asian Grilled Chicken w/ dressing	410	7	59
Southwest Chicken Salad w/ Salsa	330	16	31
Sweet Berry Chicken w/o dressing	370	19	21

Dressings: Honey Mustard

	290	27	13
Ranch	270	27	4

Soups: Per Bowl

Boston Clam Chowder	280	15	29
Broccoli Cheese	240	16	20
Chicken Tortilla	150	6	16
Homemade Chili	320	15	23
Wisconsin Cheese	340	23	29

Kids:

Junior: Cheeseburger, plain	250	13	18
Hamburger, plain	200	9	16
Swiss Cheese Mushroom Burger	300	17	17
Runza Way: Cheeseburger	270	13	22
Hamburger	220	9	20

Desserts:

Ice Cream Cones, all flavors	260	7	40
Ice Cream Dish, all flavors	230	7	34
Sundaes: Caramel; Chocolate	300	7	51
Turtle	360	13	53

Shakes: Per Regular, 16 oz

Cappuccino	490	12	82
Chocolate	480	12	81
Vanilla	430	12	66

Ryan's Grill Buffet & Bakery® (Jan '15)

Entrees: Without Sides

	C	F	Cb
Beef: BBQ'd, 4 oz	140	5	16
Country Fried Steak, w/ gravy, 2.6 oz	220	13	16
Meatloaf, 3 oz	180	11	7
Perfect Pot Roast, 5 oz	160	7	9
Salisbury Steak, 3.5 oz	150	9	8
Chicken:			
Breasts: Country BBQ, 5.8 oz	310	16	6
Rotisserie, 5.3 oz	310	17	1
Traditional, Baked, 5.3 oz	310	17	1
Chicken & Dumplings, 5 oz	160	5	17
New Orleans Bourbon Street, 3 oz	180	8	9
Orange Chicken, 3 oz	340	22	26
Fish/Seafood: Baked Fish, 2 oz	90	4.5	0
Butter Crumb Alaskan Pollock, 1.8 oz	110	5	2
Butterfly Shrimp (6), 2.3 oz	210	9	24
Carved Salmon Filet, 3 oz	190	11	0
Clam Strips, 3 oz	320	20	28
Fried: Fish, 3 pieces, 3 oz	240	12	27
Shrimp (22), 3 oz	240	11	24
Wood Seared Salmon, 1 pce, 3 oz	220	16	0
Pasta/Spaghetti: *Per 5 oz Serving*			
Country Pasta Gratine	160	4	24
Creamy Penne Carbonara	260	17	17
Fire Grilled Chicken Alfredo	220	14	14
Grilled Italian Sausage Penne	180	11	14
Pork:			
Carved: Grilled Loin, 3 oz	140	10	0
Ham, 3 oz	100	5	0
Honey Glazed Baked, 1 sl, 3 oz	120	5	1
Ribs, BBQ/County-Style (3), 3.5 oz	420	27	15
Steak: Grilled, 2 oz	140	9	0
BBQ, grilled, 2 oz	150	9	3
Salads: *Without Dressing*			
Asian Chopped, 3.5 oz	90	4	13
Caesar, 1 cup, 2.5 oz	70	6	4
Greek, 2.6 oz	120	8	10
Seafood, 4.2 oz	310	26	15
Sides:			
Baked Potato, plain, 4.3 oz	150	0	36
BBQ Baked Beans, 3 oz	130	3	26
Cauliflower Au Gratin, 3 oz	50	2	8
French Fries, 3 oz	170	9	23
Fried Okra, 3 oz	220	12	28
Mashed Potatoes, 4 oz	70	0.5	13
Desserts: Cheesecake, plain, 1 sl.	230	12	28
Key Lime Pie, scratch, 1 sl., 2.5 oz	220	9	31
Lemon Meringue Pie, 2.3 oz	130	4.5	23

7-Eleven® (Jan '15)

7-Select Burritos:

	C	F	Cb
Bean and Cheese, 5 oz	320	10	47
Beef & Bean, 5 oz	360	16	44
Beef, Bean & Green Chile, 5 oz	360	15	44
Red Hot Beef, 5 oz	340	15	41
Big Bites: Without Bun or Toppings			
Big Bite Hot Dog, 2 oz	180	17	1
Breakfast Bite Sausage, 3 oz	250	21	2
Cheeseburger Bite Link, 4.2 oz	440	38	2
Qtr Pound Big Bite Hot Dog, 4 oz	360	34	2
Breakfast Sandwiches:			
Biscuits: Egg, Cheese & Ssg, 5.5 oz	460	32	31
Sausage, 3.3 oz	330	22	28
Croissant, Egg, Cheese & Ssg, 4.8 oz	410	30	20
Eng. Muffin, Egg, Chse & Ssg, 5 oz	390	25	24
Fresh:			
Cilantro Lime Chicken Flatbread	570	25	51
Southwest Turkey Sandwich	560	28	48
Very Berry Salad	210	15	12
Yoplait Yogurt Parfait	230	2.5	47
Other Selections:			
Chicken Tenders (1), 3.3 oz	160	5	11
Maple Pancake Sausage (1), 2.6 oz	270	19	19
Pepperoni Pizza, 1 slice, 3.9 oz	300	14	30
Rollers: Buffalo Chicken (1), 3 oz	190	7	16
Corn Dog (1), 3.4 oz	320	21	23
Taquitos: Per 1.3 oz Taquito			
Bacon, Egg, Cheese & Potato	190	8	23
Jalapeno Cream Cheese	240	13	27
Monterey Jack & Chicken	280	14	30
Steak & Cheese	210	11	22
Wings, Bone In, Spicy Wing Zings,			
1 wing	80	4.5	3
Sides: Hash Browns (1), 2 oz	100	5	12
Potato Wedges (6), 0.7 oz	240	4.5	27
Slurpees, average all flavors:			
12 oz cup	95	0	26
22 oz cup	175	0	44
28 oz cup	220	0	56
Sugar Free, 12 oz cup	30	0	9

Updated Nutrition Data ~ www.CalorieKing.com
Persons with Diabetes ~ See Disclaimer (Page 22)

Saladworks® (Jan '15)

Salads: Without Dressing

	C	F	Cb
Autumn Harvest	300	12	40
Bently	245	10	11
Buffalo Bleu	250	7.5	24
Chicken Caesar	285	4	19
Cobb	270	16	13
Fire Roasted Cabo Jack	390	19	31
Greek	185	10	18
Nuevo Nicoise	230	4	31
Sophie's Salad	310	14	35
Tivoli	430	19	31

Focaccia Fusion: Without Spread

	C	F	Cb
BLT	295	14	23
Chicken Monterey	335	12	25
Fajitalicious	330	12	24
Turkey Ranch	320	11	24

Dressings & Spreads: Per 1 oz Ladle

	C	F	Cb
Balsamic: Regular	170	18	4
Classic French; Green Goddess, av	140	14	5
Honey Mustard Spread	20	0.5	4
Mayonnaise	45	5	2
Oriental Sesame	90	4.5	12
Parmesan Caesar: Thousand Isl., av.	145	15	3
Salsa Mayo Spread	20	1	2

Extra Menu Items ~ See CalorieKing.com

Sandella's® (Jan '15)

Grilled Flatbread: With Standard Toppings

	C	F	Cb
Brazilian Bacon	560	17	79
Brazilian Chicken	510	10	73
Pesto Chicken	610	28	56
Spinach & Bacon	660	39	52

Paninis: With Standard Toppings

	C	F	Cb
Philly Cheese	590	25	55
Spin., Ham & Swiss	550	20	61
Tuscan Chicken	540	21	55

Quesadillas: With Standard Toppings

	C	F	Cb
California	500	23	53
Mediterranean	400	16	53

Salads: Includes ½ Flatbread & Dressing

	C	F	Cb
Fiesta	360	8	54
Greek	310	15	37

Rice Bowls: Includes Flatbread & Standard Toppings

	C	F	Cb
Black Bean & Rice	840	20	130
Chicken Fajita	750	20	104

Wraps: With Standard Toppings

	C	F	Cb
California Turkey	410	10	55
Chipotle Chicken	350	7	55
Pesto Turkey	460	15	54
Sweet & Spicy Chicken	400	7	64

Sarku Japan® (Jan '15)

D'Lite Meals:

	C	F	Cb
Rice & Chicken Tempura, 15 oz	970	58	81
Rice & Shrimp Tempura, 11 oz	540	21	70
Vegetarian, 14 oz	360	0.5	79
Vegetarian Soba Noodle, 14 oz	710	24	106

Combos:

	C	F	Cb
Tempura: Chicken, 23 oz	1270	78	102
Chicken & Shrimp, 20 oz	980	53	95
Teriyaki: Beef, 19 oz	690	26	81
Beef & Shrimp, 21 oz	630	11	85
Chicken, 22 oz	640	13	90
Chkn & Shrimp, 24 oz	700	14	90
Shrimp, 19 oz	500	2.5	83
Sauce, Teriyaki, 1.5 oz	45	0	9
Sides: Maki Roll, 2 oz	140	11	9
Rice: Steamed, 9 oz	290	0	64
Fried, 9 oz	330	4.5	62
Tempura Chicken, 1 piece, 2 oz	230	19	8
Tempura Shrimp, 1 piece, 0.8 oz	90	7	4

Schlotzsky's® (Jan '15)

Oven-Toasted Sandwiches: Per Medium Size

Angus:

	C	F	Cb
Beef & Provolone	770	28	85
Corned Beef	510	9	72
Corned Beef Reuben	890	38	81
Pastrami Reuben	900	40	84
Pastrami & Swiss	830	33	79
BLT	540	17	74
Chicken & Pesto	560	11	79
Chicken Breast	490	3	82
Chipotle Chicken	530	9	78
Homestyle Tuna	580	16	75
Santa Fe Chicken	660	19	78
Smoked Turkey Reuben	850	35	83
Turkey & Guacamole	520	11	78
Turkey Bacon Club	770	29	81

Original Style:

	C	F	Cb
The Original	780	33	79
Deluxe	980	46	81
Ham & Cheese	730	25	81
Turkey	820	33	82

Wraps: Per Medium Size

	C	F	Cb
Chicken & Pesto	510	18	54
Homestyle Tuna	540	22	55
Santa Fe Chicken	590	24	55

Continued Next Page...

Fast - Foods & *Restaurants*

Schlotzsky's® cont... (Jan '15)

10" Pizzas: Per Pizza

	C	F	Cb
BBQ Chicken & Jalapeno	920	19	148
Combination Special	960	37	119
Double Cheese	830	326	115
Fresh Veggie	920	34	118
Grilled Chicken & Pesto	910	28	114
Pepperoni & Double Cheese	980	40	16
Smoked Turkey & Jalapeno	880	25	120

Salads: Without Dressing or Breadsticks

Cranberry, Apple, Pecan & Chicken	640	27	68
Hearts of Romaine, Chicken Caesar	400	17	29
Garden	40	2	9
Potato	240	13	29
Turkey Avocado Cobb	610	33	42
Turkey Chef	415	25	17
Garlic Breadsticks, entree portion (2)	60	2	10

Dressings: Per 3 oz

Buttermilk Ranch	320	33	4
Chunky Blue Cheese	455	49	3
Red Wine Vinaigrette	425	43	9
Robusto Italian	285	28	3
Tuscan Caesar	425	45	2

Soup: Per Bowl

Broccoli Cheddar	170	10	17
Chicken & Wild Rice	270	15	20
Chicken Enchilada	300	15	22
Loaded Baked Potato	340	27	34
Timberline Chili	450	22	33
Tomato Basil	310	24	24

Chips:

Baked: Regular; BBQ, average	130	3	26
Other varieties, average	230	14	24

Kid's Meals: Without Cookie or Drink

Cheese Pizza	540	16	78
Cheese Sandwich	390	14	49
Ham & Cheese S'wich	420	15	50
Pepperoni Pizza	590	21	78
Turkey Sandwich	290	3	50

Desserts:

Brownie (1)	370	19	49
Creamy Cheesecake, 1 slice	540	33	50
Cookies: Per Cookie			
Chocolate/Fudge Choc. Chip, av.	160	7	23
Oatmeal Raisin; Sugar, average	150	6	24
Macadamia Nut	170	9	22

Second Cup® ~ see CalorieKing.com

Shakey's® (Jan '15)

Pizzas: Per Slice, ½ Large Pizza

	C	F	Cb
Cheese:			
Pan Crust	185	6	26
Thin Crust	150	5.5	18
Firehouse: Pan Crust	255	12	27
Thin Crust	220	12	19
Garden Veggie: Pan Crust	185	5.5	27
Thin Crust	150	5	19
Margherita:			
Pan Crust	175	5	26
Thin Crust	135	4.5	18
Rustic Garlic Chicken: Pan Crust	190	5.5	26
Thin Crust	155	5.5	18
Shakey's Special: Pan Crust	210	6.5	31
Thin Crust	195	10	18
Texas BBQ Chicken: Pan Crust	205	5	29
Thin Crust	170	5	21
Ultimate Meat: Pan Crust	280	14	26
Thin Crust	245	13	18
Additional Toppings: Beef	35	3	0
Cheese	15	1	1
Chicken	15	0.5	0
Pepperoni	25	2.5	0
Sausage	45	4	1

Shareables: Per Serving, Unless Indicated

Chicken Strips (5)	620	31	48
Mojo Potatoes (5)	215	11	25
Mojo Supreme, serves 4-6	1950	120	160
Shakey's Spicy Wings (6)	495	29	27

Shakey's Famous Chicken: Per Piece

Fried Chicken: Breast	475	26	16
Leg	170	19	6
Thigh	350	24	10
Wing	130	9	4

Shari's® (Jan '15)

Breakfast:

	C	F	Cb
Favorites:			
Farmhouse Platter	1170	73	94
The Breakfast Sampler Platter	1060	74	55
Traditional Eggs Benedict, with Hashbrowns	810	46	61
Fruit Crepes: Apples; Strawb., av.	685	36	79
Burst O Berry	630	36	68
Omelettes:			
BMP	930	77	8
Chicken Fajita	720	52	13
Denver; Spring Spinach, average	655	52	11
Pancakes: Buttermilk	370	5	73
Potato Pancakes	570	17	96

Continued Next Page...

Shari's® cont... (Jan '15)

Breakfast (Cont):

	C	**F**	**Cb**
Specialties:			
Breakfast Panini	930	60	64
Classic Quiche: BMP	550	28	57
Lorraine	590	30	56
Meat Lover's Skillet,			
without side choices	1140	91	34

Lunch:

Flame-Grilled Burgers: *Without Sides*			
Bavarian	1030	47	59
Cheddar Cheesebuger	660	34	46
Garlic-Mushroom Swiss	1030	72	50
Hamburger	600	29	46
Pepperjack Cheese	700	38	46
Sriracha Burger	730	40	50
Trail Boss	1030	57	54
Flatbread Paninis: *Without Sides*			
All American	740	33	62
Pastrami	760	32	58
Salads: *Entrée Size*			
American Chopped, w/o Dress.	590	28	39
Northwest Steak	660	30	53
Spinach Cobb	780	44	46
Sandwiches: *Per Whole Sandwich, w/o Side Choices*			
Baja Chipotle Chicken	870	49	59
Cuban, on Ciabatta	600	27	46
Prime Rib Dip	670	37	48

Dinner:

Distrinctive: Chicken Penne Alfr.	1100	55	94
Chimichurri Chicken	1110	65	87
Sthn Style Chicken & Waffles	1430	86	113
Flame Grilled Classics: *With Garlic Herb Bread &*			
Onion Rings			
Center Cut NY Strip Steak	940	64	33
T-Bone Steak, 16 oz	1100	67	35
Steak: W/ Golden Fried Shrimp	1040	50	89
With Shrimp Scampi	930	62	36
With Shrimp Skewers	760	43	35
Homestyle Favorite,			
Country Fried Steak & Gravy	1250	71	119
Seafood Favorites: *As Served*			
Alaskan Cod with Shrimp & Chips	1280	79	119
Hand Cut Alaskan Cod & Chips	1220	77	111

Shari's® cont... (Jan '15)

Sides:

	C	**F**	**Cb**
Baked Potato w/ Butter& Sour Crm	280	13	38
Country Vegetables	120	9	8
French Fries	390	25	40
Rice Pilaf	90	4.5	10
Tater Tots	370	26	33
Desserts:			
Classic Pies: *Per Slice, as Served*			
Banana Cream Dream	410	19	55
Chocolate Cream Supreme	590	33	67
Gourmet Pies: *Per Slice, As Served*			
Creamy Caramel Pecan Crunch	710	45	71
Peanut Butter Chocolate Silk	660	45	60
S'mores Galore	570	31	68
Velvet Chocolate Silk	640	46	55

Sheetz® (Jan '15)

Breakfast Sandwiches:

	C	**F**	**Cb**
Walker Breakfast Ranger	680	29	74
Burgerz:			
Atomic Burger	380	20	22
Big Mozz Burger	520	27	32
Boss Bacon Burger	530	33	23
Carolina Slaw Burger	400	19	27
Twisted Brunch Burger	660	35	52
Hot Dogz:			
BLT	450	27	34
Firehouse	390	22	35
Junkyard	340	15	39
Philly	350	17	38
Smokehouse	380	18	40
Sides:			
Coleslaw	80	3.5	11
Crispy Chicken Strips: 3 pieces	390	19	33
5 pieces	650	31	55
Fried Pickles: Regular	170	9	19
Large	340	18	38
Fryz, 1 cup	730	36	95
Jalapeno Poppers, 1 order	350	19	37
Loaded Fryz	870	43	113
Mac & Cheese, 1 order	130	6	15
Popcorn Chicken: Regular	330	15	30
Large	660	30	59

Continued Next Page...

Fast - Foods & *Restaurants*

Sheetz® cont... (Jan '15)

	C	F	Cb
Donuts:			
Apple/Blueberry Fritter, average	485	24	61
Chocolate Cake Donut	530	33	54
Cotton Candy Pink/Blue Donut	400	19	52
Cream Filled: Chocolate Iced Donut	400	18	56
Glazed Donut	360	16	48
Custard Filled Chocolate Iced D'nut	350	15	50
Glazed Ring Donut	300	14	37
P'nut Butter Filled Choc Iced D'nut	380	19	50
Sour Cream Cake Donut	480	26	57
Muffin, Blueberry (1)	460	26	56
Beverages:			
Cupo'ccino: Cake Batter, 16 oz	260	6	54
Creme Brulee, 16 oz	280	8	50
French Vanilla, 16 oz	285	10	50
Hot Chocolate, 16 oz	250	4	52

Sizzler® (Jan '15)

	C	F	Cb
Burgers:			
Mega Bacon Cheeseburger, ½ lb	1010	61	48
Sizzler Burger: ⅓ lb	620	30	47
½ lb	760	40	47
Sandwiches:			
Grilled Chicken Club	645	28	48
Malibu Chicken	705	37	59
Hot Entrees: Without Condiments, Sides or Sauces Unless Indicated			
Chicken: Hibachi Chicken, Single	180	4	7
Lemon-Herb Chicken, Single	170	6	0
Malibu Chicken, Single	360	25	11
Pasta: Fettuccine Alfredo	995	64	73
Cajun Fettuccine Alfredo	1035	64	82
Pork Chop, Single, w/ Apple Sauce	420	27	15
Ribs:			
Half Rack	625	39	37
Full Rack	1155	79	51
Seafood:			
Grilled Salmon with Rice Pilaf	530	20	40
Ultimate Shrimp Platter	1010	39	103
Steaks: Bacon Wrapped Sirloin Filet	555	35	5
Burgundy M'shroom Sirloin Tips, with Rice Pilaf	870	36	85
Chopped Steak, 8 oz	520	30	17
Classic, 8 oz	395	21	1
NY Strip, 12 oz	810	57	1
Combos: Classic Trio	860	47	36
Steak & Hibachi Chicken	475	20	7
Steak & Lobster Tail	410	17	2
Steak & Malibu Chicken	660	41	12

Sizzler® cont... (Jan '15)

	C	F	Cb
Prepared Salads: W/out Dressing			
Seafood, 4 oz	160	11	11
Sicilian Pasta, 2 oz	65	4	6
Three Bean, 1 oz	25	1	5
Tuna Pasta, 4 oz	205	19	1
Waldorf, 4 oz	130	8	16
Salad Dressings: Per 1 oz			
Blue Cheese	105	11	1
Honey Mustard	110	8	9
Italian	80	8	2
Ranch	115	12	2
Thousand Island	95	9	5
Sides:			
Baked Potato, plain	265	4	51
Broccoli, 5 oz	50	0.5	7
French Fries, 5 oz	285	13	42
Rice Pilaf, 5 oz	225	4	39
For Complete Menu & Data ~ see CalorieKing.com			

Skyline Chili® (Jan '15)

	C	F	Cb
Burritos:			
Chili Burrito Deluxe	640	33	44
Vegetarian Black Bean Deluxe	700	32	73
Ways: Per Regular Serving			
Chili & Cheddar Cheese Spaghetti:			
3 Way	730	47	49
4 Way Onion	750	47	53
4 Way Bean	820	48	65
5 Way	830	48	69
Bowls: Coney	780	61	8
Loaded Chili	480	29	21
Vegetarian Black Beans & Rice	400	15	49
Chili, Deluxe	640	33	44
Potatoes:			
3-Way Potato	610	25	65
Cheddar Potato	700	42	61
Sour Cream Potato	460	19	66
Salads: Without Dressing Unless Indicated			
Buffalo Chicken	200	10	11
Garden, with Croutons	80	5	5
Greek, regular size, with dressing	390	37	9
Dressings: Blue Cheese, 1.5 oz	210	21	2
Buttermilk Ranch, 1.5 oz	210	22	2
Greek, 1.5 oz	260	28	1
Thousand Island, 1.5 oz	220	21	6
Wraps:			
Buffalo Chicken, w/ Ranch Dress.	720	40	59
Classic Chkn w/ Chili Ranch Dress.	650	36	56
Greek Chicken, w/ Greek Dressing	680	36	56
Sides:			
Fries: Chili Cheese	750	40	66
French	390	13	63

Smoothie King® (Jan '15)

Fruit Smoothies: Per 20 oz Cup **C** **F** **Cb**
Figures Include Turbinado. Without Turbinado, deduct 100 calories and 23 carbs.

	C	F	Cb
Energy Blends: Berry Punch	360	0	91
Pure Recharge, Mango Strawb.	210	0	52
Super Punch Plus	395	0	100
Fitness Blends:			
High Protein: Almond Mocha	345	9	42
Chocolate	365	9	42
Peanut Power Plus:			
Chocolate	700	26	98
Strawberry	680	21	112
The Activator: Chocolate	340	1	67
Strawberry	495	1	105
Vanilla	345	1	67
The Hulk: Chocolate	800	31	108
Strawberry	965	32	145
Vanilla	800	32	105
Take A Break Blends:			
Banana Boat	475	4	101
Muscle Punch	360	1	84
Yogurt D-Lite	275	4	46
Wellness Blends: Acai Adventure	435	5	92
Mangosteen Madness	380	0	94
Orange Ka-BAM	470	0	117

32 fl.oz Cup: Multiply 20 fl.oz figures by 1.5
40 fl.oz Cup: Multiply 20 fl.oz figures by 2

Kids Cup Smoothies: *Per 12 fl.oz Cup*

	C	F	Cb
Apple Kiwi Bunga	155	0	37
Choc-A-Laka	210	4	32
Lil' Angel	210	0	52
Strawberry Bluegurt Blitz	175	0	70

Snappy Tomato (Jan '15)

Pizza: Per Slice, ⅛ of Large Pizza **C** **F** **Cb**

	C	F	Cb
Buffalo Grilled Chicken	250	5	32
Cheese	220	7	30
Hawaiian	370	18	33
Pepperoni	340	17	31
Ranch	370	21	31
Snapperoni	390	22	31
Snappy Ultimate	460	26	33
Supreme	340	17	32
Veggie	240	8	33

Snappetizers, Snappy Wings (3),
Plain, without sauce, 2.6 oz   160 | 11 | 0

Sonic Drive-In® (Jan '15)

Burgers: With Standard Toppings **C** **F** **Cb**

	C	F	Cb
Cheeseburger, with Mustard	710	43	42
Green Chile Cheeseburger	710	43	43
Jr.	330	17	30
Jr. Deluxe	360	20	32
Sonic:			
With Mayonnaise	690	42	43
With Mustard	640	37	42
Bacon Cheeseburger, with Mayo	820	54	43
Super Sonic: *With Mayo*			
Bacon Double Cheeseburger	1240	87	44
Double Cheeseburger	1160	81	44
Coneys:			
Chili Cheese	420	26	30
Footlong, ¼ pound	830	55	54
Toaster Sandwiches:			
Chicken Club	690	36	58
Bacon Cheeseburger	850	50	59
Wraps: Crispy Chicken	510	22	57
Grilled Chicken	430	14	42
Chicken:			
Super Crunch Chicken Strips (5)	550	26	42
Jumbo Popcorn Chicken:			
Small, without Sauce, 4 oz	380	22	27
Large, without Sauce, 6 oz	640	37	47
Sides: *Per Medium Serving*			
Natural Cut Fries:			
Medium	370	18	50
With Cheese	500	27	54
With Chili & Cheese	570	32	58
Mozzarella Sticks, without sauce	440	22	40
Tater Tots: *Per Medium*			
Plain	360	19	43
With Cheese	450	28	43
With Chili & Cheese	540	34	48
Breakfast:			
Burritos: Bacon	480	26	39
Ham	460	22	40
Sausage	500	29	39
SuperSonic	580	32	49
Ultimate Meat & Cheese	800	56	46
Cinnasnacks, without frosting (3)	340	15	44
French Toast Sticks: With Syrup (4)	590	31	71
Without Syrup (4)	500	31	49
Sandwiches:			
Breakfast Bagel: With Bacon	600	24	68
With Sausage	680	32	68
CroisSonic, Sausage	650	49	28

Continued Next Page...

Fast - Foods & *Restaurants*

Sonic Drive-In® cont... (Jan '15)

	C	F	Cb
Banana Split	490	18	76
Real Ice Cream Sundaes:			
Chocolate	500	22	69
Hot Fudge	520	26	64
Pineapple	440	22	55
Strawberry	430	22	53
Sonic Blasts: *Per Small Size*			
Small: M&M's	900	48	106
Oreo	900	47	106
Beverages: Per Small Size			
Floats/Blended:			
Coca-Cola; Dr Pepper, average	330	14	49
Fanta	340	14	51
Malts: Chocolate	630	31	80
Strawberry	580	31	69
Vanilla	550	31	61
Shakes: Banana	620	31	80
Chocolate	670	31	89
Pineapple; Strawberry, average	575	31	67

For Complete Nutritional Data ~ see CalorieKing.com

Souplantation® (Jan '15)

Soups: Per Cup	C	F	Cb
Chesapeake Corn Chdr, non veget.	290	17	30
Classical Minestrone	120	2	20
Cream of Mushroom	280	22	15
New Orleans Jambalaya	210	11	18
Vegetarian Harvest	200	10	23
Pasta: Per 1 Cup			
Arizona Marinara	360	11	47
Carbonara Pasta, with Bacon	290	10	43
Creamy Bruschetta	360	16	43
Chicken Tetrazzini	480	23	47
Creamy Cilantro Lime Pesto	360	20	37
Fettuccine Alfredo	390	18	41
Fire-Roasted Tomato Basil Alfredo	370	14	44
Garden Vegetable with Meatballs	310	10	44
Vegetarian Marinara with Basil	260	4	44
Prepared Salads: Per ½ Cup			
BBQ Potato	170	9	21
Carrot Raisin	90	3	17
Dijon Potato with Garlic Dill Vinegar	150	12	9
Greek Couscous w/ Feta & Pinenuts	210	10	25
Thai Noodle w/ Chkn & Peanut Sce	190	10	19

Souplantation® cont... (Jan '15)

Bakery:	C	F	Cb
Muffins: Chocolate Brownie	180	8	26
Chocolate Chip	170	8	22
French Quarter Praline	250	10	35
Fruit Medley Bran	130	0.5	29
Breads: Per Piece			
Buttermilk Cornbread	190	7	28
Garlic Asiago Focaccia	70	2	11
Sourdough	150	0.5	27
Desserts: Per ½ Cup			
Apple Medley	70	0	18
Banana Royale	80	0	20
Caramel Apple Cobbler	390	12	68
Rice Pudding	110	2	20

For Complete Nutritional Data ~ see CalorieKing.com

Southern Tsunami® (Jan '15)

Rolls:	C	F	Cb
Hybrid: *With White Rice*			
Berry, 6 oz	230	5	44
Blueberry: Salmon, 8 oz	350	15	45
Shrimp, 8 oz	330	12	45
Done Deal, 7 oz	370	17	39
Happy Mango, 8 oz	440	21	53
Jalapeno, 8 oz	310	7	48
Mango Shrimp, 6 oz	370	19	41
Red Rock Fujisan, 7 oz	400	15	42
Spicy Mango Roll, 8 oz	400	17	46
Ultimate Chili Combo, 6 oz	290	9	41
Hybrid Rolls: *With Brown Rice*			
Berry, 6 oz	200	6	33
Blueberry: Salmon, 8 oz	320	15	34
Steelhead, 8 oz	310	14	34
Crunchy: Dragon, Hot, 6 oz	270	10	30
Tempura, 6 oz	260	7	37
Jalapeno, 8 oz	270	7	35
Mango Shrimp, 6 oz	350	19	33
Red Rock Fujisan, 7 oz	370	16	31
Ultimate Chili Combo, 6 oz	250	1	30
Chef Samplers: A, 9.5 oz	410	2	65
B, 7.5 oz	360	6	57

Continued Next Page... ...

Updated Nutrition Data ~ www.CalorieKing.com
Persons with Diabetes ~ See Disclaimer (Page 22)

Southern Tsunami® cont... (Jan'15)

Rolls (Cont):

		C	F	Cb
Plus Rolls: *Per 6 oz Servings*				
California		230	4	44
Cream Cheese Plus: Salmon		290	11	39
Shrimp		260	8	39
Tuna		280	8	39
Eel		300	9	46
Seaside Plus: Eel		380	15	47
Salmon		290	7	45
Shrimp		230	1	45
Steelhead		270	7	39
Tuna		280	1	45
Spicy Plus: Salmon		280	9	45
Shrimp		240	5	39
Steelhead		270	7	39
Tuna		270	5	39
Vegetable		230	4	46
Wraps: Avocado Salad Roll, 4.6 oz		130	5	21
Berry, 4.6 oz		180	8	25
California, 6.6 oz		270	17	28
Smoked Salmon Salad, 4.6 oz		210	3	13
Salads: *Without Dressing*				
Edamame, 4 oz		120	7	9
Seared Tuna, 9 oz		210	8	18
Dressings/Sauces: Eel Sauce, 1 T.		40	0	8
Ginger Dressing, 2 Tbsp		50	2	8
Peanut Sauce, 2 Tbsp		30	1	6
Sweet Chili, 3 fl.oz		300	0	72
Wasabe Dressing, 2 Tbsp		30	2	2

Starbucks® (Nov'14)

Brewed Coffee: *Figures based on 16 fl.oz Grande without Whipped Cream*

		C	F	Cb
Caffe Misto (Au Lait): W/ Whole Milk		130	7	10
With Nonfat Milk		70	0	10
With Soy Milk		100	3	13

Chocolate: *Per Grande, 16 fl.oz Without Whipped Cream*

		C	F	Cb
Hot Chocolate:				
With Whole Milk		330	13	47
With 2% Milk		290	9	47
With Soy		290	7	51
Peppermint Hot Chocolate:				
With Whole Milk		390	13	65
With 2% Milk		360	9	65
With Soy Milk		360	7	69

Starbucks® cont... (Nov'14)

Hot Espresso Beverages:

	C	F	Cb
Caffe Latte: With Whole Milk	220	11	18
With Nonfat Milk	130	0	19
With Soy Milk	170	4.5	23
Cappuccino: With Whole Milk	140	7	12
With Nonfat Milk	80	0	12
With Soy Milk	120	3.5	16
Caramel Macchiato: W/ Whole Milk	270	11	34
With Nonfat Milk	190	1	35
Cinn. Dolce Latte: With Whole Milk	300	10	40
With Nonfat Milk	210	0	40
Espresso: 1 Doppio, 2 fl.oz	10	0	2
1 Solo, 1 fl.oz	5	0	1
Espresso Con Panna, 1 Solo, 1 fl.oz	30	2.5	2

Iced Espresso: Per 16 fl.oz Grande without Whipped Cream

	C	F	Cb
Caffe Latte:			
With Whole Milk	150	7	13
With Nonfat Milk	90	0	13
With Soy Milk	130	3.5	17
Vanilla Latte:			
With Whole Milk	210	6	30
With Nonfat Milk	160	0	31
With 2% Milk	190	4	30

Fizzios: Per Grande, 16 fl.oz

	C	F	Cb
Ginger Ale; Lemon Ale,			
Spiced Root Beer	100	0	27

Frappuccino: *Cold, Per 16 fl.oz Grande With Whole Milk, With Whipped Cream*

	C	F	Cb
Caffe Vanilla	430	14	72
Caramel	410	15	66
Cinnamon Dolce	380	14	60
Hazelnut	390	14	62
Java Chip	460	18	72
Mocha	400	15	64
White Chocolate Mocha	440	16	69

Frappuccino Creme: *Cold, Per 16 fl.oz Grande with Whole Milk and Whipped Cream*

	C	F	Cb
Double Chocolaty Chip	410	20	57
Strawberries & Creme	380	15	57
Tazo Chai	360	15	52
Vanilla Bean Creme	400	16	59

Smoothies: *Per16 fl.oz Grande with 2% Milk, without Whipped Cream*

	C	F	Cb
Orange Mango	270	1.5	53
Strawberry	300	2	60

Continued Next Page... . . .

Starbucks® cont... (Nov'14)

Teas: Grande, With Whole Milk **C** **F** **Cb**

Hot Tea Latte:

	C	F	Cb
Chai	270	7	45
Earl Grey	200	7	29
Iced Tea Latte: Awake	120	2	24
Chai	260	7	44

Drink Extras:

	C	F	Cb
Caramel Drizzle, 1 teaspoon	15	0.5	2
Flavored Syrup: 1 Pump	20	0	5
Sugar-Free, 1 Pump	0	0	0
Mocha Syrup, 1 Pump	25	0.5	6

Sweetened Whipped Cream:

Grande/Venti, cold drinks, average	115	11	3
Grande/Venti, hot drinks	70	7	2

Breakfast, Hot:

Bacon, Gouda & Parmesan Frittata, on Artisan Roll	350	18	30
Egg & Cheddar Sandwich	400	17	45
Oatmeal, without Sugar, 1.4 oz	160	2.5	28
Sausage & Cheddar Sandwich	500	28	41

Bistro Boxes:

Chicken & Hummus	270	7	29
Protein	380	19	37

Paninis:

Chicken Santa Fe	410	12	45
Ham & Swiss	340	10	42
Roasted Tomato & Mozzarella	390	18	44
Turkey Rustico Panini	480	18	53
Sandwich, Turkey & Havarti	450	33	31

Brownie,

Double Chocolate Brownie	410	24	46

Cakes: Per Slice

Banana Walnut Bread, 4.4 oz	420	21	52
Pound: Iced Lemon, 4.4 oz	470	20	68
Marble, 3.75 oz	350	13	54
Starbuck's Classic Coffee, 3.5 oz	390	16	57

Reduced Fat Cakes:

Banana Chocolate Chip Coffee	400	8	80
Cinnamon Swirl Coffee	340	9	62
Very Berry Coffee	350	10	59

Cookies:

Chocolate Chunk	370	19	50
Outrageous Oatmeal	360	15	52

Starbucks® cont... (Jan '15)

	C	F	Cb
Croissants: Butter	310	18	32
Chocolate	300	17	34

Doughnuts,

Chocolate Old-Fashioned Glazed	420	21	57

Muffins:

Bountiful Blueberry	350	12	55
Morning Glory, 4.2 oz	380	18	51

Sweet Rolls & Danish:

Apple Fritter	420	20	59
Cheese Danish	420	25	39
Morning Bun, Small	350	16	45

Yogurt Parfaits:

Greek Yogurt with Berries	220	3	36
Greek Raspberry Puree , and Lemon Curd & Granola	310	7	49

Bottled Drinks ~ See Page 37
Coffee Mix (VIA) ~ See Page 35
Ice Cream ~ See Page 107

Steak Escape® (Jan '15)

Sandwiches: With Menu Board Toppings

Regular: Cajun Chicken	660	23	68
Grand: Chicken	620	19	68
Escape	660	19	68
Gobbler	530	13	68
Turkey Club	550	14	65
Vegetarian	550	20	71
Wild West BBQ	700	20	75

Wraps: With Menu Board Toppings

Cajun Chicken	470	17	50
Grand: Chicken	490	18	51
Escape	520	18	50
Gobbler	440	14	51
Turkey Club	440	15	49
Vegetarian	430	17	52
Wild West BBQ	550	19	56

Salads:

Grilled: Chicken	410	25	14
Ham	360	22	17
Steak	440	24	15
Turkey	360	21	15
Without Meat	280	20	13
Loaded Potatoes: Bacon & Ranch	670	46	51
Cheddar & Bacon	430	17	56

For Complete Nutritional Data ~ see CalorieKing.com

Updated Nutrition Data ~ www.CalorieKing.com
Persons with Diabetes ~ See Disclaimer (Page 22)

Steak 'n Shake® (Jan '15)

The Original Steakburgers:

	C	F	Cb
Single, without Cheese	280	11	30
Double: With Cheese	440	25	31
Bacon 'n Cheese	480	28	31
Cheesy Cheddar	480	27	32
Guacamole	670	44	47
Wisconsin Buttery	700	47	45
Triple, without cheese	510	30	30

Chili:

	C	F	Cb
3-Way (1)	830	36	94
5-Way (1)	1170	63	99
Deluxe, bowl	1220	74	81

Sandwiches:

	C	F	Cb
Guacamole Gr. Chicken	550	28	59
Jalap. Crunch Chicken	580	28	66
Spicy Chicken	460	18	51

Signature Steak Franks:

	C	F	Cb
Regular	380	27	22
Cheesy Cheddar	490	36	24
Chicago Style	420	27	30
Chili Cheese	620	44	31

Salads: Without Dressing

	C	F	Cb
Apple Harvest Grilled Chicken	480	19	56
Fried Chicken	470	26	34
Grilled Chicken	270	10	13

Sides:

	C	F	Cb
French Fries:			
Regular	440	21	60
Large	640	30	87
Onion Rings: Regular	440	25	48
Large	880	50	95

Breakfast:

	C	F	Cb
Bagels Sandwich: With Bacon	450	16	51
With Sausage	570	29	50
Biscuits: Bacon, Egg & Cheese	520	35	32
Egg & Cheese	450	30	31
Sausage & Egg	600	44	31
Sausage, Egg & Cheese	650	48	31
With Sausage Gravy: Half order	540	37	43
Full Order	1070	74	86
Hash Browns: Shredded	320	26	19
Side order, 5 pieces	260	17	23
Perfect Start Oatmeal	340	11	57
Skillets: Country	1240	94	63
Portobello & Swiss	1020	83	28

Hand Dipped Milk Shakes: Per Regular

	C	F	Cb
Banana; Mocha	630	21	103
Butterfinger	850	30	138
Chocolate	650	21	106
Oreo Cookies 'n Cream	780	26	107

Subway® (Jan '15)

6" Sandwich: 6g Fat Or Less

Figures Based on 9 grain wheat bread, lettuce, tomatoes, onions, green peppers and cucumbers. Oil or mayo not included.

	C	F	Cb
Black Forest Ham	290	4.5	46
Oven Roasted Chicken	320	5	45
Roast Beef	320	5	45
Subway Club	310	4.5	46
Sweet Onion Chicken Teriyaki	370	4	57
Turkey Breast	280	3.5	46
Turkey Breast & Black Forest Ham	280	4	46
Veggie Delite	230	2.5	44

6" Sandwiches: Figures based on 9-grain wheat bread, lettuce, tomatoes, onion, green peppers, cucumbers. Oil or mayo not included.

	C	F	Cb
Big Phhilly Cheesesteak	500	17	51
BLT	320	9	43
Chkn & Bacon Ranch Melt w/ Chse	570	28	47
Cold Cut Combo	360	12	46
Italian B.M.T.	410	16	46
Meatball Marinara	480	18	59
Spicy Italian	480	24	46
Steak & Cheese	380	10	48
Subway Melt, with Cheese	370	11	47
Tuna	480	25	44

Kids Meal Sandwiches: Figures based on 9-grain wheat bread, lettuce, tomatoes, onions, green peppers and cucumbers. Oil or mayo not included.

	C	F	Cb
Black Forest Ham	180	2.5	30
Roast Beef	200	3	30
Turkey Breast	180	2	30
Veggie Delite	150	1.5	29

Condiments & Sauces: For 6" Sandwiches

	C	F	Cb
Chipotle Southwest, 0.8 oz	100	10	1
Honey Mustard, Fat-Free, 0.8 oz	30	0	7
Mayonnaise: 1 Tbsp, 0.5 oz	110	12	0
Light, 1 Tbsp, 0.5 oz	50	5	1
Mustard, Yellow or Deli Brown. 2 tsp	5	0	1
Olive Oil Blend, 1 tsp	45	5	0
Ranch Dressing	110	11	1
Sweet Onion, Fat-Free, 0.8 oz	40	0	9

Extras: For 6" Sandwiches

	C	F	Cb
Bacon Strips (2)	45	3.5	0
Cheese: American, 2 triangles, 0.3 oz	40	3.5	0
Cheddar, 2 triangles, 0.3 oz	60	5	0
Swiss, 2 triangles, 0.3 oz	50	4.5	0

Continued Next Page....

Fast - Foods & *Restaurants*

Subway® cont... (Jan '15)

Breakfast:

6" Egg White Omelet Sandwiches: *Figures based on 9-grain*

	C	F	Cb
Bacon, Egg White & Cheese	370	11	45
Egg White & Cheese	320	8	44
Egg White & Cheese with Ham	350	9	45
Mega Melt	260	12	22
Steak, Egg White & Cheese	390	10	47

6" Omelet Sandwiches: *Figures based on 9-grain bread, cheese & regular egg*

	C	F	Cb
Bacon, Egg & Cheese	410	16	45
Egg & Cheese	360	12	44
Egg & Chse with Ham	390	13	45
Mega Melt	510	22	46
Steak, Egg & Cheese	430	15	47

Egg White on 3" Flatbread: *Figures based on flatbread, cheese and egg whites.*

	C	F	Cb
Bacon, Egg White & Cheese	190	7	21
Egg White & Cheese	170	5	21
Egg White & Cheese with Ham	180	5	22
Mega Melt	260	12	22
Steak, Egg White & Cheese	190	6	22

Regular Egg On 3" Flatbreads: *Figures based on flatbread, cheese and regular egg.*

	C	F	Cb
Bacon, Egg & Cheese	210	9	21
Breakfast B.M.T. Melt	250	12	22
Egg & Cheese	190	7	21
Mega Melt	280	14	22
Steak, Egg & Cheese	210	8	22

Salads (6g Fat or Less): *Figures based on lettuce, tomatoes, onions, green peppers, olives & cucumbers. Dressing or croutons not included.*

	C	F	Cb
Black Forest Ham	110	3	12
Oven Roasted Chicken	130	2.5	10
Roast Beef; Subway Club, av.	140	3.5	11
Sweet Onion Chicken Teriyaki, with Sweet Onion dressing	240	3	34
Turkey Breast & Ham	110	2.5	12
Veggie Delite	50	1	9

Salad Dressings:

	C	F	Cb
Chipotle Southwest, 1.5 oz	190	20	2
Ranch, 1.5 oz	220	23	2

Subway® cont... (Jan '15)

Soups: *Per 8 oz Bowl*

	C	F	Cb
Beef Chili	350	24	17
Chicken Noodle	100	1	12
Clam Chowder	200	11	20
Loaded Baked Potato	220	11	23
Minestrone	90	1	17
Poblano Corn Chowder	150	7	18
Vegetable Beef	90	2	15

Cookies & Desserts:

	C	F	Cb
Apple Slices, 1 package, 2.5 oz	35	0	9
Chocolate Chip Cookie, 1.5 oz	220	10	30
Oatmeal Raisin Cookie, 1.5 oz	200	8	30
Raspberry Cheesecake, 1.6 oz	200	9	29

Sweet Tomatoes®
Same Menu & Data as Souplantation ~ See Page 242

Swiss Chalet® (Jan '15)

Starters:

	C	F	Cb
Caesar Salad without Dressing	90	3	13
Chalet Chicken Wings (8), with sauce	550	34	23
Cheese Perogies (7)	420	10	69
Garlic Cheese Loaf, 10.5 oz	910	58	16

From The Grill: *Without Sides*

	C	F	Cb
Burgers: Classic Hamburger	710	39	43
Classic Bacon & Cheese	890	54	46
Veggie	470	13	57
BBQ Ribs: Half Rack	650	42	17
Full Rack	1300	85	34

Rotisserie Chicken: *Meat Only*

	C	F	Cb
Double Leg, with Skin	490	31	0
Half Chicken, with Skin	530	27	0
Quarter Chicken:			
Dark meat, without Skin	160	8	0
Dark meat, with Skin	240	16	0
White meat, without Skin	220	6	0
White meat, with Skin	290	11	0
Chicken Pot Pie, 1 pie	560	32	39

Sandwiches: *Without Sides*

	C	F	Cb
Classic Hot Chicken, white meat	520	11	51
Flatbread: Hickory Chicken	700	32	70
Southwest Chicken	710	37	64

Updated Nutrition Data ~ www.CalorieKing.com
Persons with Diabetes ~ See Disclaimer (Page 22)

Swiss Chalet® cont...(Jan '15)

	C	F	Cb
Wrap,			
Rotisserie Chicken Club	710	32	57
Entree Salads: Without Dressing			
Spinach Chicken Salad	410	16	28
Sweet Heat Salad with Chicken	340	9	30
West Coast Salad with Chicken	460	21	21
Dressings/Sauces:			
Caesar Dressing, 1 oz	180	18	2
Chalet Dressing, 1 Tbsp, 1 oz	160	14	6
Chalet Dipping Sauce, 3.5 oz	25	0.5	1
Sides:			
Gravy, 4 oz	45	1.5	7
Mashed Potatoes, 5 oz	150	4	27
Sauteed Mushrooms, 6 oz	140	1	30
Seasoned Rice, 6 oz	240	3.5	48
Desserts/Pies:			
Apple Pie	440	19	65
Coconut Cream Pie	540	33	57
Lemon Meringue Pie	400	11	73
Pecan Pie	590	29	79
Sticky Toffee Pudding with Ice Crm	540	20	88

Taco Bell® (Jan '15)

	C	F	Cb
Burritos:			
½ lb Cheesy Potato	510	24	56
½ lb Combo	450	18	51
7-Layer	430	16	57
Beefy 5-Layer	510	20	64
Chicken	400	18	45
Chili Cheese	370	16	39
Supreme: Beef	410	16	51
Chicken; Steak, average	395	13	49
XXL Grilled Stuft:			
Beef	870	41	91
Chicken; Steak, av.	830	35	88
Cantina Power:			
Bowl: Chicken	490	20	49
Steak	500	22	47
Veggie	460	19	58
Burrito: Chicken	460	20	43
Steak	470	22	41
Veggie	430	19	52
Chalupas:			
Supreme: Beef	370	21	31
Chicken	350	18	31
Steak	350	19	30
Fresco: Crunchy Taco	150	8	13
Soft Tacos: Original	160	7	17
Chicken; Grilled Steak, av.	145	4	17

Taco Bell® cont... (Jan '15)

	C	F	Cb
Gorditas:			
Cheesy Crunch	490	28	40
Supreme: Beef	290	13	31
Chicken	270	9	30
Steak	280	10	30
Nachos: Regular	310	17	34
BellGrande	760	39	85
Supreme	450	24	46
Specialities:			
Cheese Roll-Up	180	9	15
Chilli Cheese Burrito	370	16	39
Crunchwrap Supreme	540	21	71
Loaded Potato Griller	450	21	54
MexiMelt	250	14	19
Mexican Pizza, 7.5 oz	550	31	48
Quesadillas: Cheese	460	26	37
Steak	520	28	38
Tacos:			
Crunchy: Regular	170	10	12
Supreme	200	12	15
Double Decker: Regular	320	14	36
Supreme	350	16	38
Soft: Beef	190	9	17
Beef Supreme	220	11	20
Chicken	160	5	16
Crispy Potato	250	12	28
Fresco Chicken	140	3.5	16
Grilled Steak	200	10	16
Taco Salads:			
Express with Chips	580	29	57
Fiesta: Beef	780	42	74
Chicken	740	35	72
Steak	750	37	71
Sides: Cheesy Fiesta Potato, 4.4 oz	270	15	31
Chips & Guacamole, 3.7 oz	320	20	32
Cinnamon Twist, 1.3 oz	170	7	26
Pintos 'n Cheese, 4.3 oz	190	7	21
Condiments & Sauces:			
Avocado Ranch Dressing, 0.5 oz	80	8	1
Creamy Jalapeno Sauce, 0.5 oz	70	7	1
Green Tomatillo Sauce, 1 oz	10	0	2
Guacamole, 0.8 oz	35	3	2
Pepper Jack Sauce, 0.5 oz	70	7	1
Sour Cream, Reduced Fat, 0.8 oz	30	2	2

Continued Next Page...

247

Taco Bell® cont... (Jan '15)

Breakfast:

	C	F	Cb
AM Crunchwrap: Bacon	660	41	51
Sausage	710	46	51
AM Grilled Taco: Bacon	230	14	15
Sausage	220	14	15
Cheesy Burritos:			
Bacon	490	28	36
Sausage	470	28	36
Cinnabon Delights, 2 pack	160	9	17
Hash Brown, 1.9 oz	160	11	14

Note: Nutritional data in New York outlets may vary slightly. Please check Taco Bell website

Taco Cabana® (Jan '15)

Cabana Burritos: *Includes Flour Burrito & Menu Set Toppings*

	C	F	Cb
Beef	980	47	97
Chicken, Stewed	900	37	98
Steak Fajita	910	39	96

Quesadillas: *Personal, with Guacamole & Sour Cream*

Cheese	710	39	61
Chicken Breast Fajita; Steak, av.	765	41	62
Shrimp Tampico	820	45	63

Sizzling Skillets: *Includes Flour Tortilla, Grilled Onion, Bell Pepper, Rice, Shredded Cheese, Sour Cream, Guacamole, Lettuce & Pico de Gallo*

½ lb, 1 serving: Brisket	960	46	95
Chicken Fajita	775	26	95
Mixed Fajita Steak & Chicken	785	28	95
Shrimp Tampico; Steak Fajita, av.	795	30	97

Tacos:

Crispy: Ground Beef	200	12	12
Stewed Chicken	160	7	12
Soft: Black Bean	190	4	34
Carne Guisada	190	6	20
Chicken, Stewed	200	7	22
Ground Beef	240	12	22

Sides & Add-Ons: *Per Serving*

Black Beans, 4 oz	80	1	15
Borracho Beans, 4 oz	140	3	20
Guacamole, 3 oz	110	9	7
Queso, 3 oz	110	8	5
Refried Beans	260	14	25
Rice	120	0.5	25
Salsa: Fuego; Roja, 1 oz	5	0	1
Verde, 1 oz	10	0	1
Sour Cream, 3 oz	160	15	3

Taco Del Mar® (Jan '15)

Baja Bowls: *Per LargeBowl with Standard Menu Toppings, without Guacamole, Sour Cream, Jalapenos or Sauce*

	C	F	Cb
Mondo: Carne Asada Steak	490	15	62
Chicken; Shredded Beef	520	17	62
Fish	590	36	47
Ground Beef	570	23	62
Pork	500	15	61

Burritos: *Small, with Standard Menu Toppings, without Guacamole, Sour Cream, Jalapenos or Sauce*

Mondito: *Per 9.6 oz Unless Indicated*

Carne Asada Steak	440	13	65
Chicken; Shredded Beef	460	14	65
Fish, 10.7 oz	520	23	61
Ground Beef	480	17	65
Pork	450	13	65

Mondo: *Per 18.45 oz Unless Indicated*

Carne Asada Steak	820	23	118
Chicken; Shredded Beef	860	25	118
Fish, 19 oz	930	45	103
Ground Beef	900	32	118
Pork	840	24	117

Platters:

Enchilada: *Per 2 Corn Tortillas and Standard Menu Toppings, without Jalapenos or Sauce*

Carne Asada Steak	780	28	104
Cheese	870	38	104
Chicken; Shredded Beef, average	820	30	104
Ground Beef	860	36	105
Pork	800	28	103

Enchilada/Taco: *Includes Corn & Flour Tortillas, Standard Menu Toppings, without Jalapenos or Sauce*

Carne Asada Steak	820	30	109
Chicken; Shredded Beef	850	32	109
Ground Beef	900	38	109
Pork	830	30	108

Quesadillas: *Includes Flour Tortilla, Standard Menu Toppings, without Jalapenos and Sauce*

Carne Asada Steak	1170	49	135
Chicken; Shredded Beef	1200	51	135
Ground Beef	1250	57	136
Pork	1180	50	134

Taco Del Mar® cont... (Jan '15)

Nachos: Includes Standard Menu **C** **F** **Cb**
Toppings, without Jalapenos and Sauce

	C	F	Cb
6 Layer Cheese	1050	62	96
Super: Carne Asada Steak	1140	65	98
Chicken; Shredded Beef, av.	1170	67	97
Ground Beef	1220	74	98
Pork	1150	66	97

Salads: Includes Standard Menu Toppings, without Guacamole, Sour Cream or Jalapenos

	C	F	Cb
Cabo: Chicken; Shredded Beef	420	19	36
Fish	450	22	47
Taco: Carne Asada Steak	610	29	59
Ground Beef	690	37	60

Note: Nutritional Information varies from state to state. Please refer to Taco Del Mar Website

Taco John's® (Jan '15)

Burritos:	C	F	Cb
Bean Burrito	370	11	53
Beef Grilled Burrito	590	32	53
Beefy Burrito	440	21	42
Chicken Grilled Burrito	590	30	50
Combination Burrito	410	16	47
Crunchy Chicken & Potato Burrito	580	27	67
Meat & Potato Burrito	520	25	57
Super Burrito	450	20	50
Tacos:			
Soft Shell, Chicken	190	6	21
Taco Bravo	330	13	38
Specialties:			
Crunchy Chicken, without sauce	370	18	29
Quesadilla Melt: Cheesy	450	24	40
Fajita Beef	550	29	46
Fajita Chicken	520	25	45
Super Nachos: Small	420	25	37
Regular	790	47	72
Super Potato Oles:			
Small	650	40	59
Regular	1090	67	98
Taco Salads: Chicken, w/o dressing	500	27	39
Crunchy Chicken, without dressing	630	36	53
Plain, without dressing	540	33	40

Taco John's® cont... (Jan '15)

Sides:	C	F	Cb
Chips & Queso	430	25	43
Cilantro Lime Rice, 6 oz	220	3	39
Potato Oles: Small	480	27	52
Medium	670	38	73
Large	860	49	94
Refried Beans: With Cheese	320	7	46
Without Cheese	260	2.5	45
Condiments:			
Bacon Ranch, 1.5 oz	120	9	10
House Dressing, 1.5 oz	70	7	2
Nacho Cheese, 3 oz	110	9	5
Salsa, 2 oz	10	0	2
Sour Cream, 2 oz	120	10	3
Dessert:			
Churro, 2 oz	200	9	29
Mexican Donut Bites, 3.2 oz	290	12	47
Mexican Ice Cream S'wich, 3.7 oz	340	15	51

Taco Mayo® (Jan '15)

Burritos:	C	F	Cb
Bean	495	16	71
Beef	490	23	41
Super: Beef	540	23	57
Chicken	405	16	39
Melts:			
Tamale	615	34	50
Tostada	525	32	35
Quesadillas:			
Chicken	675	37	46
Fajita Chicken	700	39	47
Fajita Steak	725	40	47
Tacos:			
Crispy Taco, Beef	160	9	10
Soft Taco: Beef	230	11	17
Chicken	185	6	16
Salads: As Per Menu Description			
Acapulco:			
Chicken	680	50	35
Steak	705	51	35
SalsaLita Steak	305	8	33
Taco Steak	445	25	30
Sides:			
Mexicali Rice	160	1	36
Refried Beans	295	9	43
Potato Locos, Small	380	24	36

249

Taco Time® (Jan '15)

	C	F	Cb
Burritos:			
Beef, Bean & Cheese	490	17	55
Chicken B.L.T.	690	39	43
Big Juan: Chicken	580	16	70
Ground Beef	630	23	73
Casita: Chicken	490	17	42
Ground Beef	540	24	46
Crisp Burrito:			
Chicken	380	17	33
Ground Beef	430	21	36
Pinto Bean	360	14	47
Soft Burrito: Ground Beef	430	16	43
Pinto Bean	370	10	54
Veggie	520	17	73
Tacos:			
Soft Tacos: Per 7 oz			
Chicken	360	9	40
Ground Beef	420	16	43
Country, 13.25 oz	720	54	20
Nacho, 15.5 oz	740	48	26
Other Favorites: Cheddar Melt	250	12	25
Nachos Grande	930	43	96
Tostada: Bean	230	13	21
Chicken	320	13	22
Ground Beef	380	20	25
Breakfast:			
Burritos: Egg & Bacon, 7.5 oz	510	24	49
Egg & Cheese, 5.75 oz	370	16	40
Ultimate, 11 oz	860	58	52
Omelet, Cheese, 8 oz	490	36	6
Sides:			
Chips, Taco, 2 oz	150	3.5	27
Fries: Cheddar, medium, 7 oz	500	35	39
Mexi, medium, 6 oz	390	26	38
Stuffed, medium, 7 oz	460	28	42
Mexi-Rice, 3.5 oz	80	0.5	17
Refritos, with Chips, 6 oz	230	7	29
Salads:			
Regular: Chicken Taco, 9.5 oz	310	13	22
Ground Beef Taco, 9 oz	370	20	24
Tostada Delight: Chicken, 9 oz	450	19	35
Ground Beef, 9 oz	490	26	36
Desserts: Crustos	290	6	58
Churro: Plain	210	16	17
With Cinnamon & Sugar	250	16	27

TCBY® (Jan '15)

	C	F	Cb
Soft Serve Froz. Yogurt: Per 4 fl.oz			
Bananas Foster	100	0	24
Black Cherry	110	0	24
Brownie Batter	100	0	24
Caramel Supreme	130	1.5	27
Cheesecake	110	2	23
Chocolate	110	1.5	23
Coffee; Golden Vanilla	120	2	23
Dutch Chocolate	100	0	24
Peanut Butter	130	2	26
Raspberry	120	2	24
No Sugar Added, Fat Free,			
average all flavors	80	0	22
Sorbet, average all flavors, 4 fl.oz	100	0	25
Hand-Scooped Frozen Yogurt:			
Butter Pecan: Kid's, 4 fl.oz	120	4	16
Small, 6.4 fl.oz	190	6.5	31
Regular, 12.8 fl.oz	385	13	51
Chunky Choc. Cookie Dough:			
Kid's, 4 fl.oz	160	5	24
Small, 6.4 fl.oz	255	8	38
Regular, 12.8 fl.oz	510	16	77
Cookies & Cream:			
Kid's, 4 fl.oz	100	3.5	19
Small, 6.4 fl.oz	160	5	30
Regular, 12.8 fl.oz	320	11	61
Peanut Butter Delight: Kid's, 4 fl.oz	170	8	20
Small, 6.4 fl.oz	270	13	32
Regular, 12.8 fl.oz	540	26	64
Pralines & Cream: Kid's 4 fl.oz	130	4	19
Small, 6.4 fl.oz	210	6.5	30
Regular, 12.8 fl oz	415	13	60
Vanilla Bean: Kid's, 4 fl.oz	110	2.5	16
Small, 6.4 fl.oz	175	4	26
Regular, 12.8 fl.oz	350	8	52
Cakes: Per ½ Cake			
Chocolate Lovers Cake	220	6	36
Red Velvet Mousse Cake	190	6	30
Pies: Per ⅒ Pie			
Cookies & Creme Pie	320	15	42
Peanut Buttery Fudge Pie	340	17	42

Updated Nutrition Data ~ www.CalorieKing.com
Persons with Diabetes ~ See Disclaimer (Page 22)

TGI Friday's® (Jan '15)

Appetiers: As Served

Individual:	C	F	Cb
Crispy Green Bean Fries	900	65	69
Mozzarella Sticks	1100	75	62
Pan Seared Potstickers	590	25	72
Sesame Jack Chicken Strips	1090	35	159
Taste & Share:			
Ahi Tuna Crisps	330	24	15
Bacon Mac & Cheese Bites	600	40	41
Corned Beef & Swiss Sliders	510	24	46
Garlic & Basil Bruschetta	350	21	33
Hibachi Skewers: Chicken	470	15	63
Sirloin	490	20	58
Parmesan Meatballs	790	61	39
Thai Pork Tacos	280	14	25

Hand-Crafted Burgers: As Served

	C	F	Cb
Cheeseburger	1240	84	78
Jack Daniel's Burger	1490	86	132
NY Cheddar & Bacon Burger	1480	100	88
Sedona Black Bean Burger	1240	76	105
Turkey Burger	930	50	77

Sandwiches: Without Sides

	C	F	Cb
California Club	750	46	41
Jack Daniel's Chicken	1230	66	109
Triple Stack Reuben	1040	55	76

Steaks: Without Sides

	C	F	Cb
Flat Iron	380	26	3
Sirloin: 6 oz	370	23	3
With Half Rack Ribs	850	43	41
Sirloin: 10 oz	590	44	3
With Grilled Lobster Tail	710	46	6

Chicken & Pasta: As Served

	C	F	Cb
Crispy Chicken Fingers	1000	66	68
Pasta:			
Bruschetta Chicken	930	45	90
Cajun Shrimp & Chicken	1110	59	86
Hibachi Chicken Skewers	1230	34	185

Jack Daniels Grill: Without Sides

	C	F	Cb
Chicken	540	15	56
Chicken & Shrimp	530	14	65
Flat Iron Steak	500	16	57
Ribs & Shrimp	1730	75	180
Sirloin & Crispy Shrimp	920	41	79

Salads: Includes Dressing

	C	F	Cb
Balsamic-Glazed Chicken Caesar	500	31	25
Chipotle Yucatan Chicken	840	60	46
Pecan-Crusted Chicken	1080	71	76

Dressing: Per 2 oz

	C	F	Cb
Balsamic Vinaigrette	300	31	7
Bleu Cheese	320	34	2
Honey Mustard	310	29	12
Ranch	210	22	2

TGI Friday's® cont... (Jan '15)

Sides:

	C	F	Cb
Ginger-Lime Slaw	80	4.5	9
Mashed Potatoes	210	10	21
Parmesan Steak Fries	660	49	47
Seasoned Fries	290	22	21

Soups: Per 10 oz Bowl

	C	F	Cb
Broccoli Cheese	290	20	18
French Onion	310	18	21
Soup Of The Day: Chicken Noodle	250	7	33
New England Clam Chowder	500	30	45
Tomato Basil	300	24	20
Tortilla	250	13	23

Desserts:

	C	F	Cb
Brownie Obsession, ½ serve	600	30	77
Oreo Madness, 1 serving	500	21	76
Vanilla Bean Cheesecake, 1 serving	920	57	88

Signature Slushes: Per 22 oz Tumbler

	C	F	Cb
Blue Raspberry	310	0	75
Mango Peach Lemonade	150	0	41
Red Bull Passion	220	0	54
Red Bull Ruby	200	0	51

Thundercloud Subs® (Jan '15)

Subs: Small, w/ Standard Toppings

	C	F	Cb
Classic: BLT	405	17	40
Smoked Chicken	295	4	40
Turkey	280	4	41
Low Fat: Hot Pastrami	430	13	41
Roast Beef	315	4	40
Signature Subs: Club	480	19	43
California Club	510	23	45
NY Italian	570	30	42
Office Favorite	850	40	81
Texas Tuna	700	45	44
Veggie Delite, with Hummus	360	10	53

T.J. Cinnamons® (Jan '15)

Bakery:

	C	F	Cb
Cinnamon Roll, Original, 5.3 oz	505	10	73
Cinnamon Twist (1), 2.5 oz	260	14	33
Sticky Bun Smear w/ Pecans, 1.3 oz	180	12	18
T.J. Cream Cheese Icing, 1 oz	115	5	18

Beverages:

	C	F	Cb
Mocha Chill, w/o Whipped Cream, 12 fl.oz	265	4	46

Tim Hortons® (Jan '15)

Breakfast:

	C	F	Cb
Bagel BELT, Plain Bagel, with Saus. Egg Omelette & Cheese	600	29	61
Homestyle Biscuit:			
Bacon Egg Omelette & Cheese	420	23	33
Sausage, Egg Omelette & Cheese	530	34	33
English Muffins:			
Bacon, Egg Omelette & Cheese	340	16	30
Turkey Ssg, Egg Omelette & Chse	350	16	31
Wraps:			
Bacon, Egg Omelette & Cheese	290	17	19
Egg Omelette & Cheese	230	12	19
Sausage, Egg Omelette & Cheese	400	28	19
Hash Brown, Regular	130	7	16
Grilled Paninis: With White Bread			
Bacon, Tomato & Cheese	560	25	60
Cheese	490	19	58
Tuscan Chicken	550	18	62
Sandwiches: Per Regular With White Bun			
BLT	370	13	46
Chicken Salad	350	9	48
Ham & Swiss	400	12	48
Turkey Bacon Club	430	11	55
Wrap Snackers: Per 3.5 oz Wrap			
Chicken Ranch	190	7	17
Chipotle Chicken	190	7	17
Donuts:			
Cake: Chocolate, glazed	280	14	37
Old Fashioned Plain	210	10	25
Sour Cream Glazed	340	16	46
Filled: Boston Cream	220	6	35
Canadian Maple	210	6	35
Strawberry	250	9	38
Honey Cruller	310	18	37
Yeast: Apple Fritter	290	8	48
Chocolate/Maple Dip	190	7	29
Vanilla Dip with sprinkles	270	9	45
Timbits:			
Cake: Chocolate, glazed	70	3	10
Old Fashion, plain	50	2.5	7
Sour Cream, glazed	90	4.5	12
Filled, all varieties	50	1	8
Yeast, Apple Fritter; Honey Dip, av.	50	1.5	9

Tim Hortons® cont... (Jan '15)

Cookies:

	C	F	Cb
Chocolate Chunk	210	9	32
Oatmeal Raisin Spice	210	8	32
Peanut Butter	250	15	24
Greek Yogurt with Berries,			
Strawberry or Vanilla	250	5	29
Beverages: Per Medium Size			
Cafe Mocha	240	9	38
Hot Chocolate	300	7	57
Iced Cappuccinos: Per Small, 12 fl.oz			
Original: With milk	180	1.5	39
With cream	310	16	40

Togo's Eatery® (Jan '15)

Sandwiches:

	C	F	Cb
Cold: Per Regular White Bread With Standard Toppings, Without Dressing			
Albacore Tuna	550	17	73
Roast Beef	580	9	66
The Italian	880	47	67
Turkey & Avocado	530	15	74
Turkey, Bacon Club	530	16	67
Turkey, Ham & Cheese	540	13	67
Vegetarian: Avocado & Cheese	630	29	73
Hummus	650	27	85
Hot: Chicken	500	8	67
Meatball	690	27	78
Pastrami	770	37	66
Roast Beef	580	9	66
Toasted Sandwiches: Per Regular With Menu Board Featured Bread			
Clubhouse	660	23	80
Pepper Jack Pastrami	1000	60	67
Triple Dip	1110	52	67
Salad Wraps: Includes Whole Wheat Wrap, Standard Toppings & Dressings			
Asian Chicken with Asian Dressing	810	45	81
Chicken Caesar w/ Caesar Dress.	610	30	65
Santa Fe Chicken with Spicy Pepitas	610	26	70
Salads: Per Full Salad, Without Dressing			
Chicken Caesar	210	8	17
Farmer's Market	160	6	20
Santa Fe Chicken	410	21	35

Tropical Smoothie Cafe® (Jan '15)

Breakfast:

	C	F	Cb
Sandwiches: Buffalo Kick Start	570	23	50
Classic Sandwich: Bacon	640	33	47
Ham	605	28	48
Sausage	810	50	48
Toasted Bagel, with Cream Chse	410	10	67
Wraps: All American, regular size	635	29	52
Early Bird, regular size	830	47	55

Toasted Sandwiches: Without Chips or Fruit

Cranb. Waln. Ckn Salad, on 9 Gr Wht	645	35	61
Turkey Bacon, w/ Lt Ranch, on Ciab.	575	20	53
Turkey Guac., on 9 grain Wheat	495	9	66

Toasted Wraps: On Garlic Herb Tortilla, Without Chips Or Fruit

Hummus Veggie	600	23	81
King Caesar, with Caesar Dressing	635	31	56
Totally Turkey, w/ Ranch Dressing	625	25	56

Fresh Salads: Includes Standard Dressing

Chicken Caesar	495	40	11
Southwest Chicken, w/ SW Ranch	495	29	31
Thai Chicken	280	8	40

Indulgent Smoothies: 24 oz with Turbinado

Beach Bum	520	4	122
Chocolate Chiller	570	7	125
Peanut Butter Cup	695	20	121
Tropi-Colada	455	2	109

Low Fat Smoothies: Per 24 oz with Turbinado

Blimey Limey	385	0	99
Blue Lagoon	310	1	78
Hawaiian Breeze	335	0	87
Rockin' Raspberry	400	0	100
Strawberry Beach	415	0	103
Sunrise Sunset	320	0	81

Supercharged: Per 24 oz with Turbinado

Health Nut, with Soy	495	5	88
Lean Machine	440	0	112
Muscle Blaster, with Whey	440	2	88
Peanut Paradise, with Whey	675	18	101

With Splenda, deduct 200 calories & 50g carbs

Tubby's® (Jan '15)

Subs: Per 8" Regular Wheat Bun, without Dressing or Sauce

Deli-Subs:

	C	F	Cb
Ham & Cheese	500	10	76
Turkey Breast & Cheese	530	12	76
Grilled Burger Subs: Big Tub	630	25	75
Burger Special	760	33	78
Cheeseburger Italiano	740	33	76
Pizza Burger	630	25	75

Grilled Chicken Subs:

Chicken, Grilled	440	4.5	73
Chicken & Broccoli	520	10	75
Chicken & Cheddar	510	10	73
Chicken Fajita	520	10	75

Grilled Steak Subs:

Portabella Mushroom Steak	600	17	80
Pepper Steak & Cheese	570	15	76
Steak & Cheese	560	15	74
Steak Special	590	16	76
Specialty Subs: BLT	580	23	73
Cold Veggie	470	9	79
Italian Sausage	630	26	77
Pulled Pork	610	25	68
Tuna	530	9	74

Uno Chicago Grill® (Jan '15)

Appetizers: Per Whole Dish

	C	F	Cb
Mozzarella Sticks, 11.4 oz	850	47	80
Pizza Skins, 25 .4 oz	2070	140	147
Shrimp & Crab Dip, 16.4 oz	1120	81	64

Burgers: Without Sides

BBQ, with Bacon & Cheddar	1100	60	33
Cheeseburger, Buffalo Cheddar	970	51	29
Uno	860	42	28

Entrees:

Chicken: *Without Sides Or Breadstick*

Baked Stuffed Spinoccoli, 11.8 oz	360	14	10
Chicken Milanese, 22.5 oz	850	56	46
Chicken Thumb Platter, 10.5 oz	480	17	34

Steak & Seafood: *Without Sides Or Breadstick*

Baked Haddock, 11.8 oz	580	35	12
Brewmasters Grill NY Sirloin	510	14	21
Grilled Shrimp & Sirloin, 11.3 oz	440	21	4
Sides: French Fries, 5.5 oz	350	27	25
Red Bliss Mashed Potatoes	270	14	34
Roasted Seasonal Veggies, 7.2 oz	80	4.5	10
Farro Salad, 7.5 oz	180	7	31

253

Villa Fresh Italian® (Jan '15)

Pizzas: Per Slice

	C	F	Cb
Neapolitan:			
Plain, 7 oz	430	15	54
Deluxe, 9 oz	510	21	56
Sausage & Pepperoni, 8.5 oz	565	26	56
Stuffed: Baked Ziti	920	37	109
Meat	910	39	96
Spinach and Mushroom	735	33	80
Entrees:			
Baked Ziti	865	40	89
Chicken Marsala	745	20	107
Chiken Parmigiana	825	25	116
Chicken Scampi	840	33	103
Fettuccini Alfredo	930	52	88
Mac & Cheese	1160	77	83
Vegetables: Roasted Potatoes	210	12	23
Sauteed, Fresh, 6oz	85	6	6

Vocelli Pizza® (Jan '15)

Pizzas:

	C	F	Cb
Artisan: *Per ⅛ of Medium Pizza*			
Basil Pesto Primavera	240	10	28
Buffalo Chicken	220	9	26
Chicken Carbonara	250	10	27
Chicken Spinaci	220	8	27
Deluxe	260	10	29
Hawaiian	280	11	30
Meat Magnifico	280	12	26
Mexican	300	15	28
Philly Steak	270	13	25
Quattro Cheese	270	11	28
Spring Veggie	210	7	28
Pasta: Chicken Alfredo, 18 oz	1080	55	100
Chicken Parmesan, 20 oz	1030	35	132
Chicken Pesto, 18 oz	1110	59	99
House Baked Subs: *On Ciabatta*			
Buffalo Chicken, 7.2 oz	310	15	28
Chicken Parmesan, 7.2 oz	440	18	45
Meatball, 7.2 oz	460	23	36
Salads: *Per Regular Size, Without Dressing*			
Antipasta, 16 oz	270	16	17
Caesar, 8 oz	130	3	5
Mediterranean, 16 oz	270	18	17
Tuscan Grilled Chicken, 14 oz	290	13	12
Wings: *Bone In*			
BBQ, hot, 3.5 oz	190	6	20
Buffalo, 3.5 oz	170	7	14
Garlic, 3.5 oz	290	19	14
Hot Vesuvius, 3.5 oz	170	7	14

Wahoo's Fish Taco® (Jan '15)

Bowls: With White Rice & Black Beans

	C	F	Cb
#7 Blackened/Charbroiled Chkn, av.	860	15	127
# 8 Charbroiled/Teriyaki Fish, av.	930	22	126
#9 Veggie	760	11	141
#10 Carnitas/Kahlua Pig, average	1025	25	131
Burritos: With Brown Rice & White Beans			
Banzai:			
Blackened or Charbroiled:			
Chicken	575	16	77
Fish, average	620	21	77
Mushroom	490	14	81
Carne Asada	565	17	79
Carnitas	685	23	79
Shrimp	475	14	77
Vegetarian	485	14	82
Side Kicks: Brown Rice	350	7	64
White Beans	285	3	54
Salads: *Chips Not Included*			
Blackened Chicken	415	22	14
Charbroiled Chicken	415	21	14
Charbroiled Fish	485	29	14
Sandwiches: *Blackened or Charbroiled*			
Chicken	510	18	51
Fish, average	555	22	51
Carne Asada	500	19	52

For Complete Nutritional Data ~ see CalorieKing.com

WAWA® (Jan '15)

Breakfast:

	C	F	Cb
Bagels: Plain	260	1	55
With Reg. Butter	310	7	55
Cinnamon Raisin	290	1	63
With Regular Cream Cheese	380	10	64
Everything	310	6	56
Bowls: *Without Syrup*			
Creamed Chipped Beef On White	230	6	36
French Toasts: Plain	340	13	54
With Bacon	420	19	55
With Sausage Crumble	540	32	55
With Turkey Sausage Patty	430	20	55
Scrambled Eggs: With Bacon	470	34	10
With Sausage Crumble	590	47	10
Burritos: *With Scrambled Egg*			
Bacon	420	23	35
Beef Steak & Cheddar Cheese	450	23	37
Chicken Steak with Cheddar Chse	450	22	37
Sizzlis: *Per Sizzli*			
Bagels: Bacon, Egg & Cheese	410	18	43
Pork Roll, Egg & Cheese	420	19	42

Continued Next Page...

Updated Nutrition Data ~ www.CalorieKing.com
Persons with Diabetes ~ See Disclaimer (Page 22)

WAWA® cont... (Jan '15)

Breaded Chicken Strips:

	C	F	Cb
3 piece	240	13	16
5 piece	400	22	27

Cold Hoagies: On Shorti Roll without Toppings

	C	F	Cb
Egg Salad	650	37	61
Tuna Salad	690	39	63
Turkey	370	5	59

Hot Dogs: Without Toppings, Mustard or Sauce

	C	F	Cb
All Beef: ¼ Pound	420	28	21
Big Bacon Cheese Dog	810	47	57

Hot Hoagies: On Shorti Roll without Toppings

	C	F	Cb
Beef Steak & Cheddar Cheese	550	19	59
Chicken Steak & Cheddar Cheese	550	17	59
Meatballs & Cheddar Cheese	730	34	75

Soups: Per Medium Serving

	C	F	Cb
Baked Potato w/ Cheddar & Bacon	450	32	28
Chicken Noodle	150	3	23
Lobster Bisque	470	38	20
Italian Wedding	210	7	21
New England Clam Chowder	330	21	24

Quesadillas: Without Toppings

	C	F	Cb
Beef & Cheddar Cheese	450	22	36
Cheddar Cheese	330	13	34
Chicken & Cheddar Cheese	450	20	36

Sides: Per Medium Serving

	C	F	Cb
Chili	350	11	43
Macaroni & Beef	350	11	43
Macaroni & Cheese	500	25	49
Mashed Potatoes	470	28	50
Meatballs in a Cup	320	21	17

Bakery:

	C	F	Cb
Croissant, Plain	280	14	35
Muffins: Banana Walnut	670	34	83
Blueberry	610	30	78
Chocolate Chip	680	34	86
Corn	640	29	87

Hot Beverages: Per 16 oz, without Extras

	C	F	Cb
Hot Cappuccino, with 2% milk	130	5	13
Mocha Latte, with 2% milk	330	7	59

Smoothie, Strawberry Banana,

	C	F	Cb
without whipped cream, 24 oz	690	0	180

Wendy's® (Jan '15)

Old Fashioned Hamburgers: With Standard Toppings

	C	F	Cb
Dave's ¼ lb Single, w/ Cheese	580	31	42
Dave's ½ lb Double w/ Cheese	820	47	42
Dave's ¾ lb Triple w/ Cheese	1090	66	43
Baconator	940	57	41
Son of Baconator	660	38	41
Double Stack	460	25	27
Jr. Bacon Cheeseburger	390	22	26
Jr. Cheeseburger	290	13	26
Jr. Cheeseburger Deluxe	350	19	28

Sandwiches: With Standard Toppings

	C	F	Cb
Asiago Ranch Club, with Homestyle Chicken	670	32	57
Crispy Chicken	350	19	34
Homestyle Chicken	510	20	54
Spicy Chicken	510	20	55
Ultimate Chicken Grill	370	7	43

Go Wraps: Grilled Chicken

	C	F	Cb
Grilled Chicken	260	10	25
Spicy Chicken	340	16	30

Chicken Nuggets:

	C	F	Cb
Regular: 6 pieces	270	18	14
10 pieces	450	30	24
Spicy: 6 pieces	260	17	14
10 piece	430	28	23

Dipping Sauce: Per 1 oz

	C	F	Cb
Barbecue	45	0	11
Buttermilk Ranch	120	12	2
Honey Mustard	80	6	7
Sweet & Sour	45	0	12

Garden Sensations Salads: Full Size, No Dressing

	C	F	Cb
Apple Pecan Grilled Chicken	350	11	28
Asian Cashew Grilled Chicken	210	3.5	14
BBQ Ranch Grilled Chicken	390	15	28
Spicy Grilled Chicken Caesar	480	27	25

Sides:

	C	F	Cb
Baked Potatoes: Bacon & Cheddar	520	20	67
Sour Cream & Chives	320	3.5	43
Chili Cheese Fries, 10 oz	520	27	53
Natural Cut Fries: Value	220	11	28
Small, 4 oz	310	15	40
Medium, 5 oz	410	20	52
Large, 6.5 oz	500	24	65
Rich Meaty Chili, small, 8 oz	170	5	16

Frosty: Per Small

	C	F	Cb
Chocolate	340	9	56
Vanilla	330	8	55

For Complete Nutritional Data ~ see CalorieKing.com

Whataburger® (Jan '15)

Burgers & Sandwiches:

	C	F	Cb
A.1. Thick & Hearty Burger	1060	62	69
Chop House Cheddar Burger	1150	73	63
Green Chili Double	1020	61	73
Honey BBQ Chicken Strip S'wich	1040	55	89
Justaburger	320	14	35
Whataburger:			
Original	620	30	61
Avocado Bacon	900	63	53
Double Meat	850	49	62
Jalapeno & Cheese	710	38	64
Jr.	330	14	37
Triple Meat	1080	68	63
Meal: Original	1310	50	192
Bacon & Cheese	1670	73	218
Triple Meat	1980	99	219
Chicken:			
Grilled: Chicken Sandwich	460	17	50
Chicken Melt	470	21	39
Whatachick'n:			
Bites: 6 pieces, without sauce	410	18	30
9 pieces, without sauce	590	25	42
Sandwich	560	27	62
Strips, 3 pieces, without sauce	580	34	39
French Fries: Small, 3 oz	260	13	31
Medium, 4.5 oz	390	20	47
Large, 6 oz	530	27	63
Onion Rings: Medium, 4.3 oz	400	25	37
Large, 6.5 oz	590	38	56
Salad, Garden, without dressing	180	9	15
Breakfast:			
Cinnamon Roll	390	9	71
Biscuits: Plain	300	17	33
With Gravy	470	29	45
Honey Butter Chicken	590	36	51
Biscuit Sandwiches:			
With Bacon	480	31	33
With Sausage	630	45	32
On A Bun: With Bacon	380	19	34
With Sausage	530	33	34

Whataburger® cont... (Jan '15)

Breakfast (Cont):

	C	F	Cb
Platters:			
With Bacon	630	41	35
With Sausage	780	55	35
Taquitos:			
With Bacon, Egg & Cheese	410	25	27
With Cheese	360	21	27
With Potato, Egg & Cheese	470	28	57
Desserts:			
Chocolate Chunk Cookie	230	11	31
Hot Apple Pie, 3 oz	270	14	34
Beverages:			
Malts: Chocolate, 20 oz	610	14	105
Vanilla, 20 oz	570	14	88
Shake, Chocolate, 20 oz	570	14	92

White Castle® (Jan '15)

Note: Nutritional Information varies from state to state. Please check instore

	C	F	Cb
Sliders:			
Original	140	6	13
Double	240	12	21
Chicken Breast with Cheese	390	28	20
Fish, with Cheese	340	24	18
Surf & Turf with Cheese, 6 oz	540	38	27
Sides:			
Chicken Rings, average:			
6 rings, 5 oz	530	47	12
9 rings , 7.5 oz	790	71	18
French Fries:			
Small, 5.6 oz	330	21	32
Medium	600	39	57
Sack	770	49	76
Cheese Fries, small	400	27	35
Fully Loaded Fries, small	460	38	20
Mozzarella Cheese Sticks, 3 sticks	440	33	22
Condiments: Per Packet			
Ketchup	10	0	2
Mayonnaise	60	7	0
Sauces: Per Packet			
BBQ	10	0	3
Tartar Sauce	25	1.5	1
Dessert:			
On A Stick: Fudge Dipped Brownie	250	12	33
Fudge Dipped Cheesecake	180	10	21

Updated Nutrition Data ~ www.CalorieKing.com
Persons with Diabetes ~ See Disclaimer (Page 22)

Wienerschnitzel® (Jan '15)

	C	F	Cb
Hot Dogs:			
Original: *On Standard Bun*			
Chili	270	12	32
Chili Cheese	320	16	32
Deluxe; Kraut, Plain, average	245	10	31
Pastrami	350	18	30
Original: *On Pretzel Bun*			
Chili	400	14	55
Kraut; Mustard; Plain	370	13	53
Relish	380	13	55
Angus All Beef: *On Pretzel Bun*			
Chicago	560	26	61
Chili Cheese	590	32	55
Mustard	510	26	52
Relish	520	26	55
Junkyard Dog, on Seeded Bun	460	24	45
Specialties:			
Corn Dogs: Regular	230	13	31
Mini (6 pack)	290	16	28
Jalapeno Poppers, (6 pack)	300	16	31
Sides:			
Chili Cheese Fries	570	32	59
Fries: Medium	440	23	54
Large	750	39	92
Breakfast:			
Biscuits: Egg, Bacon, Cheese	450	25	36
Egg, Sausage, Cheese	540	34	40
Burritos: Egg, Bacon, Cheese	370	19	29
Egg, Sausage, Cheese	460	28	33
French Toast Sticks	530	28	61
Syrup, 1 oz	120	0	31
Desserts:			
Banana Split	820	24	148
Cones, regular:			
Plain, 5 oz	250	9	41
Chocolate Dipped, 5 oz	450	27	50
Freezees:			
Chocolate Caramel Crunch	880	39	133
Chocolate Covered Strawberry	980	56	120
Oreo; M&M	630	25	99
Reese's Pnut Butter Cup	630	26	97
Shakes, average all flavors	650	23	110
Sundaes:			
Caramel; Hot Fudge, average	400	15	64
Chocolate	390	14	64
Strawberry	370	14	59

Winchell's® (Jan '15)

	C	F	Cb
Donuts: Per Donut			
Buttermilk Bars, Choc Iced; Glazed	420	19	61
Jelly Filled:			
Apple with Cinnamon Crumb	370	15	53
Raspberry with Glaze	390	13	61
Strawberry with Sugar	380	13	60
Old Fashioned, Glazed; Maple Iced	410	17	60
Raised Ring: Chocolate Iced	270	10	41
Sugared	230	9	34

WingStreet (Jan '15)

	C	F	Cb
Chicken:			
Crispy Bone In Wings: *Per 2 Pieces*			
Buffalo, Mild/Med./Hot, 2.6 oz	220	12	19
Garlic Parmesan, 2.5 oz	290	23	12
Honey BBQ, 3 oz	250	12	28
Honey Sriracha, 2.5 oz	200	10	20
Spicy BBQ, 3 oz	230	12	24
Bone Out Wings: *Per 2 Pieces*			
Buffalo, Mild/Medium, 2.5 oz	200	9	18
Garlic Parmesan, 2.5 oz	260	20	11
Honey BBQ, 3 oz	230	9	27
Naked	160	9	11
Traditional Wings: *Per 2 Pieces*			
Buffalo, Medium/Hot, 2 oz	130	7	8
Garlic Parmesan, 2 oz	200	17	1
Spicy BBQ, 2.3 oz	140	6	12
Sweet Chili, 2.3 oz	150	6	13

Woody's Bar-B-Q® (Jan '15)

	C	F	Cb
Starters:			
Breaded Wings (10)	700	47	13
Beef Chili Cheese Fries	805	38	63
Dinner Entrees: Without Sides			
½ Chicken	840	56	0
Baby Back Ribs	520	40	2
Beef Prime Rib	760	62	1
Sandwiches: Per Regular, Without Sides			
Beef	390	14	28
Pork	490	26	29
Wraps: Without Sides			
Beef BBQ	380	13	31
Pork	440	21	30
Extras: BBQ Beans	170	8	20
Cobettes	80	1	18
French Fries	185	7	28
Garlic Toast	120	6	14
Green Beans	50	2.5	6
Okra	95	1	21
Squash	140	1	28

For Complete Nutritional Data ~ see CalorieKing.com

Fast - Foods & *Restaurants*

Yoshinoya® (Jan '15)

Appetizers: As Served

	C	F	Cb
Asian BBQ Wings: 4 pieces	410	25	21
6 peces	620	37	32
Entrees: As Served			
Bento: Beef	880	25	131
Teriyaki Chicken	1010	29	137
Beef Bowl: *With Sauce*			
Regular	730	27	91
Large	1040	38	131
With Vegetables: Regular	650	20	95
Large	960	29	141
Beef & Teriyaki Chicken Combo:			
Large, with skin	1190	36	151
Large, without skin	1150	33	151
Breaded Shrimp:			
Regular bowl, 4 pieces	690	16	119
With Beef, large	1090	34	164
With Teriyaki Chicken, large	1040	24	160
Teriyaki Chicken Bowl:			
Regular, with skin	790	18	110
Large, with skin	1140	25	165
Grilled Tilapia: With Rice & Slaw	570	13	91
With Rice & Veggies	540	12	88
With Rice, Slaw & Teriyaki Sauce	620	13	103
With Rice, Veggies & Teriyaki Sce	590	12	100
Sides, Clam chowder Soup	210	7	34
Desserts:			
Cheese Cake, 3.5 oz	330	19	35
Chocolate Cheesecake, 3.5 oz	370	22	37

Please note: Relates only to Northern California Menu

Z Pizza® (Jan '15)

Pizzas: Small, Per Slice

	C	F	Cb
Creations: Berkeley Vegan	150	5	21
California	140	4.5	18
Casablanca	180	8	17
Greek	140	5	17
Italian; Mexican, average	165	7	17
Provence; Santa Fe	150	6	17
Thai; ZBQ, average	165	5	19
Rusticas: *Per Slice*			
Chicken Sausage	100	3.5	12
Curry Chicken & Yam	130	3.5	16
Mediterranean; Moroccan, av.	140	8	13
Pear & Gorgonzola	130	6	14
Calzones: Meat Calzone	790	36	82
Veggie Calzone	630	22	86
Salads: *Small*			
Arugula, with Balsamic Vinaigrette	450	36	24
Caesar Side, with Caesar Dressing	200	16	8
California, with Chipotle Ranch	180	13	16

Zaxby's® (Jan '15)

Zappetizers: With Sauce

	C	F	Cb
Fried White Cheddar Bites w/ sce	820	51	62
Onion Rings, 5 oz	780	58	59
Spicy Fried Mushroom, 5.7 oz	620	48	43
Tater Chips, 5.2 oz	940	69	72
Meal Dealz: Without Drink			
Big Zax Snak, with Sauce	950	53	82
Buffalo Wings, without sauce	900	57	51
Chicken Finger Nibbler, w/ sauce	1330	72	137
Most Popular: As Served			
Chicken Finger Plate: Regular	1260	72	99
Large	1990	114	158
Wings & Things, regular	1490	94	85
Sandwich Baskets: Includes Fries			
Cajun Club	1020	50	90
Club	1250	74	99
Wings & Fingerz: With Sauce			
Buffalo Fingerz:			
5 pieces	630	43	15
10 pieces	1270	87	30
Buffalo Wings:			
5 pieces	540	41	3
10 pieces	880	61	4
Chicken Fingerz:			
5 pieces	610	39	19
10 pieces	1230	79	36
Zax Kidz: Without Drink			
Kiddie Cheese	800	51	69
Kiddie Finger	570	36	40
Kiddie Nibbler	550	29	59
Zalads: With Texas Toast, Without Dressing			
Blue, with Blackened Chicken	580	35	28
Caesar:			
With Fried Chicken	730	39	39
With Grilled Chicken	540	25	31
House Zalad: With Fried Chicken	760	42	44
With Grilled Chicken	570	28	36
Salad Dressings:			
Blue Cheese, 1 packet, 1.3 oz	180	19	2
Honey French, 1.3 oz	150	12	9
Honey Mustard, 1.3 oz	150	13	6
Lite Ranch, 1.3 oz	90	8	3
Mediterranean, 1.3 oz	140	14	4
Ranch, 1.3 oz	160	16	2
Thousand Island	230	24	3
Sides: Celery Basket,			
with 2 cups Ranch Sauce	420	42	10
Cole Slaw, 2.2 oz	140	11	12
Crinkle Fries, regular, 5 oz	360	16	48
Texas Toast, basket, 3 wedges, 4.3 oz	440	20	60

Zero Sub's® ~ *see CalorieKing.com*

Notes on Cholesterol

- **Cholesterol** is a white waxy substance produced mainly by our liver. It is also found in animal food products. Plant foods have no cholesterol.

- **Cholesterol is essential to life.** It is a structural part of every body cell wall and is the building block for vitamin D, sex hormones, and bile acids which help in the digestion of dietary fats.

- **The body makes sufficient cholesterol for its needs and does not rely on cholesterol in the diet.** Dietary fats have a major influence on blood cholesterol levels - more so than dietary cholesterol.

- **A high blood cholesterol level increases** the risk of atherosclerosis - the thickening of arteries that can reduce or block blood flow to the heart, brain, eyes, kidneys, sex organs and other body parts.

  This in turn increases the risk of heart attack, stroke, blindness, kidney failure, impotence and other blood circulatory problems.

  Other risk factors which increase the risk of atherosclerosis include high blood pressure, smoking, obesity and uncontrolled diabetes.

BLOOD CHOLESTEROL

CHECK YOUR RISK!

Total Cholesterol Level (mg/dl) ▼	Risk of Heart Attack ▼
240 and above	~ High Risk
200 - 239	~ Borderline/High
Below 200	~ Desirable

♥ **Know your cholesterol level, particularly if there is a family history of heart disease or stroke. If level is high, see your doctor.**

♥ **All adults should have their cholesterol, HDL and triglycerides tested at least every 5 years.**

HEART ATTACK WARNING SIGNALS

Many victims die before reaching the hospital by ignoring warning signals and delaying medical help.
Symptoms vary and commonly include:

- **Chest pain,** vice-like squeezing or burning sensation in center of the chest or between the shoulder blades, or in the mid-back. Pain may even feel like severe indigestion.

- **Pain** may be felt in the arms, shoulders, neck or jaw.

- **Shortness of breath** often occurs with or before chest discomfort.

- **Other signs,** with or without pain, include a cold sweat, nausea or light-headedness.

If you experience any of the above symptoms call IMMEDIATELY for medical help. Every minute counts.

Call 9-1-1 or your emergency number

▲ **Atherosclerosis can clog arteries and impede blood flow to the heart or other body organs.**

▼ **A thrombus (blood clot) can form on unstable, festering atherosclerotic plaque and rapidly block blood flow. A heart attack or stroke can result.**

Fats & Cholesterol Guide

The amount and type of dietary fat has the greatest influence on blood cholesterol levels.

Fats in food are a mixture of 3 basic types: saturated, monounsaturated, and polyunsaturated. Animal fats are mainly saturated while plant oils and fish oils are mainly mono- and polyunsaturated.

Saturated fats have subgroups known as long-chain, medium-chain, and short-chain fats. Most of the long chain fats raise blood cholesterol, and increase the risk of blood clots and thrombosis leading to artery blockage.

Long-chain saturated fats are found mainly in full-cream milk, cheese, butter, cream, fatty meats and sausages, and processed foods.

Monounsaturated fats tend to more selectively lower 'bad' LDL cholesterol and maintain the protective 'good' HDL cholesterol in the bloodstream – but only if they replace saturated fats in the diet.

Foods rich in monounsaturates include canola and olive oils, canola margarine, peanuts, and avocados.

Polyunsaturated fats consist of two main classes. **Omega-6** polyunsaturates tend to lower blood cholesterol. Rich sources include safflower, sunflower and corn oils.

Omega-3 polyunsaturated fats can lower blood cholesterol; significantly lower blood triglycerides; and reduce the rise of thrombosis, heart arrythmmia, and artery spasm.

Best practical omega-3 sources include canola oil and margarine, soybean oil and fish.

A balanced intake of the two omega classes is important for optimal health. For most Americans, slightly increasing omega-3 intake would help attain a more ideal balance.

Trans fats from hydrogenated vegetable oils and shortenings should also be avoided. They are common in commercial baked and fried food products such as cakes, muffins, pastries, doughnuts, fried snacks and french fries.

> Note: All fats are high in calories and need to be limited for weight control.

DIETARY FATS COMPARISON

- ■ Saturated Fat   ■ Monounsaturated Fat
- Polyunsaturated Fats:
- ■ Linoleic (Omega-6)   ■ Alpha-Linolenic (Omega-3)

OILS — PERCENTAGE CONTENT

OILS	Saturated	Monounsaturated	Linoleic (Omega-6)	Alpha-Linolenic (Omega-3)
CANOLA OIL	7	63	20	10
LINSEED/FLAX OIL	9	19	17	55
SAFFLOWER OIL	9	14	77	
GRAPESEED OIL	10	22	68	
SUNFLOWER OIL	11	23	66	
CORN OIL	14	32	52	2
OLIVE OIL	14	76		10
SOYBEAN OIL	15	23	54	8
PEANUT OIL	19	45	34	2
COTTONSEED OIL	26	16	58	
PALM OIL	51	39		10

SPREADS & FATS

Saturated Fat includes 'Trans Fats'   ☐ WATER CONTENT

	Saturated	Monounsaturated	Linoleic	Alpha-Linolenic	Water
LIGHT MARGARINE	14	14	21		51
CANOLA MARGARINE	18	45	12	6	19
POLYUNSATURATED MARG	24	20	36		20
BUTTER	57	18	2		24
LARD	41	47	12		
BEEF FAT	44	37	4		15

GOOD SOURCES Of OMEGA-3 FATS

Plant Sources	Omega-3 Fats (Grams)
Canola Oil, 1 Tbsp, ½ fl.oz	1.5g
Flaxseed Oil, 1 Tbsp	8g
Soybean Oil, 1 Tbsp	1.2g
Canola Margarine, 1 Tbsp, ½ oz	1g
Soybeans, cooked, ½ cup, 4 oz	0.5g
Walnuts, ½ oz	0.5g

FISH - *Per 4 oz Serving*
High Content: Salmon (Chinook), Tuna,
Trout (Lake), Sardines, Herring, Mackerel — 3g, 3g
Medium Content:
Salmon, (Pink/Red/Coho), 4 oz — 2g
Fair Content: *Per 4 oz Serving*
Bass, Catfish, Cod, Grouper, Hake, Halibut, Kingfish, Perch, Pollock, Shark, Trout (Rainbow), Tuna, Crab, Oysters, Blue Mussels, Shrimp, Squid — 0.5-1g

How Much Is Needed?

As little as 1-2 grams daily of omega-3 fats may benefit general health. High doses of fish-oil supplements should only be taken as directed by your doctor.

Dietary Cholesterol

Cholesterol in food varies in its effect on blood cholesterol level (BCL) from person to person. Much depends on the amount and type of fat and fiber eaten at the same meal.

Any elevating effect of dietary cholesterol on BCL is more likely to occur when the diet is high in saturated fat. Little elevation, if any, generally occurs when dietary fats are balanced in favor of monounsaturated and polyunsaturated fats (including omega-3 fats).

For example, while fish does contain cholesterol, the omega-3 fats can prevent any increase in BCL. Conversely, a meal containing no cholesterol but rich in saturated fat may result in a significant increase in BCL.

Consequently, the need to be overly concerned about dietary cholesterol is being de-emphasized in favor of the approach of limiting total fat, saturated fat, and trans fat in particular – and substituting unsaturated fats.

The liver usually cuts back its own cholesterol production in response to cholesterol in the diet. Many people can consume normal amounts of high-cholesterol foods without concern.

However, it is difficult to identify just who is at risk - the so-called 'hyper-responders'. Because over 50% of Americans have a BCL above ideal levels, the **American Heart Association** advises all Americans to be prudent and limit their cholesterol intake to less than 300mg daily, as well as to adopt a heart-healthy diet.

This limitation still allows the inclusion of most foods that are regularly eaten – even the overly maligned egg.

Eggs contain a modest 5 grams of fat per large egg. Barely 2 grams is saturated, the rest being monounsaturated or polyunsaturated.

By comparison, a cup of whole milk has 8g fat of which almost 5g is saturated.

CHOLESTEROL COUNTER

Cholesterol is found only in foods of animal origin. Plant foods contain no cholesterol.

	Cholesterol mg
Meat - Average all types:	
Lean Meat, cooked, 120g	100
Fatty Meat, cooked, 120g	100
Fat, thick strip, 60g	40

Note: While lean meat and fat have similar amounts of cholesterol, choose lean meat to limit fat intake.

	mg
Chicken/Turkey, average, 120g	100
Organ Meats: Liver, fried, 4 oz	500
Brains, beef, pan fried, 3 oz	1700
Sausages: Frankfurter, 40g	25
Salami, 2 slices, 55g	40
Bacon: 3 slices, cooked, 30g	20
Fish: Fish fillets, average, ckd, 120g	70
Tuna/Salmon, canned, 100g	50
Scallops, 9 medium, 3 oz	30
Prawns, raw, 100g	110
Oysters, raw, 6 medium, 85g	45
Crayfish, Crab, cooked, 100g	70
Eggs (Chicken), 1 large	210
1 medium	180
Egg White, *Scramblers*	0
Milk/Yoghurt: Whole, 1 cup, 250ml	30
Light/low-fat Milk (1%), 1 cup	10
Skim/Non-fat, 1 cup	10
Soy Milk, Tofu, Tempeh	0
Cheese: Natural/Hard/Cream, 30g	30
Cottage, low-fat, 2 Tbsp, 40g	5
Cream Cheese, 30g	25
Fats: Butter, 1 Tbsp, 20g	45
Margarine, Oils (vegetable)	0
Mayonnaise, 1 Tbsp	10
Cream: Heavy, whipping, 2 Tbsp, 40g	40
Light/Sour, 2 Tbsp	10
Ice Cream: Full-fat (10-11%), 100ml/50g	20
Low-fat (less than 4%), 50g	5
Fruit, Vegetables, Avocados	0
Nuts, Seeds, Grains	0
Coffee, Tea, Beer, Wine	0

For Comprehensive Food Listings ~ see CalorieKing.com

Blood Cholesterol ~ Diet Hints

DIETARY HINTS TO LOWER BLOOD CHOLESTEROL

1. Maintain a healthy weight.
If overweight, lose weight with a sensible, low-fat meal plan and daily exercise.

2. Reduce saturated fat intake by:
(a) eating less dairy fat. Choose low-fat or fat-reduced varieties of milk, yogurt, soy drinks, cheese, and ice cream.

(b) replacing saturated fats with fats and oils rich in monounsaturated and polyunsaturated fats. Choose vegetable oils such as canola, olive, sunflower and soybean. Avoid solid frying fats.

Note: *Promise Active* and *Benecol* spreads contain plant stanol esters which can lower total and LDL cholesterol.

(c) eating less fat from meat and poultry. Choose lean cuts of meat and skinless chicken. Go easy on lunch meats, salami and fatty sausages. Enjoy fish.

(d) eating less saturated and trans fats from baked and fried fast-foods. Avoid deep-fried foods. Avoid donuts, cakes, pastries and cookies unless made with healthier fats and oils.

3. Increase your soluble fiber intake.
Foods rich in soluble fiber include beans, lentils, chick peas, hummus, nuts, seeds, psyllium-seed husks and psyllium-fiber supplements. Oat bran, rice bran and barley are also good sources, as are fruit, vegetables and avocados.
(See Fiber Guide - Page 264-269).

4. Eat more soy bean products such as: soy drinks, tofu, tempeh (cultured soy beans), soy flour, soy vegetarian foods and edamame (fresh green soybeans).

Soy protein in place of animal protein can significantly decrease high blood cholesterol levels as well as 'bad' LDL cholesterol and blood triglycerides while 'good' HDL cholesterol is maintained. For best results, eat at least 25g of soy protein per day (from 3-4 servings).

5. Eat more fruit, vegetables, and whole grains in place of high-fat foods. Aim for 2 fruits and 5 servings of vegetables per day. They also contain valuable antioxidants. The fat of avocados (and most nuts) is mainly unsaturated and can lower blood cholesterol levels.

6. Limit cholesterol to 300mg per day.
(Extra Notes ~ See Previous Page)

7. Avoid brewed unfiltered coffee (espresso; plunger-style). Several cups per day may raise blood cholesterol. Filtered coffee is fine.

8. Spread your food intake over the day.
Have 5-6 small meals per day rather than just 2-3 large meals. Nibbling, versus gorging, favors lower blood cholesterol.

ALCOHOL – WINE

Alcohol is a mixed bag. Moderate amounts of 1-2 drinks daily appear to reduce the risk of heart attack and ischemic stroke in older persons.

However, larger amounts increase the risk of high blood pressure, obesity, heart failure and hemorrhagic stroke, and can aggravate hypertriglyceridemia: as well as many other health hazards. *(See Alcohol Guide – Page 23)*

The speculative benefits of moderate alcohol intake have been overstated in the media. The overriding harmful effects of excess alcohol do not allow its recommendation for any aspects of health promotion.

Fruit, Vegetables & Tea Also Protect:
Red wine and red grapes (more so than white) contain antioxidants which may help protect cholesterol in the blood from becoming oxidized.

Many fruits, vegetables, grains, nuts and tea also contain protective antioxidants.

Fats in the diet affect more than blood cholesterol levels. They can also strongly influence blood clot formation and thrombosis, as well as blood flow and ultimate oxygen delivery to body parts and organs.

While advanced atherosclerosis can impede blood flow to the heart and other organs, it is thrombosis (complete blockage by blood clots) or arterial spasm which commonly results in a heart attack or stroke.

Plant and fish oils rich in omega-3 fats lessen the risk of blood clots, thrombus formation, and artery spasm by reducing platelet stickiness and adhesion to artery walls. This reduces the risk of atherosclerotic plaque becoming unstable and reactive.

Omega-3 fats also improve blood flow by reducing blood viscosity and increasing the flexibility of red blood cells (RBC) that need to flex and twist on themselves in order to squeeze through tiny narrow capillaries often half their diameter.

A diet high in saturated fats has the opposite effect by stiffening RBC membranes and increasing blood viscosity, thereby hindering blood flow. The stiffening of the RBC membrane also reduces its ability to release vital oxygen to body cells and take up carbon dioxide.

Stiff red blood cells may also form aggregates that resemble coin stacks. In narrow blood vessels, this further impedes blood flow and impairs oxygen release through the much-lessened surface area of red blood cell membranes exposed to blood. (Smoking, lack of exercise, and stress can have similar adverse effects on thrombosis, red blood cell flexibility, and blood flow.).

▲ Picture of Healthy Blood Flow

Flexible red blood cells twist and slide through tiny capillaries - often half the diameter of red blood cells.

▲ A Not-So-Healthy Picture!

Red blood cells have lost their flexibility and ability to twist and slip through capillaries. They are stacked up, thereby impeding blood flow.

A diet high in saturated fats can contribute to this picture - as can smoking, lack of exercise, and stress.

Stay Fit Don't Quit!

Eat Light Eat Right!

Be Smart Don't Start!

Fiber Guide

Introduction

Fiber is the general term for those parts of plant food that we cannot digest (although bacteria in the large bowel partly digests fiber through fermentation). It is not found in foods of animal origin (meats, dairy products).

Fiber promotes intestinal health, bowel regularity, can benefit diabetes and blood cholesterol levels, and may help prevent colon cancer. High-fiber foods also assist weight control.

Most Americans don't eat enough fiber – less than 20 grams/day - instead of a healthier 25 to 35 grams/day.

Types of Fiber

Plant foods contain a mixture of different fibers in varying proportions. Insoluble and soluble fiber categories are based on their solubility in water. All types of fiber are beneficial to the body.

♦ **Insoluble fibers** (cellulose, hemi-celluloses, lignin) make up the structural parts of plant cell walls.

Best food sources are wheat bran, corn bran, rice bran, wholegrain cereals and breads, beans and peas, nuts, seeds, and the skins of fruits and vegetables.

These fibers absorb many times their own weight in water. They create a soft bulk and hasten the passage of waste products through the intestines.

They promote bowel regularity, and aid in the prevention and treatment of uncomplicated forms of **constipation, diverticulosis and hemorrhoids.**

The risk of colon cancer may also be reduced by fiber's diluting effect on potentially harmful substances.

♦ **Soluble fibers** (pectin, gums, mucilages) are found mainly within plant cells, soy milk (whole bean) and products.

Fiber promotes good health, and better control of diabetes and cholesterol.

'An apple a day keeps the doctor away.'
... it just might!

Types of Fiber (Cont)

Best Sources of Soluble Fiber:
Fruits and vegetables, oat bran, barley, beans and peas, prunes, psyllium and flax seed.

These fibers form a gel which slows both stomach emptying and the absorption of sugars from the intestines. **This helps to control blood sugar levels.**

Weight control is also aided by the slower emptying of the stomach and the feeling of **fullness provided by soluble fiber.**

Some soluble fibers can lower **blood cholesterol** by binding bile acids and excreting them. More body cholesterol must then be broken down to supply bile acids for emulsification of dietary fats. **Rice bran, while not high in soluble fiber, can also lower blood cholesterol.**

♦ **Resistant starch** is that part of starchy foods (approx. 10%) which is tightly bound by fiber and resists normal digestion. Friendly bacteria in the large bowel ferment and change the resistant starch into short-chain fatty acids, which are important to bowel health and may protect against colon cancer.

Starchy foods include bread, cereals, rice, pasta, potatoes and legumes.

Fiber & Weight Control

Fiber can assist weight control in several ways. Fiber-rich foods such as fresh fruit and vegetables, potatoes and wholegrain bread contain few calories for their large volume (due to their low-fat, high-water content).

Their bulk fills the stomach and satisfies the appetite much sooner than fiber-depleted foods. The extra chewing time also contributes to satiety, and gives the stomach time to register a feeling of fullness. Excessive calories are less likely to be consumed.

Fiber-depleted foods and drinks are more concentrated in calories; e.g. fats, sugar, candy, soft drinks, fruit juices, alcohol. They require little or no chewing. Large amounts with excessive calories can be consumed before the appetite is satisfied.

Example: Whereas one fresh apple might satisfy the appetite, an apple juice drink with the equivalent sugars and calories of 2-3 apples only minimally satisfies the appetite. (See illustration below.)

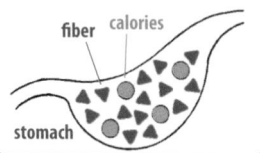

High-fiber foods fill the stomach. Fewer calories are consumed.

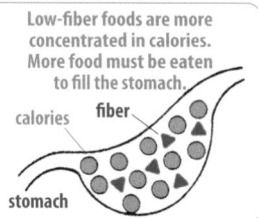

Low-fiber foods are more concentrated in calories. More food must be eaten to fill the stomach.

EFFECTS OF REMOVING FIBER FROM FOOD

2-3 pieces of fresh fruit produces 1 glass of fruit juice. The removal of fiber concentrates the sugar and calories.

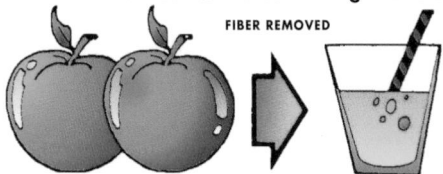

FIBER REMOVED

Fresh Fruit		Fruit Juice
High Fiber	←	Negligible Fiber
Low Calorie Density	←	High Calorie Density
Long Eating Time	←	No Eating Time (Drink)
Satisfies Hunger	←	Does Not Satisfy Hunger
Sugar Slowly Absorbed	←	Sugar More Quickly Absorbed
Less Insulin Required	←	More Insulin Required

Fiber Guide ~ Constipation

Constipation

Constipation can reasonably be defined as a failure to have a bowel movement at least every second day – and just as importantly, without straining or pain.

Typically, constipated stools are too hard, too narrow and too small.

The **main cause** is simply a lack of dietary fiber. Other contributing factors include insufficient fluids, too little exercise, emotional stress, gastrointestinal disease, lack of proper dentition to chew high-fiber foods, and some medications (e.g. some antacids, antidepressants, pain medications).

Note: Check with your doctor to rule out any underlying medical problem – especially if you have a change in bowel habits in middle-age or later years.

DESIRABLE FIBER INTAKE

Adults: 25-35gm per day
Children (under 18): Age + 5gm
Example: 6-year old (6 + 5)= 11gm

SAMPLE FOOD QUANTITIES
For 35 Grams of Fiber/Day

	Fiber
Breakfast Cereal (higher-fiber)	5g
plus 4 slices wholegrain Bread	6g
plus 3 servings fresh Fruit	9g
plus 1 medium Potato (w. skin)	
or 1 cup Brown Rice	4g
or ½ cup wholegrain Pasta	
plus 3-4 servings Veggies/Salad	6g
plus 1 cup Bean Soup	
or ¼ cup Baked/Soy Beans	
or ½ cup Corn/Peas/Lentils	5g
or 1¼ oz Almonds (natural)	
or 3 medium Figs	

HINTS TO INCREASE FIBER AND AVOID CONSTIPATION

1 **Breakfast is an important contributor** to daily fiber intake. Eat high-fiber breakfast cereals (bran-based cereals, oatmeal etc.). Add 1-2 tablespoons of unprocessed bran.

Dried fruits, chopped nuts, soy grits, and seeds are also excellent additions to cereals.

Note: A gradual increase in fiber will prevent bloating, gas or pain. People intolerant to bran may benefit from psyllium-based fiber supplements and cereals.

2 **Drink adequate water daily.** Fiber works by absorbing many times its own weight in water.

3 **Eat wholegrain breads,** or fiber-enriched breads. They have over double the fiber of regular white bread.

4 **Enjoy fruit as fresh fruit** with skin rather than as fruit juice. Enjoy wholegrain pasta, barley, brown rice, nuts and seeds.

5 **Eat more vegetables,** salads and legumes – especially cooked beans, lentils, potatoes with skins, avocado, broccoli, brussels sprouts, cabbage, carrots, celery, and peas.

6 **Add bran** (barley/rice/wheat) or soy grits to soups, casseroles, stews, desserts, cookies, cakes. Also use whole-meal flour or soy flour in place of white flour. Use nuts, seeds, and ground linseed.

7 **Snack** on fresh or dried fruits, carrot or celery sticks, popcorn, nuts or seeds, wholegrain crackers, high-fiber bars (low-fat). Limit amounts if overweight.

8 **Exercise regularly** to strengthen abdominal muscles and stimulate the gut. Keep up water intake, especially in warm weather.

9 **Avoid** indiscriminate and regular use of harsh laxatives. They can overstimulate the intestinal muscles and may make normal bowel activity impossible. It may take several weeks to restore normal bowel function.

Fiber Counter

FOODS WITH ZERO FIBER

- **Dairy Products (Milk, Cheese, etc)**
- **Meats, Poultry, Fish, Eggs**
- **Fats/Oils, Sugar/Syrups**
  (Only foods of plant origin contain fiber.)

Breakfast Cereals ~ Fiber

General Mills:

Basic 4, 1 cup, 2 oz	3
Cheerios (Honey Nut; Multigrain), 1 c., 1 oz	2
Fiber One, ½ cup, 1.1 oz	14
Multi-Bran Chex, 1 cup, 2 oz	7
Oatmeal Crisp Almond, 1 cup, 2 oz	4
Raisin Nut Bran, 1¼ cup, 2 oz	6
Total, average all types, ¾ cup, 1 oz	3
Wheat Chex, 1 cup, 2 oz	6
Wheaties ¾ cup, 1 oz	3

Health Valley:

Amaranth Flakes, ¾ cup, 1 oz	3
Crunches & Flakes, ¾ cup, 1.9 oz	4
Fiber 7 Flakes, ¾ cup, 1 oz	7
Golden Flax, ¾ cup, 1.9 oz	6
Granola (Low-Fat), ⅔ cup, 2 oz	6
Healthy Fiber Flakes, ¾ cup, 1.1 oz	4
Oat Bran Flakes, all types, ¾ cup, 1 oz	2
Oat Bran O's, ¾ cup, 1 oz	3
Real Oat Bran, ½ cup, 1.7 oz	5

Kellogg's:

All-Bran, ½ cup, 1.1 oz	10
All-Bran w. Extra Fiber, ½ cup, 1 oz	13
All-Bran Bran Buds, ⅓ cup, 1.1 oz	13
Corn Flakes, Fruit Loops, Smacks 1 cup, 1 oz	1
Cocoa/Rice Krispies Treats, 1¼ cup, 1 oz	0
Complete: Wheat Flakes, ¾ c., 1 oz	5
Oat Bran Flakes, ¾ cup, 1.1 oz	4
Corn Pops, 1 cup, 1.1 oz	0
Cracklin' Oat Bran, ¾ cup, 1.7 oz	6
FiberPlus Antioxidants:	
Berry Yogurt Crunch, 1 c., 1.9 oz	10
Cinnamon Oat Crunch ¾ c., 1.1 oz	9
Frosted Mini Wheats, 24 bisc., 2 oz	5
Granola w. Raisins, ⅔ cup, 2.1 oz	3
Raisin Bran, 1 cup, 2.1 oz	7
Smart Start, Strong Heart,	
Cinnamon Raisin, 1 cup, 1.8 oz	4
Special K, 1 cup, 1.1 oz	0.5

Fiber ~ Fiber (grams)

Breakfast Cereals (Cont) Fiber

Kashi:

GoLEAN Cereal, 1 cup, 1.8 oz	10
GoLEAN Crunch!, 1 cup, 1.9 oz	8
GoLEAN Bars, avg. (1)	6
Good Friends: Original, 1 cup, 1.9 oz	12
Cinna-Raisin Crunch, 1 cup, 1.8 oz	8
Heart to Heart, ¾ cup, 1.2 oz	5
7 Whole Grain Pilaf, ½ cup, cooked, 5 oz	7
7 Whole Grain Puffs, 1 cup, 0.7 oz	1

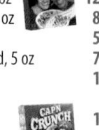

Quaker:

Cap'n Crunch, ¾ cup, 1 oz	1
100% Natural Granola,	
avg., ½ cup, 1.8 oz	3
Crunchy Corn Bran, 1 cup, 1 oz	5
Life Cereal, ¾ cup, 1.1 oz	2
Oat Bran, ½ cup, 1.4 oz	6
Oatmeal, average, 1 packet	3

Post:

100% Bran, ⅓ cup, 1 oz	9
Alpha Bits, 1 cup, 1 oz	2
Blueberry Morning, 1 cup, 1.9 oz	5
Cranberry Almond Crunch, 1 cup, 1.8 oz	3
Fruit & Bran, 1 cup, 1.9 oz	6
Grape-Nuts, ½ cup, 2 oz	7
Great Grains, ⅔ cup, 1.9 oz	5
Honey Bunches of Oats, ¾ cup, 1.1 oz	2
Shredded Wheat & Bran, ½ cup, 2 oz	8

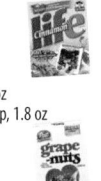

Brans & Supplements, Metamucil

Oat Bran: 1 Tbsp (level)	1
½ cup, (5½ Tbsp), 1 oz	5
Rice Bran, raw, ¼ cup, 1 oz	6
Wheat Bran, Unprocessed:	
Raw, 1 Tbsp	1.5
2 Tbsp (level), ¼ oz	3
¼ cup, (4 Tbsp), ½ oz	6
Wheat Germ, Raw, ¼ cup, 1 oz	4
Psyllium Seed Husks, 2 Tbsp	8
Fibersure, 1 heaping tsp	5
Metamucil: Orange, 1 rnd Tbsp, 11g	3
Fiber Wafers (2)	6

Hot Cereals, Oatmeal

Bulgur (cracked Wheat), ckd, 1 cup	8
Corn/Hominy Grits, dry, 3 Tbsp, 1 oz	0.5
Cream of Wheat, cooked, ¾ cup	1
Oatmeal (uncooked ⅓ cup), ckd, ⅔ cup	3

Fiber Counter

Breads & Crackers

	Fiber
Bread: White, 1 slice, 1 oz	0.6
Whole-wheat, 1 slice, 1 oz	1.5
Wholegrain, 1 slice, 1 oz	2
Rye, Pumpernickel, 1 oz	1.5
Bagel/Roll/Bun, 1 medium, 2 oz	1.5
Pita, whole wheat, 6.5" pocket	4.5
Crackers: Graham, average, 2	0.4
Saltine, 4 crackers	0.4
Crispbreads, average, 2	4
Matzo, 1 board, 1 oz	1
Rice Cakes, average, 1 cake	0.3
Tortilla: Regular, 6"	0.5
Whole-wheat, 6"	1.3

Barley, Pasta, Rice & Flours

	Fiber
Barley, pearled, raw, ¼ cup, 1.7 oz	8
Rice:	
White, cooked, 1 cup	0.6
Brown, cooked, 1 cup	3.5
Rice-A-Roni, average, 1 cup, prepared	1.5
Spaghetti/Noodles: Cooked, 1 cup	2
Whole-Wheat, cooked, 1 cup	4
Flour: Wheat, All-purpose, 1 cup, 4.5 oz	3.5
Whole-Wheat, 1 cup, 4.5 oz	15
Cornmeal, stone ground, 1 cup, 4.5 oz	13
Carob Flour, 1 cup, 3.5 oz	41
Rye Flour, 1 cup, 3.5 oz	15
Soy Flour: Defatted, 1 cup, 3.5 oz	17
Full-fat, raw, 1 cup, 3 oz	8
Soy Meal, defatted, 1 cup, 4.5 oz	14

Frozen Entrees & Dinners

Average All Brands: Per Serving

	Fiber
Beans/Chili base, average	6-10
Potato/Pasta base, average	4-6
Vegetable base, average	3
Meat/Chicken base, average	2-3
Pizzas, ¼ large, average	3
Vegetarian Soy Burgers, 1 pattie	4

Soups

	Fiber
Chicken Noodle, 1 cup	0.5
Tomato Soup, average, 1 cup	0.5
Vegetable Soup, average, 1 cup	3
Health Valley: *Per 1 Cup*	
Black Bean; Minestrone	8
Tomato	1
5 Bean Vegetable; Lentil & Carrots	10
Mushroom Barley; Vegetable	4
Split Pea	8
Progresso, High Fiber, all flavors, 1 cup	7

Fast Foods & Restaurants

	Fiber
Hamburgers: Small, average	1.5
Large/Whopper, average	2.5
Hot Dog, Regular	1.5
French Fries: Small serving, 2.5 oz	2.5
Regular/Medium, 3.5 oz	3.5
Chicken Nuggets, 6 pack	0.5
Chicken Sandwich, average	2
Taco, average	2
Sundaes, Shakes, Soft Drinks	0
Arby's, Classic Roast Beef Sandwich	1
Denny's: Grilled Chicken Salad, no bread	4
Classic Burger, no fries	4
Club Sandwich, no fries	2
Grilled Chicken Sandwich, no fries	4
Domino's: 12", Classic/Thin, 1 slice	1
Deep Dish, 1 slice	3
Feast Pizza, Classic/Thin, 1 slice	2
McDonald's: Big Mac	3
Hamburger; Quarter Pounder	3
Egg McMuffin	2
Grilled Chicken Caesar Salad	4
Pizza Hut: *Per 1 Slice, Medium*	
Pan Pizza: Cheese, Pepperoni	1
Supreme	2
Thin 'n Crispy, Supreme	2
Hand-Tossed, average all varieties	2
Subway: Sandwich, white roll, av.	4
With Honey Wheat Roll, average	4
Salads, average	4

Cakes, Cookies, Snack Bars

	Fiber
Apple/Fruit Pie, 1 serving, 4 oz	2
Cake: With plain flour, 1 serving, 3.4 oz	1.5
With whole-wheat flour, 1 serving	3
Carrot Cake, 4 oz	3
Cookies, oatmeal, (3 small/1 large)	1
Donuts, medium, 1.7 oz	0.7
Fruit Cake, 1 serving, 1.5 oz	2
Fig Bars, 1 cookie, 0.5 oz	0.7
Muffins, Oat Bran (2 small, 1 large), 4 oz	5
Granola Bars, average, 1 bar	2
Atkins Advantage Bars, average	7
Clif Bars, 2.5 oz	5
Curves, Chocolate Peanut Bar, 1 oz	5
Fi-Bar Chewy & Nutty, 1 bar	1
Fiber One (Gen. Mills), 1.4 oz bar	9
FiberPlus, all bars, 1.2 oz	9
Health Valley: Fruit/Granola Bars	3
Cereal Bars	1
Luna Bars, avg., 1.7 oz	3
Special K, Protein Meal Bar, 1.6 oz	5

Fiber Counter

Chocolate, Chips, Popcorn | Fiber
Cheese Balls/Curls/Twists 1
Chocolate, Hard Candy, 1 oz 0
Chocolate with nuts/fruit, 2 oz bar 1.5
Mars Bar, 1.8 oz 1
Potato Chips; corn chips, 1 oz 1
Popcorn, 3 cups 3
Pretzels, Twists (6) 1

Nuts, Seeds
Almonds: Natural, 25 nuts, 1 oz 3.5
  Blanched (skins removed), 1 oz 3
Cashews, Filberts, Pecans, 1 oz 1.7
Peanuts, Mixed Nuts, Coconut, 1 oz 2.5
Peanut Butter, 2 Tbsp, 1 oz 2
Pistachio Nuts, dried, shelled, 1 oz 3
Walnuts, Black/English, dried, 1 oz 2
Seeds: Amaranth, 2½ Tbsp, 1 oz 3.5
  Flax Seeds, 3 Tbsp, 1 oz 7
  Psyllium Seed Husks, 5 Tbsp, 1 oz 20
  Quinoa Seeds, 3 Tbsp, 1 oz 1.7
  Sesame Seeds, whole, 1 oz 3.4
  Sesame Butter/Tahini, 2 Tbsp, 1.1 oz 1.4
  Sunflower kernels, ¼ cup, 1 oz 3.8
  Teff Seeds, 1 oz 3.8

Fruit – Fresh
Apples: 1 medium, 5½ oz (whole)
  with skin + core 3.7
  with skin, no core 3.2
  without skin, no core 1.7
Apricots, 2 medium, 4 oz 1.5
Avocado, average, ½ medium 6
Banana, 1 medium, 6 oz (w. skin) 3
Blueberries, raw, ½ cup, 2.5 oz 1.7
Cherries, sweet, raw, 8 fruits, 1.6 oz 1
Grapefruit, average, ½ fruit, 10 oz 1.4
Grapes, 1 medium bunch, seedless, 7 oz 2
Kiwifruit, 1 medium, 2.7 oz 2.3
Mango, 1 medium, 11 oz (whole) 1.6
Melons, Cantaloupe, 4 oz (edible) 1
Nectarine, 1 medium, 4 oz 1.9
Olives, average all types, 7 jumbo, 2 oz 1.5
Oranges, 1 medium (7-8 oz w. skin)
  5½ oz (peeled) 3.8
Passionfruit, 2 medium, 2.5 oz 5
Peaches, 1 large, 6 oz 2
Pears, raw, 1 medium, 6 oz 4.5
Pineapple, 1 slice, 3 oz 1.2
Plums, 2 medium, 6 oz 1.8
Strawberries, 6 medium/3 large, 2 oz 1
Watermelon, 4 oz (edible) 0.5

Fruit – Dried, Juice | Fiber
Dried Fruit: Apricots, 8 halves, 1 oz 2.2
  Dates (3 med); Raisins (2 Tbsp), 1 oz 1.5
  Figs, 3 medium,1½ oz 5
  Prunes, 4 medium, 1 oz 2
Fruit Juice: Orange/Apple etc, 1 glass <0.5
  Prune Juice, 5 oz 1.4
  Carrot Juice, 8 oz 1.8

Vegetables
Asparagus, 4 medium spears 1.3
Bean Sprouts, ½ cup, 2 oz 1
Beans: Snap/Green, ½ cup, 2 oz 2
  Baked Beans in Tom Sce, ½ c, 4.5 oz 5
  Dried Beans, ckd, average, ½ cup 7
Beets, ckd, slices, ½ cup, 3 oz 1.7
Broccoli, cooked, ½ cup, 3 oz 2.4
Brussels Sprouts, ckd, ½ cup, 3 oz 3.5
Cabbage: White, ckd, ½ cup, 2.5 oz 1
  Red, ckd, ½ cup,2.5 oz 2
Carrots, 1 medium (7½"), ½ cup, 3 oz 2.5
Cauliflower, cooked, 3 flowerets, 2 oz 1.5
Celery, raw, diced, 1 cup, 3.5 oz 1.6
Chickpeas (Garbanzos), ckd, ½ c., 3 oz 6.5
Corn: Kernels, cooked, ½ cup, 2½ oz 2.5
  Corn on the Cob, 1 ear, 5 oz 4
Cucumber/Lettuce/Mushrooms, 2 oz 0.5
Eggplant, raw, sliced, ½ cup, 1.5 oz 2
Lentils, cooked, ½ cup, 3.5 oz 8
Mixed Vegetables, frozen, cooked, ½ cup 3
Onions: Raw, 1 medium, 4 oz 1.5
  Spring Onions, chop., ¼ cup, 1 oz 0.7
Peas: Green, raw, ½ cup, 2.5 oz 3.7
  Cowpeas (Black-eyed), ckd, ½ cup 10
  Split Peas, cooked, ½ cup, 3.5 oz 8
Peppers, sweet, raw, 1 large, 6 oz 3
Potatoes: 1 medium, with skin, 5 oz 3
  1 medium, without skin 2.5
  ½ cup mashed, 3.5 oz 1.5
  French Fries, small, 2.6 oz 2
Spinach, cooked, ½ cup, 3 oz 2.2
Squash: Summer, cooked, ½ cup, 3 oz 2.5
  Winter, cooked, ½ cup, 3.5 oz 2.4
Tomatoes: 1 medium, 4.5 oz 1.5
  Tomato Sauce, 1 cup 0.3
Soybean Products: Miso, ½ c., 5 oz 7.4
  Tempeh, cooked, 1 piece, 3 oz 4
  Tofu, ½ cup, 4.4 oz 0.4

Salads
Side Salad, average 1
Bean Salad, ½ cup 5
Coleslaw, ½ cup 1
Potato Salad, ½ cup 2

Protein Guide

General Notes

- **Protein has many important body functions.** It builds and repairs muscle, and is the basis of our body's organs, hormones, enzymes, and antibodies to fight infection.

- **Protein is also an emergency fuel** in the absence of sufficient carbohydrate and fats. For this reason, weight loss should be gradual so as to preserve protein levels in muscle, the heart and other body organs.

- **It is easy to obtain sufficient protein,** even if vegetarian. **Plant proteins are not inferior to animal proteins.** In fact, eating more soy and other plant proteins, and less animal protein, may help to build stronger bones and prevent osteoporosis, and may help to control blood cholesterol levels.

- **When changing to a vegetarian diet,** include soybeans, and other beans, soy milk drinks (calcium-enriched), lentils, tofu, tempeh, nuts and wholegrain breads and cereals. Milk, yogurt, cheese and eggs can enhance nutrient intake.

Protein & Muscle

- Although muscles are built of protein, protein is not a special fuel for working muscle cells – carbohydrates and fats are.

- In fact, a diet high in protein (and fat) and low in carbohydrate can significantly reduce the performance of endurance sports athletes. **Carbohydrates** are the best fuel for muscles exercised for long periods.

- Any **extra protein** required by athletes and body-builders can easily be obtained from the extra food eaten to satisfy hunger and energy needs.

- Remember, **excessive protein** intake will not build bigger muscles. Any excess is converted and stored as fat. Excess protein can also strain the kidneys, which excrete the waste products of protein metabolism.

Elderly people (and dieters) must eat sufficient food to ensure adequate protein intake.

Inadequate protein leads to a drop in immune response with greater susceptibility to illness and infections. Muscle strength and muscle mass also drop.

Protein needs are easily met with sensible eating. Athletes who eat enough food for their energy needs can obtain sufficient protein.

RECOMMENDED DAILY PROTEIN INTAKE ~ HEALTHY RANGE ~
(Lower figure is RDA)

		PROTEIN
Children:	1-3 yrs	13g-26g
	4-8 yrs	19g-38g
	9-13 yrs	34g-64g
Males:	14-18 yrs	52g-120g
	19+	56g-120g
Females:	14+	46g-110g
Pregnancy:		71g-120g
Breastfeeding:		71g-120g

Note: On lower-calorie diets, aim for higher amounts of protein within the Healthy Range.

Pro ~ Protein (grams)

Meat   **Pro**

	Pro
Steak: Average all cuts, lean (no fat)	
Small (4 oz raw/3 oz cooked)	23
Medium (6 oz raw/4¼ oz cooked)	34
Large (10 oz raw/7¼ oz cooked)	57
Roast Beef, lean, 2 slices, 3 oz	24
Ground Beef patty, lean, cooked, 3 oz	21
Lamb chop, broiled, 3 oz	22
Liver, cooked, 3 oz	23
Veal cutlet, 1 medium	23
Pork, cooked, lean, 3 oz	24
Bacon, 3 medium slices	6
Ham, roasted, 2 pieces, 3 oz	18
Ham, luncheon, 2 slices, 1½ oz	7
Pastrami, 3 sl., 1¾ oz	10
Sausages: Bologna, 2 sl., 2 oz	7
Braunschweiger, 2 sl., 2 oz	8
Pork link, thick, 2 oz	6
Frankfurter, 1⅓ oz	5
Salami, hard, 3 slices, 1 oz	7
Vegetarian, 1 pattie	13

Chicken/Turkey: *Without Skin*

	Pro
Chicken, cooked: Breast, Roasted, 4 oz	36
Leg/Thigh,Roasted, 2 oz	14
½ Whole Chicken	60
Drumstick, Rstd 1 med., 3 oz	13
Turkey: Light meat, cooked, 3 oz	28
Dark meat, lean, 3 oz	24

Fish

	Pro
Fresh Fish: *Per 4 oz, cooked*	
Cod, Flounder/Sole, Pollock	28
Catfish, Haddock, Halibut, M/Mahi	28
Ocean Perch, Swordf., Orange Roughy	28
Canned Fish: Tuna, Light, 3 oz	25
White, 3 oz	23
Salmon, pink, 3 oz	17
Salmon, red, 3 oz	17
Sardines, 3 whole (3"), 1¼ oz	9
Anchovies, 1 can, 1½ oz	13
Shellfish: Crabmeat, 3 oz	17.5
Clams, raw, 4 large/9 sml, 3 oz	11
Crayfish, cooked, 3 oz	20
Lobster, cooked, 3 oz	17
Oysters, raw, 6 medium, 3 oz	7
Scallops, 2 lge/5 small, 1 oz	5
Shrimp, raw, 6 large, 1½ oz	8.5
Fish Products: Fish Sticks, 4 sticks	10
Fish Portions, in batter, 4 oz	13
Gefilte Fish, 1 medium ball, 2 oz	8

Eggs   **Pro**

	Pro
1 Large Egg, whole	6
Egg Yolk	3
Egg White	3
Omelet: Plain, 2 eggs	13
Ham & cheese	17
Egg Substitutes, (liquid):	
Egg Beaters, ¼ cup, 2 oz	4.5
Better 'n Eggs/Scramblers, ¼ cup, 2 oz	6

Milk, Yogurt, Ice Cream

	Pro
Milk: Whole: 2%, 1 cup	8
Low-Fat (1%); Fat-Free, 1 cup	8.5
Chocolate Milk, 1 cup	8
Thick Shake: Chocolate, 10 oz	9
Vanilla, 10 oz	11
Soymilk, (fortified), average, 1 cup	7
Soy Dream, Enriched, shelf-stable, 1 cup	7
Yogurt, average all brands:	
Plain, 6 oz	8
Fruit flavors, 6 oz	7
Chobani, Greek, Plain, 6 oz	14
Soy, fruit flavors, 6 oz	7
Ice Cream: Rich, ½ cup	2
Regular, Vanilla, ½ cup	2.5
Sherbet, ½ cup	1
Custard, baked, ½ cup	7

Cheese

	Pro
Hard Cheeses, average, 1 oz	7
Cottage Cheese, ½ cup	13
Cream Cheese, avg., 1 oz	2
Ricotta, part skim, ½ cup	14

Bread, Bagels, Biscuits

	Pro
Bread: *With enriched flour*	
1 slice, 1 oz	2
4 thin slices, 4 oz	8
4 thick slices, 6 oz	1.2
Bagel, plain 2 oz	6
Biscuits, 1 oz	2
Pita Bread, 1 pita, 1½ oz	4
Pumpernickel, 1 slice, 1 oz	3

Infant/Baby Foods   **Pro**

	Pro
Infant Formula Milk:	
Enfamil/Gerber/Similac,	
Regular/Low Iron , 5 fl.oz	2.2
Isomil/Nursoy/ProSobee,	
Baby Cereals: *Average all brands*	
Dry, 4 Tbsp, ½ oz	1
Jars, with fruit, 4½ oz	1

Protein Counter

Breakfast Cereals · Pro

Hot Cereals ~ *Cooked:*
Bulgur, cooked, 1 cup, 5 oz — 9
Oatmeal: Reg., non-fortified, 1 cup — 6
  Instant, fortified, avg., 1 pkt — 4
  Quaker, all flavors, ½ cup — 5
Corn/Hominy Grits: 1 cup — 3
  Quaker: Reg., 3 Tbsp, 1 oz — 2
    Instant White, 1 packet — 2
Cream of Wheat, 1 cup — 4
Brands ~ *Ready-To-Eat*

General Mills:
  Cheerios, Original, 1 cup, 1 oz — 3
  Chex, Corn, 1 cup, 1.1 oz — 2
  Kix, Original, 1¼ cups, 1 oz — 2
  Lucky Charms, Original, ¾ cup, 1 oz — 2
  Total, Raisin Bran, 1 cup, 1.8 oz — 3
  Wheaties, ¾ cup, 1 oz — 2

Health Valley:
  Amaranth Flakes, 1¼ cups, 2 oz — 6
  Bran Flakes, with Raisins, 1 cup, 1.8 oz — 5
  Corn Crunch-Ems, 1 cup, 1 oz — 2
  Oat Bran Flakes, with Raisins, 1 cup, 1.9 oz — 5
  Rice Crunch-Ems, 1¼ cups, 1 oz — 2

Kashi:
  Good Friends, 1 cup, 1.9 oz — 5
  GoLean Crunch!, 1 cup, 1.9 oz — 9
  7 Whole Grain Flakes, 1 cup, 1.75 oz — 6

Kellogg's:
  All-Bran, Original, ½ cup, 1 oz — 4
  Apple Jacks, 1 cup, 1 oz — 1
  Corn Flakes, 1 cup, 1 oz — 2
  Low-fat Granola
    with Raisins ⅔ cup, 2.1 oz — 5
  Product 19, 1 cup, 1 oz — 3
  Rice Krispies, 1¼ cup, 1.2 oz — 2
  Smart-Start Strong Heart, 1 c., 1.75 oz — 4
  Special K: All flavors, 1 c., 1.1 oz — 2
    Protein, ¾ cup, 1.1 oz — 10

Post:
  Grape Nuts, Original, ½ cup, 2 oz — 8
  Raisin Bran, 1 cup, 2 oz — 5

Quaker:
  Corn Bran Crunch, ¾ cup, 1 oz — 2
  Granola, ½ cup, 1.7 oz — 5
  Honey Graham Oh's, ¾ cup, 1 oz — 1
  Life, Original, ¾ cup, 1.1 oz — 3

Brans & Wheatgerm · Pro

Oat Bran, raw, 1 Tbsp — 2
Rice Bran, raw, 2 Tbsp — 1
Wheat Bran, unprocessed, 2 T. — 1
Wheat Germ, 2 Tbsp, ½ oz — 4

Grains & Flours, Yeast

Amaranth, ½ cup, 3.4 oz — 14
Barley, ½ cup, 3.2 oz — 12
Buckwheat Flour, Whole-groat, 1 cup — 15
Carob Flour, 1 cup, 3.6 oz — 5
Corn Flour, 1 cup, 4 oz — 11
Corn Meal, 1 cup, 4½ oz — 8
Flour: White, 1 cup, 5.6 oz — 9
  Wholegrain, 1 cup, 4¼ oz — 16
Millet, wholegrain, 1 cup, 3½ oz — 12
Rye Flour: Dark, 1 cup, 4½ oz — 18
  Light, 1 cup, 3½ oz — 9
Soy Flour, full fat, 1 cup, 3 oz — 29
Yeast: Brewers, 2 Tbsp, ½ oz — 8
  Nutritional Yeast Flakes *(Red Star),*
    1 heaping Tbsp, ½ oz — 8

Rice, Spaghetti, Macaroni

Rice: Brown/White, average
  1 cup cooked, 6½ oz — 5
Spaghetti/Macaroni/Noodles (enriched):
  Cooked, 1 cup, 4½ oz — 7
  Canned: in Tomato Sce, ½ cup — 2
    with Meatballs, 1 cup, 8 oz — 10
  Macaroni & Cheese, 1 cup, 9 oz — 8

Soups

With Noodles/Vegetables, 1 cup — 3
With Meat/Beans/Peas, 1 cup — 8

Fruit

Fresh/Canned:
  Average, all types,
    1 medium/2 small fruit — 1
Avocado, ½ medium — 2
Dried Fruit: Apricots, 8 halves, 1 oz — 1
  Dates, 6 dates, 2 oz — 1.5
  Figs, 4 medium figs, 2 oz — 2
  Prunes, 5 medium, 1½ oz — 1
  Raisins, 1 oz — 1
Fruit Juice: Average, 1 cup — 0.5
  Prune Juice, 6 fl.oz — 1
  Tomato Juice, 1 cup, 8 fl.oz — 1.5

Vegetables | Pro

	Pro
Beans: Snap/green, ½ cup, 2 oz	1
Dried: Average all types, cooked, ½ cup	7
Baked Beans, ½ cup 4½ oz	5
Bean Sprouts, mung, 1 c., 4 oz	3
Broccoli, 3raw, ½ cup, 1½ oz	1.5
Cabbage; Cauliflower, raw, 1 c. 3 oz	1.5
Corn: Raw, ½ cup kernels, 3 oz	2.5
1 ear trimmed to 3½"	2
Lentils, cooked, ½ cup, 3½ oz	9
Mushrooms, raw, ½ c., sliced	1
Peas: Green, raw, ½ c., 2½ oz	4
Split Peas, cooked, 1 cup, 7 oz	16
Potatoes: *Cooked:*	
1 medium, with skin, 5 oz	3.3
without skin, 4 oz	2.3
French Fries, small, 2.6 oz	2
Potato Salad, ½ cup, 4 oz	3.5
Pumpkin, ½ cup mashed, 4.3 oz	1
Seaweed, kelp, 1 oz	<1
Spinach, cooked, ½ cup, 3 oz	2.7
Squash, ckd, all types, ½ cup	1
Tomatoes, 1 medium, 4½ oz	1
Vegetables, mixed, ckd, 1 cup	2.5
Soybeans, cooked, ½ cup, 3 oz	14

Tofu, Tempeh, Miso

Tofu, raw, firm, ½ cup, 4½ oz	10
Tempeh, ½ cup, 3 oz	16
Miso, ½ cup, 5 oz	16
Miso Soup, 1 cup	3
Soybean Protein *(TVP),* 1 oz	18

Cakes, Pastries, Pies

(Made with enriched flour)

Carrot w. cream cheese frosting, 4 oz	4
Cheesecake, 1 piece, 4 oz	6
Chocolate, 1 piece, 2 oz	2
Fruitcake, 1 piece, 3 oz	4
Plain, 1 piece, 3 oz	4
Croissant, plain, 2 oz	5
Danish Pastry, 1 pastry, 2¼ oz	4
Donuts, average, 2 oz	4
Muffins, average, 1 med., 1½ oz	4
Pancakes, 4" diam., two, 2 oz	4
Pies: Fruit, 1 piece, 5½ oz	4
Pecan, 1 piece, 5 oz	7
Puddings, average, ½ cup, 4½ oz	4
Waffles, 1 large, 2½ oz	7

Peanut Butter | Pro

	Pro
Regular: 2 Tbsp, 1.1 oz	8
Peter Pan Plus, 2 Tbsp, 1.1 oz	8

Sugar, Honey, Jam

Sugar: White	0
Brown, 1 Tbsp	0
Molasses: Light/Med., 1 Tbsp	0
Blackstrap, 1 Tbsp, ¾ oz	0
Corn Syrup, 1 Tbsp, ¾ oz	0
Honey, Jams, Jelly	0

Candy, Chocolate, Carob

Candy, sugar-based	0
Chocolate: Plain, 2 oz bar	4
with nuts, 2 oz bar	6
Carob, plain, 2 oz	6

Cookies, Crackers, Chips

Cookies, average, 4 cookies	2
Crackers, Graham, 2½" sq., (2)	1
Rice Cakes, average, one	1
Corn/Potato Chips, 1 oz	2

Nuts:

Almonds, shelled, 20-25 nuts	6
Brazil Nuts, 7-8 medium nuts, 1 oz	4
Cashews, 12-16 nuts, 1 oz	5
Macadamias, 1 oz	2
Peanuts, dry rsted, 40 nuts, 1 oz	6
Pecans, 24 halves, 1 oz	2
Walnuts, 15 halves, 1 oz	4

Seeds:

Sesame Seeds, dry, 1 Tbsp	2
Pumpkin Kernels, dry, hulled, 1 oz	7
Sunflower Seeds, dried, hulled, 1 oz	6
Tahini, 1 Tbsp, ½ oz	2.5

Granola & Food/Protein Bars

Granola Bars, average, 1 bar, 2 oz	2
Anytime Health,	
Meal Repl. Bars, 80g	20
Snack Bars, 50g	12
Balance Bars, Original, average all, 1.76 oz	14
Bariatrix, Proti-Bars (1), 1.4 oz	15
Dr Soy, Protein Bars, 1.76 oz	10
GeniSoy, Protein Bar, 1.6 oz	15
Jenny Craig, Bars, av., 1.8 oz	5
Met-Rx, "Big 100", av., 3.5 oz	27
Myoplex 30, all flavors, 3 oz	30
Optifast 800, all flavors, 2 oz	14
PowerBar, Energize, 2 oz	6
Slim-Fast, Protein Meal Bars, 1.7 oz	10
Special K: Protein Meal, 1.6 oz	10
Protein Snack, 0.9 oz	4

Protein Counter

High Protein Drinks | Pro

Anytime, Health,
  Whey Prot. Isolate, all flav., 1 oz — 25
Atkins, Shakes, 11 fl.oz — 18
Boost, High Protein, 8 fl.oz bottle — 15
Carnation, B'fast Essentials, 11 fl.oz — 10
Curves, Protein Drink, 2 scoops, dry — 15
dotFIT, First String,
  Choc., 2 scps, 2.65 oz — 21
Ensure, Plus, 8 fl.oz bottle — 13
Gatorade, Protein Recovery Shake, 11 oz — 20
GeniSoy, Protein Shake, 1 scoop, 1.2 oz — 14
Met-Rx, Meal Replacement, RTD — 40
Myoplex, Original Nutrition Shake, 1 pkt — 42
Optifast 800, prepared, 8 fl oz — 14
Slim-Fast Shakes: Meal, 10 oz can — 10
  High Protein Meal, 10 fl.oz bottle — 20
Special K₂0, Protein Water, 16 fl.oz — 5
Weider, Mass 1000, 4 scoops, 7 oz — 34

Coffee, Tea, Soda

Coffee, Coffee Substitutes, 1 cup, 8 fl.oz — 0
Coffee, with 2 oz milk, 1 cup, 8 fl.oz — 2
Caffe latte, large, 16 fl.oz — 12
Cappuccino, large, 16 fl.oz — 8
Frappuccino, average, 16 fl.oz — 6
Hot Chocolate, with milk, 1 cup, 8 fl.oz — 8
Soft Drinks/Soda — 0
Tea, all types — 0

Beer, Wine, Spirits

Beer, 12 fl.oz — 1
Wines, red/white, 1 glass — 0
Spirits/Liquor — 0

Fast-Foods/Burgers

Pancakes, average all outlets, 3 — 8
Shakes, Chocolate, 16 fl.oz — 12
Sundaes, Average all outlets — 7
Arby's:
  Chopped Farmhouse Salad, Crispy Chicken — 30
  Roast Beef Sandwich: Classic — 23
    Max — 45
Burger King: Big Fish Sandwich — 18
  Double Bacon Cheeseburger — 17
  Whopper Sandwich — 22

Fast Foods/Burgers (Cont) | Pro

Carl's Jr:
  Charbroiled Chicken Club Sandwich — 36
  Famous Star Hamburger with Cheese — 28
  Super Star Hamburger with Cheese — 48
Domino's Pizza: Hand Tossed (12")
  Feast, Ultimate Pepperoni, 1 slice — 11
  Legend: Buffalo Chicken, 1 slice — 13
    Honolulu Hawaiian, 1 slice — 8
KFC: Original, Breast — 36
  Extra Crispy Tenders, 3 strips — 33
  Grilled, Breast — 40
McDonald's: Big Mac — 25
  Cheeseburger — 15
  Chicken McNuggets (6) — 13
  Crispy Chicken Classic Sandwich — 24
  Filet-O-Fish — 15
  Hamburger — 12
  Quarter Pounder with Cheese — 30
  French Fries: Small, 2.5 oz — 3
    Large, 5.4 oz — 6
  Salad, with Chicken, average — 26
  Shake, McCafe, average, 12 fl.oz — 12
  Breakfast: Egg McMuffin — 18
    Bacon, Egg & Cheese McGriddles — 19
    Sausage Burrito — 12
    Sausage McMuffin with Egg — 21
Pizza Hut: *Per Medium, 1 slice, ⅛ Pizza*
  Thin 'n Crispy, Supreme — 10
  Pan Pizzas, average — 11
  Hand Tossed: Pepperoni Lover's — 12
    Ultimate Cheese Lover's — 10
Subway : *6" Subs with standard toppings, no oil*
  Applewood Pulled Pork — 25
  Meatball Marinara — 21
  Spicy Italian — 20
  Subway Melt — 23
  Turkey Jalapeno Melt — 21
Taco Bell: Bean Burrito — 15
  Cheesy Gordita Crunch — 20
  Chicken Quesadilla — 27
  Chicken/Steak Chalupas — 16
  Steak Burrito Supreme — 20
  Taco Supreme — 9
Wendy's:
  Asiago Ranch Chicken Club — 38
  Dave's ¼ lb Single Burger — 30
  Jr Hamburger — 14

High Blood Pressure

Many American adults have hypertension (high blood pressure), and are unaware of it. It is generally symptomless, so **have your blood pressure checked annually** – particularly if it runs in the family.

Untreated hypertension overworks the heart, damages arteries and promotes atherosclerosis. This in turn greatly increases the risk of heart disease, stroke, blindness, kidney disease and impotence. The earlier hypertension is detected, the sooner it can be brought under control.

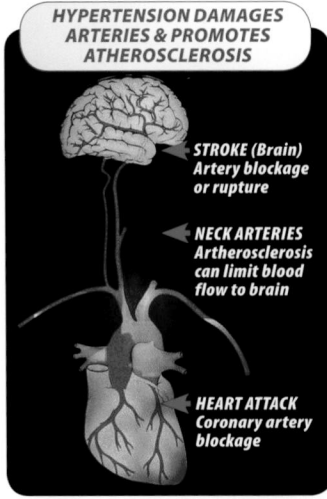

HYPERTENSION DAMAGES ARTERIES & PROMOTES ATHEROSCLEROSIS

STROKE (Brain) Artery blockage or rupture

NECK ARTERIES Artherosclerosis can limit blood flow to brain

HEART ATTACK Coronary artery blockage

BLOOD PRESSURE CLASSIFICATION

For Adults Age 18 & Older ~ Not Acutely ill or on Medication (American Heart Association)

	DIASTOLIC		SYSTOLIC
Normal ➤	Below 80	and	Below 120
Prehypertension ➤	80-89	or	120-139
Hypertension:			
Stage 1 ➤	90-99	or	140-159
Stage 2 ➤	100 or more	or	160 or more

Treating Hypertension

Prehypertension (in the chart above) means you don't have high blood pressure now but are likely to develop it in the future.

You can take steps to lessen the risk by adopting healthy lifestyle habits such as:
- reducing sodium intake
- eating adequate fruit and vegetables
- losing weight if overweight
- limiting alcohol to 2 drinks or less daily
- quitting smoking
- exercising regularly, managing stress.

Stage 1 hypertension can often be treated with the above lifestyle changes.

Stage 2 hypertension usually requires drug therapy. However, salt restriction, abstaining from alcohol, and the above lifestyle changes will improve the success of drug therapy, and enable smaller drug doses to be prescribed.

STROKE
KNOW THE WARNING SIGNS

Stroke is a medical emergency! If you notice one or more of these signs, call 9-1-1 or your doctor immediately.

These signs may be signalling a possible stroke or transient ischemic attack:

- **Sudden weakness** or numbness in your face, arm, or leg on one side of your body.
- **Sudden confusion,** trouble speaking or understanding. Slurred speech.
- **Sudden trouble seeing,** in one or both eyes.
- **Sudden trouble walking,** dizziness, loss of balance or coordination.
- **Sudden severe headache** - 'a bolt out of the blue' – with no apparent cause.

Extra Info: www.stroke.org

Salt & Sodium Guide

Salt & Sodium

- **Sodium is a mineral element** most commonly found in salt (sodium chloride). It also occurs naturally in much smaller amounts in animal and plant foods, and water – normally sufficient for our needs without having to add salt to our diet.

- **Sodium is required** for nerve and muscle function, as well as to balance the amount of fluid in our tissues and blood. Sodium acts like a sponge to attract and hold fluids in body tissues.

- **Excess sodium** can cause water retention, and increase the risk of developing hyper-tension. Very high salt intake may also increase the risk of stomach cancer.

- **Too little sodium** may cause low blood pressure (hypotension), and decrease blood flow to the heart, brain and kidneys – especially during exercise. (A certain blood volume is required to sustain the blood pressure needed for adequate blood flow in the capillaries).

Salt-Sensitive Persons

- **Normally, our kidneys** excrete excess dietary sodium. The thirst we feel after a salty meal is the body calling for water to dilute the sodium, and enable the kidneys to flush out excess sodium.

- **However, 'salt - sensitive'** persons (up to 70% of adults) tend to retain excess sodium (above approximately 3000mg daily) instead of excreting it. Such persons are more likely to develop hypertension and would benefit most from sodium restriction. Assume you are susceptible if there is a family history of hypertension.

- **Although not everyone will benefit, all Americans are being asked to moderate their salt and sodium intake** as a public health measure – particularly because so many do not know whether or not they have hypertension, and also because we do not know just who is salt-sensitive.

On average, **less than one third of our sodium intake comes from the salt shaker.** The rest is hidden in processed foods that have salt added during manufacture.

Sodium compounds added to food or medicinals can also contribute significant sodium.

Sodium bicarbonate in particular is widely used in antacid tablets (such as *Alka Seltzer*) and powders. Sodium bicarbonate contains 27% sodium by weight. Each gram contributes 270mg sodium. Large amounts of sodium can be unwittingly consumed – up to 600mg per tablet. (See Antacids ~ Page 280)

Example: 2 *Alka-Seltzer* Tablets = 1000mg sodium

Other sodium compounds include monosodium glutamate (MSG), sodium ascorbate, sodium nitrite, and sodium citrate.

POTASSIUM BALANCES SODIUM

Potassium helps to balance sodium by helping the kidneys to excrete excess sodium. Fruit and vegetables are rich sources of potassium - another reason to ensure you have your 5-7 servings every day.

Nuts also provide potassium as well as magnesium and other heart-healthy nutrients and anti-oxidants. Eat them unsalted.

Note: This info is only for people with normal kidney function. Also not for persons on potassium-sparing diuretics.

ALCOHOL DANGER

Excessive alcohol intake contributes to hypertension. Susceptible persons should limit alcohol intake to 1-2 drinks per day.

> Sodium accounts for only 40% of the weight of salt (sodium chloride). Examples:
> **1 gram (1000mg) Salt has 400mg Sodium**
> **1 teaspoon (5g) Salt has 2000mg Sodium**

HINTS TO REDUCE SODIUM

- **Cut down use of the salt shaker.** Start with an easy 50% cut in sodium by using Lite Salt (*Morton*) or *Cardia* Salt. Then gradually cut back until you can leave the salt shaker off the table. Sea salt is still high in sodium.

- **Use fresh herbs,** and salt-free seasonings to add flavor to food.

- **Choose low-sodium,** sodium-free, and reduced-sodium products in place of regular, salted products.

- **Check food labels for sodium levels.**
  FDA Guidelines for sodium descriptors are:
  - **Reduced Sodium:** At least 25% less sodium than the original product
  - **Low Sodium:** 140 mg or less/serving
  - **Very Low Sodium:** 35mg or less/serving
  - **Sodium Free:** Less than 5mg/serving
  - **No Salt Added:** Made without the salt normally added, but still contains the sodium that is a natural part of the food

- **Use reduced-sodium breads,** butter and margarine. Regular varieties are considered high in sodium in view of their significant contribution to our diet.

- **Go easy on salty condiments and sauces** such as ketchup, mustard, soy sauce, spaghetti sauces, and salad dressings. Use low-sodium varieties.

- **Limit pizzas and salty fast-foods.**
  Check the *CalorieKing.com* food database.

- **Avoid salty snack foods** such as potato chips, corn chips, salted nuts, pretzels and cheesy-flavored snacks. **Choose unsalted** popcorn, nuts or seeds. Eat more fruit.

- **Don't salt children's food** to your taste.

- **Avoid antacids** with sodium bicarbonate (such as *Alka-Seltzer*). They are high in sodium. Look for low-sodium alternatives.

HIGH SODIUM

- Cheese, Butter, Margarine
- Pickles, Sauerkraut, Olives
- Condiments, Sauces
- Salad Dressings
- Canned vegetables/salads/beans
- Deli Salads (with dressing)
- Frozen/Packaged Meals/Entrees
- Soups: Canned/dry; bouillon cubes
- Meats: Ham, bacon, sausage, luncheon meats, smoked meats
- Canned Fish (in brine/salt)
- Sea Salt, Garlic/Celery Salt
- Snack Foods (potato chips, pretzels)
- Tomato Juice (Canned), V8 Vegetable Juice
- Fast Foods: Pizza, Burgers, Chicken
- *Alka-Seltzer* Antacid
- Bread (regular)

MODERATE SODIUM

- Meat, Fish, Poultry - Unprocessed
- Milk, Yogurt, Soy Drinks, Eggs
- Peanut Butter
- Breakfast Cereals (less than 200mg/serving)
- Chocolate Candy, Fruit/Nut Bars
- *Reduced Sodium & Low Sodium Products*

FOODS LOW IN SODIUM

- Products labelled *Very Low Sodium*, or *Sodium Free*
- Bread (No Salt Added)
- Fresh fruits and vegetables
- Canned and Dried Fruits
- Potatoes, Rice, Pasta
- Dried Beans & Lentils, Tofu
- Nuts & Seeds (unsalted)
- Corn & Popcorn (unsalted)
- Pepper, Spices, Herbs
- Jam, Honey, Syrup
- Candy, Gum
- Hard & Jelly Candy
- Coffee, Tea, Alcohol
- Fresh Fruit Juices, Water

Sodium Counter

Milk & Dairy Products

	Sodium
Milk: Whole/lowfat/skim, average	
1 glass, 8 fl.oz	120
Whole, low sodium, 1 cup	5
Choc Milk, 1 cup	130
Soy Milk, 8 fl.oz	30
Buttermilk, cultured, 8 fl.oz	250
Dry/Powder, skim, ¼ cup, 1 oz	110
Yogurt, with fruit average, 8 oz	130
Cheese: Bleu, 1 oz	330
Cottage Cheese, Creamed, ½ cup, 4 oz	450
Kraft: Cheddar Singles, 2% milk, 0.7 oz	290
Philadelphia Cream Cheese Brick, Orig.,1 oz	105
Parmesan, 1 oz	450
Process Cheese., average,1 oz	430
Ricotta Cheese, ½ cup, 4 oz	150
Swiss, Deli Style, 1 oz	60

Ice Cream, Frozen Yogurt

Icecream, average, ½ cup	50
Frozen Yogurt, ½ cup	50

Fats/Oils

Butter/Margarine:	
Regular, 2 Tbsp, 1 oz	230
Unsalted, reg., 2 Tbsp, 1 oz	5
Mayonnaise, avg., 2 Tbsp, 1 oz	160
Oils/Lard/Drippings	0
Cream, average, 1 Tbsp	5
Coffee-Mate: Powdered, 1 tsp	2
Liquid, 1 Tbsp	5

Eggs

Whole, 1 large	70
Omelet: 2 egg, plain	220
With 1 oz Cheddar Cheese	400
Egg Beaters: Original, ¼ cup	115
Flavors, average, ¼ cup	230

Meats

Meat, average all types, cooked	
Beef/Lamb/Veal/Pork, 4 oz	80
Corned Beef, cooked, 3 oz	800
Bacon, cooked, 2 slices, 0.5 oz	270
Ham, 3 oz	1100

Chicken & Turkey

Chicken/Turkey, cooked, unsalted, 4 oz	80
Stuffing Mixes, average., ½ cup	500

Sodium ~ Sodium (mg)

Sausages & Meats

	Sodium
Bologna, 1 oz	280
Frankfurter, 2 oz	640
Ham, chopped, 0.8 oz slice	290
Liverwurst (Braunschweiger), 1 oz	320
Pepperoni, 5 slices, 1 oz	570
Salami: Cooked, 1 oz	350
dry/hard, 1 oz	600
Sausage, 1 oz link	220
Pork, 2 oz patty	260
Spam: Classic, 2 oz	790
25% Less Sodium, 2 oz	580
Turkey Roll, 1 oz	160

Fish:

Fresh Fish: average, plain	
Cooked, 4 oz, without bone	60
Broiled w. butter, 4 oz	150
Breaded & fried, 4 oz	320
Fish fillets, batter-dipped 3 oz	350
Fish sticks, 1 oz stick	160
Gefilte Fish, with broth, 1 pce, 1.5 oz	220
Herring, pickled, 2 pces, 1 oz	260
Lobster, meat only, 4 oz	180
Oysters, fresh, 6 med., 3 oz	95
Salmon: Canned, 3 oz	460
No Salt Added, 3 oz	65
Smoked fish, average, 3 oz	650
Tuna: Canned, drained, 3 oz	160
Light, drained, 3 oz	200
No Added Salt, 3 oz	40
Spicy Flavored, 5 oz	260

Entrees & Meals

Frozen Meals, average	600-900
Lean Cuisine, average	700
Stouffer's, average	580
Dinners, average	900-1200
Side Dishes, average	400-600
Pizza, frozen, ¼ large, 6 oz	800-1200
Microwave, Cup Meals	900-1200
Cup O'Noodles, average	1500

More Sodium Counts:
www.CalorieKing.com

Sodium Counter

Soups

	Sodium
Condensed: Average, 1 cup, 8 oz	800-1000
Low Sodium, average	70
Chicken Noodle, average, 1 cup	900
Bouillon Cube, average	950
Ramen Noodle Soup, av., 3 oz pkg	1500
Soup Cups, average	850
Soup Mixes, average, 1 cup	900

Condiments, Sauces, Dressings

	Sodium
A-1 Sauce, 1 Tbsp	280
Barbecue Sauce, 1 Tbsp	130
Bragg's Liquid Aminos, 1 tsp	220
Chili Sauce, 1 Tbsp	230
Ketchup: Tomato, 1 Tbsp	180
Low Sodium, 1 Tbsp	20
Mayonnaise, 1 Tbsp	80
Mustard, 1 tsp	70
Pizza Sauce, ½ cup	700
Salad Dressings, 2 Tbsp, 1 oz	160-400
Spaghetti Sauce, ½ cup	500
Soy Sauce: 1 Tbsp	900
Lite, 1 Tbsp	600
Sweet & Sour, ½ cup	250
Tabasco, 1 tsp	25
Vinegar, Lemon Juice	0
Worcestershire, 1 Tbsp	65
Tomato: Sauce, 1 cup	1200
Paste/Puree (salted), ½ cup	1000
No Salt Added, ½ cup	75

Salt & Salt Substitutes

	Sodium
Table Salt: 1 teaspoon, 6g	2400
Single Serve package, 1 g	400
Cardia Salt, 1 teaspoon	1080
Lite Salt, 1 teaspoon, 6g	1200
Morton, No Salt Substitute, 1 tsp	5
Garlic/Onion/Seasoned Salt, 1 tsp, 4g	1350
Garlic/Seasoned Salt 1 teaspoon, 4g	1300
Sea Salt, 1 teaspoon, 5g	2250

Seasonings, Herbs & Spices

	Sodium
Baking Powder, 1 tsp, 3g	340
Baking Soda (Sodium bicarb), 1 tsp, 3g	810
Accent, Flavor Enhancer, 1 tsp	600
Chili Powder, 1 tsp, 3g	25
Curry Powder	1
Lemon Pepper 1 tsp	340
Meat Tenderizer, 1 tsp, 5g	1750
MSG (Monosodium Glutamate), 5g	500
Mrs Dash, Blends/Marinades	0
Old Bay, Seasoning (Less Sodium), 1 teaspoon, 2.4g	380
Pepper, Mustard (dry), 1 tsp	1.2
Yeast, Nutritional, 1 Tbsp	10

Breakfast Cereals

	Sodium
Kellogg's:	
All-Bran, Original, ½ cup, 1 oz	80
Special K, Original, 1 cup, 1.1 oz	220
Corn Flakes, 1 cup, 1 oz	200
Frosted Mini Wheats, Blueb./Strawb., (25)	0
Raisin Bran, 1 cup	210
Quaker:	
Corn Bran Crunch, ¾ cup, 1 oz	210
Natural Granola, average, ½ cup, 1 oz	30
Oh's, ¾ cup, 1 oz	170
Puffed Rice/Wheat, 2 cups, 1 oz	1
General Mills, Total, ¾ cup, 1 oz	140
Oatmeal: Regular, ¾ cup	1
Quaker, Instant, ⅔ cup (1 pkt)	260

Breads, Bagels, Crackers

	Sodium
Bread: Thin Slice, average 1 oz	140
Thick Slice, 1.5 oz	210
Low Sodium, 1 oz	10
Bagels: Plain, medium, 2 oz	200
Large, take-out, average, 4 oz	550
Panera Bread, 3.8 oz	460
Biscuits, average, 1 oz	180
Bun/Roll: 1 medium, 1.5 oz	200
Large, 4 oz	560
Crackers: Saltine, 2 crackers	70
Low Salt, 2	25
Graham, 2 regular	50
Croissant, Plain, average, 2 oz	280
Rice Cakes, average	25
Ritz Crackers, Low-Sodium, 1 oz	60
Ry-Krisp, Crispbread, Sesame, 2	90

Cookies, Cakes, Desserts

	Sodium
Cookies: Average, 2-3 cookies, 1 oz	100
Average, 1 cookie, 2.5 oz	180
Baked Custard, ½ cup	100
Brownie, 1.5 oz	130
Carrot Cake, 8 oz	650
Cheesecake, 7 oz	350
Cinnamon Sweet Roll, 2 oz	250
Danish, Apple/Fruit	250
Donut, average	150
Muffins: 1 medium, 2 oz	150
1 extra large, 4 oz	300
Pancakes, (4"), x 3	360
Fruit Pies, average, 7 oz	600
Pudding: Average, ½ cup	160
Jell-O (Mix), Instant, 0.9 oz	350
Waffles: Home-made, 7", 2.5 oz	350
Frozen: Average, 1.2 oz	260
Aunt Jemima, av., 2.5 oz	336

Sodium Counter

Fruit & Juices
	Sodium
Fresh Fruit, average all types, 1 serving	1
Dried/Canned Fruit, ½ cup	1
Fruit Juice: Fresh, sqz'd, 6 fl.oz	1
Commercial, aver., 6 fl.oz	20
Tomato Juice (Campbell's), 6 fl.oz	570
Low Sodium (No Salt Added)	20
V8 Vegetable (Campbell's): 5.5 fl.oz can	290
12 fl.oz bottle	630
Low Sodium, 5.5 fl.oz can	95

Vegetables
Fresh/Frozen (No Salt Added): Per ½ Cup
Asparagus, Bean Sprouts, Corn	3
Beets, Carrots, Celery, ½ cup	40
Broccoli, Cabbage, Cauliflower	10
Cucumber, Green Beans, Mushroom, Okra	3
Onions, Peas, Potato, Pumpkin, Squash	3
Peppers, Hot Chili, raw, each	3
Spinach, Turnips, ½ cup, cooked	40
Tomato, 1 medium, 5 oz	10
Canned: Asparagus, 4 spears	300
Beans, baked in tomato sauce	450
Beets, ½ cup, 3 oz	240
Corn Kernels, ½ cup, 3 oz	190
Creamed, ½ cup, 4.5 oz	330
Mushrooms w. butter sce, 2oz	550
Peas, ½ cup, 3 oz	250
Sauerkraut, ½ cup, 4 oz	750

Pickles, Olives
Olives: pickled: Green, 1 large	90
Ripe/black, 1 large	40
Pickles: Bread & Butter, 4 slices, 1 oz	200
Dill, 1 pickle, 2.5oz	900
Sweet, 1 gherkin, 0.5 oz	130

Soybean Products
Miso (Soy Paste), ¼ c., 2.5 oz	2500
Soybean Protein Isolate, 1 oz	280
Tempeh, Natural, ½ cup, 3 oz	5
Tofu, average, ½ cup, 4 oz	5

Jam, Honey, Syrups
Jam/Jelly, 1 Tbsp	2
Honey/Maple Syrup, 1 Tbsp	1
Log Cabin, Syrup, 1 fl.oz	35
Lite, 1 fl.oz	90

Peanut Butter
Peanut Butter: Regular, 2 Tbsp, 0.5 oz	190
Jif, Low Sodium, 2 Tbsp	65
Trader Joe's, Unsalted, 2 Tbsp	5

Snacks, Nuts
	Sodium
Cheese Balls/Curls, 1 oz	280
Cheetos, 1 oz	290
Corn/Tortilla Chips: average, 1 oz	220
Fritos, Lightly Salted, 1 oz	80
Granola bars, average, 1 bar	80
Nuts: Plain, unsalted, 1 oz	1
Lightly salted, 1 oz	80
Salted or Honey Roasted, 1 oz	160
Popcorn: Plain (unsalted), 1 cup	1
Flavored, average, 1 cup	60
Salt added, 1 cup	180
Potato Chips: Plain, 1 oz	160
Lay's, Lightly Salted, 1 oz	90
Flavored, average, 1 oz	250
Pretzels: Regular, 3, 1 oz	450
Soft, salted, large	1000

Candy, Chocolate
Chocolate, milk, 1 oz	30
Fudge, chocolate, 1 oz	55
Candy Bars, average, 1.5 oz	60
Hard Candy, 1 oz	10
Licorice, 1 oz	30

Beverages, Alcohol
Coffee or Tea, 1 cup	1
Cocoa: Dry, plain, 1 Tbsp	0
Mix, average, 1 envelope	120
Quik, 2 tsp	35
Soft Drinks, average, 8 fl.oz	20
Mineral Water: Perrier, 8 fl.oz	5
Gatorade, Thirst Quencher, 8 fl.oz	110
Red Bull, 8½ fl.oz can	200
Water, Average, 1 cup, 8 fl.oz	5
Alcohol: Beer, average, 12 fl.oz	15
Wines, average, 4 fl.oz	10
Spirits (distilled), 1.5 fl.oz	1

Antacids ~ Alka-Seltzer
Alka-Seltzer: Per Tablet
	Sodium
Original; Heartburn	570
Extra Strength	590
Lemon Lime	500
Gold	310
Alka-Mints, chewable	0
Bromo Seltzer, ¾ capful	760
Picot, 1 packet, 5g	670
Rolaids, All types	0
Tums, Regular/Extra Strength	0

Cold & Flu ~ Alka-Seltzer Plus
Effervescents, average, 1 tablet	480
Fast Crystal Packs; Liquid Gels	0

Fast-Foods & Restaurants | Sodium

Burger King:
Burgers: Cheeseburger — 690
Double Bacon Cheeseburger — 940
Hamburger — 460
Whoppers: Original — 980
  With Cheese — 1380
  Whopper Jr. with Cheese — 730
Chicken Sandwich, Original — 1390
Sides: French Fries, medium, salted — 570
  Onion Rings, medium — 1080
Breakfast, Ham, Egg & Cheese Croissan'wich — 1030

Denny's:
Burgers: Bacon Avocado Cheeseburger — 1830
  Macho Nacho Burger — 1980
Sandwiches: Club — 1850
  Prime Rib Philly Melt — 2000
Dinner: Brooklyn Spaghetti & Meatballs — 2460
  Sirloin Steak with bread — 1590
  Sides: Broccoli — 20
    French Fries, salted, 6 oz — 110
    Red-Skinned Potatoes — 627
Soup: Chicken Noodle, 12 oz bowl — 1130
  Clam Chowder, 12 oz bowl — 1870
Breakfast: Buttermilk Pancakes (2) — 1170
  Moons Over My Hammy Omelette, w/ Hash — 2530
  Hearty Breakfast Skillet — 2130
  Sides: Hash Browns, 1 serving — 650
    Hearty Breakfast Sausage — 830
Desserts: Apple Pie, 7 oz — 580
  Hot Fudge Brownie al a Mode, 9 oz — 520

Jack In The Box:
Burgers: Bacon Untimate Cheeseburger — 2190
  Hamburger — 680
  Jumbo Jack with Cheese — 1310
  Sandwiches: Homestyle Ranch Chicken Club — 2010
    Sourdough Grilled Chiken Club — 1490

KFC:
Chicken Breast: Original — 1130
  Extra Crispy — 1140
  Grilled — 730
Popcorn Chicken,
  Value Box — 2160
Sandwich, Crispy Twister — 1260
Strips, Extra Crispy Tenders, 3 pieces — 940
Sides: Macaroni & Cheese — 830
  Mashed Potatoes with Gravy — 530
  Potato Wedges — 810
Wings, HBBQ Hot (1) — 160

Fast-Foods & Restaurants | Sodium

McDonalds:
Burgers: Big Mac — 970
  Cheeseburger — 680
  Double — 1050
  Hamburger — 480
  Quarter Pounder with Cheese — 1100
Chicken McNuggets: 6 pieces — 540
  Chipotle BBQ Sauce, 1 package, 1 oz — 190
Sandwich, Prem. Grilled Chicken Ranch BLT — 1210
French Fries: Small, 2.5 oz — 160
  Medium, 4 oz — 270
  Large, 5.4 oz — 350
  Ketchup, 1 package, 10g — 100
Breakfast: Egg McMuffin — 780
  Big Breakfast, reg. size Biscuit — 1560
  Hash Browns, 2 oz — 310
  Hotcakes, with Syrup & Whipped Margarine — 665
  Sausage Burrito — 790
  Southern Style Chicken Biscuit, regular bisc. — 1180
Desserts/Shakes: Hot Fudge Sundae — 170
  Strawberry McCafe Shake, 12 fl.oz — 240

Pizza Hut:
Pan Pizza: 12", Per ½ Pizza, 4 Slices
  Meat Lovers — 3280
  Cheese; Chicken Supreme; average — 2110
  Pepperoni; Supreme, average — 2560
  Pepperoni Lover's: Super Supreme, av. — 3120

Subway:
6" Lowfat Sandwich: W/ Set Menu Board Toppings, no oil
  Chicken, oven roasted — 610
  Roast Beef — 660
  Subway Club — 850
  Sweet Onion Chicken Teriyaki — 840
6" Sandwiches: With Set Menu Board Toppings, no Oil
  BLT; Tuna, average — 625
  Meatball Marinara — 920
  Spicy Italian — 1490
12" Footlong ~ Double above figures

Taco Bell:
Burritos: Combo, 8.2 oz — 1380
  Supreme, Chicken; Steak, average — 1065
Chapulas: Chicken; Steak, average — 515
Gorditas, Cheesy Crunch — 830
Nachos: Regular — 420
  BellGrande — 1270
Specialties: Cheese Quesadillas — 990
Tacos: Chicken, Soft — 480
  Crunchy Supreme — 340

A-1 Steak Sauce 144
A&W Cream Soda 51
Agave Nectar 157
Ahi Tuna 95
Albertson's Sodas 51
Alcoholic Drinks 24
Alcohol Guide 23
Al-Bran Bkfast Cereal 60
Alligator 168
Almond Breeze 49
Almond Butter 131
Almond Dream 49
Almond Joy 68
Almond Paste 30
Almonds 130
Aloe Vera Juice 156
Alouette Cheese 76
Alpina: Oat Smoothies 49
   Greek ogurt 162
Alta Dena Yogurt 162
Amaranth Flour 98
Amazake 49
AMP Energy Drink 38
Anchovies 95
Ant Eggs/Larvae 174
Antacids 156
Apple Danish 62
   Dunkin Donuts 197
Apple Fritter,
   Dunkin Donuts 197
Apple Pie 134
Apple Sauce 80, 102
Applebee's 176
Apples 99
Apricots 99
Arbor Mist Blenders 26
Arbor Mist Wine 26
Arby's 177
Arizona Teas 53
Arroz Con Pollo 174
Asian Foods 168
   Panda Express 222-223
   Pei Wei 225
Asparagus 158
Atkins Bars 31
Au Bon Pain 178-179
Aunt Jemima:
   Pancakes 132
   Waffles 132
Austin S'wich Crackers 151
Avocado 99

Baba Ghannouj 172
Baba Ghanoush 79
Baby Ruth 68
Babybel 76
Bacardi & Coke 28
Bacardi Silver 27
Bacon 126
Bacon Bits 126
Bagels:
   Chips 56
   Dogs 128
   S'wiches:
      Dunkin Donuts 198
   Spreads 56
Big Apple Bagels 182
Bruegger's Bagels 185
   Manhattan Bagel 215
Baileys Irish Cream 29
Baking Ingredients 30
Baking Mix 30
Baking Powder 30
Baklava 62

Balance Bars 31
Ball Park Franks 127
Balsamic Vinaigrette 142
Banana 99
Banana Chips 102
Banana Flakes 102
Banquet Meals 111
Barbecue Sauce 80
Bariatrix: Shakes 38
   Proti-Bar 34
Barley 98
Bars: Granola 31-34
   Meal/Nutrition 31-34
   Sports & Diet 31-34
Bartles & Jaymes 27
Baskin-Robbins 181
Beans 158
Bear Claw 62
Beaver Tails 169
Bee Maggots 174

Beef 124
   Beef Ribs 124
   Franks 127
   Ground Beef 124
   Jerky 128
   Roast Beef 124
   Tallow 94
Beer: Alcoholic 24-25
   Non-Alcoholic 25
Beerwurst 128
Beiglach 171
Ben & Jerry's:
   Ice Cream 104
   Ice Cream Bars 108
Benecol Spread 93
Bernstein's Dressings 142
Best Foods Dressings 142
Betty Crocker::
   Cake Mixes 65
   Muffin Mixes 67
Biggest Loser:
   Entrees 112
   Shakes 38
Big Mac 216
Birds Eye Frozen Veg. 160

FAST-FOODS INDEX
~ PAGE 175 ~

Biscotti 81
Biscuits Packaged 55
Burger King 186
Hardee's 204
Jack in the Box 207
McDonald's 216
Bison Steak 126
Blintzes 171
Bloody Mary 28
Bloomin' Onion 222
BLT Sandwich 165
Blue Bunny: Novelties 108
   Ice Cream 104
Blue Cheese Dressing 142
Blue Sky Sodas 51
Bob Evans 183
Boca Burgers 112
Bok Choy 158
Bologna 128
Bolthouse Juice 41
Boost Drinks 38

Borscht Soup 152
Boston Market 184
Boston's Pizza 184-185
Brach's Candy 68
Brain 126
Bran 57
Brandy 27-29
Bratwurst 128
Braunschweiger 128
Brazil Nuts 130
Bread 54
Bread Crumbs 55
Bread: Buns/Rolls 55
Breadsticks 55
Breakfast Cereals 57-61
Breakfast Meals,
   Denny's 194
Breakfast Sausages 127
Brewer's Yeast 156
Breyers: Ice Cream 104
   Ice Cream Bars 108
Brioche Cake 168
Broccoli 158
Brownies 62-65
Brownie Mixes 65
Bruegger's 185
Bruschetta 170
Brussels Sprouts 158
Bubble Tea 168
Bubble Yum 75
Buckwheat: 98
   Groats 57
Budweiser Beer 24
Buffalo Wings,
   Domino's 196
Buitoni Pasta 133
Bulgur: Grain 57, 98
   Salad 141
Bumble Bee Tuna 95
Burger King 186
Burritos: Qdoba 230
   Taco Bell 247
   Taco John's 249
   Taco Mayo 249
   Taco Time 249
Butter & Margarine 93
Butter Balls, deep fried 166

Butter Substitutes: 93
   Butter Buds 93
   Molly McButter 93
Butterfinger 69
Buttermilk 47
Butterscotch 69
Butter Tart 69
Cabbage 158
Cabbage Rolls 171
Cactus Fruit 99
Cactus Leaf 158
Caesar Dressing 142
Cadbury Candy 69
Cafeteria Foods 165
Cajun Foods 168
Cake Frosting/Mixes 65
Cakes 62
Calamari: Fried 95, 169
   Macaroni Grill 214
Calcium Chews 156
California Pizza Kitchen 136
Calorie Countdown 47
Camembert 76
Canada Dry Sodas 51
Canadian Bacon 126
Canadian Foods 168
Candied Apple 167
Candied Fruit 102
Candy 68-74
Cannelloni 170
Cannoli 62
Cantaloupe 99
Cappuccino 36
Capri Sun 42
Caramello 69
Caramels 69
Carb Smart: Ice Cream 104
   Ice Cream Bars 108
Cardini's Dressings 142
Caribou 126
Carob 75
Carrots 158
Cashews 130
Caterpillars 174
Catfish 95
Caviar 95
Cereal Drinks 49
Challah Bread 54
Champagne 26
Chapati 54
Cheerios Cereal 59
Cheese 76-79
   Balls 76, 150
   Cheese Whiz 76

Cheese Fries,
Nathan's Famous 219
Cheese Puffs 150
Cheeseburgers::
Burger King 186
Hardee's 204
Jack in the Box 207
McDonald's 216
Cheesecake 62
Cheesecake Factory 188
Cheetos 150
Cheez-It Crackers 150
Chef Boyardee 113
Chef's Salad 141
Cherries 99
Chestnuts 130
Chex Breakfast Cereal 59
Chex Mix 150
Chia Seeds 131
Chi Chi's 29
Chick Peas 158
Chicken Alfredo 170
Chicken 138
Chik-fil-A 189
Church's Chicken 190
KFC 210
S'wich, McDonald's 216
Chicken Buffalo Wings:,
KFC 210
Chicken Helper 112
Chicken Katsu 169
Chicken Korma 170
Chicken Kung Pao:
P.F. Chang's 226
Panda Express 223
Chicken McNuggets 216
Chicken of the Sea 97
Chicken Strips:
KFC 210
McDonald's 216
Chili Sauce 80
Chili: Con Carne 113
Gold Star Chili 202
Stagg Meals 120
Trader Joe's Meals 121

Chili's 189
Chimichangas 172
Chinese Food 168
P.F. Chang's 226
Chipotle 190
Chips Ahoy! 85
Snacks 150
Chocolate Candy 68-74
Chocolate Baking Chips 30
Chocolate Chip Cookies 81
Chocolate Milk 48
Chocolate Cake 62
Chocolate Éclair 62
Cholent 171
Chopped Liver 171
Chorizo 127
Churros 62
Ciabatta 54
Cider, Alcoholic 26
Cinnabon 67
Cinnamon Rolls 62
T.J.Cinnamons 252
Claim Jumper 191
Clam Chowder 152
Long John Silver's 213
Clamato Juice 42
Clams 95
Clif Bars 31
Coca-Cola 51
Coca-Cola Zero 51
Cocktail Mixers 27
Cocktails 28
Premixed 27
Cocoa 35
Cocoa Powder 30
Coconut: Desiccated 130
Fresh 99, 130
Drink 50
Milk 89
Water 89
Zico 40

Coffee: 35-37
Biggby Coffee 182
Caribou Coffee 187
Creamers 89
Espresso 36
Flavored Mixes 35
Instant 35
Iced 35,
McCafe 217
Ready To Drink, Cold 37
Starbucks 37, 243
Coffee-Mate 89
Cola Drinks 51-52
Coldstone Creamery 191
Coleslaw Dressing 142
Combos 150
Concha 62
Condensed Milk 47
Condiments/Sauces 80
Cookie Dough,
Toll House 88
Cookies 81-88
Cooking Sprays Pam 94
Cool Whip 89
Coors Beer 24
Coq au Vin 168
Corn 158
Corn Chips 149
Corn Dog 128
Corn Flakes 58
Corn Grits 98
Corned Beef 128
Cornmeal 98
Cornstarch 98
Cosmopolitan 28
Cottage Cheese 76
Cough/Cold Syrups 156
Cough Drops 75
Country Choice Cookies 82
Cous Cous 98, 172
Crab 95
Crab Cakes 95
Cracker Jack 148
Crackers 81-88

Cranberries: Dried 102
Fresh 99
Cranberry Sauce 80-102
Crawfish 168
Cream 89
Cream Cheese 79, 84
Cream of Wheat 57
Creamers, Bailey's 89
Creamsicle 108
Creole Foods 168
Crepe Suzette 169
Crispbreads 88
Croissant-Donuts 66
Croissants: Plain 134
Sandwiches 165
Dunkin Donuts 198
Sweet 134
Cronuts 66
Croutons 55
Crunch 'N Munch 148
Crystal Light 52
Cup-a-Soup 154
Cupcakes 62
Curves, Protein Drinks 38
Custard, Frozen 103
Custard 90
Daiquiri 28
Dairy Ease 47
Dairy Queen 193
Danish Pastry 62
Dates 99
Deer 126
Del Taco 194
Deli Meats 128
Denny's 194-195
Desserts/Puddings 90
Dibs 110
Diet Drinks/Shakes 38
Diet Sodas 51-52
DiGiorno Pizzas 136
Dill Pickle 80
Dippin' Dots 105, 195
Dips/Spreads 79

Dolmades 169
Domino's Pizza 196
Donnairs 168
Donuts 66
Tim Horton's 252
Winchell's 257
dot.FIT:
Bars 31
FirstString 274
Dove: Candy 69
Ice Cream 105
Ice Cream Bars 108
Dr Pepper Sodas 51
Dried Fruit 102
Dried (Powdered) Milk 47
Drippings 94
Duck 139
Dumplings 168
P.F. Chang's 226
Duncan Hines,
Cake Mixes 65
Dunkin' Donuts 197
Ears, Pork 126
EAS Bars 31
Edamame 158, 171
Eel 95
Eggplant 159
Egg Roll Wrappers 133
Egg Rolls 92
Eggs: Egg Whites 91
Better'n Eggs 91
Egg Beaters 91
Egg Nog 91
Eggs Benedict 91
Eggo: French Toast 132
Pancakes 132
Empanadas 173
Enchilada 172
Endive 159
Energy Drinks 38-40

English Muffins	56
Ensure Drinks	38
Entenmann's: Cakes	63
Cinnamon Bun	63
Equal	157
Espresso Coffee	36
Starbucks	243
Evaporated Milk	47
Extra Gum	75
Fair/Carnival	166-167
Fajitas	172
Chili's	189
Falafel	166
Famous Amos	82
Fanta	51
Feet, Pork	126
Feta Cheese	77
Fettuccine Alfredo	170
Fiber One: Bars	31
Cereal	59
Muffin Mix	67
Fibersure	156
Fiddle Faddle	148
5th Avenue	70
Fig Bars	62
Figs	100
Filet Mignon Steak	123
Fish	95
Fish & Chips	95
Fish Oil	94
Capsules	156
Flame Broiler	201
Flaxseeds	131
Fleischmann's Spread	93
Flours	98
Fortune Cookie	168
Franks	127
Frappuccino,	
Starbucks	243
French Fries	168-169
Burger King	186
McDonald's	216
Fr./Italian Dressing	142
French Stick	54
French's Fried Onions	161
Fresca	51
Freschetta Pizzas	136
Freshens	201
Fried Dough	167
Fried Oreos	167

Fried Rice,	
Panda Express	223
Fried Twinkie	167
Frissants	66
Fruit Snacks	151
Fruit Spreads	157
Frog Legs	168
Froot Loops	60
Frosting, cake	65
Frozen Custard	103
Frozen Vegetables:	
Birds Eye	160
Green Giant	161
Ore-Ida	161
Frozen Yogurt	103
FrozFruit	108
FRS Energy Drink	38
Fruit Juices	41-46
Fruit Leather	102
Fruit Pies	134
Fruit Sauces	102
Fruit Smoothies	48
Orange Julius	221
Fruit Snack Cups	102
Fruit: Fresh	99-101
Candied	102
Canned/Bottled	102
Dried	102
Fruit Leather	101
Sauces	102
FryBread	167
Fudge	70
Fudgesicle	109
Full Throttle Energy	38
Funnel Cake	167
Fuze: Energy Drinks	38
Iced Teas	53
GardenBurger	114
Garlic	159
Garlic Bread	54
Gazpacho Soup	152
Gatorade	38
Gefilte Fish Balls	171
Gelati-da	105
Gelatin: Parfait	90
Snacks	90
Gelato	103
GeniSoy	32
Genisoy Powder Shakes	38
German Foods	169
Ghee	93

Ghirardelli	70
Gin	27
Ginger	159
Glaceau Drinks	38
Glowelle	156
Gluhwein	26
GNC: Bar	32
Protein Drinks	39
Gnu Foods	32
Goat Meat	126
Goat's Milk	47
Goat's Milk Cheese	77
Goldfish	150
Goldvia Candy	70
Goober P'nut Butter	131
Good Humor	109
Goose	139
Gorditas, Taco Bell	247
Graham Crackers	81
Grains	98
Grandma's Cookies	82
Granola	58
Granola Bars	31-34
Grapefruit	100
Grapes	100
Gravy	144
Great Value: Bars	32
Meals	114
Greek Foods,	
Daphne's Café	193
Ground Pork	126
Guacamole	172
Guava	100
Gum	75
Gum Drops	70
Gummi Bears	70
Gyros	169
Haagen-Dazs:	
Ice Cream	105, 204
Ice Cream Bars	109
Haggis	174
Half & Half	89
Halls Drops	75
Ham:Roasted/ Sliced	128
Ham Steak	126
Lunch/Deli	128

Hamburger:	
Carnival/Fair	166
Jack in the Box	207
McDonald's	216
Hamburger Helper	112
Hansen's:	
Energy Drinks	39
Iced Teas	53
Juices	42
Sodas	51
Hardee's	204
Hash Browns:	92
Burger King	186
McDonald's	217
Hawaiian Foods	169
Healthy Choice: Meals	114
Heart	126
Hebrew National Links	127
Heineken Beer	24
Herring	96
Hershey's: Candy/Choc.	70
Chocolate Mix	35
Hidden Valley Dressings	142
Hissho Sushi	205
Hoagies, Davanni's	193
Honey	157
Honeycomb	71
Honeydew	100
Horchata	172
Horseradish	80
Hostess: Cup Cakes	63
Ding Dongs	63
Donettes, Mini	66
Fruit Pies	134
Twinkies	63
Hot & Sour Soup	155
Hot Chocolate	35
Hot Dogs/Franks:	128
Carnival	166
WAWA	255
Wienerschnitzel	257

Hot Dog On A Stick	205
Hot Dog Toppings	128
Hot Pockets	115
Hummus	79, 172
Hunt's Snack Pack	90
Hushpuppy,	
Long John Silver	214
Ice Cream	103-107
Ice Cream Novelties	108-110
Butterfinger	108
Drumstick	109
Klondike	109
Oreo	109
Slim-a-Bear	109
Ice Cream: Carvel	188
Dippin' Dots	195
Starbucks	107
Ice Cream Toppings	157
Iced Tea	53
Mixes	53
Icee Drinks	51
IHOP	206
Indian Foods	170
Italian Dressing	142
Italian Foods:	170
Fazoli's	200
Macaroni Grill	214
Italian Sausage	128
Jack In The Box	207
Jam	157
Jamba Juice	208
Jambalaya	168
Japanese Foods:	171
Edo Japan	199
Yoshinoya	258
Java Monster Energy	39
Jellies	71
Jell-O: Gel Snacks	90
Gelatin Mixes	90
No Bake Cheesecake	65
Puddings	90
Jelly Beans	71
Jif Peanut Butter	131
Jolly Rancher	71
Junior Mints	71

FAST-FOODS INDEX
~ PAGE 175 ~

Kahlua 29
Kahlua Mudslide 28
Kaiser Roll 55
Kalua Chicken 169
Kashi: Bars 32
   Cereal 59
   Cookies/Crackers 83
Keebler: Cookies 83
   Crackers 83
Kefir Milk 47
Kellogg's:
   Bars 32
   Breakfast Cereals 60
   To Go B'Fast Shakes 39
KFC 210
Kid Cuisine 115
Kidneys 126
Kielbasa 121, 128
Kimchee 172
Kind Bars 32
Kisses 71
Kit Kat 71
Kiwifruit 100
Knish 171
Kombucha Drink 39
Kool-Aid 52
Korean Foods 172
Kosher Deli Foods 171
Kozy Shack 90
Kraft: Cheese 76-78
   Dressings 143
   Mayonnaise 94
   Meals 116
Krispy Kreme Donuts 66
Kudos Bars 32

Lactaid 100 47
Lactose-Free Drinks 47
Lamb 125
Lamb Pilaf 169
Land O'Lakes Spread 93
Lard 94
Lasagna: Villa Pizza 254
   Chicken, Fazoli's 200
Latkes, Potato Patty 171
Lau Lau 169
Lean Cuisine: 116-117
   Pizza 137
Lean Pockets 117
Lebanese Foods 172
Lecithin Granules 57
Lemons 100
Lemon Cake 62
Lemon Crème 134
Lettuce 159

Lettuce Wraps:
   P.F.Chang's 226
   Pei Wei 224
Licorice 71
Life Breakfast Cereal 61
Lifesavers 71
Lighter Bake 93
Limes 100
Lindora Bars 32
Lindt 72
Linguine 133
Lipton: Brisk 53
   Green/Iced Tea 53
Liqueur, Coffee 29
Liqueurs 29
Liquor 29
Little Caesar 213
Little Debbie: Cakes 63
   Cookies 84
   Donut Stick 66
   Honey Buns 67

Liver: 126
   Liver Pate 128
   Liver, Chopped 171
Liverwurst 128
Lobster 96
Lochshen 171
Locusts 174
Lollipops 72
Lox 96
Luna Bar 32
Lunchables 117
Lunchmakers 117

M & M's 72
Macadamia Nuts 130
Macaroni & Cheese 133
Macaroni Salad 141
Mamey Apple 100
Manapua 169
Mandarin 100
Mandelbrot 171
Mango 100
Manhattan Clam Chowder,
   Campbell's 153
Manischewitz 84
Marathon Bars 32
Marble Cake 62
Margarita 27

Marie Callender's,
   Dinners 117
Marie's Dressings 143
Marsala 117
Marshmallows 72
Maruchan Noodles 117
Masa 172
Matzos: 88
   Balls 171
   Ball Soup 152
Mayonnaise 94
Mazola Spray 94
McDonald's: McCafe 217
   McMuffin 217
Meals:
   Amy's 111
   Betty Crocker 112
   Gorton's 114
   Hungry Man 115
   Thai Kitchen Meals 121
   Trader Joe's 121
   Worthington 122

FAST-FOODS INDEX
~ PAGE 175 ~

Meat Snacks 128
Meat Spreads 129
Meats 123-126
Melons 100-101
Mentos 72
Meringues 90
Met-Rx: Bars 33
   Energy Drinks/Shakes 39
Metamucil 156
Mexican:
   Carnival 166
   Cheese 76
Mexican Foods 172
Michelob Beer 25
Middle Eastern Foods 172
Mike's Hard Lemonade 27
Milk: Canned 47
   Dried 47
   Flavored 48
   Plain 47
Milky Way 72
Miller Beer 25
Millet 98
Minestrone Soup 152
Mint Julep 28
Mints 72

Minute Maid: Juices 43
   Lemonade; Punch 43
Minute Rice 118
Miracle Whip 94
Miso Soup 171
Mojo Bar, Clif 32
Molasses 157
Morningstar Farms 118
Mounds 71
Mountain Dew 52
Moussaka 169
Mozzarella Cheese 77
Mr Goodbar 72
MRM Protein Drinks 39
Mrs Dash Seasonings 146
Mrs Fields Cookies 219
Mud Cake 62
Muffin Mixes 67
Muffins 67
Dunkin Donuts 197
Mulled Wine 26

Munchies 150
Muscle Milk: Powders 39
   Ready To Drink 39
Mushrooms 159
Mussels 96

Naan Bread 55
Nachos: 166, 172
   Chili's 189
   Qdoba 230
   Taco Bell 247
Naked Juice 43
Nanaimo Bar 169
Nathan's Famous 219
Nature's Path Bars 33
Nayonaise 94
Nectarines 100
Nesquik 35, 48
Nestea, Iced Tea 53
Nestle Crunch: Bar 72
   Ice Creams Bars 110
New England,
   Clam Chowder,Blimpie 182
Newman's Own:
   Cookies 86
   Dressings 143

Juice 44
Newtons Cookies 85
Nissin Noodles 118
No Fear Energy 39
Noni Juice 39
Noodles 133
   Pei Wei 224
Noodles & Company 220
Nopal Cactus Salad 172
Nopales 159
NOS Energy 39
Nothing But Noodles 220
Nut Spreads 131
Nutella 131
Nutri-Grain Bars 33
Nutrilite: Bars 33
   Protein Drinks 39
NutriSystem: Bars 33
   Breakfast Cereals 61
Nuts 130

Oat Bran 57
Oatmeal 57
Oatmeal Raisin Cookies 81
Oats 98
Ocean Spray, Juice 44
Odwalla Bars 33
Oils: Fish 94
   Vegetable 94
Okra 159
Old El Paso:
   Dinner Kits 118
   Dip 79
   Refried Beans 118
   Salsa 79
Olive Garden 221
Olive Loaf 128
Olives 100
Omelets: 91
   Ham & Cheese 92
   Western 92
   Bob Evans 183
Onion Flower 166
Onions 159
Onion Rings:
   Burger King 186
   Dairy Queen 193
   Jack in the Box 207
   Zaxby's 258
Optifast: Bars 33
   Shakes 40
Orange Juice 41
Orange Julius 221
Oranges 100

Orangina 44
Oreo: Cakesters 64
  Cookies 85
  Snacks 150
Ostrich 126
Outback Steakhouse 222
Ovaltine 35
Oyster & Soup Crackers 81
Oysters 96
Pad Thai 174
Paella 174
Palmier Cookie 62
Pancakes 132
  IHOP 206
Pancreas 126
Panda Express 223
Panera Bread 223
Paninis:
  Hot Pockets 115
  Lean Cuisine 116
Papaya 100
Pappadum 170
Parfait 90
Parkay Spread 93
Parmesan Cheese 78
Parsnip 159
Passionfruit 100
Pasta: Fresh 133
  Macaroni Grill 214
  Pizza Hut 227
Pasta Roni 118
Pasta Sauces 144-147
Pastrami 129
Pastries 62-64
Pastry Crust 134
Pate 134
PayDay Bar 72
Peach Melba 62
Peaches 100
Peanut Butter Cookie 81
Peanut Butter Cups:
  Newman's Own 72
  Reese's 73
Peanut Butter
  & Jelly S/wich 131
Peanuts 130
Pears 100
Peas 159
Pecan Pie 134
Pecans 130
Pepperidge Farm: Cakes 64
  Cookies 86
Peppermints 73
Peppers 159
Pepsi 52
Persimmons 100

Pez 73
Philadelphia Cheese 78
Pickles & Relish 80
Pie Crust 134
Pie Fillings 30, 134
Pies 134
Pilaf 140
Piloncillo Sugar Cone 157
Pina Colada 28
Pine Nuts 130
Pineapple 101
Pinkberry 106
Pirate's Booty 150
Pistachios 130
Pizza Hut 227
Pizzas: Frozen 136, 137
  Ready-To-Eat 135
Planters, Peanuts 130
Plums 101
Poi 169
Poke Salad 173
Polenta 98
Polish Foods 173
Pom Wonderful: Juices 44
  Pomegranate Teas 53
Pomegranate 101
Popcorn: Plain 148
  Caramel 148
  Orv. Redenbacher's 148
Popcorners 148
Popcorn Chicken: KFC 210
  Sonic Drive-In 241
Popchips 149
Pop Tarts, Kellogg's 64
Pops, Ice Cream 108-110
Pork: Meat 125
  Cracklings 173
  Rinds/Skins 150
  Sausages 127
  Spareribs 125
Port Wine 26
Porterhouse Steak 123
Post Cereals 61
Potato Salad 141
Potatoes: 159
  Carnival 166
  French Fries 166
Poutine, Canadian 168
PowerAde ION4 40
PowerBar: Bars 33
  Shakes 40
Pretzelmaker 229
Pretzels: Flipz 149
  Rold Gold 149
Prickly Pear 101
Probiotics 164

Progresso Soup 154
Promise Spread 93
Proscuitto 129
Protein Drinks/Shakes 38
Prunes 101
Psyllium Husks 57, 98
Puddings 90
Pumpkin Pie 134
Pumpkin Seeds 131
Pumpkin 160
Qdoba 230
Quail 139
Quaker: Bars 34
  Breakfast Cereals 57, 61
Quakes Rice Snacks 151
Quarter Pounder 175
Quesadilla 166, 172
  Qdoba 230
Quiche 91
Quinoa 98
Rabbit 126
Radish 160
Raisin Bran 58
Raisin Bread 54
Raisinets 73
Raisins 101
Rambutan 101
Ranch Dressing 142
Raspberries 101
Ravioli 112-119
  Fazoli's 200
Red Bull & Vodka 28
Red Bull Energy 40
Reddi-Wip 89
Red Mango,
  Frozen Yogurt 106
Reese's 73
Refried Beans 112, 118-120
Relishes 80
Reuben Sandwich 165
Revival Soy Shakes 50
Rice: 140
  Bran 57, 98
  Cakes 56
  Crackers 81
  Drinks 49
  Snacks 151
Rice Dream 49
Rice Krispies 58
Rice Noodles 133
Rice, Sticky Thai 169
Rice-A-Roni 119
Ricola 75
Ricotta Cheese 78

Ritz Crackers 86
Rockstar Energy 40
Rogan Josh 170
Rolo 73
Root Beer 51
Rugulah 62
Rum 27-28
Russell Stover Candy 73
Rye Bread 54
Rye Flour 57
Sabritones Snacks 151
Sake 26
Salad Dressings 142
Salad Toppings:
  Bacon Bits 141
Salads: Deli 141
  Packaged 141
Salami 129
Salmon 96
Salsa 79, 80
Saltines 81
Sandwiches: Cosi 191
  D'Angelo's 192
  Denny's 194
  Einstein Bros 199
  Mr. Hero 218
  Schlotzsky's 237
  Subway 245
Sara Lee: Bagels 134
  Croissants 134
  Frozen Cakes 64
  Pies 134
Sardines 97
Sashimi 171
Sausages 127
Sauces: 144
  Prego Pasta Sauces 144
  Ragu 147
  Worcestershire 145
Sarku Japan 237
Scallops 97
Scone, Fruit 62
Scotch 27
Screwdriver 28
Seagram's Coolers 27
Seaweed 156
See's Candies 73
Seeds 131
Semolina 98
Sesame Butter 131
Sesame Seeds 131
7-Eleven 236
7-UP Soda 52
Shakes 48
Shasta Sodas 52

Shaved Ice 103
Shellfish 95-97
Shawourma 172
Sherry 26
Shooters 28
Shish Taouk 168
Shrimp 97
Silk: Creamer 89
Soy Drinks 50
Simply Asia Meals 119
Sirloin Steak 123
Sizzler 240
Skippy Peanut Butter 131
Skittles 73
Skyline Chili 240
Slim-Fast: Bars 34
  Shakes 40
Slurpees, 7-Eleven 236
Smart Balance Spread 93
Smarties 73
Smirnoff Ice 27
Smoked Sausage 127
Smoothies: 41
  Freshens 201
  Jamba Juice 208
  Smoothie King 241
  Tropical Smoothie 253
Smucker's Goober 131
Snacks 148-151
Snow Cone 167
Snackwell's Cookies 85
Snails 169
Snake 174
Snapple 45, 53
Snickers 74
So Delicious: Yogurt 163
  Coconut Milk 50
SoBe: Energy Drinks 40
  Green Tea 53
Soft Drink Mixes 52
Soft Drinks/Soda 51-52
Sonic Drive-In 240-241
Sopapillas Pastry Puffs 173
Soul Foods 173
Soup: 152-155
  Campbell's 152-153
  Progresso 154
Sour Cream 89
Sourdough Bread 54

Southern Comfort 27
Souvlaki 169
Soy Dream: Drinks 50
  Ice Cream 107
Soy Flour 98
Soy Milk/Drinks 49
Soy Nuts 130, 151
Soy Powder Mix 50
Soybeans 160
Spaghetti:
  & Meat Sauce 117-119
  & Meatballs 111, 113
  Cooked 133
  Dry/Fresh 133
  Old Spagh. Factory 221
Spam: Canned 129
  Musubi 169
Spanish Foods 174
Spareribs 174
  P.F. Chang's 226
Sparks 27
Special K: Bars 34
  Cereals 60
Spreads 79
Spices & Herbs 147
Spinach 160
Spirulina 156
Splenda 157
Spring Roll: Chinese 168
  Panda Express 222
  Pei Wei Asian Diner 224
Sprite 52
Squash 160
Squaw Bread 54
Squid 97
Stadium Foods 174
Stagg Chili Meals 120
Starbucks: Coffee 243
  Bottled Coffee 37
  Cakes/ Bakery 244
  VIA Mix 35
Starburst 74
Starkist 97
Steak Subs Mr. Hero 218
Steaks 123
  Chili's 189
  Lone Star 213
  Outback Steakhouse 222
  Ruby Tuesday 234
Steaz: Energy Drink 40
  Green Teas 53
Stella D'Oro Cookies 87
Stevia 157
Stouffer's 120

Strawberries 101
String Cheese 77
Stromboli:
  Stouffers 120
  Villa Fresh Italian 254
Stonyfield Farm Yogurt 163
Strudel 62
Stuffing Mix 55
Subway 245-246
Succotash 160
Sugar 157
Sugar Substitutes 157
Sukiyaki 171
Sundaes 103
  McCafe 217
Sunflower Seeds 131
Sunkist: Sodas 52
SunnyD 45
Sunsweet: Lighter Bake 93
  Prune Juice 44
Supplements 156
Surimi 97
Sushi 171
Southern Tsunami 242
Swanson Pot Pies 120
Sweet 'N Low 157
Sweet Buns/Rolls 67
Sweetbreads 126
Sweet Potatoes 160
Swiss Miss: Drinks 35
  Pudding Snacks 90
Swordfish 97
Syrups 157

TAB Soda 52
Tabouli 141
Tacos 172
  Qdoba 230
  Taco Bell 247
Taco Salad Qdoba 230
Taco Shell 56, 172
Tahini 131
Tahini Sauce 172
Take 5 74
Tamales 172
Tamarillo 101
Tamarind 101
Tandoori Chicken 170
Tang 52

Tangelo 101
Tangerine 101
Tapioca 90
Taramosalata 169
Tartar Sauce 80
Tassot, Beef/Goat 168
Tasti D-Lite 107
TCBY 250
Tea 53
Tempura 171
Teppan Yaki 171
Tequila 27
Tequila Sunrise 28
Teriyaki: Beef 171
  Chicken 171
  Salmon 171
TGI FRiday 250-251
  Frozen Meals 120
Thai Foods 174
Thai Kitchen Meals 121
Thousand Is. Dressing 142
3 Musketeers 68
Tia Maria 29
Tilt Energy 27
Tim Hortons 252
Tiramisu 62
Toblerone 74
Tofu Fresh/Packaged 156
Tofurky Meals 121
Tofutti 107
Tofutti Cheese 78
Tomatillos 101, 160
Tomato: Fresh 101
  Ketchup 144
  Paste/Puree/Sauce 144
  Sundried 144
Toaster Streudel 64
Tombstone Pizzas 137
Tongue 126
Tony's Pizzas 137
Torte 169
Tortellini 133
Tortillas: Chips 149
  Dorritos 149, 151
  ...Shells 56
Tostada 172
Tostitos 149, 151

Tostitos Dip 79
Toutiere 168
Trader Joe's: Bars 34
  Breakfast Cereals 61
  Cakes 64
  Cookies 87
  Juices 45
  Meals 121
  Yogurt 163-164
Trail Mix 130, 151
Tripe 126
Tuna 97
Turkey 139
  Breast, Deli 129
  Loaf; Pastrami 129
Turnip 160
Turnovers, Fruit 62
Twinkies 63
Twix 74
Twizzlers 74

Udon Noodles 133
Uncle Ben's Meals 121

V8 Juice 46
Veal 125
  Veal Parmigiana 170
Vegetable Juices 41-46
Vegetable Oils 94
Vegetable Shortening 94
Vegetables 158-160
  Frozen 160-161
  Canned/Bottled 161
Vending Machine Snacks 151
Vermouth 26
Via® Iced Coffee 35
Vienna Sausage 129
Vietnamese Foods 174
Vinegar 30, 80
Vitamins 156
VitaMuffins 67
Vodka 27

Waffles 132
Walgreens Sodas 52
Walnuts 130
Wasabi Peas 151
Water Crackers 81
Water Chestnuts 160
Watermelon 101
  Seeds 131
WAWA 254-255
Weetabix 61

Weight Watchers:
  Candy 74
  Pizzas 137
  Smart Ones::
    Cakes 64
    Meals 119
Weiners 127
Wendy's 255
Werther's 75
WestSoy: Rice Drinks 49
  Soy Milk 50
Wheat Germ 57, 98
Wheat Thins 85
Whipped Toppings 89
Whipping Cream 89
Whiskey 27
Whitman's Chocolates 75
Wienerschnitzel 257
Wine 26
Wishbone Dressings 143
Wonton Wrappers 133
Wonder Bread 55
Wonka 75
Worthington 122
Wraps, Sandella's 236
Wrigley's 75
Wyder's Cider 26

Yams: 160
Yakult 164
Yeast 30
Yogurt 162-164
Yogurt Drinks 164
Yogurt Raisins 151
Yonique Yogurt 164
Yoo-Hoo 48
York Peppermint Pattie 75
Yorkshire Pudding 124
Yucca Root 160
Yves Veggie Cuisine 122

Zatarain's 122
Ziti, Fazoli's 200
Zola Acai Drink 46
Zone Perfect Bars 34
Yoplait 164
Zucchini 160

FAST-FOODS INDEX
~ PAGE 175 ~